Perspectives in Exercise Science
and Sports Medicine: Volume 9

Exercise and the Female—
A Life Span Approach

Edited by

Oded Bar-Or
McMaster University

David R. Lamb
The Ohio State University

Priscilla M. Clarkson
University of Massachusetts

COOPER

Publishing
Group

Library of Congress Cataloging in Publication Data:
LAMB, DAVID R., 1939–
PERSPECTIVES IN EXERCISE SCIENCE AND SPORTS MEDICINE
VOLUME 9: EXERCISE AND THE FEMALE—A LIFE SPAN APPROACH

Cover Design: Gary Schmitt

Library of Congress Catalog Card number: 88-70343

ISBN: 1-884125-28-X

Printed in the United States of America by Cooper Publishing Group, 1048 Summit Drive, Carmel, IN 46032
10 9 8 7 6 5 4 3 2 1

Contents

Contributors

Donald Bailey, Ph.D.
College of Physical Education
University of Saskatchewan
Saskatoon, SK S7N 0W0

Oded Bar-Or, M.D.
Chedoke Hospital
McMaster University
Hamilton, Ontario L8N 3Z5
CANADA

Cameron Blimkie, Ph.D.
Department of Kinesiology
McMaster University
Hamilton, ON L8S 4K1
CANADA

P.D. Chilibeck, M.Sc.
Faculty of Kinesiology
University of Western Ontario
London, ON
CANADA

James Clapp III, M.D.
MetroHealth Medical Center
Cleveland, OH 44109-1998

Priscilla M. Clarkson, Ph.D.
Department of Exercise Science
University of Massachusetts
Amherst, MA 01003

Edward F. Coyle, Ph.D.
Department of Kinesiology and Health
Education
University of Texas
Austin, TX 78712

K.S. Davison, M.Sc.
Department of Kinesiology
McMaster University
Hamilton, ON L8S 4K1
CANADA

J. Mark Davis, Ph.D.
Department of Exercise Science
University of South Carolina
Columbia, SC 29208

Loretta DiPietro, Ph.D.
John B. Pierce Laboratory
Yale University School of Medicine
New Haven, CT 06519

Jean-Pierre Despres, Ph.D.
Laval University Medical Research
Center
Ste-Foy, PQ G1V 4G2
CANADA

E. Randy Eichner, M.D.
Health Sciences Center
University of Oklahoma
Oklahoma City, OK 73190

Patty Freedson, Ph.D.
Department of Exercise Science
University of Massachusetts
Amherst, MA 01003

Carl V. Gisolfi, Ph.D.
Department of Exercise Science
University of Iowa
Iowa City, IA 52242

Scott Going, Ph.D.
Department of Exercise and Sport
Sciences
University of Arizona
Tucson, AZ 85721

Steven Gregg, Ph.D.
Gatorade Exercise Physiology
Laboratory
The Gatorade Company
Barrington, IL 60010

William Haskell, Ph.D.
Division of Cardiovascular Medicine
Stanford University
Palo Alto, CA 94304

Craig A. Horswill, Ph.D.
Gatorade Exercise Physiology
Laboratory
The Gatorade Company
Barrington, IL 60010

Mitch Kanter.
Gatorade Exercise Physiology
Laboratory
The Gatorade Company
Barrington, IL 60010

W. Larry Kenney, Ph.D.
Exercise and Sport Science Department
Pennsylvania State University
University Park, PA 16802

Howard Knuttgen, Ph.D.
Center for Sports Medicine
Pennsylvania State University
University Park, PA 16082

Andrea Kriska, Ph.D.
Department of Epidemiology
University of Pittsburgh
Pittsburgh, PA 15261

David R. Lamb, Ph.D.
Sport and Exercise Science Faculty
The Ohio State University
Columbus, OH 43210

Anne Loucks, Ph.D.
Department of Zoological and
Biomedical Sciences
Ohio University
Athens, OH 45701

Ronald J. Maughan, Ph.D.
Dept. of Environmental and
Occupational Medicine
University of Aberdeen
Foresterhill, Aberdeen AB9 2ZD
SCOTLAND

Robert Murray, Ph.D.
Gatorade Exercise Physiology
Laboratory
The Gatorade Company
Barrington, IL 60010

Ethan R. Nadel, Ph.D.
John B. Pierce Foundation Laboratory
Yale University School of Medicine
New Haven, CT 06519

Neil Oldridge, Ph.D.
Department of Health Sciences
University of Wisconsin
Milwaukee, WI 53201

Hélène Perrault, Ph.D.
Physical Education Department
McGill University
Montreal, PQ H2W 1S4

Digby Sale, Ph.D.
Department of Kinesiology
McMaster University
Hamilton, ON L8S 4K1
CANADA

Xiaocai Shi, Ph.D.
Gatorade Exercise Physiology
Laboratory
The Gatorade Company
Barrington, IL 60010

Angela Smith, M.D.
Department of Orthopedics
University Hospitals
Cleveland, OH 44106

Lawrence Spriet, Ph.D.
Human Biology & Nutritional Sciences
University of Guelph
Guelph, Ontario N1G 2W1

John R. Sutton, M.D.
Cumberland College of Health Sciences
New South Wales 2141
AUSTRALIA

Ronald L. Terjung, Ph.D.
Department of Physiology
SUNY Health Science Center
Syracuse, NY 13210

Clyde Williams, Ph.D.
Department of Physical Education,
Sports Science, & Recreation
Management
Loughborough University
Loughborough, Leicestershire LE11 3TU
UNITED KINGDOM

Jack Wilmore, Ph.D.
Department of Kinesiology and Health
Education
University of Texas
Austin, TX 78712

Robert Wiswell, Ph.D.
Department of Exercise Sciences
University of Southern California
Los Angeles, CA 90089

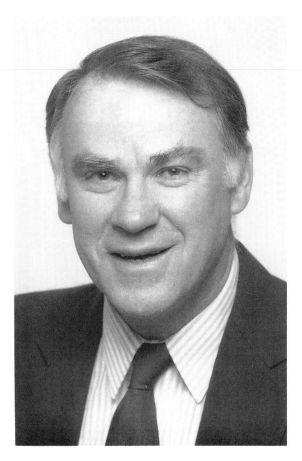

John R. Sutton

Dedication

This book is dedicated to the memory of Professor John R. Sutton, M.D., a dear friend and colleague, who died unexpectedly in his sleep on February 7th of this year. John contributed to each of the nine volumes of this *Perspectives* series, and all who attended the conferences associated with the development of these books came to know him as an outstanding scientist and clinician. He was widely known as one who put his own body on the line in extreme environments, from the hottest deserts to the coldest mountain tops, in the interest of science. He was also known as one of the most friendly and enthusiastic of human beings; he would greet each of us at the *Perspectives* conferences as though we were his long-lost brothers and sisters. In fact, John was so enthusiastic at pumping one's arm during a handshake, it is rumored that he left a trail of injured elbows around the world.

John's tendency to overcommit himself was legendary, and he coupled that overcommitment with a sense of humor that at times was a bit trying. An example that comes to mind goes back to the first Perspectives conference in 1987. John had agreed to write a chapter on endocrine responses to prolonged exercise but had not delivered his manuscript up to the day before the meeting. David Lamb, the conference coordinator, was in his hotel room the night before John was to present his chapter to the conference attendees and received a phone call from Professor Sutton. John was, as always, effusive in his greeting and indicated that Lamb had nothing to worry about because Sutton's manuscript was ready. Sutton said, "I dictated the paper on the plane flight here, and it's all on audio tape. Is there someone in the hotel who can transcribe it for me?" Lamb turned white and then red and began sweating profusely before Sutton finally told him that the manuscript was, in fact, ready in print form for distribution to the participants.

There will be stories that circulate about John Sutton for years to come, and they will celebrate his wisdom, his work ethic, his contributions to science and medicine, his friendship, his sense of humor, and his joy of living. We will miss him greatly.

Oded Bar-Or
David Lamb
Priscilla Clarkson

Acknowledgement

As part of our continuing commitment to research and education in sports science and sports nutrition, Gatorade is proud to sponsor the series, *Perspectives in Exercise Science and Sports Medicine*. As with the previous eight volumes of the series, this book resulted from our annual Gatorade Sports Science Institute *Perspectives* Conference at which invited scientists of international repute discuss a variety of scientific issues related to an annual theme; in this case, the participants enthusiastically discussed the role and effects of exercise across the life span of females.

We hope that you will find this volume to be a valuable addition to your professional library. Congratulations to the authors, reviewers, and editors for a job extremely well done.

James F. Doyle
President
Quaker Oats Beverages

Preface

We undertook the publication of this book because we believed that a life-span perspective on the associations between gender and exercise would make an important contribution to exercise science and sports medicine. We think this volume of the *Perspectives* series has accomplished what we intended, and we are eager to hear if you agree.

Many people made this book possible, especially, of course, the authors and reviewers. The manuscripts were reviewed in advance of a conference in Santa Barbara, California, in June of 1995, and the chapters were fine-tuned at that meeting. The presentations by the authors at the conference were stimulating, and the chapter discussions were thoroughly engaging; we believe the quality of this volume will attest to the success of the meeting. We are especially grateful to Kathryn Bowling and her colleagues at McCord Travel Management who made the conference arrangements and organized the travel with superb skill. We greatly appreciate the efforts of Joan Seye and Betty Dye, who efficiently and accurately transcribed all the chapter discussions at the conference so that the meeting participants could edit their contributions before leaving California.

Finally, we wish to recognize the contributions of the Gatorade Company, which so generously sponsor the *Perspectives* series. We believe that Gatorade has established a model for the interaction between science and the corporate world that should be emulated by other corporations. Many representatives of the Gatorade Company attend the *Perspectives* conference presentations, and we hope they have come away with an enhanced appreciation for the problems scientists face in trying to meld theory with practice. In turn, the scientists have a better understanding of how important it is that they articulate the knowledge they produce from their research in ways that are useful, not only to the corporate world, but especially to trainers, coaches, athletes, and physicians.

Oded Bar-Or
David Lamb
Priscilla Clarkson

1

Introduction to Exercise and the Female: A Life Span Approach

PRISCILLA M. CLARKSON, Ph.D.

ODED BAR-OR, M.D.

INTRODUCTION

"It was the best of times; it was the worst of times." Although Dickens used this phrase to describe the situation just before the French Revolution, it can be applied as well to current events related to women's health. In the past decade, the explosion of interest in this area has produced the Office of Research in Women's Health at the National Institutes of Health. New research centers are focusing on various aspects of women's health.

At the same time there are growing health concerns for females of all ages (Finn, 1993). In young girls the incidence of eating disorders, restriction of dietary energy, and overexercise have made them vulnerable to early osteoporosis. Adolescent girls and adult women face the challenge of increased weight gain. After menopause, women's risk of cardiovascular disease increases precipitously, yet they are less likely to receive proper medical care than men.

1

EXERCISE AND NUTRITION

Exercise and nutrition can play significant roles in reducing health risks in women. For example, peak bone mass is formed in the first three decades of life, when it is especially important to consume adequate calcium and to have sufficient circulating estrogen (Cooper et al., 1995; Matkovic et al., 1990; Recker et al., 1992). Too much exercise and too little energy intake may result in menstrual irregularities that contribute to lower overall concentrations of estrogen in the blood (Constantini & Warren, 1994; Loucks, 1994). After menopause the loss in bone can be reduced by exercise and diet interventions (Lohman, 1995; Silver & Einhorn, 1995; Wardlaw, 1993). There is a strong positive association between obesity and the risk of coronary heart disease and between estrogen and blood cholesterol and lipoproteins (Despres et al.,1989; Kris-Etherton & Krummel, 1993). Obesity increases the risks of diabetes, some types of cancer, stroke, and atherosclerosis (Manson et al., 1990; Pasquali et al., 1990; St Jeor, 1993). Accumulating evidence suggests that breast cancer may be related to exercise status (Bernstein et al., 1994), and results of animal studies and correlational research suggest a causal relationship between fat intake and breast cancer (Hankin, 1993).

If proper amounts of exercise and good nutrition will prevent or reduce the risk of several debilitating diseases among women, why aren't all women exercising and choosing low-fat, nutrient-rich diets? One reason may be insufficient knowledge among laypersons about the benefits of exercise and nutrition, which may stem from conflicting information in the media. Also, some of the available evidence on these issues is contradictory or flawed, so physicians and other opinion leaders are reluctant to aggressively recommend exercise and diet as preventive measures. Societal, cultural, or economic "roadblocks" may make it difficult for some women to make healthy choices.

Public Knowledge Base

A Gallup survey (Gallup, 1993) of 1021 women revealed that many had inadequate knowledge of factors regarding health, or they had the knowledge but chose to ignore it. For example, 80% of the women knew about the relationship between diet and health but one third said they did nothing to lower their risk of heart disease, cancer, or osteoporosis. Only 4% of the respondents were concerned about heart disease. One third reported that they did nothing on a regular basis to keep fit, and two-thirds believed a physical fitness test would show them to be in fair or poor shape.

Research findings are quickly picked up by the media and almost instantaneously available to the public. The media often do not have the scientific background required to interpret these findings adequately, sometimes leaving the mistaken impression that study results change from day to day. An important example involves the widely publicized statement by the Centers for Disease Control and Prevention (CDC) and the American College of Sports Medicine (ACSM) recommending that even moderate exercise has substantial health benefits (Pate et al., 1995). Several months later the news media covered the Harvard Alumni Study, which found that only vigorous exercise was associated with reduced mortality (Lee et al., 1995). The latter news coverage made it seem that two conclusions were completely different, leaving the public with more questions and much doubt about whether any type of exercise was worthwhile. What the media did not point out was that the former paper addressed many health benefits such as lowering blood lipid levels, whereas the latter assessed only mortality.

Similar problems exist in the nutrition arena. Although the data regarding benefits of antioxidant supplementation are equivocal, the popular press does not provide the public with the most complete information. In 1994, the news media widely reported results of a study showing that male smokers who took beta carotene supplements had a greater incidence of lung cancer (Heinonen & Albanes, 1994). What the news media did not report was the author's own caveat in that publication "in spite of its formal statistical significance, . . . this finding may well be due to chance." Moreover, there was no mention of the fact that many of the patients were in end-stage cancer; there was probably no reason to believe that an antioxidant would help in this circumstance. In fact, many scientists would have predicted the results.

The public is often confused about the relationships among physical activity, nutrition, physical fitness, and health. In Chapter 2, DiPietro describes exercise-related terminology. While physical activity and exercise are classified as behavioral, physical fitness is an outcome related to the achievement of certain performance standards. Fitness could mean achieving a given aerobic capacity or muscle strength, both of which may have little meaning when assessing health benefits. Yet how much exercise is enough to ensure health? Although consensus statements (CDC/ACSM) have been based largely on data from men, the public needs to be aware that overall physical activity, not just formal exercise, is important to gain health benefits.

It may be difficult for many laypersons to understand how exercise and diet in childhood and young adulthood can affect health in later life. For example, osteoporosis is considered a disease of old women. Yet, peak bone mass is formed in the first three decades of life. The greater the peak levels, the greater the bone mass at menopause, and the less likely a woman will be to suffer premature bone loss and osteoporosis. Thus, delayed menarche and amenorrhea, which compromise estrogen levels and thereby bone mass, may have profound implications for bone health after menopause (Ito et al., 1995).

Scientists and educators are faced with the challenge of correctly interpreting research and getting that information to the public. The public needs guidance in how to evaluate research findings so they do not rely on inadequate or even misleading information.

Scientific Knowledge Base

The chapters in this book have covered the state of knowledge of the physiology of the responses of females to exercise and training over the life span. Although there appears to be a wealth of information, each chapter identifies numerous gaps in the knowledge base.

An overall concern in all areas covered in this book is in the relative strength of the experimental designs used in many of the studies cited. For example, there is often a heavy reliance on cross-sectional versus longitudinal research. The interest in women's health has been rather recent, so there are few longitudinal studies. Cross-sectional studies cannot conclusively prove a causative or temporal relationship. This is particularly critical when assessing maturational or aging effects because of the vast array of changes that occur over the course of time.

Methodologies used in several areas are flawed, or adequate technology has not been developed. For example, Blimkie in Chapter 4 has addressed problems associated with measurement of bone mineral density. If we are to fully understand the effects of exercise and nutrition on bone health in growing and older females, improvement is needed in the normalization of traditionally used absorptiometric techniques to various populations. As another example of methodological concerns, Clarkson and Going point out in Chapter 5 that many studies of body composition have not used state-of-the-art imaging techniques to describe changes in internal (visceral) and external (subcutaneous) fat depots. Therefore, it is difficult to derive meaningful models for the accurate determination of body composition. Also, they criticize methods of assessing both dietary intake and disordered eating. Finally, accurate measurement of an individual's participation in physical activity is problematic, as addressed both by DiPietro and by Haskell and Pruitt in Chapters 2 and 9, respectively.

The specific effects of gender on physiological functions are often hard to evaluate because factors such as body adiposity, size, and aerobic fitness affect these same functions. For example, the relatively lower thermoregulatory effectiveness of women may reflect their lower maximal aerobic power and larger adiposity, rather than gender *per se*. Likewise, maturational and aging effects on the responses of females to exercise may be masked (or enhanced) by differences in body size and composition and by fitness levels. As shown in several chapters of this volume, such constraints have hindered our understanding of the effects of exercise and physical activity on females across the life span.

There is little information on how women participate over lifetimes in various forms of physical activity. Keeping in mind that physical activity includes "informal" exercise, there is almost no information on the long-term benefits of the types of daily activity that women do, such as carrying and tending to children or elderly parents. The extent to which habitual activity is underestimated in women is not known (Shephard, 1995).

In many cases there is simply a lack of important information, and scientists are often forced to rely on anecdotal information. For example, hot flashes in women have been suggested to be due to a change in the thermal setpoint, yet data to confirm this or explain a mechanism do not exist. Similarly, although suggestions have been made that swimming is a valuable exercise for pregnant women, there is insufficient research available to substantiate this recommendation.

Barriers To Physical Activity And Proper Nutrition

Today's woman is often balancing family, home, and career activities. Although she may desire to participate in recreational activity there may not be time or convenient access to such activity. Inconvenience and cost are two of the top reasons for dropping out of exercise programs (Foreyt & Goodrick, 1995).

While urban life may offer the convenience of local gyms, health centers, or fitness centers, there may be a lack of safe access for common outdoor activities such as jogging, walking, or biking. Only those women who can afford both the time and the money can take advantage of exercise programs offered by health clubs, and women in lower socioeconomic groups are least likely to have access to this type of exercise participation. Thus, for economic and cultural reasons, women and girls of minority status probably have the lowest levels of physical activity (Aaron et al., 1993). However, there is a serious lack of information on physical activity and contributing factors in minority populations. For example, the extent to which lower levels of activity reflect cultural influences and pressures is not known.

A LIFE SPAN APPROACH

Although several conferences have been conducted and books published on women and physical activity, this is the first book to provide an evaluation of the roles of exercise and nutrition in health over the life span of females. Each chapter offers a comprehensive examination of the literature pertaining to nutritional and physiological factors that alter the responses and adaptations of females to exercise. The overwhelming need for more research in this field has prompted the authors to conclude each chapter with specific challenges for future research.

BIBLIOGRAPHY

Aaron, D.J., A.M. Kriska, S.R. Dearwater, R.L. Anderson, T.L. Olsen, J.A. Cauley, and R.E. Laporte (1993). The epidemiology of leisure physical activity in an adolescent population. *Med. Sci. Sports Exerc.* 25:847–853.

Bernstein, L., B.E. Henderson, R. Hanisch, J. Sullivan-Halley, and R.K. Ross (1994). Physical exercise and reduced risk of breast cancer in young women. *J. Nat. Cancer Inst.* 86:1403–1408.

Constantini, N.W., and M.P. Warren (1994). Special problems of the female athlete. *Bailliers's Clin. Rheumatol.* 8:199–219.

Cooper, C., M. Cawley, A. Bhalla, P. Egger, F. Ring, L. Morton, and D. Barker (1995). Childhood growth, physical activity, and peak bone mass in women. *J. Bone Mineral Res.* 10:940–947.

Despres, J.P., S. Moorjani, A. Tremblay, M. Ferland, P.J. Lupien, A. Nadeau, and C. Bouchard (1989). Relation of high plasma triglyceride levels associated with obesity and regional adipose tissue distribution to plasma lipo-protein-lipid composition in premenopausal women. *Clin. Invest. Med.* 12:374–380.

Dickens, C. (1985). In: G. Woodcock (ed.) *The Tale of Two Cities.* New York: Penguin Books, p. 35.

Finn, S.C. (1993). ADA's nutrition & health campaign for women. *J. Am. Diet. Assoc.* 93:986.

Foreyt, J.P., and G.K. Goodrick (1995). Living without dieting: motivating the obese to exercise and eat prudently. *Quest* 47:262–273.

Gallup, G. (1993). Women's knowledge and behavior regarding health and fitness. Conducted for Weight Watchers and the American Dietetic Association. Princeton, NJ: The Gallup Organization, pp. 1–108.

Hankin, J.H. (1993). Role of nutrition in women's health: Diet and breast cancer. *J. Am. Diet. Assoc.* 93:994–999.

Heinonen, O.P., and D. Albanes (on behalf of the Alphatocopherol, Beta Carotene Cancer Prevention Study Group) (1994). The effect of vitamin E and beta carotene on the incidence of lung cancer and other cancers in male smokers. *New Engl. J. Med.* 330(15):1029–1035.

Ito, M., M. Yamada, K. Hayashi, M. Ohki, M. Uetani, and T. Nakamura (1995). Relation of early menarche to high bone-mineral density. *Calc. Tiss. Int.* 57:11–14.

Kris-Etherton, P.M., and D. Krummel (1993). Role of nutrition in the prevention and treatment of coronary heart disease in women. *J. Am. Diet. Assoc.* 93:987–993.

Lee, I.M., C.C. Hsieh, and R.S. Paffenbarger, Jr. (1995). Exercise intensity and longevity in men. The Harvard Alumni Health Study. *J.A.M.A.* 273:1179–1184.

Lohman, T.G. (1995). Exercise training and bone-mineral density. *Quest* 47:354–361.

Loucks, A.B. (1994). Physical activity, fitness, and female reproductive morbidity. In: C. Bouchard, R.J. Shephard, and T. Stephens (eds.) *Physical Activity, Fitness, and Health.* Champaign, IL: Human Kinetics, pp. 943–954.

Manson, J.E., G.A. Colditz, M.J. Stamfer, W.C. Willett, B. Rosner, R.R. Monson, F.E. Speizer, and C.H. Hennekens (1990). A prospective study of obesity and risk of coronary heart disease in women. *New Engl. J. Med.* 322:882–889.

Matkovic, V., D. Fontana, C. Tominac, P. Goel, and C.H. Chesnut (1990). Factors that influence peak bone mass formation: a study of calcium balance and the inheritance of bone mass in adolescent females. *Am. J. Clin. Nutr.* 52:878–888.

Pasquali, R., F. Casimirri, L. Plate, and M. Capelli (1990). Characterization of obese women with reduced sex hormone-binding globulin concentrations. *Horm. Metab. Res.* 22:303–306.

Pate, R.R., M. Pratt, S.N. Blair, W.L. Haskell, C.A. Macera, C. Bouchard, D. Buchner, W. Ettinger, G.W. Heath, and A.C. King (1995). Physical activity and public health. A recommendation from the Centers for Disease Control and Prevention and the American College of Sports Medicine. *J.A.M.A.* 273:402–407.

Recker, R.R., K.M. Davies, S.M. Hinders, R.P. Heaney, M.R. Stegman, and D.B. Kimmel (1992). Bone gain in young adult women. *J.A.M.A.* 268:2403–2408.

Shephard, R.J. (1995). Physical activity, fitness, and health: The current consensus. *Quest* 47:288–303.

Silver, J.J., and T.A. Einhorn (1995). Osteoporosis and Aging—Current Update. *Clin. Orthopaed. Rel. Res.* 316:10–20.

St Jeor, S.T. (1993). The role of weight management in the health of women. *J. Am. Diet. Assoc.* 93:1007–1012.

Wardlaw, G.M. (1993). Putting osteoporosis in perspective. *J. Am. Diet. Assoc.* 93:1000–1006.

6   PERSPECTIVES IN EXERCISE SCIENCE

2

Habitual Physical Activity Among Women

LORETTA DIPIETRO, Ph.D., M.P.H.

INTRODUCTION
  Definitions
  Physical Activity Assessment
  Measurement Issues
DEMOGRAPHICS OF PHYSICAL ACTIVITY
  Children and Adolescents
  Adults
DETERMINANTS OF PHYSICAL ACTIVITY
  Physiological
  Psychosocial
    Personality
    Beliefs and Attitudes
    Social Support
  Environmental
    Safety and Accessibility
    Time Constraints
PHYSICAL ACTIVITY, CHRONIC DISEASE, AND DISABILITY
  Dimensions of Physical Activity
  How Much is Enough?
    Breast Cancer
    Noninsulin-Dependent Diabetes Mellitus
  Overweight, Regional Adiposity and Metabolic Indicators
    Overweight and Adiposity
    Lipid Metabolism
    Glucose/Insulin Metabolism
  Blood Pressure
  Bone Growth
  Musculoskeletal Function
DIRECTIONS FOR FUTURE RESEARCH
SUMMARY
ACKNOWLEDGEMENTS
BIBLIOGRAPHY
DISCUSSION

INTRODUCTION

Definitions

Physical activity is a complex behavior and difficult to define operationally (Caspersen, 1989). The problems in the definition and measurement of physical activity limit the ability to assess activity properly and, therefore, to determine the health consequences associated with an active lifestyle.

The terms "physical activity," "exercise," and "physical fitness" are often used interchangeably. Caspersen (1989) and Caspersen et al. (1985) defined physical activity as any bodily movement produced by the skeletal muscles that results in energy expenditure, whereas exercise is described as a subcategory of physical activity behavior. Accordingly, exercise is defined as "any physical activity which is planned, structured, repetitive, and results in improvements or maintenance of one or more facets of physical fitness." Thus, physical activity and exercise are classified as behaviors, whereas physical fitness is classified as an outcome related to the ability to achieve certain performance standards or traits (Caspersen, 1989; Caspersen et al. 1985).

In the past, exercise of sufficient frequency, duration, and intensity (i.e., ≥ 20 min/session; ≥ 3 times/wk; $\geq 60\%$ maximal aerobic capacity [$\dot{V}O_2$max]) to promote cardiopulmonary fitness (American College of Sports Medicine, 1990) was thought necessary to achieve various health benefits. Recent public health recommendations, however, have focused on regular, moderate physical activity as a sufficient stimulus for a wide array of physiological and psychological benefits (Pate et al., 1995). The guidelines of the Centers for Disease Control and of the American College of Sports Medicine call for at least 30 min of *accumulated* moderate-intensity activity on most days of the week for every adult. Indeed, this broader model of physical activity for health enhancement augments the traditional and more specific model of exercise for fitness improvement and underscores the importance of standardizing both the definition and the measurement of physical activity.

Physical Activity Assessment

Physical activity can be achieved through school (e.g., physical education class or recess) or occupational activity, home maintenance activity (e.g., housework or yardwork), or as part of leisure-time pursuits (play, sports participation, conditioning, walking, gardening). Techniques for assessing physical activity range from very crude current or historical self-reported surveys to very objective, precise, and specific laboratory-based measures, such as calorimetry or doubly-labeled water. The time for the assessment generally ranges from current (past 24 h, wk, or mon) to historical (past y, age ranges, or lifetime) (LaPorte et al., 1985). Direct observation (Bailey et al., 1995; Klesges et al., 1984) or objective monitoring (Bray et al., 1994; Freedson, 1989, 1991; Sallis et al. 1990, 1995) of physical activity is the assessment method most often used with infants and young children, whereas self-reported activity diaries, surveys, and structured interviews have been used with adequate reliability and validity in samples of older children and adolescents (Sallis et al., 1993; Saris, 1985). It follows that the more precise and valid the measurement technique, the less potential there is for misclassification of physical activity level, which may result in an attenuation of the strength of the association between physical activity and various health outcomes. The more precise measures, however, generally are not feasible in large-scale epidemiologic research, which tends to rely on less costly and less labor-intensive survey instruments. Among survey instruments, physical activity may be measured as the frequency (times/wk) and the duration (min/session) of participation in various types of activity (e.g., sports, house/yardwork, walking) or various intensities of activity (e.g., light, moderate, vigorous) (Jacobs et al., 1991). Simple ways of expressing physical activity levels are as the proportion (%) of the population engaged in or as the time (e.g., h/wk) spent in various types or intensity classifications of activities. A simple summary score can be calculated by summing the reported amount of time spent in a given activity over all reported activities. Similarly, a more complex energy expenditure score can be calculated by assigning an energy cost ($kcal \cdot kg^{-1} \cdot h^{-1}$) to the different activities, based on their relative intensities (Ainsworth et al., 1993a; Taylor et al., 1978), and then summing over all reported activities. The total time or the energy expenditure summary scores then can be expressed relative to a daily, weekly, or yearly category.

Measurement Issues

Physical activity assessed by questionnaire is usually limited to that which requires an energy expenditure above that of daily living. The questionnaire method assumes that factors such as bathing and feeding are similar among most people in a population and that accurate measurement of such activities is neither feasible nor necessary (Kriska et al., 1994). Moreover, basal metabolic rate and the thermic effect of a meal are not considered with survey methods, and, therefore, energy expenditure estimates do not reflect total energy expenditure for a given individual. Nonetheless, these total time and energy expenditure estimates are quite useful for ranking individuals according to their reported activity levels to determine the association between relative activity level and various health or disease endpoints (Kriska et al., 1994). Unfortunately, information on the important components such as frequency, duration, and intensity may be difficult to gather in large-scale studies. One or two simple questions about typical physical activity often are used to classify individuals into crude (e.g., low, moderate, high) levels of participation.

It is important to consider that the identification of a population sub-group as active or inactive is dependent upon the types of activities queried. Typically, physical activity surveys have been geared towards white populations of middle to upper socioeconomic status (SES) and may not be sensitive to activity patterns of less affluent or minority (e.g., African- or Hispanic-American) populations. For example, certain lower SES segments of the population may not walk specifically for exercise or leisure-time recreation but may walk a great deal for transportation or as part of their occupational activities. Similarly, women often appear less active than men when vigorous or sport activities are assessed; however, when light or moderate activities, particularly those associated with household maintenance or care giving, are included in the assessment, gender differences often are attenuated (Ainsworth, 1993b; King et al., 1992). An additional challenge to measuring physical activity among women with children, particularly among those who work outside the home and are also care providers, is in categorizing activities carried on *simultaneously*. Current survey techniques that attempt to distinguish among discrete categories of exercise, transportation, and house/yardwork behavior may not be appropriate.

Therefore, activity surveys need to be sensitive to the wide spectrum of physical activities prevalent in the population, in order to accurately describe these behavioral patterns. This is especially important for women of lower socioeconomic status, who may spend a large proportion of their total activities walking, doing housework, and caring for children.

Small or negligible correlations between physical activity and various health outcomes may also be a consequence of measurement error due to inaccurate recall of habitual low-intensity behaviors more common among women. Accuracy in recalling physical activity may vary with gender (Sallis et al., 1985). Several studies (Baranowski, 1987; DiPietro et al., 1993a; Hopkins et al., 1991; Jacobs et al. 1991; Sallis et al., 1986) have demonstrated low accuracy in recalling low-intensity behaviors but higher accuracy with hard or very hard activities. Moreover, structured exercise activities may lend themselves to more accurate and reliable recollection because they are performed within a stable, scheduled time-frame that can be readily referred to (Caspersen et al., 1985).

In addition, physical activity (especially that of lower intensity) may display a great deal of intra-individual variation. Even if a survey or monitor assesses these types of behaviors, their usual pattern may not be adequately characterized with a one-time assessment (Kriska et al., 1994; Sallis et al., 1995). Dannenberg and colleagues (1989) reported substantial seasonal variation in activity patterns of adults in the Framingham Offspring cohort. Moreover, Durant's group (1992, 1993) reported substantial within-day variability in physical activity in samples of young children. Activity levels in these young children, estimated by heart rate monitoring, were different during the morning, early afternoon, and late afternoon. Other studies of children have demonstrated variability of physical activity over time periods ranging from 1 d (Durant et al., 1992, 1993) to 1 wk (Sallis et al., 1990, 1995) to 6 mon (Durant et al., 1992, 1993; Sallis et al., 1995).

Stability or tracking of physical activity refers to the maintenance of a relative position in rank of the behavior over time. Only a few studies have assessed the tracking of physical activity over longer periods of time in children and adolescents (Bild et al., 1993; Kelder et al., 1994; Mechelen et al., 1993; Pate et al., 1993; Sallis et al., 1995). In a 3-y study of preschool children, physical activity data from heart rate monitors were strongly correlated over 1 (r = 0.66) and 2 (r = 0.57) y (Pate et al., 1993), suggesting that young children's relative activity levels remained fairly stable during this time period. Recent data from adolescents in the Minnesota Heart Health community (Kelder et al., 1994) and from young women in the CARDIA Study (Bild et al., 1993) corroborate these findings from the preschool children. In contrast, Sallis and colleagues (1995) reported considerably smaller tracking estimates within a sample of young children and, in addition, found that less than 20% of the variance in physical activity was stable over 2 y. Also, longitudinal data from the Amsterdam Growth and Health Study on a selected sample of younger Dutch people (ages 13–28 y) suggest adequate tracking over 4 y but substantially lower tracking estimates over 9 and 15 y of follow-up in both male and female respondents (Mechelen et al., 1993). Indeed, the Amsterdam data show that activity level at age 13 did not predict activity level at age 28.

Thus, because of the short-term variability in physical activity behavior (especially in children), activities more easily reported or assessed for the past 24 hours, a week, or even in a typical week in the past month may not be representative of a habitual year-long or, certainly, a life-long pattern. The time-frame of the physical activity assessment becomes extremely important when correlating behavioral patterns to health or disease status. Therefore, multiple assessments over an entire lifetime may be necessary to accurately describe the contribution of physical activity to outcomes with a long developmental course, such as cancer, CHD, bone integrity, or long-term weight regulation.

DEMOGRAPHICS OF PHYSICAL ACTIVITY

The Healthy People 2000 Objectives (U.S. Dept. Health and Human Services, 1991) aim "to increase to at least 30% the proportion of people aged 6 and older who engage in light- to moderate-physical activity for at least 30 min/day." Approximately 22% of the U.S. adult population currently meets this goal, with 54% reporting some activity, but not meeting the objective, and 24% reporting no leisure-time activity in the past month.

Surveillance data from 29 states in the U.S. (Caspersen & Merritt, 1992; Merritt & Caspersen, 1992) suggest an overall decline in inactivity (i.e., no reported leisure-time physical activities in the past month) between 1986 and 1990 (Figure 2-1), although this decline in inactivity was not apparent among non-white adults or adults of lower educational attainment (Caspersen & Merritt, 1994). Data from the University of Minnesota (Jacobs et al., 1991) collected between 1957–1960 and 1985–1987 with the Minnesota Leisure-time Physical Activity (LTPA) survey (Taylor et al., 1978) also suggest that leisure-time physical activity has been increasing for three decades among both white- and blue-collar men and women living in the Upper Midwest.

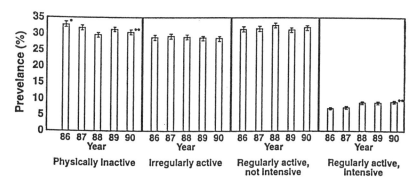

FIGURE 2-1. *Trends in physical activity patterns in the United States between 1986 and 1990 (Caspersen & Merritt, 1995).* **P<0.05 for 1990 vs. 1986.

Children and Adolescents

Data from the National Children and Youth Fitness Study, Phase I, (NCYS-I) (Ross & Pate, 1985) indicate that, on average, U.S. children engage in about 1.5–2.0 h/d of physical activity in both physical education class and extramural activity. In general, girls are purported to be less active than boys (Aaron et al., 1993; Centers for Disease Control, 1992; Pate et al., 1994; Ross & Pate, 1987). This gender disparity is possibly due to differences in socialization, body composition, and motor development, and it continues throughout early and older adulthood (Stephens et al., 1985). Results of the 1990 Youth Risk Behavior Survey (YRBS)(Centers for Disease Control, 1992) suggest that 66% of adolescent boys and 50% of adolescent girls reported participating in activity of at least moderate intensity three or more times per week in the past month. In addition, approximately 50% of the boys and 25% of the girls reported vigorous exercise three or more times per week (Table 2-1). While it is difficult to make direct comparisons with the findings of other studies because survey

TABLE 2-1. *Mean percentages and 95% confidence intervals (CI) of high-school students who participated in vigorous physical activity three or more days per week (N = 11,631; unweighted sample size).* Data are from the 1990 U.S. Youth Behavioral Risk Factor Survey (Centers for Disease Control, 1992).

Category	Female %	Female 95%CI	Male %	Male 95%CI
Race				
White	27.5	±2.9	51.4	±2.7
Black	17.4	±3.5	42.7	±6.7
Hispanic	20.9	±4.5	49.9	±6.1
Grade				
9th	30.6	±2.9	51.1	±5.1
10th	27.1	±4.7	54.6	±4.1
11th	23.4	±3.1	50.2	±3.9
12th	17.3	±2.9	43.8	±6.1

methodologies vary, this prevalence of regular (i.e., ≥ 3/wk) participation in moderate and/or vigorous physical activity among U.S. adolescents is quite similar to that recently found using the National Fitness Survey in England (Sports Council and Health Education Authority, 1993), but it is lower than that found among Canadian male (74%) and female (67%) adolescents (Stephens, 1993).

Participation in physical activity declines substantially with age even during childhood and adolescence (Aaron et al., 1993; Centers for Disease Control, 1992; Sallis, 1993). This decline is considerably greater among girls than boys (7.4% vs. 2.7% per y, respectively) (Sallis, 1993) and may result in as much as a 50% decrease in reported activity between ages 6 y and 16 y (Rowland, 1990).

There is also evidence of important racial differences in reported activity levels among children and youth, with girls of minority populations reporting the lowest activity levels (Aaron et al., 1993; Centers for Disease Control, 1992; Pate et al. 1994). Aaron et al. (1993) reported median levels of 23.3 vs. 18.9 h·wk^{-1} (P < 0.05) for white vs. nonwhite males and 7.0 vs. 4.9 h·wk^{-1} (P < 0.05) for white vs. nonwhite females, respectively, in a cohort of 1245 adolescents, 12–16 y old (Figure 2-2). These race-specific data are corroborated by data from the YRBS (Centers for Disease Control, 1992) and the NCYS-I (Ross & Pate, 1985).

There is a paucity of information on the actual choices or types of physical activity among children in the U.S. In general, bicycling, swimming, and ball sports are the more prevalent activities; however, these choices may vary by age, gender, race, season, and setting (e.g. physical education class vs. outside of school) (Pate et al., 1994; Ross & Pate, 1985; Ross et al., 1985). Of increasing public health concern for children and ad-

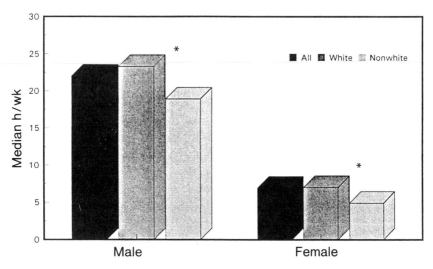

FIGURE 2-2. *Median leisure physical activity (h/wk) by gender and race (Aaron et al., 1993).* *P<0.05 for white vs. nonwhite groups

olescents is the promotion of "lifetime physical activities" (i.e., activities that can be readily continued into adulthood), such as walking, running, swimming, and tennis (Ross & Pate, 1985). Among the U.S. adolescent population, girls report a higher prevalence of lifetime activities than boys (71% vs. 56%, respectively). Forty-eight percent of the activities reported within physical education classes are lifetime activities compared to 63% of the reported activities outside of school (Ross et al., 1985).

It is also important to consider that the sum of passive leisure-time activities among children, such as television viewing and video/computer games, displaces time available for physical activities and exercise. Most of the reported physical activity among children takes place outside of school (Ross et al., 1985) when television is a viable option, so the relationship between active and passive leisure-time activities is of considerable interest (Pate et al., 1994).

Adults

In 1991 nearly 60% of the U.S. adult population reported little or no leisure-time physical activity (Centers for Disease Control, 1993). Levels of leisure-time activity also appear to vary by gender and race among adults in the U.S. (Centers for Disease Control, 1995; U.S. Dept. Health and Human Services, 1991). Women are less likely than men to report regular leisure-time activity (Caspersen et al., 1986; Folsom et al., 1985), and the lowest activity levels typically are reported among women of Hispanic or African-American descent (Bild et al., 1993; Centers for Disease

Control, 1995; DiPietro & Caspersen, 1991; Folsom et al., 1991). Among adults, racial comparisons tend to be distorted by the influence of socioeconomic status and education, however. Results from several studies (Bild et al., 1993; Folsom et al., 1985; Matthews et al., 1989; Stephens et al., 1985) show a strong positive correlation between years of educational attainment and level of habitual physical activity in both men and women, particularly with regard to the prevalence of regular (i.e., $\geq$20 min/session; $\geq$3 times/wk) and regular/intense activity (i.e., $\geq$60% $\dot{V}O_2$max) (Caspersen & Pollard, 1987; Centers for Disease Control, 1993; DiPietro & Caspersen, 1991; Yeager et al., 1991).

A report using Behavioral Risk Factor Surveillance System (BRFSS) data (Centers for Disease Control, 1995) shows that in 1992, approximately 27% of adult women in the U.S. met the newly recommended level of physical activity (i.e., either $\geq$20 min/d of vigorous activity on $\geq$3 d/wk, or $\geq$30 min/d of moderate activity on $\geq$5 d/wk), and this proportion remained somewhat consistent by age category. Reported participation varied substantially by race, income, and education level, with African-American women being the least likely to participate in these recommended levels of physical activity (Figure 2-3).

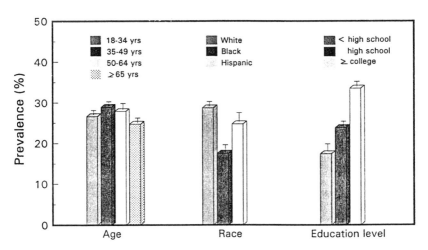

FIGURE 2-3. *Prevalence in 1992 of regular leisure-time physical activity among women by selected sociodemographic characteristics (Centers for Disease Control, 1995).* Regular activity was defined as $\geq$ 20 min/d of vigorous activity 3 d/wk or $\geq$ 30 min/d of moderate activity during $\geq$ 5 d/wk.

The prevalence of specific higher intensity activities decreases with age among adults, while the prevalence of reported inactivity shows an age-related increase (Caspersen et al., 1990; Stephens et al., 1985) that is especially evident among women (Caspersen & DiPietro, 1991; Centers for Disease Control, 1995; DiPietro et al., 1993b). Based on data from the BRFSS, more than 40% of U.S. women ≥65 y reported no leisure-time activity in 1992 (Centers for Disease Control, 1995).

Walking is the most prevalent activity reported among adults of all sociodemographic strata in the United States (Bild et al., 1993; DiPietro & Caspersen, 1991; DiPietro et al., 1993b; Stephens & Craig, 1985; Stephens et al., 1985), Canada (Stephens & Craig, 1985; Stephens et al., 1985), and Europe (Caspersen et al., 1991). Running, team sports, and weightlifting are the next most common activities among younger men, while participation in aerobics is more prevalent among younger women (DiPietro et al, 1993b). The most prevalent activities among older adults tend to be lower intensity but sustained activities such as walking, yardwork/gardening, or golf (Caspersen & DiPietro, 1991; Caspersen et al., 1991; DiPietro et al., 1993b) (Figure 2-4).

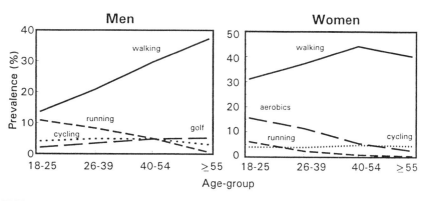

FIGURE 2-4. *Prevalence in 1989 of participation in popular activities among persons trying to reduce body weight (DiPietro et al., 1993b).*

In summary, physical activity is a complex behavior and is often difficult to describe. Relative to adults, children and adolescents tend to be more active, with more than 80% accumulating at least 30 min of activity on most days and 50% engaging in 20 min or more of moderate to vigorous activity three or more times per week (Pate et al., 1994). However, declining age trends in physical activity participation suggest that many adolescents are at risk of becoming sedentary adults. Important gender and race differences in reported physical activity patterns emerge in children and continue through adulthood. Typically, reported levels of leisure-time physical activity appear lowest among girls and women of minority status and older adult women. The ever-widening racial disparity in activity levels may well be explained by socioeconomic status among children and by level of educational attainment among adults, although data from the CARDIA Study show that important racial differences remained among women even after adjustment for several important sociodemographic factors (Bild et al., 1993). Encouraging, albeit limited, evidence indicates that the prevalence of reported inactivity is decreasing over time among some sectors of the general U.S. population, with an increasing trend in the prevalence of regular leisure-time activity. It is important to consider, however, that leisure-time physical activity is only a portion of total activity. The other components of total activity involve school or occupational activity, household activity, and transportation. Although surveillance data are not available on these other components, one can reasonably assume that energy spent in occupational and household tasks, as well as in transportation, has progressively declined with increasing automation. It therefore is possible that overall physical activity has declined in spite of increases in leisure-time activity (Powell, 1991).

The decline in overall physical activity has tremendous public health implications because there is increasing evidence that the health effects of physical activity are linked specifically to the total amount of energy expenditure or activity time accrued per day or week, rather than to the actual duration or intensity of the exercise bout (see Pate et al., 1995). Recommendations for children (Sallis & Patrick, 1994) and adults (Pate et al., 1995) call for a lifestyle approach to increasing activity levels among the public, by incorporating any activity of at least moderate intensity into the day. Indeed, the new Centers for Disease Control/American College of Sports Medicine recommendations are unique and especially useful for women in that they emphasize the value of moderate-intensity activity, as well as the daily accumulation of physical activity in intermittent bouts, as sufficient to achieve the CDC/ACSM recommendations and the associated health benefits (DeBusk et al., 1990; Ebisu, 1985; Leon et al., 1987; Paffenbarger et al., 1986). Thus, the recommended accumulated expenditure of 200 kcal/d can be achieved easily by most women through short bouts of activities such as stair climbing, gardening, brisk walking, playing with children, or housework (Pate et al., 1995).

DETERMINANTS OF PHYSICAL ACTIVITY

Of recent interest in the study of physical activity and exercise among the general population are the determinants of regular participation (Dishman et al., 1985; King et al., 1992; Sallis et al., 1992). These determinants (e.g., physiological, psychosocial, or environmental), which may vary by age, gender, and socioeconomic status, must be clearly identified and subsequently managed before the public health potential of physical activity can be fulfilled (Dishman et al., 1985; King et al., 1992).

Physiological

Heredity, or genetic predisposition, is an important component of physical fitness (Bouchard et al., 1986), which may contribute to physical activity level as well (Perusse et al., 1989). Among young children, central nervous system development provides the basis for the coordination necessary to perform activities and games. Cardiovascular fitness may also be an important determinant of activity; however, cross-sectional data suggest that fitness level is only modestly associated with physical activity level among children and adolescents (Pate et al., 1990; Taylor & Baranowski, 1991). (See Morrow & Freedson, 1994, for additional references.) Before puberty, girls may be better in balance and coordination whereas boys may excel at kicking and throwing (Thomas & French, 1985). Following puberty, however, the greater increase in muscle mass relative to fat mass seen in boys may partially explain the observed gender differences in motor skills (Shvartz & Reibold, 1990). It is difficult to determine if observed gender differences in motor skills reflect physiological or social differences. One can hypothesize that these gender differences will attenuate as more girls receive equal access to athletic programs at younger ages.

Among adults, especially older adults, speed, flexibility, balance, strength, and aerobic capacity may also be important determinants of participation in a particular activity (Sallis et al., 1989). Thus, physiological differences may be associated with gender and age differences in physical activity because they may act as incentives for persons to participate in activities at which they are more competent (Eaton & Enns, 1986).

Psychosocial

Personality. Characteristics such as motivation, stress tolerance, social adequacy, and independence do not strongly influence children's participation in physical activity (Butcher, 1985), but self-motivation has consistently been correlated with physical activity level in several adult populations (Dishman & Steinhardt, 1988; Knapp, 1988; Raglin et al., 1990). On the other hand, as reviewed by Dzewaltowski (1994), self-efficacy, or confidence in one's abilities, is strongly associated with both the adoption of and adherence to physical activity among both adolescents (Ferguson et al., 1989; Godin & Shephard, 1986) and adults (McAuley & Jacobson, 1991; Sallis et al., 1989).

Affective disorders such as anxiety and depression tend to be inversely associated with participation in physical activity (Emery & Blumenthal, 1992; Taylor et al., 1985). Although limited data show that various mood disturbances and depressive personality are associated with inactivity or can actually predict adherence to fitness or rehabilitation programs (Lobstein et al., 1983; Oldridge & Streiner, 1990; Ward & Morgan, 1984), it remains unclear whether affective states are determinants or consequences of physical activity behavior.

Beliefs and Attitudes. Knowledge about the health effects of exercise does not necessarily translate into increased physical activity among children and adolescents (Krucera, 1985); however, knowledge about how to be physically active may be quite influential (Gottlieb & Chen, 1985). Various other measures of attitudes towards physical activity in children typically show low to moderate correlations with activity behaviors (Desmond et al., 1990; Ferguson et al., 1989; Godin & Shephard, 1986), although it is possible that these attitudes may have a delayed, rather than an immediate, impact on activity levels (Sallis et al., 1992).

Studies of these same factors among adults suggest that knowledge and beliefs about the health effects of physical activity are positively associated with current physical activity levels (Sallis et al., 1989). Conversely, a less than favorable perception of one's own health status is associated with reduced participation in cardiac rehabilitation programs (Oldridge & Spencer, 1985) and at the community level as well (Sallis et al., 1986). Perceived enjoyment and satisfaction are positive predictors of physical activity in both men and women (King et al., 1988); however, intentions to be physically active do not necessarily predict subsequent participation (Godin et al., 1987).

With regard to intentions, the decision to exercise may not be an all-or-none phenomenon. Marcus and colleagues have presented a more dynamic model of exercise behavior that focuses on the different transitions an individual makes in the adoption and maintenance of exercise-related behavior (Marcus & Owen, 1992; Marcus & Simkin, 1993, 1994; Marcus et al., 1992). Indeed, this model suggests that an individual may move forward and backward in a cyclical manner through different stages of change (i.e., precontemplation, contemplation, preparation, action, and maintenance). Thus, persons may make several attempts at behavioral change before reaching the maintenance stage and then may return to a previous stage before moving forward again (Marcus & Simkin, 1994). The stages-of-change model is especially applicable to women who may stop exercising due to certain life changes (e.g., parity with increased child care responsibilities, new job, illness, or death of a spouse) with the intention to later resume an exercise program.

Social Support. Social influences on physical activity patterns appear to be strong throughout the life span. Peer reinforcement is especially important to physical activity patterns in youth (Sallis et al., 1992), and social support from friends has been correlated with vigorous activity in adult populations (King et al., 1990; Sallis et al., 1992). There appears to be a modest aggregation of physical activity levels within families (Bouchard & Malina, 1983; Perusse et al., 1989), but the specific behavioral mechanisms underlying this effect are not clear (King et al., 1992). Parents are strong influences on physical activity levels in children and adolescents (Klesges et al., 1990; Sallis et al., 1988), especially with regard to encouragement (Klesges et al., 1986; McKenzie et al., 1991) and modeling of an active lifestyle (Ross & Pate, 1985, 1987; Sallis et al., 1988). The extent to which children influence their parents' levels of activity, however, has not been determined (King et al., 1992).

Environmental

Safety and Accessibility. Safety and accessibility are two important environmental factors associated with activity participation, but these two factors have not been studied extensively (Bild et al., 1993; King et al. 1992). Paths for walking, running, or bicycling, and recreational areas that are set away from traffic, patrolled, and well-lighted, are especially important for females of all ages. Supervision among first-time participants in the skill-building phase of an activity is an important concern, especially for many of the underserved minority sectors of the population. Most of the organized activity for children takes place outside of school (Ross et al., 1985), and many youth programs are directed specifically towards the elite athlete (Sallis et al., 1992) or those able to pay dues and equipment and travel costs. Similarly, among adults, membership fees or lack of transportation often present insurmountable barriers to activity in health clubs or other training facilities. Thus, unequal access to safe exercise programs and facilities may serve as an important mediating factor in the relationship between age or socioeconomic status and physical activity.

Time Constraints. An important barrier to participation in leisure-time activity reported among adults is lack of time. This is especially true for working mothers or working women caring for infirm parents. Indeed, the lives of dual-career women have been characterized by role conflict and overload (Bird, 1979; Bodin & Mitelman, 1983), which is most alarming for single working mothers, who comprise an overwhelming majority of all single heads of households. "Leisure-time" is a value-ladened term, and its meaning may vary by social group and by gender. Deem (1982) and others (Bird, 1979; Shank, 1986; Witt & Goodale, 1981) suggest that women have unequal access to leisure and free time, often constrained by domestic labor, caregiving, the behavior of a male partner, and/or lack of financial resources or transportation.

An important issue for the promotion of physical activity among women is that of integrating exercise with an already saturated life. Such promotion would encourage activities that could be done simultaneously with domestic, parenting, and/or caregiving duties. Such activities might include walking with a child in a stroller or backpack rather than driving; doing housework or yardwork to music or in such a way as to maximize the calorigenic or aerobic benefit; and as always, climbing stairs at every opportunity (preferably while carrying a heavy briefcase, load of groceries, or a child).

Thus, an array of physiological, psychological, and environmental factors may determine physical activity behavior among young girls and women. Many of these determinants, particularly some of the psychosocial and environmental factors, are particularly amenable to change and should be the focus of community intervention efforts. Strategies for increasing physical activity levels among females include: increased public education about the health effects of moderate physical activity; more school, work-site, and community center programs that provide social support, child care, and other incentives for exercise; and greater community availability and accessibility of safe physical activity and recreational facilities such as hiking, biking, and fitness trails, public swimming pools, and acres of park space.

PHYSICAL ACTIVITY, CHRONIC DISEASE, AND DISABILITY

Physical activity and fitness have been associated with a lower incidence of morbidity and mortality from a number of major chronic diseases affecting women, namely, coronary heart disease (CHD) (Blair et al., 1989; Leon et al., 1987; Paffenbarger et al., 1993; Powell et al., 1987), breast cancer (Bernstein et al., 1994; Frisch et al., 1985; Vena et al., 1987), and noninsulin-dependent diabetes mellitus (NIDDM) (Helmrich et al., 1991; Kriska et al., 1994; Manson et al., 1991). Physical activity also has an independent protective effect on the risk of becoming overweight (Berkowitz et al., 1985; DiPietro, 1995; Williamson et al., 1993), losing bone mass (Drinkwater, 1994; Snow-Harter & Marcus, 1991), suffering hip fracture (Farmer et al., 1989; Paganini-Hill et al., 1991; Wickham et al., 1989), and falling (Stones & Kozma, 1987; Tinetti et al., 1994), as well as on the rate of functional decline so common with aging (Haskell & Phillips, 1995; Pescatello & DiPietro, 1994). There is evidence to suggest that current activity is more protective than past activity; however, cumulative, lifetime activity patterns may be more influential factors for most of these diseases, especially those with a long developmental period, such as cancer, bone integrity, or long-term weight regulation.

Indeed, the evidence clearly indicates that sedentary behavior is a major risk factor for chronic disease morbidity and mortality. Because such a large proportion (60%) of the general adult population reports no activity, the public health impact of a sedentary lifestyle may be considerable. This inverse association between physical activity and disease or decline is consistently strong, graded, and independent, and it is biologically plausible and specific (Blair et al., 1992a, 1992b), thereby meeting most criteria for inferring a causal relationship. However, the challenge often encountered in epidemiologic research relying on self-reported measures of physical activity is that of establishing temporal sequencing, i.e., does sedentary behavior truly precede the onset of decline or disease?

Dimensions of Physical Activity

It is difficult to determine the characteristics of physical activity related most specifically to different aspects of health because there are several dimensions of physical activity behaviors. These dimensions, which are neither exclusive to any one type of activity nor to each other, include aerobic intensity, energy expenditure, weight-bearing, flexibility, and muscular strength (Laporte et al., 1985). Certainly the dimensions are interrelated since, for example, activities that increase aerobic capacity also require energy expenditure; any sustained weight-bearing activity will also expend energy, and if done vigorously enough, will increase aerobic capacity.

The relative importance of each of these dimensions to health may shift with age. For example, among adolescent girls and younger women, dimensions of physical activity related to muscle and bone growth may be of primary interest, whereas among middle-aged women, the influence of energy expenditure on weight regulation or of aerobic intensity on cardiovascular health becomes more important. Among older women, the influences of weight-bearing, strength, and flexibility on bone and lean mass preservation and balance assume highest priority with regard to maintaining functional ability and independence.

How Much is Enough?

The level of exercise both necessary and sufficient to achieve health benefits has become of recent interest (Blair et al., 1992b; Haskell, 1985; King, 1991; LaPorte et al., 1984). Historically, experts had proposed that exercise of sufficient frequency, intensity, and duration to achieve improvements in physical fitness was necessary to promote resistance to disease. Although the effects of physical activity on health status may be mediated primarily by the physiologic changes that accompany increased aerobic fitness (Sobolski et al., 1987), recent data suggest that biological changes with increased physical activity can lead to positive changes in various health indicators independent of the changes responsible for increased fitness (Blair et al., 1989, 1992b; Haskell, 1985; Pescatello et al., 1994). Indeed, a growing literature of epidemiologic data shows significant relationships between low- and moderate-intensity activities and all-cause mortality, as well as mortality from cardiovascular disease, stroke, cancer, and respiratory disease (Blair et al., 1989; Ekelund et al., 1988;

Kiely et al., 1994; Leon et al., 1987; Morris et al., 1990; Paffenbarger et al., 1993; Sandvik et al., 1993).

The exercise prescription (i.e., frequency, duration, intensity) optimal in achieving one type of health outcome (e.g., weight loss) may be very different from the prescription necessary to achieve another (increased bone mineral content or muscular strength). Age may also be an important variable in modifying the effects of a given exercise stimulus on health and functioning. That is, the amount of exercise related to disease-specific morbidity in middle age may be very different from the amount related to successful aging and longevity. Overall, there is a paucity of information on the exercise prescriptions for health outcomes other than aerobic fitness or CHD; this is especially true among women and children (Blair et al., 1992b).

Breast Cancer. Most epidemiologic studies of physical activity and breast cancer risk have been equivocal. Whereas some data demonstrate an inverse relationship (Bernstein et al., 1994; Frisch et al., 1985; Vena et al., 1987), others indicate a null (Paffenbarger et al., 1987) or even a positive relationship (Albanes et al., 1989; Dorgan et al., 1994), suggesting that women who are more active are at higher risk for breast cancer. Most of the research to date, though, has used only a single assessment of current physical activity, rather than multiple assessments of habitual lifetime activity. However, in a recent case-control study using 545 cancer cases with matched controls, along with a measure of lifetime physical activity (h/wk), Berstein et al., (1994) found a 60% lower risk of breast cancer among women in the highest category of reported lifetime activity (i.e., ≥3.8 h/wk) compared to inactive women. The lower relative risk of breast cancer among more active women was independent of a number of influential variables and suggests that about 4 h of activity per week from menarche onward was a sufficient protective factor.

Noninsulin Dependent Diabetes Mellitus. Physical activity is inversely associated with both the prevalence (Dowse et al., 1991; Kriska et al., 1993; Taylor et al., 1984) and incidence (Helmrich et al., 1991; Manson et al., 1991) of noninsulin dependent diabetes mellitus (NIDDM) (Kriska et al., 1994). Although data are limited, they also suggest that it is *regular lifetime* physical activity that is most protective against NIDDM (Kriska et al., 1993; Laws & Reaven, 1991). Moreover, data from the Harvard Alumni Study (Helmrich et al., 1991) support the notion that overall activity (i.e., energy expenditure per week) is the important factor in the prevention of NIDDM. Although vigorous activities (e.g., sports, running, swimming, etc.) were most protective, moderate activities were also associated with decreased risk. Therefore, since moderate activities can be sustained regularly for longer periods of time, thereby maximizing total energy expenditure, their merits should be encouraged in the prevention and/or management of NIDDM.

Excess adiposity is an important predictor of NIDDM (Dowse et al., 1991; Helmrich, 1991) and is a primary condition for insulin resistance and glucose intolerance (Bjorntorp, 1981, 1991); these relationships may be stronger among women than among men (Dowse et al., 1991; Haffner et al., 1991). Thus, the protective effects of increased physical activity on NIDDM may be due in part to the relationships among exercise, adiposity, and glucose/insulin metabolism. Special consideration should be given to the study of how this relationship may vary by gender.

Overweight, Regional Adiposity, and Metabolic Indicators.

Overweight and Adiposity. The inverse association between physical activity and body weight or body fat has been reported in several cross-sectional observational studies of both children (Davies et al., 1995; Johnson et al., 1956; Waxman & Stunkard, 1980) and adults (DiPietro, 1995), in two meta-analyses (Ballor & Keesey, 1991; Epstein & Wing, 1980), and in numerous intervention studies (Despres et al., 1988a; Stefanick, 1993). However, the data linking habitual physical activity to the risk of weight gain among the general population remain inconclusive (Rissanen et al., 1991; Voorrips, 1991; Williamson et al., 1993).

Following a drop in sex hormone levels with menopause, women have an increased tendency to deposit fat more centrally (Rebuffe-Scrive et al., 1986). There is important evidence that abdominal adiposity is the more specific risk factor for a number of metabolic complications (Kissebah & Krakower, 1994; Sjoestrom, 1993). Unlike femoral/gluteal adiposity, however, abdominal fat, especially that composed of hypertrophied fat cells, is much more responsive to exercise interventions (Bjorntorp, 1990; Despres et al., 1989). Although younger women with excess abdominal adiposity appear to respond to exercise training with fat loss and improved lipid and carbohydrate metabolism (Despres et al., 1989), further investigation is needed to establish the association between sex hormone levels, regional fat distribution, and exercise-related changes in weight or fat among children, adolescents, and women of older ages.

With sustained exercise of low to moderate intensity (i.e., <50% $\dot{V}O_2max$), fats may provide up to 90% of the fuel source; work of higher intensity relies more on carbohydrate as the primary fuel source (Stefanick, 1993). With regard to reducing total body fat stores, however, total energy expenditure during exercise may be the more important variable than the fuel source. Regular (i.e., ≥3 times/wk) physical activity of low to moderate intensity but of relatively long duration (i.e., at least 50–60 min) usually is most efficacious in maximizing total energy expenditure and emphasizing fat utilization during exercise.

Lipid Metabolism. Improvements in lipid metabolism with exercise also may be gained in the absence of weight or fat loss (Hardman et al., 1992; Hardman & Hudson, 1994; Tran & Weltman, 1985; Tremblay et al.,

1991). The increased lipoprotein lipase (LPL) activity in adipose and muscle tissue that is stimulated by regular exercise facilitates the clearance of circulating triglycerides (Durstine & Haskell, 1994; Haskell, 1984; Stefanick, 1993). In cross-sectional studies of children, physical activity or fitness has been associated with lower serum levels of triglycerides and higher levels of HDL-cholesterol (Durant et al., 1983; Thorland & Gilliam, 1981); however, the limited data from controlled training studies are less conclusive (Gilliam & Burke, 1978; Gilliam & Freedson, 1980; Savage et al., 1986). Baronowski et al. (1992) and Despres et al. (1990) have also provided excellent reviews of this literature. The results of many cross-sectional and longitudinal studies among men and women suggest the presence of higher concentrations of HDL-cholesterol in the blood of persons who exercise than in sedentary controls; however, exercise appears to have only a minor influence on lowering LDL-cholesterol (Durstine & Haskell, 1994; Haskell, 1986). Furthermore, lipoprotein responses to exercise may be less dramatic among women than among men (Brownell & Stunkard, 1981; Frey et al., 1982; Hardman & Hudson, 1994; Hardman et al., 1989). Indeed, menopausal status may modify exercise-induced changes in lipoproteins, with pre-menopausal women being less responsive (Lokey & Tran, 1989). Nonetheless, studies by Hardman and colleagues (1989, 1994) have demonstrated that a program of regular, brisk walking ($\geq$60% $\dot{V}O_2$max) is a sufficient stimulus in improving the HDL-cholesterol concentrations of previously sedentary women.

Recent studies suggest that the duration of the exercise bout is more important than the intensity to acutely change HDL-cholesterol (Hughes et al., 1990). Generally, a single, sustained bout of aerobic exercise evokes a 4–6 mg/dL increase in plasma HDL-cholesterol in both men and women (Gordon & Cooper, 1988). Chronic exercise training has resulted in approximately 5–15% increases in plasma HDL-C levels, which appear to be directly related to both the intensity of the exercise and the total amount of weekly energy expenditure in men (Wood et al., 1983). Evidence also suggests that it is the HDL_2 subfraction that increases with exercise, while the HDL_3 subfraction decreases (Dengel et al., 1994; Rauramaa et al., 1984; Williams et al., 1992). These reciprocal changes in HDL subfractions may explain why some longitudinal studies fail to demonstrate increases in HDL-cholesterol with exercise training (Coon et al., 1990; Despres et al., 1988b; Moll et al., 1979).

Glucose/Insulin Metabolism. In normal children, physical fitness and glucose tolerance may not be related (Montoye et al., 1978); however, children's physical activity level was inversely associated with glucose tolerance in both the Bogalusa Heart Study (Voors et al., 1982) and the Tecumseh Study (Montoye et al., 1977). Similarly, exercise training does not affect glucose tolerance in lean nondiabetic adults who already have normal glucose tolerance (Bjorntorp, 1981; Despres et al., 1988b; Tremblay et al., 1987). However, among obese children and adults with diabetes or glucose intolerance, both acute exercise bouts and routine exercise training increase insulin sensitivity and glucose tolerance and improve glucose disposal by enhancing glucose uptake by muscle (Kirwan et. al, 1993; Mikines et al., 1988; Reaven, 1995; Rosenthal et al., 1983). Because insulin resistance and hyperinsulinemia are independently associated with dyslipidemia and hypertension (DeFronzo & Ferrannini, 1991), interventions that prevent or reverse insulin resistance may also have a substantial impact on the other two metabolic indicators (Douglas et al., 1992; Laws & Reaven, 1992). In adults, reversal of insulin resistance through exercise has indeed been associated with decreased concentrations of triglycerides and VLDL-cholesterol and increased concentrations of HDL-cholesterol plus improvements in moderate hypertension (Laws & Reaven, 1992; Seals et al., 1984). Similar results have been observed in cross-sectional studies of children (Burke et al., 1986). The exercise-induced improvements in glucose and insulin metabolism may last from hours to days; thus, it is unclear whether such improvements are due to the effects of individual bouts of exercise or to training (Vranic & Wasserman, 1990).

Blood Pressure. There is little evidence that aerobic physical activity affects resting blood pressure in children with normal blood pressure (Baranowski et al., 1988; Eriksson & Koch, 1973), but regular activity may lower blood pressure in obese children who begin training with elevated resting blood pressures (Dansforth et al., 1990; Hagberg et al., 1983; Ylitalo, 1981). (See Baranowski et al. (1992) and Despres et al. (1990) for additional references.) Most of the epidemiologic research on physical activity and blood pressure (conducted primarily among adult male populations) has documented a lower occurrence of hypertension among active relative to inactive populations (Blair et al., 1984; Gordon et al., 1990; Paffenbarger et al., 1983), a relationship that is independent of factors such as age, smoking, body weight, or family history. A meta-analysis of 25 training studies showed the effectiveness of aerobic exercise on lowering elevated systolic and diastolic blood pressure (Hagberg, 1990). On average, observed reductions in systolic and diastolic blood pressure among these studies were 10.8 and 8.2 mm Hg, respectively; moreover, moderate-intensity exercise appeared to be as effective as high-intensity exercise in lowering blood pressure.

Bone Growth. Regular physical activity is associated with greater peak bone mass in adolescents and in young women and with an attenuated reduction of bone mineral density in middle-aged and older women (Dalsky et al., 1988; Marcus et al., 1992; Snow-Harter & Marcus, 1991). Among women, childhood physical activity (Fehily et al., 1992; McColloch et al., 1990) and lifetime physical activity (Halioua & Anderson, 1989; Tylavsky et al., 1992) have been shown to be more important than current levels of activity in affecting bone integrity. The type and amount of exercise that best promotes bone growth has not been established (Marcus et al., 1992), although weight-bearing exercise (e.g., walking, jogging, dancing) has been the type most often prescribed to women following menopause. The effects of exercise on bone growth may be heterogenous, with greater loads at specific bone sites providing a more effective osteogenic stimulus than lesser loads that are generally distributed. For example, the loads placed on the lumbar vertebrae with brisk walking and jogging are up to 1.75 times body weight (Capozzo et al., 1983), whereas weightlifting may produce loads on the lumbar vertebrae that are as much as 5–6 times body weight (Granhad et al., 1987). Muscle strength actually may be a better correlate of bone mineral density than age (Pocock et al., 1989; Snow-Harter et al., 1990). Strength of individual muscle groups seems to be related specifically to the mineral density of the bones supported by the muscle, e.g., hip strength predicts mineral density of the bones at the hip joint (Hughes et al., 1995; Sinaki & Offord, 1988). Therefore, programs of regular, sustained, resistance exercises that overload the muscular system at specific sites may provide the optimal stimuli for bone growth.

Musculoskeletal Function. Musculoskeletal weakness and disability are especially common among older women and, along with compromised flexibility and balance, contribute substantially to functional disability and the risk of falling (Nevitt et al., 1989; Tinetti et al., 1988). Two landmark studies by Frontera (1988) and Fiaterone (1990) heralded a growing body of evidence of the benefits of higher intensity (e.g., 80% of the maximal load that can be correctly lifted only once) resistance training for inducing muscle hypertrophy and increasing strength in older persons (Haskell & Phillips, 1995). Indeed, these studies demonstrate that older people can safely tolerate relatively high-intensity strength training and experience muscular improvements comparable on a relative basis to those seen among younger persons.

The epidemiologic data linking physical activity or specific exercise training to outcomes of activities of daily living (ADL) (e.g., basic self-care activities) (Katz et al., 1963) or more necessary components of independent living (e.g., shopping) (Fulton et al. 1989) are equivocal. Prospective, observational studies suggest an inverse relationship between reported physical activity and risk of disability, with several studies finding that moderate to high levels of recreational activity are necessary for risk reduction (Kaplan et al., 1987; Mor et al., 1989; Simonsick et al., 1993). Intervention studies, however, which tend to focus more on the impact of strength training on gait and balance, report conflicting results (Judge, 1993; Lichtenstein et al., 1989; Sauvage et al., 1992). More randomized controlled interventions are needed to determine the exercise prescription sufficient to cause the adaptations in aerobic capacity, muscular strength, muscular endurance, flexibility, and balance that translate into improved daily functioning for older persons.

In summary, there is limited information on the amount of exercise needed to promote optimal health and function in women through their life spans. Prescribing levels of exercise necessary to achieve aerobic fitness may no longer be appropriate; rather, public health policy should focus on *sufficient levels* when promoting physical activity among the more sedentary female sectors of the general population. Given that health benefits may accrue that are independent of the fitness effects achieved through sustained vigorous exercise, a new lifestyle approach should be emphasized from childhood through older adulthood. This approach calls for incorporating at least 30 min of any activity (sustained or accumulated) into the daily schedule. Thus, regular participation in activities of moderate intensity, e.g., walking, climbing stairs, biking, or yardwork/gardening, that increase accumulated daily or weekly energy expenditures and maintain muscular strength, even though they may not improve aerobic fitness, should be encouraged in the community (King, 1991; Pate et al., 1995; Sallis & Patrick, 1994). This is especially important for members of the population who may risk injury or illness if they participate in more vigorous exercise.

DIRECTIONS FOR FUTURE RESEARCH

The areas of focus for future research on physical activity epidemiology among women include, but certainly are not limited to the following.

1. **Surveillance and tracking studies.** Studies that follow large, representative female cohorts for 5, 10, or 20 y would provide valuable longitudinal information on how physical activity patterns of a generation change over time and how these patterns persist or change throughout a woman's life span. There is some evidence of persistence of physical activity patterns among adolescents (Kelder et al., 1994) and young adults (Bild et al., 1993). Kelder and colleagues (1994) propose that if children diverge at early ages into higher and lower activity groups and maintain their relative activity rankings through adolescence and into adulthood, then intervention efforts should be targeted early, before the diversion in activity patterns occurs.

Also, by selecting subsamples of families for study, questions on the inheritability of physical activity patterns can be addressed. In addition, twin and/or adoption studies provide valuable information on the unique contributions of genetics and environment to physical activity behaviors.

2. **Energy expenditure studies.** Field studies of 24-h energy expenditure that use doubly-labeled water would provide objective, precise, and useful information on energy expenditure patterns among samples of girls and women. These data could be compared to those of boys and men, and within gender comparisons could also be made to determine whether age or race differences actually exist among women. An additional valu-

able comparison would be the energy expenditures of mothers working outside the home to those of "at home" mothers.

3. **Community interventions.** These interventions would focus on assessing the impact of public policy strategies for increasing physical activity among females. These strategies could range from increasing the number of safe playgrounds and walking/biking paths or work-site exercise programs in a community to changing building and transportation codes to make stair climbing or walking more attractive to the public. Further, providing on-site daycare at the work place or exercise facility may ease some of the time constraints that often hinder the ability of working mothers to exercise in healthful ways.

4. **Large-scale epidemiologic studies of women.** These studies would link physical activity with health outcomes specific to girls and women in particular ranges of age. Such ranges might include: a) *Birth through 2 y or pre- through post-adolescence* for studying how activity influences bone growth and muscle development as well as the onset of menarche and subsequent menstrual function; b) *Pre-through post-parity (i.e., 18–40 y)* for studying how physical activity influences menstrual function, pregnancy, and weight control; and c) *Pre-, peri-, post-menopause through older age (>65 y)* for investigating the associations between physical activity and a) the development of metabolic disorders and consequent cardiovascular disease, b) bone and lean mass preservation, and c) physical, psychological, and cognitive function. Given the demographic trends in the older adult population, enormous public health benefits would accrue if one could identify factors that not only influence longevity but also promote independent, highly functional survival. Interest in the determinants of successful aging has led to the investigation of the heterogeneity in both physical and cognitive function within healthier, higher functioning groups of older people. A primary goal of such studies would be to determine the modifiable factors related to the plasticity of higher functional abilities, as opposed to the mere presence or absence of disease or disability. Prospective studies and especially randomized controlled interventions offer the best opportunity to determine the true impact of exercise on the prevention or attenuation of various disorders and dysfunction throughout older adulthood.

SUMMARY

Physical activity is complex and often difficult to describe in women. Consequently, the prevalence of reported activity tends to be lower among women than among men, and it may be lowest among African-American or Hispanic-American women and those of lower socioeconomic status. Sedentary behavior is an important risk factor for chronic disease morbidity and mortality; however, there is encouraging evidence that moderate levels of physical activity may provide protection from certain chronic diseases. More research is needed to determine the exercise prescriptions likely to lead to optimal health for women throughout their life spans. Physical activity choices and the physiological, psychosocial, and environmental determinants of activity participation vary by the sociodemographic characteristics of age, gender, and education level. Therefore, these characteristics should be fully considered by professionals when educating the public about the health effects of daily, accumulated activity. Similarly, *healthy public policy* (WHO, 1986) should focus on ways of increasing volitional activity among the public, as well as on increasing the availability and accessibility of school, worksite, and community center programs for promoting physical activity.

ACKNOWLEDGEMENTS

I wish to thank Andrea M. Kriska, Patty S. Freedson, Ethan R. Nadel, and Clyde Williams for their valuable comments on the manuscript. This work was supported by NIH Grant AG-09872.

BIBLIOGRAPHY

Aaron, D.J., A.M. Kriska, S.R. Dearwater, R.L. Anderson, T.L. Olsen, J.A. Cauley, and R.E. Laporte (1993). The epidemiology of leisure physical activity in an adolescent population. *Med. Sci. Sports Exerc.* 25:847–853.

Ainsworth, B.E., W.L. Haskell, A.S. Leon, D.R. Jacobs, Jr., H.J. Monyoye, J.F. Sallis, and R.S. Paffenbarger, Jr. (1993a). Compendium of physical activities: classification of energy costs of human physical activities. *Med. Sci. Sports Exerc.* 25:71–80.

Ainsworth, B.E., M. Richardson, D.R. Jacobs, and A.S. Leon (1993b). Gender differences in physical activity. *Women in Sports and Activity Journal.* 2:1–16.

Albanes, D., A. Blair, and P.R. Taylor (1989). Physical activity and risk of cancer in the NHANES I population. *Am. J. Pub. Health* 79:744–750.

American College of Sports Medicine (1990). Guidelines for the recommended quantity and quality of exercise for developing and maintaining cardiorespiratory and muscular fitness in healthy adults. *Med. Sci. Sports Exerc.* 22:265–274.

Bailey, R.C., J. Olson, S.L. Pepper, J. Porszasz, T.J. Barstow and D.M. Cooper (1995). The level and tempo of children's physical activities: an observational study. *Med. Sci. Sports Exerc.* 27:1033–1041.

Ballor, D.L., and R.E. Keesey (1991). A meta-analysis of the factors affecting exercise-induced changes in body mass, fat mass in males and females. *Int. J. Obes.* 5:717–726.

Baranowski, T. (1987). Validity and reliability of self-report measures of physical activity: an information processing perspective. *Res. Q. Exerc. Sport.* 59:314–327.

Baranowski, T., C. Bouchard, O. Bar-Or, T. Bricker, G. Heath, S.Y.S. Kimm, R. Malina, E. Obarzanek, R.R. Pate, and W.B. Strong (1992). Assessment, prevalence, and cardiovascular benefits of physical activity and fitness in youth. *Med. Sci. Sports Exerc.* 24(Suppl.):S237–247.

Baranowski, T., Y. Tsong, J. Henske, J.K. Dunn, P. Hooks, and P. Davis (1988). Ethnic variation in blood pressure among preadolescent children. *Pediatr. Res.* 23:270–274.

Berkowitz, R.I., W.S. Agras, A.F. Korner, H.C. Kraemer, and C.H. Zeanah (1985). Physical activity and adiposity: a longitudinal study from birth to childhood. *J. Pediatr.* 106:734–738.

Bernstein, L., B.E. Henderson, R. Hanisch, J. Sullivan-Halley, and R.K. Ross (1994). Physical exercise and reduced risk of breast cancer in young women. *J. Nat. Cancer Inst.* 86:1403–1408.

Bild, D.E., D.R. Jacobs, Jr., S. Sidney, W.L. Haskell, N. Anderssen, and A. Oberman (1993). Physical activity in young black and white women. The CARDIA Study. *Ann. Epidemiol.* 3:636–644.

Bird, C. (1979). *The Two-Paycheck Marriage.* New York:Rawson-Wade.

Bjorntorp, P. (1990). Adipose tissue adaptation to exercise. In: C. Bouchard, R.J. Shephard, T. Stephens, J.R. Sutton, and B.D. McPherson (eds.) *Exercise, Fitness, and Health: A Consensus of Current Knowledge.* Champaign, IL: Human Kinetics, pp. 315–323.

Bjorntorp, P. (1991). Adipose tissue distribution and function. *Int. J. Obes.* 15:67–81.

Bjorntorp, P. (1981). The effects of exercise on plasma insulin. *Int. J. Sports Med.* 2:125–129.

Blair, S.N., N.N. Goodyear, L.W. Gibbons, and K.H. Cooper (1984). Physical fitness and incidence of hypertension in healthy normotensive men and women. *J.A.M.A.* 252:487–490.

Blair, S.N., H.W., Kohl, III, and N.F. Gordon (1992a). Physical activity and health: a life-style approach. *Med. Ex. Nutr. Health* 2:54–57.

Blair, S.N., H.W. Kohl, III, N.F. Gordon, R.S. Paffenbarger, Jr. (1992b). How much physical activity is good for health? *Ann. Rev. Publ. Health* 13:99–126.

Blair, S.N., H.W. Kohl, III, R.S. Paffenbarger, Jr., D.G. Clark, K.H. Cooper, and L.W. Gibbons (1989). Physical fitness and all-cause mortality. A prospective study of healthy men and women. *J.A.M.A.* 262:2395–2401.

Bodin, J., and B. Mitelman (1983). *Mothers Who Work: Strategies for Coping.* New York:Random House.

Bouchard, C., and R.M. Malina (1983). Genetics of physiological fitness and motor performance. *Exerc. Sport Sci. Res.* 11:306–339.

Bouchard, C., R. Lesage, G. Lortie, J.A. Simoneau, P. Hamel, M.R. Boulay, L. Perusse, G. Theriault, and C. Leblanc (1986). Aerobic performance in brothers, dizygotic and monozygotic twins. *Med. Sci. Sports Exerc.* 18:639–646.

Bray, M.S., W.W. Wong, J.R. Morrow, Jr., N.F. Butte, and J.M. Pivarnik (1994). Caltrac versus calorimeter determination of 24-hour energy expenditure in female children and adolescents. *Med. Sci. Sports Exerc.* 26:1524–1530.

Brownell, K.D., and A.J. Stunkard (1981). Differential changes in plasma high-density lipoprotein-cholesterol levels in obese men and women during weight reduction. *Arch. Intern. Med.* 141:1142–1146.

Burke, G.L., L.S. Webber, S.R. Srinivasan, B. Radhakrishnamurthy, D.S. Freedman, and G.S. Berenson (1986). Fasting plasma glucose and insulin levels and their relationship to cardiovascular risk factors in children: Bogalusa Heart Study. *Metabolism* 35:441–446.

Butcher, J. (1985). Longitudinal analysis of adolescent girls' participation in physical activity. *Sociol. Sport J.* 2:130–142.

Capozzo, A. (1983). Force actions in the human trunk during running. *J. Sports Med.* 23:14–22.

Caspersen, C.J. (1989). Physical activity epidemiology: concepts, methods, and applications to exercise science. *Exer. Sport Sci. Rev.* 17:423–473.

Caspersen, C.J., and L. DiPietro (1991) National estimates of physical activity among older adults. (abstract). *Med. Sci. Sports Exerc.* 23:S106.

Caspersen, C.J., and R.K. Merritt (1994). Leisure-time physical activity trends by race and social status. The Behavioral Risk Factor Surveillance System Survey, 1986–1990. (abstract). *Med. Sci. Sports Exerc.* 26:S80.

Caspersen, C.J., and R.K. Merritt (1992). Trends in physical activity patterns among older adults. The Behavioral Risk Factor Surveillance System Survey, 1986–1990. (abstract). *Med. Sci. Sports Exerc.* 24:S26.

Caspersen, C.J., and R.A. Pollard (1987). Prevalence of physical activity in the United States and its relationship to disease risk factors. (abstract). *Med. Sci. Sports Exerc.* 19:S6.

Caspersen, C.J., B.P.M. Bloemberg, W.H.M. Saris, R.K. Merritt, and D. Kromhout (1991). The prevalence of selected physical activities and their relation with coronary heart disease risk factors in elderly men: the Zutphen Study, 1985. *Am. J. Epidemiol.* 133:1–15.

Caspersen, C.J., G.M. Christenson, and R.A. Pollard (1986). The status of the 1990 Physical Fitness Objectives—Evidence from NHIS, 1985. *Pub. Health Rep.* 101:587–592.

Caspersen, C.J., and R.K. Merritt (1995). Physical activity trends among 26 states, 1986–1990. *Med. Sci. Sports Exerc.* 27:713–720.

Caspersen, C.J., R.K. Merritt, G.W. Heath, and K.K. Yeager (1990). Physical activity patterns of adults age 60 years and older. (abstract). *Med. Sci. Sports Exerc.* 22:S79.

Caspersen, C.J., K.E. Powell, and G.M. Christenson (1985). Physical activity, exercise, and physical fitness: definitions and distinctions for health-related research. *Pub. Health Rep.* 100:126–131.

Centers for Disease Control (1995). Prevalence of recommended levels of physical activity among women—Behavioral Risk Factor Surveillance System, 1992. *Morbid. Mortal. Weekly Rep.* 44:105–113.

Centers for Disease Control (1993). Prevalence of sedentary life-style—BRFSS, United States, 1991. *Morbid. Mortal. Weekly Rep.* 42:576–579.

Centers for Disease Control (1992). Vigorous physical activity among high school students—United States, 1990. *Morbid. Mortal. Weekly Rep.* 41:33–35.

Coon, P.J., E.R. Bleeker, D.T. Drinkwater, D.A. Meyers, and A.P. Goldberg (1990). Effects of body composition and exercise capacity on glucose tolerance, insulin, and lipoprotein lipids in healthy older men: a cross-sectional and longitudinal intevention study. *Metabolism* 38:1201–1209.

Dalsky, G., K.S. Stocke, and A.A. Ehsani (1988). Weight-bearing exercise training and lumbar bone mineral content in postmenopausal women. *Ann. Int. Med.* 108:824–828.

Dannenberg, A.L., J.B. Keller, P.W.F. Wilson, and W.P. Castelli (1989). Leisure-time physical activity in the Framingham Offspring Study. Description, seasonal variation, and risk factor correlates. *Am. J. Epidemiol.* 129:76–88.

Dansforth, J.S., K.D. Allen, J.M. Fitterling, et al. (1990). Exercise as a treatment for hypertension in low-socioeconomic-status black children. *J. Consult. Clin. Psychol.* 58:237–239.

Davies, P.S.W., J. Gregory, and A. White (1995). Physical activity and body fatness in pre-school children. *Int. J. Obes.* 19:6–10.

DeBusk, R.F., U. Stenestrand, M. Sheehan, and W.L. Haskell (1990). Training effects of long versus short bouts of exercise in healthy subjects. *Am. J. Cardiol.* 65:1010-1013.

Deem, R. (1982). Women, leisure, and inequality. *Leisure Studies* 1:29-46.

DeFronzo, R.A., and E. Ferrannini (1991). Insulin resistance: a multifaceted syndrome responsible for NIDDM, obesity, hypertension, dyslipidemia, and atherosclerotic cardiovascular disease. *Diabetes Care* 14:173-194.

Dengel D.R., J.M. Hagberg, P.J. Coon, D.T. Drinkwater, and A.P. Goldberg (1994). Comparable effects of diet and exercise on body composition and lipoproteins in older men. *Med. Sci. Sports Exerc.* 26:1307-1315.

Desmond, S.M., J.H. Price, R.S. Lock, D. Smith, and P.W. Stewart (1990). Urban black and white adolescents' physical fitness status and peceptions of exercise. *J. Sch. Health* 60:220-226.

Despres, J-P., C. Bouchard, and R.M. Malina (1990a). Physical activity and coronary heart disease risk factors during childhood and adolescence. *Exerc. Sport Sci. Rev.* 18:243-261.

Despres, J-P., S. Moorjani, A. Tremblay, E.T. Poehlman, P.J. Lupien, A. Nadeau, and C. Bouchard (1988a). Heredity and changes in plasma lipids and lipoproteins after short-term exercise training in men. *Arteriosclerosis* 8:402-409.

Despres, J-P., M.C. Pouliot, S. Moorjani, A. Nadeau, A. Tremblay, P.J. Lupien, G. Theriault, and C. Bouchard (1991). Loss of abdominal fat and metabolic response to exercise training in obese women. *Am. J. Physiol.* 261:E159-E167.

Despres, J-P., A. Tremblay, and C. Bouchard (1989b). Sex differences in the regulation of body fat mass with exercise training. In: P. Bjorntorp and S. Rossner (eds.) *Obesity in Europe, I.* London: Libbey, pp. 297-304.

Despres, J-P., A. Tremblay, A. Nadeau, and C. Bouchard (1988b). Physical training and changes in regional adipose tissue distribution. *Acta Med. Scand., Suppl.* 723:205-212.

DiPietro, L. (1995). Physical activity, body weight, and adiposity: an epidemiologic perspective. *Exerc. Sport Sci. Rev.* 23:275-303.

DiPietro, L., and C.J. Caspersen (1991). National estimates of physical activity among white and black Americans. (abstract). *Med. Sci. Sports Exerc.* 23:S105.

DiPietro, L., C.J. Caspersen, A.M. Ostfeld, and E.R. Nadel (1993a). A survey for assessing physical activity among older adults. *Med. Sci. Sports Exerc.* 25:628-642.

DiPietro, L., A.M. Ostfeld, and G.L. Rosner (1994). Adiposity and stroke among older adults of low socioeconomic status: The Chicago Stroke Study. *Am. J. Pub. Health* 84:14-19.

DiPietro, L., D.F. Williamson, C.J. Caspersen, and E. Eaker (1993b). The descriptive epidemiology of selected physical activities and body weight among adults trying to lose weight: The Behavioral Risk Factor Surveillance System Survey, 1989. *Int. J. Obes.* 17:69-76.

Dishman, R.K., and M. Steinhardt (1988). Reliability and concurrent validity for a seven-day recall of physical activity in college students. *Med. Sci. Sport Exerc.* 20:14-25.

Dishman, R.K., J.F. Sallis, and D.R. Orenstein (1985). The determinants of physical activity and exercise. *Pub. Health Rep.* 100:158-171.

Dorgan, J.F., C. Brown, M. Barrett, G.L. Splansky, B.E. Kreger, R.B. D'Agostino, D. Albanes, and A. Schatzkin (1994). Physical activity and risk of breast cancer in the Framingham Heart Study. *Am. J. Epidemiol.* 139:662-669.

Douglas, P.S., T.B. Clarkson, N.C. Flowers, K.A. Hajjar, E. Horton, F.J. Klocke, J. LaRosa, and C. Shively (1992). Exercise and atherosclerotic heart disease in women. *Med. Sci. Sports Exerc. (Suppl.)* 24:S266-S276.

Dowse, G.K., P.Z. Zimmett, H. Gareeboo, K.G. Alberti, J. Tuomilehto, C.F. Finch, P. Chitson, and H. Tulsidas (1991). Abdominal adiposity and physical inactivity are risk factors for NIDDM and impaired glucose tolerance in Indk of breast cancer in the Framingham Heart Study. Indian, Creole, and Chinese Mauritians. *Diabetes Care* 14:271-282.

Drinkwater, B.L. (1994). Physical activity, fitness and osteoporosis. In: C. Bouchard, R.J. Shephard, and T. Stephens (eds.) *Physical Activity, Fitness, and Health: International Proceedings and Consensus Statement.* Champaign, IL: Human Kinetics.

Durant, R.H., T. Baranowski, H. Davis, T. Rhodes, W.O. Thompson, K.A. Greaves, and J. Puhl (1993). Reliability and variability of indicators of heart-rate monitoring in children. *Med. Sci. Sports Exerc.* 25:389-395.

Durant, R.H., T. Baranowski, H. Davis, W.O. Thompson, J. Puhl, K.A. Greaves, and T. Rhodes (1992). Reliability and variability of heart rate monitoring in 3-, 4-, or 5-yr-old children. *Med. Sci. Sports Exerc.* 24:265-271.

Durant, R.H., C.W. Linder, and O.M. Mahoney (1983). Relationship between habitual physical activity and serum lipoprotein levels in white male adolescents. *J. Adolesc. Health Care* 4:235-240.

Durstine, J.L., and W.L. Haskell (1994). Effects of exercise training on plasma lipids and lipoproteins. *Exerc. Sport Sci. Rev.* 22:477-520.

Dzewaltowski, D.A. (1994). Physical activity determinants: a social cognitive approach. *Med. Sci. Sports Exerc.* 26:1395-1399.

Eaton, W.O., and L.R. Enns (1986). Sex differences in human motor activity level. *Psychol. Bull.* 100:19-28.

Ebisu, T. (1985). Splitting the distance of endurance running on cardiovascular endurance and blood lipids. *Jpn. J. Phys. Educ.* 30:37–43.

Ekelund, L., W.L. Haskell, J.L. Johnson, F.S. Whaley, M.H. Criqui, and D.S. Sheps (1988). Physical fitness as a predictor of cardiovascular mortality in asymptomatic North American men: The Lipid Research Clinics Mortality Follow-up Study. *N. Engl. J. Med.* 319:1379–1384.

Emery, C.F., and J.A. Blumenthal (1991). Effects of physical exercise on psychological and cognitive function of older adults. *Ann. Behavior. Med.* 13:99–107.

Epstein, L.H., and R.R. Wing (1980). Aerobic exercise and weight. *Addict. Behav.* 5:371–388.

Eriksson, R.O., and G. Koch (1973). Effect of physical training on hemodynamic response during submaximal and maximal exercise. *Acta Physiol. Scand.* 87:27–39.

Farmer, M.E., T. Harris, J.H. Madans, R.B. Wallace, J. Cornoni-Huntley, and L.R. White (1989). Anthropometric indicators and hip fracture. The NHANES I epidemiologic follow-up study. *J. Am. Geriatr. Soc.* 37:9–16.

Fehily, A.M., R.J. Coles, W.D. Evans, and P.C. Elwood (1992). Factors affecting bone density in young adults. *Am. J. Clin. Nutr.* 56:579–586.

Ferguson, K.V., C.E. Yesalis, P.R. Pomrehn, and M.B. Kirkpatrick (1989). Attitudes, knowledge, and beliefs as predictors of exercise intent and behavior in school children. *J. Sch. Health.* 59:112–115.

Fiaterone, M.A., E.C. Marks, N.D. Ryan, C.N. Meredith, L.A. Lipsitz, and W.J. Evans (1990). High intensity strength training in nonagerians. *J.A.M.A.* 263:3029–3034.

Folsom, A.R., C.J. Caspersen, H.L. Taylor, D.R. Jacobs, Jr., R.V. Luepker, O. Gomez-Marin, R.F. Gillum, and H. Blackburn (1985). Leisure time physical activity and its relationship to coronary risk factors in a population-based survey: The Minnesota Heart Survey. *Am. J. Epidemiol.* 121:570–579.

Folsom, A.R., T.C. Cook, J.M. Sprafka, G.L. Burke, S.W. Norsted, and D.R. Jacobs (1991). Differences in leisure-time physical activity levels between blacks and whites in a population-based sample: The Minnesota Heart Survey. *J. Behav. Med.* 14:1–9.

Freedson, P.S. (1991). Electronic motion sensors and heart rate as measures of physical activity in children. *J. School Health* 61:220–223.

Freedson, P.S. (1989). Field monitoring of physical activity in children. *Pediatr. Exerc. Sci.* 1:8–18.

Frey, M.A.B., B.M. Doerr, L.L. Laubach, B.L. Mann, and C.J. Glueck (1982). Exercise does not change high-density lipoprotein cholesterol in women after 10 weeks of training. *Metabolism* 31:1142–1146.

Frisch, R.E., G. Wyshak, N.L. Albright, L. Schiff, K.P. Jones, J. Witschi, E. Shiang, E. Koff, and M. Marguglio (1985). Lower prevalence of breast cancer and cancers of the reproductive system among former college athletes compared to non-athletes. *Br. J. Cancer* 52:885–891.

Frontera, W.R., C.N. Meredith, K.P. O'Reilly, H.G. Knuttgen, and W.J. Evans (1988). Strength conditioning in older men: skeletal muscle hypertrophy and improved function. *J. Appl. Physiol.* 64:1038–1044.

Fulton, J.P., S. Katz, S.S. Jack, and G.E. Hendershot (1989). Physical functioning of the aged: United States, 1984. *Vital and Health Statistics, Series 10, No. 167. Department of Health and Human Services pub. (PHS) 89-1595.* Hyattsville, MD: National Center for Health Statistics.

Gilliam, T.B., and M.B. Burke. (1978). Effects of exercise on serum lipids and lipoproteins in girls, ages 8 to 10 years. *Artery* 4:203–213.

Gilliam, T.B., and P.S. Freedson (1980). Effects of a 12-week school physical fitness program on peak VO_2, body composition, and blood lipids in 7- to 9-year old children. *Int. J. Sports Med.* 1:73–78.

Godin, G., and R.J. Shephard (1986). Psychosocial factors influencing intentions to exercise of young students from grades 7 to 9. *Res. Q. Exerc. Sport* 57:41–52.

Godin, G., P. Valois, R.J. Shephard, and R. Desharnais (1987). Prediction of leisure-time exercise behavior: a path analysis (LISREL V) model. *J. Behav. Med.* 10:145–158.

Gordon, N.F., and K.H. Cooper (1988). Controlling cholesterol levels through exercise. *Comprehensive Ther.* 14:52–57.

Gordon, N.F., C.B. Scott, W.J. Wilkinson, J.J. Duncan, and S.N. Blair (1990). Exercise and mild essential hypertension. Recommendations for adults. *Sports Med.* 10:390–404.

Gottlieb, N.H., and M. Chen (1985). Sociocultural coorelates of childhood sporting activities: their implications for heart health. *Soc. Sci. Med.* 21:533–539.

Granhad, H., R. Jonson, and T. Hansson (1987). The loads on the lumbar spine during extreme weight lifting. *Spine* 12:146–149.

Haffner, S.N., B.D. Mitchell, H.P. Hazuda, and M.S. Stern (1991). Greater influence of central distribution of adipose tissue on incidence of non-insulin-dependent diabetes in women than men. *Am. J. Clin. Nutr.* 53:1312–1317.

Hagberg, J.M. (1990). Exercise, fitness, and hypertension. In: C. Bouchard, R.J. Shephard, T. Stephens, J.R. Sutton, and B.D. McPherson (eds.) *Exercise, Fitness, and Health: A Consensus of Current Knowledge.* Champaign, IL: Human Kinetics, pp. 455–466.

Hagberg, J.M., D. Goldring, A.A. Ehsani, G.W. Heath, A. Hernandez, K. Schechtman, and J.O. Holloszy (1983). Effect of exercise training on the blood pressure hemodynamic features of hypertensive adolescents. *Am. J. Cardiol.* 52:763–768.

Halioua, L., and J.J.B. Anderson (1989). Lifetime calcium intake and physical activity habits: independent and combined effects on the radial bone of healthy premenopausal Caucasian women. *Am. J. Clin. Nutr.* 49:534–541.

Hardman, A.E., and A. Hudson (1994). Brisk walking and serum lipid and lipoprotein variables in previously sedentary women—effect of 12 weeks of regular brisk walking followed by 12 weeks of detraining. *Br. J. Sp. Med.* 28:261–266.

Hardman, A.E., P.R.M. Jones, N.G. Norgan, and A. Hudson (1992). Brisk walking improves endurance fitness without changing body fatness in previously sedentary women. *Eur. J. Appl. Physiol.* 65:345–349.

Hardman, A.E., A. Hudson, P.R.M. Jones, and N.G. Norgan (1989). Brisk walking and plasma high density lipoprotein cholesterol concentration in previously sedentary women. *Br. Med. J.* 299:1204–1205.

Haskell, W.L. (1984). The influence of exercise on the concentrations of triglycerides and cholesterol in human plasma. *Exerc. Sport Sci. Rev.* 12:205–244.

Haskell, W.L. (1986). The influence of exercise training on plasma lipids and lipoproteins in health and disease. *Acta. Med. Scand. (Suppl.).* 711:25–37.

Haskell, W.L. (1985). Physical activity and health: Need to define the required stimulus. *Am. J. Cardiol.* 55:4D–9D.

Haskell, W.L., and W.T. Phillips (1995). Exercise training, fitness, health, and longevity. In: D.R. Lamb, G.V. Gisolfi, and E.R. Nadel (eds.) *Perspectives in Exercise Science and Sports Medicine. Volume 8: Exercise in Older Adults.* Carmel, IN: Cooper Publishing Group, pp. 11–52.

Helmrich, S.P., D.R. Ragland, R.W. Leung, and R.S. Paffenbarger, Jr. (1991). Physical activity and reduced occurrence of non-insulin-dependent diabetes mellitus. *N. Engl. J. Med.* 325:147–152.

Hopkins, W.G., N.C. Wilson, and D.G. Russell (1991) Validation of the physical activity instrument for life in the New Zealand National Survey. *Am. J. Epidemiol.* 133:73–82.

Hughes, V.A., W.R. Frontera, G.E. Dallal, K.J. Lutz, E.C. Fisher, and W.J. Evans (1995). Muscle strength and body composition: associations with bone density in older subjects. *Med. Sci. Sports Exerc.* 27:967–974.

Hughes, R.A., W.G. Thorland, T.J. Housh, and G.O. Johnson (1990). The effect of exercise intensity on serum lipoprotein responses. *J. Sports Med. Phys. Fitness* 30:254–260.

Jacobs, D.R., Jr., L.P. Hahn, A.R. Folsom, P.J. Hannan, J.M. Sprafka, and G.L. Burke (1991). Time trends in leisure-time physical activity in the upper midwest 1957–1987: University of Minnesota Studies. *Epidemiology* 2:8–15.

Johnson, M.L., B.S. Burke, and J. Mayer (1956). Relative importance of inactivity and overeating in the energy balance of obese high school girls. *Am. J. Clin. Nutr.* 4:37–44.

Judge, J.O., C. Lindsey, M. Underwood, and D. Winsemius (1993). Balance improvements in older women: Effects of exercise training. *Phys. Ther.* 73:254–265.

Kaplan, G.A., T.E. Seeman, R.D. Cohen, L.P. Knudsen, and J. Guralnick (1987). Mortality among the elderly in the Alameda County Study: behavioral and demographic risk factors. *Am. J. Publ. Health* 77:307–312.

Katz, S.C., A.B. Ford, R.W. Moskowitz, et al. (1963). Studies of illness in the aged. The index of ADL: a standardized measure of biological and psychosocial function. *J.A.M.A.* 185:914–919.

Kelder, S.H., C.L. Perry, K.I. Klepp, and L.L. Lytle (1994). Longitudinal tracking of adolescent smoking, physical activity, and food choice behaviors. *Am. J. Public Health* 84:1121–1126.

Kiely, D.K., P.A. Wolf, L.A. Cupples, A.S. Beiser, and W.B. Kannel (1994). Physical activity and stroke risk: The Framingham Study. *Am. J. Epidemiol.* 140:608–620.

King, A.C. (1991). Community intervention for promotion of physical activity and fitness. *Exerc. Sport Sci. Rev.* 19:211–259.

King, A.C., S.N. Blair, D.E. Bild, R.K. Dishman, P.M. Dubbert, B.H. Marcus, N.B. Oldridge, R.S. Paffenbarger, Jr., K.E. Powell, and K.K. Yeager (1992). Determinants of physical activity and interventions in adults. *Med. Sci. Sports Exerc. (Suppl.)* 24:S221–S236.

King, A.C., C.B. Taylor, W.L. Haskell, and R.F. DeBusk (1990). Identifying strategies for increasing employee physical activity levels: findings from the Stanford/Lockheed exercise survey. *H. Educ. Q.* 17:269–285.

King, A.C., C.B. Taylor, W.L. Haskell, and R.F. DeBusk (1988). Strategies for increasing early adherence to and long-term maintenance of home-based exercise training in healthy middle-aged men and women. *Am. J. Cardiol.* 61:628–632.

Kirwan, J.P., W.M. Kohrt, D.M. Wojta, R.E. Bourey, and J.O. Holloszy (1993). Endurance exercise training reduces glucose-stimulated insulin levels in 60- to 70-year-old men and women. *J. Gerontol.* 48:M84–M90.

Kissebah A., and G. Krakower (1994). Regional adiposity and morbidity. *Physiol. Rev.* 74:761–811.

Klesges, R.C., T.J. Coates, L.M. Klesges, B. Holzer, J. Gustavson, and J. Barnes (1984). The FATS: an observational system for assessing physical activity in children and associated parent behavior. *Behav. Assess.* 6:333–345.

Klesges, R.C., L.H. Eck, C.L. Hanson, C.K. Haddock, and L.M. Klesges (1990). Effects of obesity, social interactions, and physical environment on physical activity in preschoolers. *Health Psychol.* 9:435–449.

Klesges, R.C., J.M. Malott, P.F. Boschee, and J.M. Weber (1986). The effects of parental influences on children's food intake, physical activity, and relative weight. *Int. J. Eating Dis.* 5:335–346.

Knapp, D.N. (1988). Behavioral management techniques and exercise promotion. In: R.K. Dishman (ed.) *Exercise Adherence: Its Impact on Public Health.* Champaign, IL: Human Kinetics, pp. 203–236.

Kriska, A.M., S.N. Blair, and M.A. Pereira (1994). The potential role of physical activity in the prevention of non-insulin-dependent diabetes mellitus: the epidemiologic evidence. *Exerc. Sport Sci. Rev.* 22:121–143.

Kriska, A.M., R.E. LaPorte, D.J. Pettitt, M.A. Charles, R.G. Nelson, L.H. Kuller, P.H. Bennett, and W.C. Knowler (1993). The association of physical activity, with obesity, fat distribution, and glucose intolerance in Pima Indians. *Diabetologia* 36:863–869.

Krucera, M. (1985). Spontaneous physical activity in preschool children. In: R.A. Binkhorst, H.C.G Kemper, and W.H.M. Saris (eds.) *Children and Exercise IV.* Champaign, IL: Human Kinetics, pp. 175–182.

LaPorte, R., L. Adams, D. Savage, G. Brenes, S. Dearwater, T. Cook. (1984). The spectrum of physical activity, cardiovascular disease, and health: an epidemiologic perspective. *Am. J. Epidemiol.* 120:507–517.

LaPorte, R.E., H.J. Montoye, and C.J. Caspersen (1985). Assessment of physical activity in epidemiologic research: problems and prospects. *Pub. Health Rep.* 100:131–146.

Laws, A., and G.M. Reaven (1992). Evidence for an independent relationship between insulin resistance and fasting plasma HDL-cholesterol, triglyceride and insulin concentrations. *J. Intern. Med.* 231:25–30.

Leon, A.S., J. Connett, D.R. Jacobs, and R. Rauramaa (1987). Leisure time physical activity levels and risk of coronary heart disease and death: The Multiple Risk Factor Intervention Trial. *J.A.M.A.* 258:2388–2395.

Lichenstein, M.J., S.L. Shields, R.G. Shiavi, and C. Burger (1989). Exercise and balance in aged women: a pilot controlled clinical trial. *Arch. Phys. Med. Rehabil.* 70:138–143.

Lobstein, D.D., B.J. Mosbacher, and A.H. Ismail (1983). Depression as a powerful discriminator between physically active and sedentary middle-aged men. *J. Psychosom. Res.* 27:69–76.

Lokey, E.A., and Z.V. Tran (1989). Effects of exercise training on serum lipids and lipoprotein concentrations in women: a meta-analysis. *Int. J. Sports Med.* 10:424–429.

Manson, J.E., E.B. Rimm, M.J. Stampfer, G.A. Colditz, W.C. Willett, A.S. Krolewski, B. Rosner, C.H. Hennekens, and F.E Speizer (1991). Physical activity and incidence of non-insulin-dependent diabetes mellitus in women. *Lancet* 338:774–778.

Marcus, B.H., and N. Owen (1992). Motivational readiness, self-efficacy, and decision-making for exercise. *J. Appl. Soc. Psychol.* 22:3–16.

Marcus, B.H., and L.R. Simkin (1993). The stages of exercise behavior. *J. Sports Med. Phys. Fitness* 33:83–88.

Marcus, B.H., and L.R. Simkin (1994). The transtheoretical model: applications to exercise behavior. *Med. Sci. Sports. Exerc.* 26:1400–1404.

Marcus, B.H., V.C. Selby, R.S. Niaura, and J.S. Rossi (1992). Self-efficacy and the stages of exercise behavior change. *Res. Q. Exerc. Sport* 63:60–66.

Marcus, R., B. Drinkwater, G. Dalsky, J. Dufek, D. Raab, C. Slemenda, and C. Snow-Harter (1992). Osteoporosis and exercise in women. *Med. Sci. Sports Exerc. (Suppl.)* 24:S301–S307.

Matthews, K.A., S.F. Kelsey, E.N. Meilahn, L.H. Kuller, and R.R. Wing (1989). Educational attainment and behavioral and biologic risk factors for coronary heart disease in middle-aged women. *Am. J. Epidemiol.* 129:1132–1144.

McAuley, E., and L. Jacobson (1991). Self-efficacy and exercise participation in adult females. *Am. J. Health Promotion* 5:185–191.

McCulloch, R.G., D.A. Bailey, S. Houston, and B.L. Dodd (1990). Effects of physical activity, dietary calcium intake, and selected lifestyle factors on bone density in young women. *Can. Med. Assoc. J.* 142:221–227.

McKenzie, T.L., J.F. Sallis, P.R. Nader, S.L. Broyles, and J.A. Nelson (1991). BEACHES: an observational system for assessing children's eating and physical activity and associated events. *J. Appl. Behav. Anal.* 24:141–151.

Mechelen, W.V., H.C.G. Kemper, J. Twisk, G.B. Post, and D. Welten (1993). Tracking of habitual physical activity from 13–28 years of age. *Med. Sci. Sports Exerc.* 25:S122.

Merritt, R.K., and C.J. Caspersen (1992). Trends in physical activity patterns among younger adults. The Behavioral Risk Factor Surveillance System Survey, 1986–1990. (abstract). *Med. Sci. Sports Exerc.* 24:S26.

Mikines, K.J., B. Sonne, P.A. Farrell, B. Tronier, and H. Galbo (1988). Effects of physical exercise on sensitivity and responsiveness to insulin in humans. *Am. J. Physiol.* 254 (Endocrinol. Metab. 17): E248–E259.

Moll, M.E., R.S. Williams, R.M. Lester, S.H. Quarfordt, and A.G. Wallace (1979). Cholesterol metabolism in non-obese women: failure of physical conditioning to alter levels of high density lipoprotein cholesterol. *Atherosclerosis* 34:159–166.

Montoye, H.J., W. Block, J.B. Keller, and P.W. Willis (1977). Glucose tolerance and physical fitness: an epidemiologic study of an entire community. *Eur. J. Appl. Physiol.* 37:237–242.

Montoye, H.J., W.M. Mikkelsen, W.D. Block, and R. Gayle (1978). Relationship of oxygen uptake capacity, serum uric acid, and glucose tolerance in males and females, age 10–69. *Am. J. Epidemiol.* 108:274–282.

Mor, V., J. Murphy, and S. Masterson-Allen (1989). Risk of functional decline among well elders. *J. Clin. Epidemiol.* 42:895–904.

Morris, J.N., D.G. Clayton, M.G. Everitt, A.M. Semmence, and E.H. Burgess (1990). Exercise in leisure time: coronary attack and death rates. *Br. Heart J.* 63:325–334.

Morrow, J.R., Jr., and P.S. Freedson (1994). Relationship between habitual physical activity and aerobic fitness in adolescents. *Pediatr. Exerc. Sci.* 6:315–329.

Nevitt, M.C., S.R. Cummings, S.R. Kidd, and D. Black (1989). Risk factors for recurrent nonsyncopal falls: a prospective study. *J.A.M.A.* 261:2663–2668.

Oldridge, N.B., and J. Spencer. (1985). Exercise habits and perceptions before and after graduation or drop-out from supervised cardiac exercise rehabilitation. *J. Cardiopul. Rehabil.* 5:313–319.

Oldridge, N.B., and D. Streiner (1990). Health belief model as a predictor of compliance with cardiac rehabilitation. *Med. Sci. Sports Exerc.* 22:678–683.

Paffenbarger, R.S. Jr., R.T. Hyde, and A.L. Wing (1987). Physical activity and incidence of cancer in diverse populations: a preliminary report. *Am. J. Clin. Nutr.* 45 (1 Suppl.):312–317.

Paffenbarger, R.S., R.T. Hyde, A.L. Wing, and C-C. Hsieh (1986). Physical activity, all-cause mortality, and longevity of college alumni. *N. Engl. J. Med.* 314:605–613.

Paffenbarger, R.S., Jr., R.T. Hyde, A.L. Wing, I-M. Lee, D.L. Jung, and J.B. Kampert (1993). The association of changes in physical activity level and other lifestyle characteristics with mortality among men. *N. Eng. J. Med.* 328:538–545.

Paffenbarger, R.S., A.L. Wing, R.T. Hyde, and D.L. Jung (1983). Physical activity and incidence of hypertension in college alumni. *Am. J. Epidemiol.* 117:245–257.

Paganini-Hill, A., A. Chao, R.K. Ross, and B.E. Henderson (1991). Exercise and other factors in the prevention of hip fracture: The Leisure World Study. *Epidemiology* 2:16–25.

Pate, R.R., M. Dowda, T. Baranowski, and J. Puhl (1993). Tracking of physical activity behavior during early childhood. *Med. Sci. Sports Exerc.* 25:S122.

Pate, R.R., M. Dowda, and J.G. Ross (1990). Association between physical activity and physical fitness in American children. *Am. J. Dis. Child.* 144:1123–1129.

Pate, R.R., B.J. Long, and G. Heath (1994). Descriptive epidemiology of physical activity in adolescents. *Pediatr. Exerc. Sci.* 6:434–437.

Pate, R.R., M. Pratt, S.N. Blair, W.L. Haskell, C.A. Macera, C. Bouchard, D. Buchner, W. Ettinger, G.W. Heath, and A.C. King (1995). Physical activity and public health. A recommendation from the Centers for Disease Control and Prevention and the American College of Sports Medicine. *J.A.M.A.* 273:402–407.

Perusse, L., A. Tremblay, C. LeBlanc, and C. Bouchard (1989). Genetic and familial environmental influences on level of habitual physical activity. *Am. J. Epidemiol.* 129:1012–1022.

Pescatello, L.S., and L. DiPietro (1994). Physical activity in older adults: an overview of health benefits. *Sports Med.* 15:353–364.

Pescatello, L.S., L. DiPietro, A.E. Fargo, A.M. Ostfeld, and E.R. Nadel (1994). The impact of physical activity and physical fitness on health indicators among older adults. *J. Aging Phys. Act.* 2:2–13.

Pocock, N., J. Eisman, T. Gwinn, P. Sambrook, P. Kelly, J. Freund, and M. Yeates (1989). Muscle strength, physical fitness, and weight but not age predict femoral neck bone mass. *J. Bone Miner. Res.* 4:441–447.

Powell, K.E. (1991). On basketballs and heartbeats. (editorial) *Epidemiology* 2:3–5.

Powell, K.E., P.D. Thompson, C.J. Caspersen, and J.S. Kendricks (1987). Physical activity and incidence of coronary heart disease. *Ann. Rev. Public Health* 8:253–287.

Raglin, J.S., W.P. Morgan, and A.E. Luchsinger (1990). Mood and self-motivation in successful and unsuccessful female rowers. *Med. Sci. Sports Exerc.* 22:849–853.

Rauramaa, R., J.T. Salonen, K. Kukkonen-Harjula, K. Seppanen, E. Seppala, H. Vapaatalo, and J.K. Huttunen (1984). Effects of mild physical exercise on serum lipoproteins and metabolites of arachidonic acid: a controlled randomised trial in middle-aged men. *Br. Med. J.* 288:603–606.

Reaven, G.M. (1995) Insulin resistance and aging: modulation by obesity and physical activity. In: D.R. Lamb, C.V. Gisolfi, and E.R. Nadel (eds.) *Perspectives in Exercise Science and Sports Medicine. Volume 8: Exercise in Older Adults.* Carmel, IN: Cooper Publishing Group. pp. 395–434.

Rebuffe-Scrive, M., J. Eldh, L-O. Hafstrom, and P. Bjorntorp (1986). Metabolism of mammery, abdominal and femoral adipocytes in women before and after menopause. *Metabolism* 35:792–797.

Rissanen, A., M. Heliovaara, P. Knekt, A. Reunanen, and A. Aromaa (1991). Determinants of weight gain and overweight in adult Finns. *Eur. J. Clin. Nutr.* 45:419–430.

Rosenthal, M., W.L. Haskell, R. Solomon, A. Widstrom, and G.M. Reaven (1983). Demonstration of a relationship between level of physical training and insulin-stimulated glucose utilization in normal humans. *Diabetes* 32:408–411.

Ross, J.G., and R.R. Pate (1987). The National Children and Youth Fitness Study II: a summary of findings. *J. Phys. Educ. Recreat. Dance* 58:51–56.

Ross, J.G., and R.R. Pate (1985). The National Children and Youth Fitness Study: a summary of findings. *J. Phys. Educ. Recreat. Dance* 56:45–50.

Ross, J.G., C.O. Dotson, G.G. Gilbert, and S.J. Katz (1985). After physical education . . . physical activity outside of school physical education programs. *J. Phys. Educ. Recreat. Dance* 56:35–39.

Rowland, T.W. (1990). *Exercise and Children's Health.* Champaign, IL: Human Kinetics, pp. 31–45.

Sallis, J.F. (1993). Epidemiology of physical activity and fitness in children and adolescents. *Crit. Rev. Food Sci. Nutr.* 33:403–408.

Sallis, J.F., and K. Patrick (1994). Physical activity guidelines for adolescents: consensus statement. *Pediatr. Exerc. Sci.* 6:302–314.

Sallis, J.F., C.C. Berry, S.L. Broyles, T.L. McKenzie, and P.R. Nader (1995). Variability and tracking of physical activity over 2 yr in young children. *Med. Sci. Sports Exerc.* 27:1042–1049.

Sallis, J.F., M.J. Buono, J.J. Roby, D. Carlson, and J.A. Nelson (1990). The Caltrac accelerometer as a physical activity monitor for school-age children. *Med. Sci. Sports Med.* 22:698–703.

Sallis, J.F., M.J. Bouno, J.J. Roby, F.G. Micale, and J.A. Nelson (1993). Seven-day recall and other physical activity self-reports in children and adolescents. *Med. Sci. Sports Exerc.* 25:99–108.

Sallis, J.F., W.L. Haskell, S.P. Fortmann, P.D. Wood, and K.M. Vranizan (1986). Predictors of adoption and maintenance of physical activity in a community sample. *Prev. Med.* 15:331–341.

Sallis, J.F., W.L. Haskell, P.D. Wood, S.P. Fortman, and K.M. Vranizan (1985). Physical activity assessment methodology in the Five-City Project. *Am. J. Epidemiol.* 121:91–106.

Sallis, J.F., M.F. Hovell, C.R. Hofstetter, P. Faucher, P. Faucher, J.B. Elder, J. Blanchard, C.J. Caspersen, K.E. Powell, and G.M. Christenson (1989). A multivariate study of determinants of vigorous exercise in a community sample. *Prev. Med.* 18:20–34.

Sallis, J.F., B.G. Simons-Morton, E.J. Stone, C.B. Corbin, L.E. Epstein, N. Faucette, R.J. Ionnotti, J.D. Killen, R.C. Klesges, C.K. Petray, T.W. Rowland, and W.C. Taylor (1992). Determinants of physical activity and interventions in youth. *Med. Sci. Sports Exerc.* 24(Suppl.):S248–S257.

Sallis, J.F., T.L. Patterson, M.J. Buono, C.J. Atkins, and P.R. Nader. (1988). Aggregation of physical activity habits in Mexican-American and Anglo families. *J. Behav. Med.* 11:31–41.

Sandvik, L., J. Erikssen, E. Thaulow, G. Erikssen, R. Mundal, and K. Rodhal (1993). Physical fitness as a predictor of mortality among healthy middle-aged Norwegian men. *N. Engl. J. Med.* 328:533–537.

Saris, W.H.M. (1985). The assessment and evaluation of daily physical in children: a review. *Acta. Paediatr. Scand. (Suppl.)* 318:37–40.

Sauvage, L.R., B.M. Myklehurst, J. Crow-Pan, S. Novak, P. Millington, M.D. Hoffman, A.J. Hartz, and D. Rudman (1992). A clinical trial of strengthening and aerobic exercise to improve gait and balance in elderly male nursing home residents. *Am. J. Phys. Med. Rehabil.* 71:33–342.

Savage, M.P., M.M. Petratis, W.H. Thompson, K. Berg, J.L. Smith, and S.P. Sady (1986). Exercise training effects on serum lipids of prepubescent boys and adult men. *Med. Sci. Sports Exerc.* 18:197–204.

Seals, D.R., J.M. Hagberg, B.F. Hurley, A.A. Ehsani, and J.O. Holloszy (1984). Effects of endurance training on glucose tolerance and plasma lipid levels in older men and women. *J.A.M.A.* 252:645–649.

Shank, J.W. (1986). An exploration of leisure in the lives of dual career women. *J. Leisure Res.* 18:300–319.

Shvartz, E., and R.C. Reibold (1990). Aerobic fitness norms for males and females aged 6 to 75 years: a review. *Aviat. Space Environ. Med.* 61:3–11.

Simonsick, E.M., M.E. Lafferty, C.L. Phillips, C.F. Mendes de Leon, S.V. Kasl, T.E. Seeman, G. Fillenbaum, P. Hebert, and J.H. Lemke (1993). Risk due to inactivity in physically capable older adults. *Am. J. Public Health* 83:1443–1450.

Sinaki, M., and K. Offord (1988). Physical activity in postmenopausal women: effect on back muscle strength and bone mineral density of the spine. *Arch. Phys. Med. Rehabil.* 69:277–280.

Sjostrom, L. (1993). Impacts of body weight, body composition, and adipose tissue distribution on morbidity and mortality. In: A.J. Stunkard and T.A. Wadden (eds.) *Obesity: Theory and Therapy, 2nd edition.* New York: Raven Press, pp. 13–41.

Snow-Harter, C., and R. Marcus (1991). Exercise, bone mineral density, and osteoporosis. In: J.O. Holloszy (ed.) *Exercise and Sport Sciences Reviews* Baltimore, MD: Williams & Wilkins, pp. 351–388.

Snow-Harter, C., M. Bouxsein, B. Lewis, S. Charette, P. Weinstein, and R. Marcus (1990). Muscle strength as a predictor of bone mineral density in young women. *J. Bone Miner. Res.* 5:589–595.

Sobolski, J., M. Kornitzer, G. DeBacker, M. Dramaix, M. Abramowicz, S. Degre, and H. Denolin (1987). Protection against ischemic heart disease in the Belgian Physical Fitness Study: physical fitness rather than physical activity? *Am. J. Epidemiol.* 125:601–610.

Sports Council and Health Education Authority (1993). Allied Dunbar National Fitness Survey. London: Belmont Press.

Stefanick, M.L. (1993). Exercise and weight control. In: J.O. Holloszy (ed) *Exercise and Sport Sciences Reviews,* Vol. 21. Baltimore, MD: Williams & Wilkins, pp. 363–396.

Stephens, T. (1993). Leisure time physical activity. In: *Canada's Health Promotion Survey, 1990: Technical Report.* T. Stephens and F.D. Graham (eds.) Ottawa, ON: Health and Welfare, Canada, pp. 139–150.

Stephens, T., and C.L. Craig (1985). Fitness and activity measurement in the 1981 Canada Fitness Survey. In: T. Stephens and C.L. Craig (eds.) *Proceedings of the workshop on assessing physical fitness and activity patterns in general population surveys.* Hyattsville, MD: NCHS, 16–20.

Stephens, T., D.R. Jacobs, and C.C. White (1985). A descriptive epidemiology of leisure-time physical activity. *Pub. Health Rep.* 100:147–158.

Stones, M.J., and A. Kozma (1987). Balance and age in the sighted and blind. *Arch. Phys. Med. Rehabil.* 68:85–89.

Taylor, C.B., J.F. Sallis, and R. Needle (1985). The relation of physical activity and exercise to mental health. *Pub. Health Rep.* 100:195-201.

Taylor, H.L., D.R. Jacobs, B. Schucker, J. Knudsen, A.S. Leon, and G. Debacker (1978). A questionnaire for the assessment of leisure time physical activities. *J. Chron. Dis.* 31:741-755.

Taylor, R.J., P. Ram, P. Zimmett, L. Raper, and H. Ringrose (1984). Physical activity and prevention of diabetes in Melanesian and Indian men in Fiji. *Diabetologia* 27:578-582.

Taylor, W., and T. Baranowski (1991). Relationship of physical activity to cardiovascular fitness among preadolescent children in three ethnic groups. *Res. Q. Exerc. Sport* 62:157-163.

Thomas, J.R., and K.E. French (1985). Gender differences in motor performance: a meta-analysis. *Psychol. Bull.* 98:260-282.

Thorland, W.G., and T.B. Gilliam (1981). Comparison of serum lipids between habitually high and low active pre-adolescent males. *Med. Sci. Sports Exerc.* 13:316-321.

Tinetti, M.E., D.I. Baker, G. McAvay, E.B. Claus, P. Garrett, M. Gottschalk, M.L. Koch, K. Trainor, and R.I. Horwitz (1994). A multifactorial intervention to reduce the risk of falling among elderly people living in the community. *N. Engl. J. Med.* 331:821-827.

Tinetti, M.E., M. Speechley, and S.F. Ginter (1988). Risk factors for falls among elderly persons living in the community. *N. Engl. J. Med.* 319:1701-1707.

Tran, Z.V., and A. Weltman (1985). Differential effects of exercise on serum lipid and lipoprotein levels seen with changes in body weight. *J.A.M.A.* 254:919-924.

Tremblay, A., J-P. Despres, J. Maheux, M.C. Pouliot, A. Nadeau, S. Moorjani, P.J. Lupien, and C. Bouchard (1991). Normalization of the metabolic profile in obese women by exercise and low fat diet. *Med. Sci. Sports Exerc.* 23:1326-1331.

Tremblay, A., E. Poehlman, A. Nadeau, L. Perusse, and C. Bouchard (1987). Is the response of plasma glucose and insulin to short-term exercise training genetically determined? *Horm. Metab. Res.* 19:65-67.

Tylavsky, F.A., J.J.B. Anderson, R.V. Talmage, and T.N. Taft (1992). Are calcium intakes and physical activity patterns during adolescence related to radial bone mass of white college-age women? *Osteoporosis Int.* 2:232-240.

U.S. Department of Health and Human Services (1991). *Healthy People 2000: national health promotion and disease prevention objectives.* Washington, D.C.: U.S. Government Printing Office. DHHS pub. (PHS) 91-50212.

U.S. Department of Health and Human Services (1989). *The Surgeon General's Report on Nutrition and Health.* Washington, D.C.: U.S. Government Printing Office. DHHS pub. (PHS) 88-50210.

Vena, J.E., S. Graham, M. Zielezny, J. Brasure, and M.K. Swanson (1987). Occupational exercise and risk of cancer. *Am. J. Clin. Nutr.* 45:318-327.

Voorrips, L.E., J.H.H. Meijers, P. Sol, J.C. Seidell, and W.A. van Staveren (1991). History of body weight and physical activity of elderly women differing in current physical activity. *Int. J. Obes.* 16:199-205.

Voors, A.W., D.W. Harsha, L.S. Webber, B. Radhakrishnamurthy, S.R. Srinivasan, and G.S. Berenson (1982). Clustering of anthropometric parameters, glucose tolerance, and serum lipids in children with high and low B- and pre-B-lipoproteins: Bogalusa Heart Study. *Arteriosclerosis* 2:346-355.

Vranic, M., and D. Wasserman (1990). Exercise, fitness and diabetes. In: C. Bouchard, R.J. Shephard, T. Stephens, J.R. Sutton, and B.D. McPherson (eds.) *Exercise, Fitness, and Health: A Consensus of Current Knowledge.* Champaign, IL: Human Kinetics, pp. 467-490.

Ward, A., and W.P. Morgan (1984). Adherence patterns of healthy men and women enrolled in an adult exercise program. *J. Cardiac. Rehabil.* 4:143-152.

Waxman, M., and A.J. Stunkard (1980). Caloric intake and expenditure of obese boys. *J. Pediatr.* 96:187-196.

Wickham, C.A.C., K. Walsh, C. Cooper, D.J. Barker, B.M. Margetts, J. Morris, and S.A. Bruce (1989). Dietary calcium, physical activity, and risk of hip fracture: a prospective study. *Br. Med. J.* 299:889-892.

Williams, P.T., R.M. Krauss, K.M. Vranizan, J.J. Albers, and P.D.S. Wood (1992) Effects of weight-loss by exercise and by diet on apolipoproteins A-I and A-II and the particle-size distribution of high-density lipoprotein in men. *Metabolism* 41:441-449.

Williamson, D.F., J. Madans, R.F. Anda, J.C. Kleinman, H.S. Kahn, and T. Byers (1993). Recreational physical activity and 10-year weight change in a U.S. national cohort. *Int. J. Obes.* 17:279-286.

Witt, P., and T. Goodale (1981). The relationships between barriers to leisure enjoyment and family stages. *J. Leisure Res.* 4:29-49.

Wood, P., W.P. Haskell, S.N. Blair, P.T. Williams, and R.M. Krauss (1983). Increased exercise level and plasma lipoprotein concentrations: a one-year, randomized controlled study in sedentary, middle-aged men. *Metabolism* 32:31-39.

World Health Organization, Health and Welfare Canada, and Canadian Public Health Association. Ottawa charter for health promotion. International Conference on Health Promotion, November, 1986. Ottawa, Ontario, CANADA.

Yeager, K.K., C.A. Macera, and R.K. Merritt (1991). Sedentary women: is it an issue of socioeconomic status? (abstract) *Med. Sci. Sports Exerc.* 23:S105.

Ylitalo, V. (1981). Treatment of obese schoolchildren with special reference to the mode of therapy, cardiorespiratory performance and the carbohydrate and lipid metabolism. *Acta Paed. Scand.* (Suppl.) 290:1-108.

DISCUSSION

COYLE: Is it clear that the declines in activity in females from 9th to 12th grade are largely sociological? In other words, if we could correct the sociologic differences between females and male adolescents will we be left with some biological reasons for increased inactivity? Do girls naturally tend toward different activity levels compared to boys?

DI PIETRO: I don't know the answer to that question.

COYLE: Do you think it would ever be possible to separate out socioeconomic effects from biological effects?

DI PIETRO: Not entirely, no.

HORSWILL: Could the data on the high schoolers be somewhat biased in that from the 9th grade to the 12th grade the school requirements for physical education may be reduced? The trend appeared to occur in the males as well as in the females.

DI PIETRO: Possibly, but these data were corroborated by studies in England; unfortunately, I am not sure what the physical education requirements are in England. There is much better access to organized activities, such as vigorous sport activities in England for girls and boys throughout different ages.

HASKELL: The CARDIA data represent four sites throughout the country and include both black and white men and women. The advantages of this data set are that the black and white populations were selected to minimize socioeconomic differences and there are data from age 18–30 at baseline with a 7-y follow-up. They are getting trend data that are consistent with the impression that it is black women whose activity declines the most, not only through high school, but up through age 25 or 50. It is just not tied to high school physical education requirements.

DESPRES: In the field of nutrition, it is pretty well accepted now that many individuals under report their energy intakes. Everybody knows that a high-fat, high-energy diet is bad for you, so it is natural to under report one's fat and energy intake. A normal individual might under report by up to 20% and an overweight individual by 40%. Most of us also know that being sedentary is bad for us. Do people over report their participation in physical activity? Do we have the appropriate tools to assess the changes in physical activity habits?

DI PIETRO: There is some controversy surrounding the accuracy of the measurement of this behavior. One may argue, for example, that the BRFSS data aren't particularly good on that score. Only 26 states are represented, and it was a telephone survey. Both under reporting and over reporting of activity are of concern.

DESPRES: It is also possible that one might take daily, 20-min brisk walks but compensate by being more sedentary between exercise bouts so that the impact of total daily energy expenditure might be trivial. Thus, the issue of the effect of exercise on total daily energy expenditure remains to be further examined.

CLAPP: What evidence is there that community action such as building a jogging path or bike trail or baseball park actually does improve physical activity for the community? I am aware of none.

DI PIETRO: There are no studies that I know of.

CLAPP: I am also interested in the relative efficacy of continuous vs. cumulative activity on people's health. What evidence is there that the cumulative model will be affective on a national basis?

DI PIETRO: That is a controversy right now concerning the issue of cumulative vs. sustained activity. There is a statement in the new ACSM/CDC recommendation paper that three 10-min bouts of exercise may be as beneficial as a 30-min sustained bout. This is based on very limited data, and I'm not prepared to comment on which is better.

LAMB: One interpretation of the epidemiological data might be that education can have a positive impact on participation in exercise. Are there educational intervention studies to support that hypothesis?

DI PIETRO: Information is a necessary determinant of physical activity, but it is certainly not sufficient.

PERRAULT: There are many constraints for women wanting to do exercise by virtue of their social roles and responsibilities. I wonder if these women really need to do more exercise. Perhaps we should give them positive reinforcement for what they are already doing throughout the day.

DI PIETRO: Barbara Ainsworth raises this same question. Is it helpful to say to women whose lives are already saturated with multiple types of activity that they need to do more? I think the big message in these guidelines is that most women can meet the recommended daily energy expenditure.

3

The Reproductive System

A.B. LOUCKS, Ph.D.

INTRODUCTION

For many years, anecdotes and case reports associated exercise training with menstrual irregularities. Then, about 20 y ago, surveys indicating a high prevalence of menstrual irregularities among female dancers and athletes began to appear as more girls and women began to participate in sports. Associations with many factors led to diverse speculations about the mechanism of these irregularities and to an argument over whether these irregularities were signs of health or disease. That argument was settled with the discovery about 10 y ago that, despite the mechanical loading of their exercise training, amenorrheic athletes had low bone densities, were losing bone over time, and suffered a higher prevalence of fractures than did regularly menstruating athletes and sedentary women (Constantini, 1994; Drinkwater, 1992). Since then, these and other morbid consequences of hypoestrogenism have motivated efforts to identify the behavioral and neuroendocrine mechanisms of athletic amenorrhea so that this disease can be effectively treated and prevented. Meanwhile, the endocrine investigation of athletic amenorrhea has revealed an asymptomatic condition, luteal suppression, which may be very common among athletes and which also raises clinical concerns.

This author (Loucks, 1990, 1994; Loucks & Horvath, 1985; Loucks et al., 1992b) and others (Bonen, 1994; Constantini, 1994) have reviewed the literature on the impact of athletic training on reproductive function in women several times. The present review summarizes the current state of knowledge on reproductive disorders in athletes, constrained as that knowledge is by our incomplete understanding of the normal regulation of the female reproductive system. It also draws attention to recent investigations of the influence of energy availability on reproductive function, and it recommends directions for future research.

CHANGES IN THE REPRODUCTIVE SYSTEM THROUGH THE LIFE CYCLE

Figure 3-1 illustrates the functional states of the reproductive system through a woman's life cycle. Only one of these states involves menstrua-

Reproductive States

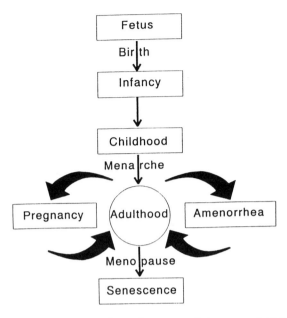

FIGURE 3-1. *The states of the human female reproductive system during a woman's life (Loucks, 1995).*

tion, but the reproductive system is highly active in all of these states except childhood and amenorrhea.

During fetal life, the mother, placenta, and fetus maintain gonadotropin and sex steroid concentrations at very high levels throughout the second and third trimesters of gestation. The contributions of the maternal-placental unit to these hormone levels disappear at birth, so sex steroid concentrations drop abruptly in the newborn, but gonadotropin levels remain as high during the first few years of infancy as they later become in the adult. Then, by unknown mechanisms, the reproductive system becomes quiescent for several years during childhood before being activated again by another unknown mechanism at puberty.

Endocrinologically, puberty extends over several years as hormone systems sequentially turn on: first, the adrenal axis at about 8 y of age, followed by the thyroid axis a year or two later, and then the reproductive axis a year or two after that. Even in the activation of the reproductive axis, menarche is a late event, following the appearance of pubic hair and early breast development, and for the next few years menses are very irregular in most females.

Although the age of menarche is reported to be later in athletes than in non-athletes, the controversies concerning the potential influence of athletic training, in general, and exercise, in particular, on the age of menarche have been reviewed several times (Loucks, 1989, 1995; Malina, 1983, 1994). None of the available evidence has been collected from girls in controlled experiments, and it has been argued that the reported differences in menarcheal age could be explained by retrospective sampling bias (Stager et al., 1990), by self-selection (Malina, 1983), by socialization processes (Malina, 1983), and by genetics (Malina et al., 1994).

During the next three decades the human female reproductive system displays the regular monthly rhythms of hormones and tissues. This is followed by another few years of menstrual irregularity before menopause when the menstrual cycle ceases permanently, despite increasing gonadotropin stimulation. As the ovaries become unresponsive to very high gonadotropin levels, sex steroid concentrations fall to very low levels, and women begin to suffer the damaging consequences of hypoestrogenism.

Of course, in most women of reproductive age the menstrual cycle is interrupted by pregnancy, and lactation also prevents gonadotropins from being secreted in the special rhythmic pattern that stimulates ovarian follicular development.

At any given time, about 3–5% of healthy women of reproductive age have not menstruated for three months or more (Bachman & Kemmann, 1982; Pettersson et al., 1973; Singh, 1981). The mechanism that turns off the menstrual cycle in these women, and which may later spontaneously turn it back on, is unknown. Like postmenopausal women, these women display chronically low estrogen levels, initiating the same damaging processes that undermine skeletal and cardiovascular health. Prompt medical intervention to supplement sex steroids may prevent these effects (Committee on Sports Medicine of the American Academy of Pediatrics, 1989; Shangold et al., 1990).

The above remarks indicate how little is known about the mechanisms that regulate the normal switching of the reproductive system from state to state during a woman's lifetime. Without an understanding of normal reproductive physiology, it is especially difficult to identify the mechanism of menstrual disorders or to treat the affected women appropriately so that their reproductive health can be recovered and so that potential long-term effects on disease processes such as osteoporosis and breast cancer can be prevented.

CROSS-SECTIONAL OBSERVATIONS OF EXERCISE-ASSOCIATED MENSTRUAL DISTURBANCES

Luteal Suppression

The term *luteal suppression* refers to a reduction in the length of the luteal phase or a reduction in progesterone levels during the luteal phase of the menstrual cycle. It is not known whether this condition represents a midpoint in a progressive condition that worsens to amenorrhea under more severe training regimens, or to the end point of successful acclimation to even the most severe regimens, or to the end point of reproductive disturbances in especially robust individuals.

The clinical consequences of luteal suppression are speculative. Estrogen levels are unimpaired during luteal suppression so skeletal integrity appears not to be a concern. However, because one category of infertile women displays luteal phases shorter than 10 d, fertility is a concern. Under estrogen stimulation during the follicular phase of the menstrual cycle, the inner lining or endometrium of the uterus proliferates and becomes highly vascularized. During the luteal phase after ovulation, progesterone secreted by the corpus luteum maintains this lining. If an egg released from the ovarian follicle during ovulation is not fertilized, the corpus luteum ages and dies, progesterone production declines, the endometrium sloughs off, and the egg is washed away in menstrual blood. If the egg is fertilized late, or if the production of estrogen and progesterone by the corpus luteum is inadequate or declines prematurely, the fertilized ovum encounters a degenerated endometrium and is again washed away with the endometrium in menstrual blood. No information on the fertility of athletes with luteal suppression is available.

A second concern is breast cancer. Epidemiological evidence associates short luteal phase and low progesterone levels with breast cancer (Cowan et al., 1981; Mauvais-Jarvis et al., 1982; Sherman & Korenman, 1974). The hypothetical physiological explanation for this association is that the unimpaired estrogen secretion in these women is not sufficiently "opposed" by progesterone. The available epidemiological evidence on the relationship between physical activity and breast cancer is conflicting and weak (Bernstein et al., 1994; Dorgan et al., 1994). This is not the place for a review of the literature on that subject, but a summary of two studies indicates the limitations of the evidence.

Data from a retrospective case-control study have been presented as indicating that physical exercise is protective against breast cancer (Bernstein et al., 1994). In this study, 545 premenopausal women between the ages of 36 and 40 diagnosed with breast cancer were matched with 545 similar women without breast cancer. "Physical exercise" was quantified in two ways: by the weekly hours of exercise during the first 10 y after menarche, and by the weekly hours of exercise between menarche and a reference date one year before the case's diagnosis. After adjustment for various confounding factors, not including diet, a progressively declining proportion of such "breast cancer" cases occurred as "physical exercise" increased (P<0.0001), but only in parous women. There was no effect among nulliparous women, perhaps, the investigators speculated, because some such women may have reproductive disorders with steroid abnormalities similar to the hypothesized effect of physical activity. Perhaps inconsistently with this study, the NHANES I (National Health and Nutrition Examination Survey) Epidemiological Follow-up Study found the risk of premenopausal breast cancer to be nonsignificantly elevated among the most active women (Albanes et al., 1989).

By contrast, prospective data from the Framingham Heart Study have been presented as not supporting a protective effect of physical activity on breast cancer (Dorgan et al., 1994). In this study "physical activity" was quantified as a weighted rating of time spent in various occupational and leisure activities at the time of the 4th biennial examination conducted between 1954 and 1956, when the 2321 women were between the ages of 35 and 68 y. Physical activity levels at the time of the 11th and 12th biennial examinations 14 to 16 y later had little correlation with the earlier ratings (rank correlation = 0.25 and 0.18, respectively) but were not included in the analysis. "Breast cancer" in the Framingham study included a total of 117 cases identified at examinations, at Framingham Union Hospital, and on death records. Almost all of these (91%) were postmenopausal cases. Thus, the premenopausal breast cancers studied by Bernstein's group may not be representative of the vast majority of breast cancers that women suffer. Very few Framingham women (5% of cases and 6% of non-cases) participated in strenuous activities, so data from women who participated in strenuous activities and moderate activities (effort greater than walking and less than running) were combined for analysis. Diet was not examined. The only suggestion of an association between "physical activity" and "breast cancer" so defined was a marginally significant (P = 0.06) 20% increase in the proportion of cases of breast cancer among women who replaced an hour of sleep and rest with an hour of moderate-to-heavy leisure activity.

Other epidemiological studies that have purported to find a relationship between physical activity and breast cancer have used less direct measures of physical activity. One such study used participation in college athletics as the index of physical activity, relied on self-reports of cancer, and excluded women who had died (Frisch et al., 1985). Another study interpreted inferred physical activity from occupations (Vena et al., 1987). A retrospective comparison of physical education and language teachers found a higher risk of premenopausal breast cancers among the language teachers but little difference in postmenopausal breast cancers (Vihko et al., 1992).

Like all observational studies, these attempts to find a relationship between physical activity and breast cancer have been highly susceptible to bias by confounding factors. In particular, as with almost all animal and human experiments that have investigated the influence of exercise on the reproductive system, these observational studies have not distinguished physical activity from its energy cost. This is a critical oversight because the hypothesized reproductively-suppressive effect of physical activity is identical to the known reproductively-suppressive effect of dietary restriction. The scientific literature contains no information about the independent effect of physical activity on the reproductive system in adequately nourished women. Our own short-term experiments indicate that exercise has no deleterious effect on the reproductive system in women beyond the impact of its energy cost on energy availability, the effect of which can be completely blocked by dietary supplementation (Loucks & Callister, 1993; Loucks & Heath, 1994; Loucks et al., 1994a, 1994b, 1995).

Prevalence. Luteal suppression is entirely asymptomatic when it is expressed as an attenuation of progesterone production and when the length of the menstrual cycle is unaffected, because abbreviation of the luteal phase is matched by extension of the follicular phase. Therefore, regularly menstruating athletes with luteal suppression are often entirely unaware that their reproductive functions are in any way unusual. The only way to detect luteal suppression is by assaying for progesterone in a series of blood, urine, or saliva samples throughout a menstrual cycle. Because such measurements have not been made on a wide scale, the prevalence of luteal suppression has not been quantified. Nevertheless, its observation in even the most regularly menstruating, competitive athletes (Loucks et al., 1989) as well as in recreational athletes (Ellison & Lager, 1986) suggests that the prevalence in the general athletic population, which also includes many women with shorter, longer, and less regular menstrual cycles, may be extremely high.

Behavioral Characterization. Cross-sectional comparisons have found regularly menstruating and amenorrheic athletes to be similar in dietary habits, exercise regimens, and body compositions. Investigations comparing reported dietary energy intake to estimated energy expenditure have found that both regularly menstruating and amenorrheic athletes report their dietary energy intakes to be much less than would be expected for their levels of physical activity (Drinkwater et al., 1984; Kaiserauer et al., 1989; Loucks et al., 1989; Marcus et al., 1985; Nelson et al., 1986). Some investigators have attributed these reports to underreporting of dietary energy intake (Edwards et al., 1993; Wilmore et al., 1992), but the author is not convinced. The very universality of such reports is an argument against this interpretation. Can no one anywhere find an honest athlete? In the author's opinion, the possibility that commonly used techniques overestimate energy expenditure in chronically energy-deficient subjects deserves investigation. The underreporting hypothesis appears to be contradicted by the metabolic and endocrine symptoms of energy deficiency, at least as observed in amenorrheic athletes as described below. Meanwhile, in contrast to a common assumption of the proponents of the underreporting hypothesis, stable body weight is *not* proof of energy sufficiency. Behavior modification and endocrine-mediated alterations of resting metabolic rate can counteract the influences of energy excess and energy deficiency on body weight (Leibel et al., 1995). Whereas many mechanisms have been hypothesized to explain the high prevalence of amenorrhea among athletes, few hypotheses have been offered to explain the regular reproductive function maintained by other athletes cross-sectionally similar in body composition, exercise training, and reported dietary intake. Thus, regularly menstruating athletes present a largely unaddressed challenge to investigators seeking to understand the relationship between physical activity and reproductive function.

Endocrine Characterization. Regularly menstruating, competitive triathletes and runners, whose menstrual cycles were symptomatically indistinguishable from those of sedentary women, i.e., occurring at regular intervals of 26–32 d, have been shown to display luteal phases that were 2 d shorter and progesterone levels that were reduced almost 50% (Figure 3-2, Cyclic Athletes) (Loucks et al., 1989). Similar observations have been made in women running as little as 20 km/wk (Broocks et al., 1990; Ellison & Lager, 1986; Pirke et al., 1990).

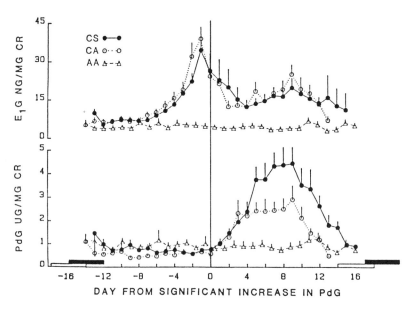

FIGURE 3-2. *Urinary estrone-glucuronide ($E_1 G$), an estradiol metabolite, and pregnanediol-glucuronide (PdG), a progesterone metabolite, over an entire menstrual cycle in cyclic sedentary women (CS) and cyclic athletes (CA), and over an entire month in amenorrheic athletes (AA).* The mass of each metabolite (ng E_1 and μg PdG) excreted in overnight urine samples was normalized to the mass (mg) of creatinine (CR) excreted in the same samples. The black and open bars at the bottom of the figure indicate the days of menses in the CS and CA women, respectively, at the beginning and end of the cycle of observation (Loucks et al., 1989).

Glands do not secrete hormones at a continuous rate. Rather, hormones are secreted in discrete pulses many times a day. For hormones like LH that are rapidly cleared from the blood, these pulses are obvious in the pattern of hormone measurements in blood samples drawn at frequent intervals throughout the day. Clinical tests have shown that it is the frequency of LH pulses that regulates ovarian follicular development. Thus, the steady infusion of GnRH fails to stimulate ovarian function in women with inadequate GnRH production, whereas the pulsatile infusion of GnRH at intervals of 60–90 min is frequently an effective treatment for infertility, resulting in many pregnancies and successful births (Liu & Yen, 1984).

The typical pulsatile pattern of the LH concentrations of a regularly menstruating, sedentary young woman (Cyclic Sedentary) during a 24-h period in the early follicular phase of the menstrual cycle is shown in Figure 3-3. Such patterns are characterized by regular, high frequency pulses

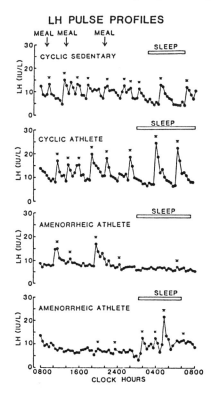

FIGURE 3-3. *The 24-hour pulsatile rhythms of luteinizing hormone (LH), expressed as international units per liter (IU/L), for a cyclic (regularly menstruating) sedentary woman, a cyclic athlete, and two amenorrheic athletes. Among amenorrheic athletes, the extensively quiescent, irregular pulsatile rhythms differed markedly. Pulsatile rhythms were considerably less variable among cyclic sedentary women and athletes (Loucks et al., 1989).*

of low amplitude. During sleep the frequency slows down, and the amplitude increases. In the luteal phase (not shown) larger pulses occur at a considerably slower, regular frequency.

In contrast to the regular pattern of high-frequency, low-amplitude LH pulses in the early follicular phase in regularly menstruating, sedentary women, larger-amplitude LH pulses occur regularly at a slower frequency in cyclic athletes with luteal suppression (Loucks et al., 1989) (Figure 3-3, Cyclic Athlete). Whether the greater amplitude of the lower-frequency LH pulses derives from increased responsiveness of the anterior pituitary to normal GnRH pulses or to normal sensitivity to larger GnRH pulses is unknown.

Amenorrhea

The term *amenorrhea* refers to the cessation of menstrual function. Two types of amenorrhea are distinguished by physicians: primary amenorrhea in which menarche is abnormally delayed, and secondary amenorrhea in which menses cease sometime after menarche. Although athletic women report retrospectively that their menarche occurred later than did those of non-athletic women, there exists no evidence that their menarche was delayed, i.e., would have occurred earlier under different circumstances. The later age of menarche among athletic women may be due to social influences, i.e., earlier maturing girls may be socialized away from athletics, and the athletic advantages of the longer limbs that develop in later maturing girls may encourage them to persist in athletics until an investigator arrives to interview them (Malina, 1983). The later age of menarche among athletic women may also be due to genetic factors, as evidenced by the following facts. The age of menarche in young athletic women is closely associated with that of their mothers, even though their mothers had fewer opportunities to participate in athletics before Title IX of the 1972 federal Education Amendment prohibited gender bias at institutions that receive federal aid (Malina et al., 1994). In addition, the age of menarche in young athletic women is also closely associated with that of their nonathletic sisters (Malina et al., 1994), although the same may not be true in dancers (Brooks-Gunn & Warren, 1988).

Experimental evidence demonstrates that dietary restriction delays puberty in other species of mammals (Bronson, 1986), but there is no evidence that exercise has this effect in adequately nourished animals. Prospective experimental evidence on the independent effects of exercise and nutrition on the age of menarche in humans does not exist.

Aside from infertility, the aspect of amenorrhea that is of the greatest concern is hypoestrogenism. Without adequate estrogen levels, amenorrheic athletes lose bone mineral, which increases their susceptibility to fractures and predisposes them to osteoporosis later in life (Constantini,

1994; Drinkwater, 1992). Hypoestrogenism also deprives amenorrheic athletes of the beneficial effects of estrogen on serum lipoproteins, potentially increasing their risk of coronary heart disease (Constantini, 1994). Because of the pathological effects of hypoestrogenism on skeletal integrity, and because amenorrhea can result from pathological conditions that are unrelated to exercise, prompt medical evaluation and intervention are warranted. Steroid replacement therapy in the form of low-dose oral contraceptives (<50 μg estrogen/d) (Committee on Sports Medicine of the American Academy of Pediatrics, 1989; Shangold et al., 1990) or conjugated estrogens and progesterones (0.625 mg/d) (Shangold et al., 1990) is specifically recommended to prevent bone loss. The former also provide contraceptive benefits, whereas the latter do not. Pharmaceutical induction of ovulation, although available, has been discouraged as a treatment for infertility in amenorrheic women until they reform their dietary and exercise habits because of an increased risk of spontaneous abortion and low birth-weight babies in treated women with hypothalamic amenorrhea who have not reformed these habits (Abraham et al., 1990; van der Spuy et al., 1988).

Prevalence. Physical, psychiatric, and endocrine examinations reveal that some cases of amenorrhea among athletes can be attributed to factors extraneous to athletic training (e.g., pregnancy, organic diseases, and eating disorders). The term *athletic* amenorrhea is reserved as a diagnosis of *exclusion* for the majority of cases that cannot be explained by anything other than athletic training. If the amenorrhea in an athlete can be attributed to anything other than athletic training, it is not athletic amenorrhea. For example, some women with anorexia nervosa exercise extensively, but, by this operational definition, no amenorrheic athlete satisfies the diagnostic criteria for anorexia nervosa as stated in the Diagnostic and Statistical Manual (DSM IV) of the American Psychiatric Association.

In contrast to luteal suppression, amenorrhea is obvious to the affected woman. Therefore, its occurrence among athletes and dancers has been widely reported and its prevalence frequently assessed through surveys. Although the results of these surveys have varied greatly because of differences in methodology, studies employing methodologies similar to those used to study the general population have found the prevalence of amenorrhea among athletes to be 4–20 times higher than in the general population (Loucks & Horvath, 1985). Among athletes, the prevalence appears to be greater among younger athletes, among athletes who train more intensively, and in sports in which leanness is thought to provide a competitive advantage.

Behavioral Characterization. Nevertheless, substantial proportions of athletes at each age group, competitive level, and body composition remain regularly menstruating, and cross-sectional comparisons have not consistently distinguished between amenorrheic and regularly menstruating athletes on the basis of their exercise regimens, dietary energy intakes, or body compositions. Psychologically, amenorrheic athletes display the vigorous, cheerful, "iceberg" profile of mood states characteristic of athletes in general (Loucks & Horvath, 1984).

As stated above, the low intake of dietary energy reported by amenorrheic athletes has been widely attributed to underreporting, but this interpretation seems to be in conflict with the metabolic and endocrine symptoms of energy deficiency described below and may not survive a close scrutiny of the techniques utilized for estimating energy expenditure.

Endocrine Characterization. Dramatic differences between amenorrheic and regularly menstruating athletes are revealed by endocrine tests. Sex steroid measurements over a period of 30 d indicate the complete absence of follicular development, ovulation, and luteal function in amenorrheic athletes (Figure 3-2, Amenorrheic Athlete) (Loucks et al, 1989; Pirke et al., 1990). Their LH pulses occur even less often than those in regularly menstruating athletes, and at irregular intervals (Figure 3-3, Amenorrheic Athlete), but their pituitary glands are capable of secreting LH when GnRH is exogenously administered (Loucks et al., 1989; Veldhuis et al., 1985; Yahiro et al., 1987). Thus, the neuroendocrine origin of the disease appears to occur at the level of the hypothalamus or higher.

Amenorrheic athletes also display a complex of abnormalities in metabolic hormones that regulate energy utilization and blood glucose levels. Regularly menstruating and amenorrheic athletes both display suppressed insulin and elevated growth hormone levels (Laughlin et al., 1994), but amenorrheic athletes also display low blood glucose levels (Laughlin et al., 1994), mildly elevated cortisol levels (De Souza et al., 1991, 1994; Ding et al., 1998; Loucks et al., 1989), Low T_3 Syndrome (Loucks et al., 1992a; Myerson et al., 1991), and high levels of insulin-like growth factor binding protein 1 (IGFBP-1) (Jenkins et al., 1993; Laughlin et al., 1994).

Because cortisol, like insulin, is a glucoregulatory hormone as well as a stress hormone, and because glucose administration suppresses the acute cortisol response to exercise in rats (Slentz et al., 1990) and in men (Tabata et al., 1991), the early interpretation of elevated cortisol levels in amenorrheic athletes as evidence of "exercise stress" may have been incorrect. These higher concentrations of cortisol may simply reflect a multifaceted endocrine response to energy deficiency. Thyroid hormones regulate the basal metabolic rate, and Low T_3 Syndrome occurs in numerous conditions, from fasting to cancer, in which dietary energy intake is insufficient to meet metabolic demand. The IGFBP-1 is a hepatic protein thought to modulate the growth-promoting actions of insulin-like growth factor 1, which has been proposed as a signal to the hypothalamus and/or ovaries that helps integrate fuel availability and reproductive control (Jenkins et al., 1993).

Amenorrheic athletes display other neuroendocrine abnormalities as well, including low prolactin levels (Loucks & Laughlin, 1992) and high melatonin levels at night (Laughlin et al., 1991), but the physiological implications of these conditions are unknown.

THE MECHANISM OF REPRODUCTIVE DISORDERS

Early hypotheses about the mechanism of reproductive disturbances in athletes derived from questionnaires finding associations between amenorrhea and other characteristics of athletes and from known causes of amenorrhea in other women. Some of these hypotheses have been investigated through cross-sectional comparisons of regularly menstruating and amenorrheic athletes; others are being tested currently through prospective experiments.

Unlikely Factors

Body Fatness. Early in the observational stage of research on menstrual disorders, an association between menstrual dysfunction first with body weight and then with body composition (Frisch & McArthur, 1974) led to speculations about how menarche and regular menstruation might depend upon the presence of particular amounts of body fat. However, later observations have not consistently verified these associations (e.g., Crist & Hill, 1990) or found the appropriate temporal relationship between changes in body weight and composition and menstrual function (For reviews, see Bronson & Manning, 1991; Loucks & Horvath, 1985; Scott & Johnson, 1982; Sinning & Little, 1987).

Hyperprolactinemia. Chronically elevated prolactin levels induce amenorrhea in women with tumors of the prolactin-secreting cells of the pituitary (Yen, 1991a). Indeed, early detection of lactotrophic tumors is one motivation for the prompt medical evaluation of any woman who becomes amenorrheic. The reproductive axis is also suppressed in nursing mothers, whose prolactin levels surge to very high levels during suckling. Early clinical speculations that amenorrheic athletes might have lactotrophic tumors or that breast motion during exercise might stimulate surges in prolactin levels were contradicted by endocrine comparisons of regularly menstruating and amenorrheic athletes. Prolactin levels are actually chronically suppressed in amenorrhea of hypothalamic origin, whether the affected women are athletes (De Souza et al., 1991; Loucks et al. 1992) or not (Berga et al., 1989), and acute prolactin responses to exercise are smaller in amenorrheic than in regularly menstruating athletes (De Souza et al., 1991; Loucks & Horvath, 1984).

Hyperandrogenism. Chronically elevated androgen levels of ovarian or adrenal origin also disrupt the female reproductive system with consequent amenorrhea, hirsutism, and masculinization (Yen, 1991b). Because exercise stimulates the adrenal gland to secrete androgens, another early hypothesis was that these surges in androgenic hormones during exercise might disrupt the female reproductive system. Androgenic effects are observed in women taking anabolic steroids, but no one has reported hirsutism or masculinization in amenorrheic athletes. Furthermore, baseline androgen levels are similar (Loucks et al., 1989) and androgen responses to exercise are smaller (Loucks & Horvath, 1984) in amenorrheic than in regularly menstruating athletes.

Psychological Stress. Several early investigators speculated that the psychological stress of athletic competition and of managing a busy lifestyle might disrupt the reproductive system in women. Occasionally, too, some investigators found that amenorrheic athletes scored higher than regularly menstruating athletes on one scale or another in a battery of psychological tests. Such scores were rarely, if ever, outside the normal range, however, and have not been a consistent observation. What has been repeatedly observed is that amenorrheic athletes display the "iceberg" profile of mood scores characteristic of athletes in general, scoring higher than the general population on vigor and lower on tension, depression, anger, fatigue, and confusion (Loucks & Horvath, 1984).

Other Factors Under Investigation

Energy Availability. The concept of energy availability is based upon the recognition that mammals partition dietary energy among six major metabolic activities: cellular maintenance, thermoregulation, locomotion, growth, reproduction, and, if any energy remains, storage (Wade & Schneider, 1992). Certainly, this partitioning varies at different stages of life and under different environmental conditions. The key insights are that dietary energy is limited and that the use of energy for one purpose makes it unavailable for others.

Exercise Stress. The stress hypothesis holds that the ovarian axis is disrupted in amenorrheic athletes by activation of the adrenal axis. To be independently meaningful, the stress hypothesis must more specifically imply that the adrenal axis is activated by some physiological consequence of exercise other than energy expenditure.

There definitely exist central and peripheral mechanisms mediated by opiate and adrenergic pathways by which the adrenal axis can disrupt the ovarian axis (Rivier & Rivest, 1991), but most animal experiments have administered adrenal agents, footshock, or immobilization to demonstrate these mechanisms. To be sure, prolonged aerobic exercise, as it is commonly practiced, does activate the adrenal axis, but whether or not this occurs in such a way as to disrupt the ovarian axis is not known.

RESULTS AND PROBLEMS OF PROSPECTIVE EXPERIMENTS

Animal Experiments

Exercise Stress. Selye (1939) induced anestrus and ovarian atrophy in rats by abruptly forcing them to run strenuously for prolonged periods. Later, others also induced anestrus in rats by forced swimming (Asahina et al., 1959; Axelson, 1987), forced running (Carlberg & Fregly, 1985; Chatterton et al., 1990), and by training animals to run for food rewards (Manning & Bronson, 1989, 1991). Elevated cortisol levels in such studies were represented as the characteristic sign of stress, and the reproductive effects were widely interpreted as evidence of the counterregulatory influence of "exercise stress" on the female reproductive system.

However, "exercise stress" was confounded in all these studies by the methods used to force animals to exercise, by training animals to run for food rewards, or by the energy cost of exercise. Electroshock, for example, is known to disrupt the reproductive system through a mechanism involving endogenous opiates and activation of the adrenal axis, and the threat of drowning probably activates a similar mechanism, the activation of which in voluntarily exercising humans is at best debatable. As mentioned above, the acute cortisol response to exercise can be prevented by glucose infusion (Slentz et al., 1990; Tabata et al., 1991). Thus, in those studies confounded by energy availability, investigators may have erred in interpreting the elevation of glucocorticoids as evidence of stress rather than of energy deficiency. At present, there is no unconfounded experimental evidence that "exercise stress" disrupts the female mammalian reproductive system.

Energy Availability. As reviewed by Bronson (1988), Bronson & Manning (1989), and by Wade & Schneider (1992), considerable evidence from biological field trials indicates that reproductive function in mammals depends upon energy availability. In general, reproductive function is characteristic of populations in particular environments rather than of species. Different populations of the same species, including humans, display seasonal or continuous breeding habits depending on local environmental conditions (Bronson, 1988). Furthermore, the mammalian dependence of reproductive function on energy availability operates principally in females, with reproductive development, for example, continuing in males under conditions in which it is entirely blocked in females (Aguilar at al., 1984; Hamilton & Bronson, 1985, 1986). Indeed, because the energetic costs of their reproductive efforts vary so greatly, when considering energy requirements, ecologists have long viewed the two sexes almost as if they were entirely different species (Trivers, 1972).

In rats, reproductive function clearly depends on energy availability and not on body fat. LH pulsatility resumes within a few hours after severely growth-restricted rats are permitted to begin ad libitum feeding and long before significant changes in body weight and composition occur in either female (Bronson, 1986; Bronson & Heideman, 1990) or male (Sisk & Bronson, 1986) rats.

A recent series of experiments on female Syrian hamsters was reviewed by Wade & Schneider (1992), and has drawn attention to the concept of energy availability and its influence on the regulation of reproductive function. In these experiments, anestrus was induced by several procedures other than food restriction that reduced the availability of oxidizable metabolic fuels for cellular metabolism. These procedures included the administration of pharmacological blockers of carbohydrate and fat metabolism (Schneider & Wade, 1989, 1990a), insulin administration that shunts metabolic fuels into storage (Wade et al., 1991), and cold exposure that consumes metabolic fuels in shivering and nonshivering thermogenesis (Schneider & Wade, 1990b). Disruptive effects on the reproductive system were independent of body size and composition (Schneider & Wade, 1990a). Clearly, the extrapolation from uncoordinated muscular contractions in shivering to coordinated muscular contractions in exercise is straightforward.

Strongly supporting an energy availability hypothesis of reproductive disorders in athletes was the demonstration that amenorrhea, induced in monkeys by their voluntarily running for prolonged periods on a motorized treadmill, could be reversed by dietary supplementation, without restricting the exercise regimens of the monkeys (Cameron et al., 1990).

Human Experiments

Long-Term Experiments. Several investigators have attempted to induce menstrual disorders through exercise training, but most (Bonen, 1992; Boyden et al., 1983; Bullen et al., 1984; Rogol et al., 1992) have been unsuccessful. In these studies, a moderate volume of exercise was applied, or the volume of exercise was increased gradually over several months, and diet was uncontrolled or unquantified. In the most recent such study (Rogol et al., 1992), subjects appear to have been physically trained and luteally suppressed before the study began (Loucks et al., 1993; Rogol et al., 1993).

The only longitudinal experiment that did induce menstrual disorders in regularly menstruating women imposed a high volume of aerobic exercise abruptly, causing a large proportion of menstrual disorders in the first month and a larger proportion in the second (Bullen et al., 1985). Both proportions were greater in a subgroup fed a controlled weight-loss diet than in another subgroup fed for weight maintenance. However, even the weight maintenance subgroup may have been substantially underfed because body weight may be an unreliable indicator of energy balance. For example, body weight is stable in amenorrheic athletes, whose endocrine status is similar to individuals in severe energy deficiency (Loucks et al., 1989, 1992a; Marcus et al., 1985; Myerson et al., 1991).

Short-Term Experiments. Experimental subjects have been rigorously screened, and energy availability and exercise volume and intensity have been precisely controlled, in a series of so-called EXCALIBUR experiments that investigated the independent short-term effects of exercise training and energy availability on metabolic and reproductive hormones in regularly menstruating, habitually sedentary women (Loucks & Callister, 1993; Loucks & Heath, 1994; Loucks et al., 1994a, 1994b, 1995). These four-day experiments suggest that poor energy availability disrupts the regulation of both metabolic and reproductive hormones and that exercise has little effect on these hormones beyond its impact on energy availability. These experiments have been too brief, though, to imply that exercise training and energy availability have similar longer-term effects on menstrual function.

In EXCALIBUR I (Loucks & Callister, 1993), subjects were assigned to six groups: energy-balanced (B) and energy-deprived (D) groups that performed zero (Z) exercise (groups ZB and ZD) or that performed 1300 kcal/d of aerobic exercise at either a light (L), 40% $\dot{V}O_2$max intensity (groups LB and LD) or heavy (H), 70% $\dot{V}O_2$max intensity, (groups HB and HD). For four days, dietary energy intake was restricted by 1300 kcal/d in the energy-deprived sedentary subjects, and dietary energy intake was supplemented by the same amount in the energy-balanced exercising groups. Figure 3-4 shows that dietary restriction suppressed T_3 levels in the sedentary women and in the exercising women whose dietary energy intake was not supplemented in compensation for their exercise energy expenditure, but not in the energy-supplemented exercising women. These results suggest that energy availability (behaviorly defined as dietary energy intake minus exercise energy expenditure), rather than exercise stress or dietary energy intake or exercise training separately, appears to be a major factor that alters metabolic hormones in athletes. The T_3 levels were suppressed in the women with low energy availability by the same proportion as had been observed in amenorrheic women (Loucks et al., 1992a; Myerson et al., 1991).

In EXCALIBUR II (Loucks & Heath, 1994), regularly menstruating, habitually sedentary women expended approximately 1300 kcal/d during exercise while being fed various amounts. Figure 3-5 shows that the suppression of T_3 occurred abruptly at a threshold of energy availability of 20–25 kcal/kg LBM per day. This result suggests that regularly menstruating and amenorrheic athletes may be very similar in energy availability, with amenorrheic athletes just below and regularly menstruating ones

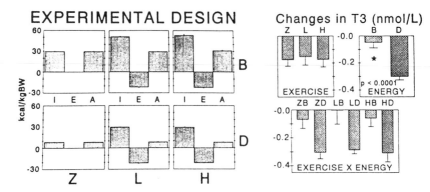

FIGURE 3-4. *Left panel:* *Experimental design for EXCALIBUR I.* Energy availability (A) was defined as dietary energy intake (I) minus exercise energy expenditure (E). Exercise treatments (Z = zero; L = 1300 kcal/d at 40% $\dot{V}O_2$max; and H = 1300 kcal/d at 70% $\dot{V}O_2$max) and energy availability treatments (B = 1750 kcal/d; and D = 500 kcal/d) were administered to regularly menstruating, untrained women for 4 d. (BW = body weight.) *Right panel:* *Changes in serum triiodothyronine (T_3) levels after 4 d of exercise and energy availability treatments.* T_3 fell 15% in the energy deficient groups (ZD, LD, and HD) and was maintained in exercising groups that received dietary supplementation in compensation for their exercise energy expenditure (LB and HB) (Loucks & Callister, 1993).

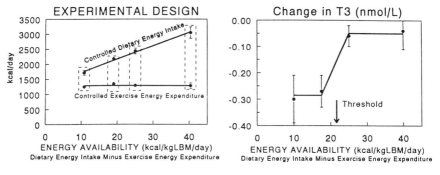

FIGURE 3-5. *Left panel:* *Experimental design for EXCALIBUR II.* Exercise treatments (1300 kcal/d at 70% $\dot{V}O_2$max) and energy availability treatments (10.8, 19.0, 25.0, and 40.4 kcal/kg LBM/d) were administered to regularly menstruating untrained women for 4 d. *Right panel:* *Changes in serum triiodothyronine (T_3) levels after 4 d of exercise and energy availability treatments.* T_3 levels fell abruptly when energy availability fell below 20-25 kcal/kg LBM/d (Loucks & Heath, 1994).

just above the threshold, i.e., too close together in energy availability to be distinguished in cross-sectional studies.

In EXCALIBUR III (Loucks et al., 1994a, 1994b, 1995), low energy availability was also found to suppress LH pulsatility. This occurred in sedentary women whose dietary energy intake was severely restricted to below the energy availability threshold, in exercising women whose energy availability fell below the threshold because they did not compensate their dietary energy intake for their high exercise energy expenditure, and in women who exercised moderately while their dietary energy intake was moderately restricted (Figure 3-6). The smaller effect in women whose low energy availability was due to exercise alone suggests that, contrary to popular belief, exercise may actually be protective against the disruption of LH pulsatility by low energy availability. In addition to also suppressing T_3 levels in these women, low energy availability suppressed insulin and IGF-1 while raising cortisol levels (Loucks et al., 1994a (P = 0.04), 1994b (P = 0.12)), also reminiscent of cross-sectional observations in amenorrheic athletes.

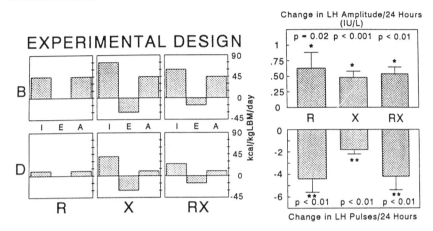

FIGURE 3-6. *Left panel: Experimental design for EXCALIBUR III.* Energy availability (A) was defined as dietary energy intake (I) minus exercise energy expenditure (E). Balanced (B = 45 kcal/kg LBM/d) and sub-threshold deficient (D = 10 kcal/kg LBM/d) energy availability treatments were administered to regularly menstruating, untrained, sedentary women through severe dietary energy restriction alone (R), through severe exercise energy expenditure alone (X: E = 1300 kcal/d at 70% $\dot{V}O_2$max), and through the combination (RX) of moderate dietary restriction (I = 25 kcal/kg LBM/d) and moderate exercise energy expenditure (E = 650 kcal/d at 70% $\dot{V}O_2$max) for 4 d. *Right upper panel:* Effects of low energy availability on luteinizing hormone (LH) pulse amplitude (IU = international units). LH pulse amplitude was increased by all three treatments. *Right lower panel:* Effects of low energy availability on LH pulse frequency. LH pulse frequency was reduced by all three treatments, but the reduction was smaller in the women whose low energy availability was due to exercise alone (P<0.05).

In general, the EXCALIBUR results support the hypothesis that menstrual function is disrupted in athletes by chronically low energy availability and that exercise training itself has little or no effect on reproductive function. If this proves to be the case in similarly controlled experiments of longer duration, athletic amenorrhea may be effectively prevented or reversed by dietary reform, without moderation of the exercise regimen. No neuroendocrine mechanism linking energy availability to reproductive disorders in physically active women has been demonstrated to date, and available evidence is insufficient to implicate thyroid or any other metabolic hormones in that mechanism.

DIRECTIONS FOR FUTURE RESEARCH

In 1991 a workshop sponsored by the National Heart, Lung, and Blood Institute developed recommendations for future research on the influence of exercise training on the female reproductive system (Loucks et al., 1992b). These and other recommendations of the author are summarized below.

The Clinical Consequences of Prolonged Hypoestrogenism

Research is needed to determine the clinical consequences of prolonged hypoestrogenism in premenopausal, physically active women. For ethical reasons prospective experiments may be possible only in animal models. In support of them, extensive observational and epidemiological studies of long-term and delayed effects on fertility, menopause, osteoporosis, and breast cancer in women are also needed.

The Neuroendocrine Mechanism of Amenorrhea

Controlled experiments are needed to reveal the precise neuroendocrine mechanism(s) by which athletic training disrupts reproductive function; this will facilitate the development of effective and specific therapeutic and preventive treatments. Such studies would include investigation of how the brain regulates the partitioning of dietary energy among competing metabolic demands. Some of these experiments may be best performed in animals or in tissue culture, but many will require human subjects.

Identification of Specific Influences on the Mechanisms Regulating Adolescent Development

Information is needed on whether or not training regimens in certain sports adversely affect growth and development in adolescent girls. Experiments are needed to distinguish the independent effects of diet, exercise, and genetics on age of menarche, reproductive function, and skeletal health. Because of the potential for irreversible skeletal damage, human subjects approval for randomized, prospective experiments on such topics may be difficult to obtain. Since retrospective studies of the influence of factors imposed before or after menarche are inherently biased (Stager et al., 1990), carefully designed, prospective, case-control studies of self-selected subjects may be the best that can be done in humans.

The Mechanism and Clinical Consequences of Luteal Suppression

At present, we have no understanding of why some women remain menstrually regular while practicing training regimens that are very similar, if not identical, as to those undertaken by amenorrheic athletes. Studies are needed to investigate the quality of follicular development and the biological activity of the steroid hormones secreted by these regularly menstruating women. Information is needed to determine if luteal suppression is an intermediate condition that may progress to amenorrhea, if it is an end point of successful acclimation to athletic training, or if it is an end point that occurs in genetically robust individuals. Information is also needed on the fertility and menopause of women who exhibit luteal suppression and on whether or not luteal suppression is a risk factor for osteoporosis, cardiovascular disease, and cancer. Since most of the available data have been collected on women with highly regular, asymptomatic menstrual cycles, comparative information is needed on athletic women with short, long, and irregular cycles.

Development of New Animal Models

Animal models will be needed for many mechanistic experiments that will not be possible in human subjects. Such experiments are necessary for important issues concerning neuroendocrine regulatory pathways in the brain, reproductive behavior, fertility, pregnancy outcome, and long-term consequences on health. Almost all animal research on the influence of exercise on reproductive function has been confounded by low energy availability and the methods used to force animals to exercise, so innovations in the control of such experiments will be needed. Species will need to be carefully selected for generalization to humans.

Documentation of Growth and Development of Physically Active Girls

Basic descriptive data are lacking on the effect of disciplined athletic training on adolescent growth and development. Large, prolonged prospective studies beginning before menarche are needed to document linear growth, body proportions and composition, bone density, sexual development, and hormonal function in girls engaging in recreational exercise, organized sports, and elite performance training. Such studies will be complicated by the high variability among and within individuals during the adolescent years.

Prevalence of Amenorrhea and Luteal Suppression

Until the prevalences of amenorrhea and luteal suppression among physically active women in different gynecological age ranges are better quantified, the scope of these problems will remain obscure. Therefore, well-controlled epidemiological studies are needed to differentiate dietary and exercise regimens and to verify menstrual status on the basis of serial measurements of multiple hormones through an entire menstrual cycle. For this purpose, LH and metabolites of estrogen and progesterone can be conveniently measured in samples of urine or saliva.

Effects of the Menstrual Cycle, Its Disturbances, and Treatments on Athletic Performance

If athletes and coaches believe that the menstrual cycle impairs athletic performance, athletic amenorrhea will be accepted and desired, especially at the most elite levels of competition. Furthermore, athletes and coaches are unlikely to comply with treatments and preventive measures that are perceived to impair performance. Therefore, experiments are needed to determine if athletic performance is affected by the menstrual cycle and by hormone supplementation and other interventions.

SUMMARY

The human female reproductive system is a complex feedback system that changes state several times during a woman's lifetime. Research into the mechanism of menstrual disorders in athletes is hindered by our ignorance of the signals triggering normal transitions between reproductive states and the mechanisms by which those signals act. A wide range of research is needed to increase our understanding of the normal physiology of human reproduction and the influence of athletic training on it.

Amenorrhea, which occurs disproportionately often among physically active women, is a disease requiring prompt medical intervention in the form of hormone replacement therapy to prevent potentially irreversible skeletal demineralization, fractures, and predisposition to osteoporosis. The clinical consequences of luteal suppression, the prevalence of which may be very high indeed, are unknown but may include infertility and an increased risk of breast cancer.

The proximal cause of athletic amenorrhea is the disruption of the GnRH pulse generator at the level of the hypothalamus or higher in the brain, but the mechanism that disrupts GnRH pulse generator and the specific behavioral factor activating that mechanism are unknown. The strongest evidence available at present appears to indicate that this behavioral factor may be low energy availability, which for athletes may be behaviorly defined as dietary energy intake minus exercise energy expenditure. Low energy availability occurs in women with frank eating disorders such as anorexia nervosa, but it also occurs in athletes consuming diets that would be described as normal and healthy for sedentary women. If the hypothesis is confirmed that low energy availability induces athletic amenorrhea, athletes may be able to reverse or prevent amenorrhea through dietary reform without moderating their exercise regimens.

ACKNOWLEDGEMENTS

The author is grateful for critical reviews of the manuscript that were provided by Randy Eichner, Xiaocai Shi, and the late John Sutton. She also thanks the conference participants for their suggestions for further improvements.

BIBLIOGRAPHY

Abraham, S., M. Mira, and D. Llewellyn-Jones (1990). Should ovulation be induced in women recovering from an eating disorder or who are compulsive exercisers? *Fertil. Steril.* 53:566–568.

Aguilar, E., L. Pinella, R. Guisado, D. Gonzalez, and F. Lopez (1984). Relation between body weight, growth rate, chronological age, and puberty in male and female rats. *Rev. Esp. Fisiol.* 40:82–86.

Albanes, D., A. Blair, and P.R. Taylor (1989). Physical activity and risk of cancer in the NHANES I population. *Am. J. Public Health* 79:744–750.

Asahina, K., F. Kitahara, M. Yamanaka, and T. Akiba (1959). Influences of excessive exercise on the structure and function of rat organs. *Jpn. J. Physiol.* 9:322–326.

Axelson, J.F. (1987). Forced swimming alters vaginal estrous cycles, body composition, and steroid levels without disrupting lordosis behavior or fertility in rats. *Physiol. Behav.* 41:471–479.

Bachmann, G.A., and E. Kemmann (1982). Prevalence of oligomenorrhea and amenorrhea in a college population. *Am. J. Obstet. Gynecol.* 144:98–102.

Berga, S.L., J.F. Mortola, L. Girton, B. Suh, G. Laughlin, P. Pham, and S.S.C. Yen (1989). Neuroendocrine aberrations in women with hypothalamic-amenorrhea. *J. Clin. Endocrinol. Metab.* 68:301–308.

Bernstein, L., B.E. Henderson, R. Hanisch, J. Sullivan-Halley, and R.K. Ross (1994). Physical exercise and reduced risk of breast cancer in young women. *J. Natl. Cancer Inst.* 86:1403–1408.

Bonen, A. (1994). Exercise-induced menstrual cycle changes: A functional, temporary adaptation to metabolic stress. *Sports Med.* 17:373–392.

Bonen, A. (1992). Recreational exercise does not impair menstrual cycles: A prospective study. *Int. J. Sports Med.* 13:110–120.

Boyden, T.W., R.W. Pamenter, P. Stanforth, T. Rotkis, and J.H. Wilmore (1983). Sex steroids and endurance running in women. *Fertil. Steril.* 39:629–632.

Bronson, F.H. (1986). Food-restricted, prepubertal female rats: Rapid recovery of luteinizing hormone pulsing with excess food, and full recovery of pubertal development with gonadotropin-releasing hormone. *Endocrinology* 118:2483–2487.

Bronson, F.H. (1988). Seasonal Regulation of Reproduction in Mammals. In: E. Knobil and J. Neill (eds.) *The Physiology of Reproduction* Volume 2. New York: Raven Press, pp. 1831–1871.

Bronson F.H., and P.D. Heideman (1990). Short-term hormonal responses to food intake in peripubertal female rats. *Am. J. Physiol.* 259: R25–R31.

Bronson, F.H., and J. Manning (1989). Food consumption, prolonged exercise, and LH secretion in the peripubertal female rat. In: K.M. Pirke, W. Wuttke, and U. Schweiger (eds.) *The Menstrual Cycle and Its Disorders*. Berlin: Springer-Verlag, pp. 42–49.

Bronson, F.H., and J. Manning (1991). The energetic regulation of ovulation: A realistic role for body fat. *Biol. Reprod.* 44:945–950.

Broocks, A., K.M. Pirke, U. Schweiger, R.J. Tuschl, R.G. Laessle, T. Strowitzki, E. Hörl, T. Hörl, W. Haas, and D. Jeschke (1990). Cyclic ovarian function in recreational athletes. *J. Appl. Physiol.* 68:2083–2086.

Brooks-Gunn, J., and M.P. Warren (1988). Mother-daughter differences in menarcheal age in adolescent girls attending national dance company schools and non-dancers. *Ann. Hum. Biol.* 15:35–44.

Bullen, B.A., G.S. Skrinar, I.Z. Beitins, D.B. Carr, S.M. Reppert, C.O. Dotson, M.deM. Fencl, E.V. Gervino, and J.W. McArthur (1984). Endurance training effects on plasma hormonal responsiveness and sex hormone excretion. *J. Appl. Physiol.* 56:1453–1463.

Bullen, B.A., G.S. Skrinar, I.Z. Beitins, G. von Mering, B.A. Turnbull, and J.W. McArthur (1985). Induction of menstrual disorders by strenuous exercise in untrained women. *N. Engl. J. Med.* 312:1349–1353.

Cameron, J.L., C. Nosbisch, D.L. Helmreich, and D.B. Parfitt (1990). Reversal of exercise-induced amenorrhea in female cynomolgus monkeys (Macaca fascicularis) by increasing food intake. *Proceedings of the 72nd Annual Meeting of the Endocrine Society*, Abstract 1042, p. 285.

Carlberg, K.A., and M.J. Fregly (1985). Disruption of estrous cycles in exercise-trained rats. *Proc. Soc. Exp. Biol. Med.* 179:21–24.

Chatterton, R.T. Jr., A.L. Hartman, D.E. Lynn, and R.C. Hickson (1990). Exercise-induced ovarian dysfunction in the rat. *Proc. Soc. Exp. Biol. Med.* 193:220–224.

Committee on Sports Medicine of the American Academy of Pediatrics (1989). Amenorrhea in adolescent athletes. *Pediatrics* 84:394–395.

Constantini, N.W. (1994). Clinical consequences of athletic amenorrhoea. *Sports Med.* 17:213–223.

Cowan, L.D., L. Gordis, J.A. Tonascia, and G.S. Jones (1981). Breast cancer incidence in women with a history of progesterone deficiency. *Am. J. Epidemiol.* 114:209–217.

Crist, D.M. and J.M. Hill (1990). Diet and insulin like growth factor I in relation to body composition in women with exercise-induced hypothalamic amenorrhea. *J. Am. Coll. Nutr.* 9:200–204.

De Souza, M.J., A.A. Luciano, J.C. Arce, L.M. Demers, and A.B. Loucks (1994). Clinical tests explain blunted cortisol responsiveness but not mild hypercortisolism in amenorrheic runners. *J. Appl. Physiol.* 76:1302–1309.

De Souza, M.J., M.S. Maguire, C.M. Maresh, W.J. Kraemer, K.R. Rubin, and A.B. Loucks (1991). Adrenal activation and the prolactin response to exercise in eumenorrheic and amenorrheic runners. *J. Appl. Physiol.* 70:2378–2387.

Ding, J.-H., C.B. Schecter, B.L. Drinkwater, M.R. Soules, and W.J. Bremner (1988). High serum cortisol levels in exercise-associated amenorrhea. *Ann. Intern. Med.* 108:530–534.

Dorgan, J.F., C. Brown, M. Barrett, G.L. Splansky, B.E. Kreger, R.B. D'Agostino, D. Albanes, and A. Schatzkin (1994). Physical activity and risk of breast cancer in the Framingham Heart Study. *Am. J. Epidemiol.* 139:662–669.

Drinkwater, B.L. Amenorrhea, body weight, and osteoporosis (1992). In: K.D. Brownell, J.Rodin, and J.H. Wilmore (eds.) *Eating, Body Weight and Performance in Athletes.* Philadelphia: Lea & Febiger, pp. 235–247.

Drinkwater, B.L., K. Nilson, C.H. Chesnut, W.J. Bremner, S. Shainholtz, and M.B. Southworth (1984). Bone mineral content of amenorrheic and eumenorrheic athletes. *N. Engl. J. Med.* 311:277–281.

Edwards, J.E., A.K. Lindeman, A.E. Mikesky, and J.M. Stager (1993). Energy balance in highly trained female endurance runners. *Med. Sci. Sports Exerc.* 25:1398–1404.

Ellison, P.T., and C. Lager (1986). Moderate recreational running is associated with lowered salivary progesterone profiles in women. *Am. J. Obstet. Gynecol.* 154:1000–1003.

Frisch, R.E., and J.W. McArthur (1974). Menstrual cycles: fatness as a determinant of minimum weight for height necessary for their maintenance or onset. *Science* 185:949–951.

Frisch, R.E., G. Wyshak, N.L. Albright, T.E. Albright, I. Schiff, K.P. Jones, J. Witschi, E. Shiang, E. Koff, and M. Marguglio (1985). Lower prevalence of breast cancer and cancers of the reproductive system among former college athletes compared to non-athletes. *Br. J. Cancer* 52:885–891.

Hamilton, G.D., and F.H. Bronson (1985). Food restriction and reproductive development in wild house mice. *Biol. Reprod.* 32:773–778.

Hamilton, G.D., and F.H. Bronson (1986). Food restriction and reproductive development: male and female mice and rats. *Am. J. Physiol.* 250: R370–R376.

Jenkins, P.J., X. Ibanez-Santos, J. Holly, A. Cotterill, L. Perry, R. Wolman, M. Harries, and A. Grossman (1993). IGFBP-1: a metabolic signal associated with exercise-induced amenorrhea. *Neuroendocrinol.* 57:600–604.

Kaiserauer, S., A.C. Snyder, M. Sleeper, and J. Zierath (1989). Nutritional, physiological, and menstrual status of distance runners. *Med. Sci. Sports Exerc.* 21:120–125.

Laughlin, G.A., C.E. Dominguez, A.J. Morales, and S.S.C. Yen (1994). Alterations of insulin/glucose and the GH-IGF-IGFBP system during the 24h metabolic clock in cycling and amenorrheic athletes. *Proceedings of the 76th Annual Meeting of the Endocrine Society,* Abstract 842, p. 411.

Laughlin, G.A., A.B. Loucks, and S.S.C. Yen (1991). Marked augmentation of nocturnal melatonin secretion in amenorrheic athletes, but not in cycling athletes: unaltered by opioidergic or dopaminergic blockade. *J. Clin. Endocrinol. Metab.* 73:1321–1326.

Leibel, R.L., M. Rosenbaum, and J. Hirsch (1995). Changes in energy expenditure resulting from altered body weight. *N. Engl. J. Med.* 332:621–628.

Liu, J.H., and S.S.C. Yen (1984). The use of gonadotropin-releasing hormone for the induction of ovulation. *Clin. Obstet. Gynecol.* 27:975–982.

Loucks, A.B. (1989). Athletics and menstrual disfunction in young women. In: G.V. Gisolfi and D.R. Lamb (eds.) *Perspectives in Exercise Science and Sports Medicine, Vol. 2: Youth, Exercise, and Sport.* Indianapolis: Benchmark Press, pp. 513–538.

Loucks, A.B. (1990) Effects of exercise training on the menstrual cycle: existence and mechanisms. *Med. Sci. Sports Exerc.* 22:275–280.

Loucks, A.B. (1994). Physical activity, fitness, and female reproductive morbidity. In: C. Bouchard, R.J. Shephard, and T. Stephens (eds.) *Physical Activity, Fitness, and Health.* Champaign: Human Kinetics, pp. 943–954.

Loucks, A.B. (1995). The reproductive system and physical activity in adolescents. In: C.J.R. Blimkie and O. Bar-Or (eds.) *New Horizons in Pediatric Exercise Science.* Champaign: Human Kinetics Publishers, pp. 27–37.

Loucks, A.B., R. Brown, K. King, J.R. Thuma, and M. Verdun (1995). A combined regimen of moderate dietary restriction and exercise training alters luteinizing hormone pulsatility in regularly menstruating young women. *Proceedings of the 77th Annual Meeting of the Endocrine Society,* Abstract #P3-360, p. 558.

Loucks, A.B., and R. Callister (1993). Induction and prevention of low-T$_3$ syndrome in exercising women. *Am. J. Physiol.* 264:R924–R930.

Loucks, A.B., J.L. Cameron, and M.J. De Souza (1993). Subject assignment may have biased experimental results. *J. Appl. Physiol.* 74:2045–2046.

Loucks, A.B., and E.M. Heath (1994). Induction of low-T$_3$ syndrome in exercising women occurs at a threshold of energy availability. *Am. J. Physiol.* 266:R817–R823.

Loucks, A.B., E.M. Heath, K. King, T.D. Law, Sr., D. Morrall, M. Verdun, and J.R. Watts (1994a). Low energy availability alters luteinizing hormone pulsatility in regularly menstruating, young exercising women. *Proceedings of the 1994 Endocrine Society Meeting,* Abstract #822, p. 406.

Loucks, A.B., E.M. Heath, T. Law, Sr., M. Verdun, and J.R. Watts (1994b). Dietary restriction reduces luteinizing hormone (LH) pulse frequency during waking hours and increases LH pulse amplitude during sleep in young menstruating women. *J. Clin. Endocrinol. Metab.* 78:910–915.

Loucks, A.B., and S.M. Horvath (1985). Athletic amenorrhea: a review. *Med. Sci. Sports Exerc.* 17:56–72.

Loucks, A.B., and S.M. Horvath (1984). Exercise-induced stress responses of amenorrheic and eumenorrheic runners. *J. Clin. Endocrinol. Metab.* 59:1109–1120.

Loucks, A.B., and G.L. Laughlin (1992). Hypoprolactinemia in amenorrheic athletes: 24-hour profiles and responses to thyrotropin-releasing hormone and metoclopramide. *Proceedings of the 74th Annual Meeting of the Endocrine Society,* Abstract #61, p. 67.

Loucks, A.B., G.A. Laughlin, J.F. Mortola, L. Girton, J.C. Nelson, and S.S.C. Yen (1992a). Hypothalamic-pituitary-thyroidal function in eumenorrheic and amenorrheic athletes. *J. Clin. Endocrinol. Metab.* 75:514–518.

Loucks, A.B., J.F. Mortola, L. Girton, and S.S.C. Yen (1989). Alterations in the hypothalamic-pituitary-ovarian and hypothalamic-pituitary-adrenal axes in athletic women. *J. Clin. Endocrinol. Metab.* 68:402–411.

Loucks, A.B., J. Vaitukaitis, J.L. Cameron, A.D. Rogol, G. Skrinar, M.P. Warren, J. Kendrick, and M.C. Limacher (1992b). The reproductive system and exercise in women. *Med. Sci. Sports Exerc.* 24 Supplement:S288–S293.

Malina, R.M. (1983). Menarche in athletes: a synthesis and hypothesis. *Ann. Hum. Biol.* 10:1–24.

Malina, R.M. (1994). Physical activity: relationship to growth, maturation, and physical fitness. In: C. Bouchard, R.J. Shephard, and T. Stephens (eds.) *Physical Activity, Fitness, and Health.* Champaign: Human Kinetics Publishers, pp. 918–930.

Malina, R.M., R.C. Ryan, and C.M. Bonci (1994). Age at menarche in athletes and their mothers and sisters. *Ann. Hum. Biol.* 21:417–422.

Manning, J.M., and F.H. Bronson (1989). Effects of prolonged exercise on puberty and luteinizing hormone secretion in female rats. *Am. J. Physiol.* 257: R1359–R1364.

Manning, J.M., and F.H. Bronson (1991). Suppression of puberty in rats by exercise: effects on hormone levels and reversal with GnRH infusion. *Am. J. Physiol.* 260: R717–R723.

Marcus, R., C. Cann, P. Madvig, J. Minkoff, M. Goddard, M. Bayer, M. Martin, L. Guadiani, W. Haskell, and H. Genant (1985). Menstrual function and bone mass in elite women distance runners. *Ann. Intern. Med.* 102:158–163.

Mauvais-Jarvis, P., R. Sitruk-Ware, and F. Kuttenn (1982). Luteal phase defect and breast cancer genesis. *Breast Cancer Res. Treat.* 2:139–150.

Myerson, M., B. Gutin, M.P. Warren, M.T. May, I. Contento, M. Lee, F.X. PiSunyer, R.N. Pierson, Jr., and J. Brooks-Gunn (1991). Resting metabolic rate and energy balance in amenorrheic and eumenorrheic runners. *Med. Sci. Sports Exerc.* 23:15–22.

Nelson, M.E., E.C. Fisher, P.D. Catsos, C.N. Meredith, R.N. Turksoy, and W.J. Evans (1986). Diet and bone mineral status in amenorrheic runners. *Am. J. Clin. Nutr.* 43:910–916.

Pettersson, F., H. Fries, and S.J. Nillius (1973). Epidemiology of secondary amenorrhea. I. Incidence and prevalence rates. *Am. J. Obstet. Gynecol.* 117:80–86.

Pirke, K.M., U. Schweiger, A. Broocks, R.J. Tuschl, and R.G. Laessle (1990). Luteinizing hormone and follicle stimulating hormone secretion patterns in female athletes with and without menstrual disturbances. *Clin. Endocrinol.* 33:345–353.

Rivier, C., and S. Rivest (1991). Effect of stress on the activity of the hypothalamic-pituitary-gonadal axis: peripheral and central mechanisms. *Biol. Reprod.* 45:523–532.

Rogol, A.D., W.S. Evans, J.Y. Weltman, J.D. Veldhuis, and A.L. Weltman (1993). Reply to "Subject assignment may have biased experimental results." *J. Appl. Physiol.* 74:2046–2047.

Rogol, A.D., A. Weltman, J.Y. Weltman, R.L. Seip, D.B. Snead, S. Levine, E.M. Haskvitz, D.L. Thompson, R. Schurrer, E. Dowling, J. Walberg-Rankin, W.S. Evans, and J.D. Veldhuis (1992). Durability of the reproductive axis in eumenorrheic women during 1 year of endurance training. *J. Appl. Physiol.* 72:1571–1580.

Schneider, J.E., and G.N. Wade (1989). Availability of metabolic fuels controls estrous cyclicity of Syrian hamsters. *Science* 244:1326–1328.

Schneider, J.E., and G.N. Wade (1990a). Decreased availability of metabolic fuels induces anestrus in golden hamsters. *Am. J. Physiol.* 258: R750–R755.

Schneider, J.E., and G.N. Wade (1990b). Effects of diet and body fat content on cold-induced anestrus in Syrian hamsters. *Am. J. Physiol.* 259: R1198–R1204.

Scott E.C., and F.E. Johnson (1982). Critical fat, menarche, and the maintenance of menstrual cycles: a critical review. *J. Adolesc. Health Care* 2:249–260.

Selye, H. (1939). The effect of adaptation to various damaging agents on the female sex organs in the rat. *Endocrinology* 25:615–624.

Shangold, M., R.W. Rebar, A. Colston Wentz, and I. Schiff (1990). Evaluation and management of menstrual dysfunction in athletes. *J.A.M.A.* 263:1665–1669.

Sherman, B.M., and S.G. Korenman (1974). Inadequate corpus luteum function: a pathophysiological interpretation of human breast cancer epidemiology. *Cancer* 33:1306–1312.

Singh, K.B. (1981). Menstrual disorders in college students. *Am. J. Obst. Gynecol.* 140:299–302.

Sinning, W.E., and K.D. Little (1987). Body composition and menstrual function in athletes. *Sports Med.* 4:34–45.

Sisk, C.L., and F.H. Bronson (1986). Effects of food restriction and restoration on gonadotropin and growth hormone secretion in immature male rats. *Biol. Reprod.* 35:554–561.

Slentz, C.A., J.M. Davis, D.L. Settles, J.R.P. Russell, and S.J. Settles (1990). Glucose feedings and exercise in rats: glycogenous, hormone responses, and performance. *J. Appl. Physiol.* 69:989–994.

Stager, J.M., J.K. Wigglesworth, and L.K. Hatler (1990). Interpreting the relationship between age of menarche and prepubertal training. *Med. Sci. Sports Exerc.* 22:54–58.

Tabata, I., F. Ogita, M. Miyachi, and H. Shibayama (1991). Effect of low blood glucose on plasma CRF, ACTH, and cortisol during prolonged physical exercise. *J. Appl. Physiol.* 71:1807–1812.

Trivers, R.L. (1972). Parental investment and sexual selection. In: B. Campbell (ed.) *Sexual Selection and the Descent of Man.* Chicago: Aldine Press, pp. 136–171.

van der Spuy, Z.M., P.J. Steer, M. McCusker, S.J. Steele, and H.S. Jacobs (1988). Outcome of pregnancy in underweight women after spontaneous and induced ovulation. *Br. Med. J.* 296:962–965.

Veldhuis, J.D., W.S. Evans, L.M. Demers, M.O. Thorner, D. Wakat, and A.D. Rogol (1985). Altered neuroendocrine regulation of gonadotropin secretion in women distance runners. *J. Clin. Endocrinol. Metab.* 61:557–563.

Vena, J.E., S. Graham, M. Zielezny, J. Brasure, and M.K. Swanson (1987). Occupational exercise and risk of cancer. *Am. J. Clin. Nutr.* 45:318–327.

Vihko, V.J., D.L. Apter, E.I. Pukkala, M.T. Oinonen, T.R. Hakulinen, and R.K. Vihko (1992). Risk of breast cancer among female teachers of physical education and languages. *Acta Oncol.* 31:201–204.

Wade, G.N., and J.E. Schneider (1992). Metabolic fuels and reproduction in female mammals. *Neurosci. Biobehav. Rev.* 16:235–272.

Wade, G.N., J.E. Schneider, and M.I. Friedman (1991). Insulin-induced anestrus in Syrian hamsters. *Am. J. Physiol.* 260: R148–R152.

Wilmore, J.H., K.C. Wambsgans, M. Brenner, C.E. Broeder, I. Paijmans, J.A. Volpe, and K.M. Wilmore (1992). Is there energy conservation in amenorrheic compared with eumenorrheic distance runners? *J. Appl. Physiol.* 72:15–22.

Yahiro, J., A.R. Glass, W.B. Fears, E.W. Ferguson, and R.A. Vigersky (1987). Exaggerated gonadotropin response to luteinizing hormone-releasing hormone in amenorrheic runners. *Am. J. Obstet. Gynecol.* 156:586–591.

Yen, S.S.C. (1991a). Chronic anovulation due to CNS-hypothalamic-pituitary dysfunction. In: S.S.C. Yen & B.B. Jaffe (eds.) *Reproductive Endocrinology: Physiology, Pathophysiology and Clinical Management.* Philadelphia: W.B. Saunders Company, pp. 631–688.

Yen, S.S.C. (1991b). Chronic anovulation caused by peripheral endocrine disorders. In: S.S.C. Yen & B.B. Jaffe (eds.) *Reproductive Endocrinology: Physiology, Pathophysiology and Clinical Management.* Philadelphia: W.B. Saunders Company, pp. 576–630.

DISCUSSION

SMITH: Is there any evidence that educational intervention is actually helpful in changing dietary restriction behaviors in ballerinas and other women athletes? Has it been proven that any type of intervention changes the way these athletes think in terms of either their energy intake or their exercise performance behavior?

LOUCKS: Not any large-scale study. The reason that I am hesitant to suggest behavior modification is my experience with some of these women athletes who have seen clinicians, and the recommendation they are given is "Stop your training program." That's not a very viable solution to an elite ballerina or professional athlete. So the frustration with not being able to provide very precise advice and conversations with athletes who have attempted to make some behavioral changes with no success has led me to be more cautious. Some clinicians have turned to what might be considered a more stop-gap approach, e.g., treating these women with some type of steroid replenishment in an effort to try to protect their bones.

WILMORE: I think that the only way to get to the athlete and probably to the coach as well, who often becomes a direct or indirect partner in this whole eating disorder problem, is by educating them concerning the potentially adverse effect of weight loss on sport performance. In the one study with which I am familiar (*Scand. J. Med. Sports Exerc.* 1:141–146, 1991) the authors showed that those elite women distance runners who underwent marked weight loss had significant decrements in $\dot{V}O_2$max and also in their running performances. This should be one way to get the attention of the athletes and their coaches.

CLARKSON: That may work with figure skaters or gymnasts, but it won't work with dancers. They would accept a decrement in performance to look better. Often dancers will not be allowed to perform if they are "over weight." Many dance companies still have contract weights.

LOUCKS: You are probably correct up to the point of experiencing stress fractures; that is a wake-up call for them.

CLAPP: How do you differentiate what you find in these women from what you would see in an overtraining syndrome? Are these women simply overtrained or do they have a low enough level of exercise performance to exclude that possibility?

LOUCKS: Unfortunately, we don t have data to suggest that these women are not performing adequately. Individual coaches of elite athletes have informed me in the last year that by observing deteriorations in performance, they can pick out the women who are regularly menstruating from the women who are amenorrheic, but this is totally anecdotal evidence.

MAUGHAN: You quoted a study reporting that even very low levels of physical activity can markedly reduce progesterone levels. What about women who have physically demanding occupations where the levels of activity can be very much greater than that? Are there similar hormonal changes in those women?

LOUCKS: We don't know how widespread this is, and we don't know whether it really is due to exercise or to energy imbalance.

MAUGHAN: In many countries in Southeast Asia, for example, most of the physically demanding jobs, e.g., the agricultural work and the construction site work, are largely done by women, often in conjunction with restricted energy intake. Is there reduced fertility in those women?

LOUCKS: The scientific evidence is very limited. In times of famine, e.g., during World War II, reduced fertility is commonly observed.

MAUGHAN: That was a very extreme situation, but it does seem that a large part of the female population can work extremely hard on a daily basis with restricted energy intake and still be fertile.

DESPRES: As an investigator working in a lipid clinic, I wish I had the plasma lipoprotein lipid profile that we see in highly trained women with low estrogen levels. From a clinical point of view, I think these amenorrheic women are far from having a dyslipidemic profile, and it is premature to raise these altered lipoprotein levels as a concern.

LOUCKS: Thank you. I wanted an expert opinion on whether these statistical differences in the lipoprotein profile represent a clinical problem, and I guess the answer is, "probably not."

WILMORE: Might one use the detraining model to study mechanisms of luteal suppression? I realize it's very difficult to get elite athletes to stop training, but it would be interesting to try to use this model to tease out which of your possible explanations is correct. You could take athletes with luteal suppression who are training at very high volumes or high intensities and have them detrain for two or three months to see if this normalizes luteal function or not.

LOUCKS: Any detraining protocol will need to carefully control dietary energy intake as well as energy expenditure both before and after detraining begins if one is to have any chance at distinguishing the effects of energy availability vs. exercise stress.

GISOLFI: What do you think is the mechanistic link between reduced energy availability and the LH pulse?

LOUCKS: LH pulsatility is indicative of alterations in GnRH pulsatility at the level of the hypothalamus. It is not clear how energy availability acts to affect the hypothalamic pulse generator. Some refeeding data in animal research report a very rapid return of LH pulsatility upon refeeding; this suggests that it is more likely to involve a neural rather than a hormonal mechanism.

GISOLFI: Aside from the primate, what do you think is the best animal model for studying amenorrhea?

LOUCKS: George Wade with his hamster model and Frank Bronson with his rat model, both manipulating energy and exercise independently, have contributed a great deal to our knowledge of the neuroendocrine mechanism.

EICHNER: Don't men who overtrain also show diminished LH pulses?

LOUCKS: We do have one study indicating that highly trained male runners (in excess of 70–80 mi/wk) have altered LH pulse frequency. From the animal literature, we have indications that lack of energy certainly inhibits LH pulsatility. What seems to be the case is that the level of energy deprivation needed to disrupt reproductive function for the male system is more severe than what is needed for the female system.

SUTTON: The Wade model of energy compartmentalization strikes me as being intuitively wrong if energy supposedly cannot be exchanged among compartments. In most biological systems there is a hierarchy of preference, and when the demand in one area is greater, during exercise for instance, energy should be able to move from one compartment to another.

LOUCKS: No. Priorities would be established. Functions such as growth and reproduction that are not necessary for survival of the individual would probably receive low priority. High priority would go to critical functions such as cellular metabolism.

TERJUNG: Except for the storage; as long as there is a surfeit of energy, than the storage has a positive side. As soon as there is an energy deficit, then you have a negative entry into storage, and energy depleted from storage can enter into the other categories, e.g., maintenance of the cell. So, it seems that there can be interchange.

HASKELL: There can be interchange, but if you stored it, you're not using it simultaneously for another function.

TERJUNG: At the moment.

LOUCKS: Yes. At the moment. The reproductive system seems to have a very short memory, as if it is constantly asking, "What have you fed me lately?" With regard to the availability to the reproductive system of dietary energy that is put into storage, several animal experiments have diverted dietary energy into storage by insulin administration with the result that GnRH pulse generator activity was suppressed. It is not clear yet whether energy from fat is as available as energy from carbohydrates.

CLARKSON: Why do you think that underreporting of energy intake isn't as large a problem as many have implied?

LOUCKS: To attribute all of what appears to be an energy imbalance to underreporting of energy consumption is too simplistic. Many investigators seem to have concluded that these women are all underreporting just because the intake and expenditure data don't add up.

WILLIAMS: There is a simple filtering technique for such data. This involves calculating the BMR of each athlete from height, weight, and age and then multiplying this BMR value by 1.4. This figure gives the energy intake necessary to sustain a sedentary lifestyle. Any energy intake data that fall below this figure are clearly unacceptable because they indicate that either the athletes are underreporting their food intakes or undereating during the period of observation. The discriminating factor can be revised to 1.6 for females and 1.7 for males to reflect the energy needs of active people.

WILMORE: Leslie Schultz's group addressed this issue in the 1991 volume of *J. Appl. Physiol.* using doubly-labeled water. They found that their athletes were undereating on days they were completing food logs. There definitely is some underreporting among such athletes, but undereating may occur as well. Dale Schoeller published a nice review on doubly-labeled water studies and showed that female athletes, along with obese women, tend to be the most likely to underreport or undereat at the time they're actually filling out their food logs.

LOUCKS: We need to repeat those studies on amenorrheic athletes. If they're in a low-T_3 state, they're different from cyclic athletes.

WILMORE: I totally agree, but I think the magnitude of the underreporting/undereating phenomenon in women athletes is not nearly as great as what the literature suggests. Some of those studies have reported energy intakes as low as 11,000 or 12,000 kcal. We have measured resting metabolic rates (RMR) in similar athletes and have found their values to be normal, even when corrected for fat-free mass. The RMR is between 1,300 and 1,400 kcal for the average size runner, and this is greater than what has been reported as the daily intake in these athletes. There definitely is an energy deficit, but not as great as the literature might suggest.

LOUCKS: I acknowledge that there may be some underreporting, but I question whether the assumptions relating height, weight, and age to metabolic rate apply to women with low-T_3 syndrome and whether the assumptions relating oxygen consumption to energy expenditure apply in indirect calorimetry. I also question whether the assumptions relating isotope concentrations to energy expenditure apply in the doubly-labeled water technique. We need to recalibrate all these techniques in the chronically energy-deficient woman, and the metabolic hormone profile of the amenorrheic athlete indicates that she belongs in this energy-deficient category.

SMITH: I have concern about completely disregarding some of the behavioral stresses that many perceive to be important factors in the menstrual disturbances in athletes. There are certainly young athletes that are in fearful situations, e.g., fearful of parents, poor performance, the media, and coaches.

LOUCKS: I have used a set of psychological inventories and have had discussions with psychiatrists and psychologists and have been unable to pick out psychological factors that I can use to differentiate amenorrheic athletes from the cyclic athletes. I know that there is a theoretical basis for the operation of psychological stress in altering menstrual function, but I have not been able to detect differences among normal and amenorrheic athletes.

DAVIS: Is energy deficit a very important mechanism of amenorrhea or the *only* mechanism?

LOUCKS: I think it may be the only or at least the predominant mechanism.

DAVIS: That says to me that you are ready to rule out many other stresses associated with heavy exercise and training that are equally as likely to cause amenorrhea but may not yet have been tested adequately. Clearly, your well-controlled experiments show very nicely that energy deficit can cause amenorrhea. However, this doesn't rule out other causes that might occur under different circumstances from your experimental paradigm.

LOUCKS: Obviously, other possibilities remain, but the most likely predominant mechanism is energy deficit. The hypothalamic-pituitary-adrenal axis responds to energy deprivation as well as other types of so-called stressors.

DAVIS: I agree that in your experimental model this seems to be the case, but I'm not convinced it will be the case in all situations in which stressful training causes amenorrhea.

LOUCKS: In our experiments, differences in exercise status do not affect LH pulse frequency, but differences in energy status clearly slow down that pulse generator. If anything, we're seeing a blunted response in exercising groups compared to the dietary restricted ones. If you think some stress not linked to energy deficiency is disrupting LH pulsatility, I say, "Prove it." Perform an experiment in which stress and energy availability are independently controlled, and show that there is a deleterious effect of stress that cannot be prevented by dietary energy supplementation. I think you will find the same thing I found. The onus is on the proponents of the stress hypothesis to show an energy-independent effect of stress on LH pulsatility, but I bet they can't.

4

Bone Mineralization Patterns: Reproductive Endocrine, Calcium, And Physical Activity Influences During The Life Span

CAMERON J.R. BLIMKIE, Ph.D.

PHILIP D. CHILIBECK, M.Sc.

K. SHAWN DAVISON, M.Sc.

INTRODUCTION

The human skeleton is composed of more than 200 bones that provide a reservoir for the body's calcium and a framework for the translation of muscle forces into movement. Bone is a specialized form of connective tissue containing bone cells or osteocytes that make up less than 2% of its volume (Teitelbaum, 1993). The remainder is an expansive matrix consisting of collagen fibers, other proteins, ground substance, and the minerals calcium, phosphorous, sodium, and potassium (Montoye, 1987; Sledge & Rubin, 1989). Although bone contains 99% of the total body calcium stores, only 37% of the total mineral content of bone is calcium. Bone tissue is organized structurally into two basic forms: cortical, or compact bone, and trabecular, or spongy bone (Figure 4-1). Cortical bone, which forms the outer layer of most bones and is found mostly in the shafts of the appendicular (limbs) skeleton, comprises about 80% of total skeletal mass (Kanis, 1991). Trabecular bone, which is found mostly in the distal portions of long bones, many flat bones, and the vertebral bodies,

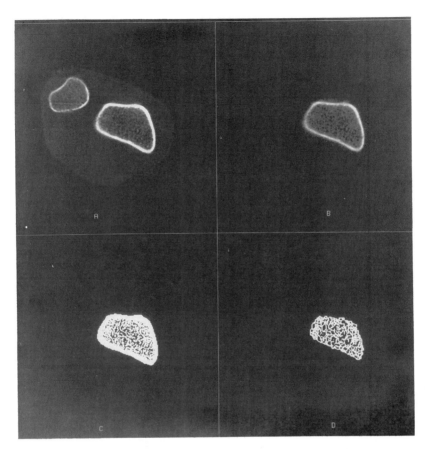

FIGURE 4-1. *The upper left panel depicts cross-sectional images of the distal ulna (smaller bone) and radius of the left arm of a 23 year old healthy woman. The thick white collar at the perimeters of the bones represents compact cortical bone; the dark spaces in the central portions of the bones represent bone marrow and fat; the thinner white lattice-like structures in the central regions (lower panels) represent trabecular bone.* Cortical, trabecular, and total bone mineral contents (BMC) and volumetric bone densities (BMD) in mg/mm³ are derived from such images. The image of the radius has been isolated (upper right panel), represented as a binary image (lower left panel), and thinned to produce a representation of trabeculae from which connectivity among trabeculae can be assessed (lower right panel). The technique used was peripheral quantitative computed tomography (pQCT) using a Stratec XCT-960 instrument (Stratic Medizintechnik, distributed by Norland Corp., U.S.A.). The image is reproduced with permission from C.L. Gordon, C.E. Webber, J.D. Adachi, and N. Christoforou, In-vivo assessment of trabecular bone structure at the distal radius from high-resolution computed tomography images, *Physics Med. Biol.*, 41:495–508, 1996.

comprises about 20% of skeletal mass (Kanis, 1991b; Parfitt, 1988; Teitelbaum, 1993). Trabecular bone is more porous than cortical bone (25% and 90% osseous mass, respectively) and has about four times the volume ratio of surface area to bone (Parfitt, 1988).

The absolute quantities of cortical and trabecular bone as well as their proportional distribution vary from bone to bone, within the same bone at different sites and stages of the life span, between genders, and among individuals and races. The first part of this chapter describes bone mineralization patterns throughout the life span, at the most commonly measured and clinically important sites of the human skeleton (Figure 4-2), with emphasis on normal healthy females. The remaining sections address the complex interaction of the mineralization process with reproductive endocrine events, calcium status, and physical activity or training for females only, at different stages of the life span. Aspects of these latter topics have been addressed in recent excellent reviews (Bailey et al., 1996; Bloomfield, 1995; Drinkwater, 1990; Snow-Harter & Marcus, 1991).

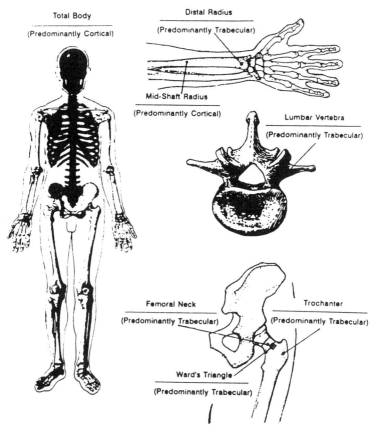

FIGURE 4-2. *Common sites for measuring bone mineral density in humans.* The relative distributions of cortical and trabecular bone tissue are indicated.

TECHNICAL CONSIDERATIONS

Numerous methods, including weighing of bone, bone morphometry, bone biopsy, radiogrammetry, photon scattering, radiographic photodensitometry, single (SPA) and dual (DPA) photon absorptiometry, dual-energy x-ray absorptiometry (DXA), and quantitative computed tomography (QCT), have been applied over the years to describe skeletal development and to quantify bone mineralization in humans (Arnold et al., 1966; Mazess, 1982; Mazess & Wahner, 1988; Mueller et al., 1966; Newton-John & Morgan, 1970; Riggs & Melton, 1986; Tothill, 1989; Trotter & Hixon, 1974). This chapter focuses on the patterns of bone mineral development derived from the more recent techniques of absorptiometry and computed tomography. These techniques provide more valid estimates of bone mineral than did some of the earlier non-invasive techniques and permit *in-vivo* determinations of bone mineral at a greater variety of sites and in larger numbers of healthy individuals than was possible in the past.

The technical underpinnings of these approaches, their relative strengths and limitations, and their comparability in relation to the determination of bone mineral in humans have been thoroughly reviewed (Borders et al., 1989; Holbrook et al., 1991; Mazess & Wahner, 1988; Pacifici et al., 1988; Shipp et al., 1988; Tothill, 1989) and are beyond the scope of this chapter. This literature supports the conclusion that the absorptiometric and computed tomography techniques provide highly accurate measures (within 1-3% of phantom or actual bone specimens) of bone mineral in humans. The precision or reproducibility varies slightly among sites within the skeleton and ranges from 0.5-2.5% when measured by an experienced technician (Mazess & Wahner, 1988; Tothill, 1989).

Effect Of Bone Size On Mineralization Patterns

Both absorptiometry and computed tomography provide measures of bone mineral mass or content and a corresponding measure of bone density. Caution is warranted, however, when interpreting the bone density measure because this variable is calculated differently for the absorptiometric and computed tomography techniques (Table 4-1). With the absorptiometric techniques, the mass equivalent (g or mg) per scanned segment (e.g., for the entire skeleton or the lumbar vertebrae) or the mass equivalent for a standard scan length (e.g., for the radius or femoral neck) is normalized for the projected scan area (segment length × bone width), resulting in areal bone density in units of $g \cdot cm^{-2}$. With computed tomography, however, the mineral mass is normalized for the bone segment volume, resulting in a true measure of volumetric bone density in units of either $g \cdot cm^{-3}$ or $mg \cdot mm^{-3}$.

Bone mineral mass or content is highly dependent on the size of the bone scanned; the larger the skeleton or skeletal segment, the greater the

TABLE 4-1. *Technical considerations in determination of bone density*

Single-Photon Absorptiometry (SPA)
- Bone mineral content of a defined segment length
- Bone mineral density is calculated as: bone mineral content/scan width × scan length
- Areal bone mineral density is expressed as g/cm^2
- SPA technique is used mostly at the distal and mid-radial sites

Dual-Photon Absorptiometry (DPA) and Dual-Energy X–Ray Absorptiometry (DXA)
- Bone mineral content is determined for specific regions of interest
- Bone mineral density is calculated as: bone mineral content/projected scan area in region of interest
- Areal bone mineral density is expressed as g/cm^2; bone mineral apparent density as g/cm^3
- Absorptiometry techniques are used for total body, spine, hip, and other regions of interest

Computed Tomography (QCT)
- Bone mineral content is determined for specific regions of interest
- Bone mineral density is calculated as: bone mineral content/volume of bone in the region of interest
- Volumetric bone mineral density is expressed as g/cm^3, mg/mm^3, mg/cm^3, or g/L
- Computed tomography differentiates between cortical and trabecular bone
- Computed tomography is used at the lumbar spine and at the radius

amount of bone mineral. The normalizing approaches described above have been applied in an attempt to remove the bone size effect, thereby facilitating fairer comparisons of mineralization levels across skeletons or segments of skeletons of variable size. However, as illustrated schematically in Figure 4-3, bone volume increases disproportionately more than projected scan area, with an increase in skeletal or bone segment size (depth). Consequently, larger individuals with the same empirically derived true bone densities will invariably have greater areal bone densities than smaller individuals when measurements are obtained by absorptiometry.

The absorptiometric techniques do not account for bone depth or thickness (with the exception of the newest generation DXA scanners that have a lateral scan mode for application at the spine) and, unlike computed tomography, are incapable of measuring true bone volume. Failure to correct absorptiometric measures of areal bone density for bone thickness provides developmental patterns of bone density that systematically underestimate the actual density of smaller, compared to larger, individuals.

This limitation of absorptiometry is most problematic during childhood and adolescence because of the dramatic growth-related changes in skeletal size that occur during this period. Thus, absorptiometric measures of areal bone density probably overestimate the true magnitude of change in mineralization that occurs during this period. This limitation may also influence both the interpretation of bone mineral density (BMD) differences between individuals of similar age but different skeletal size

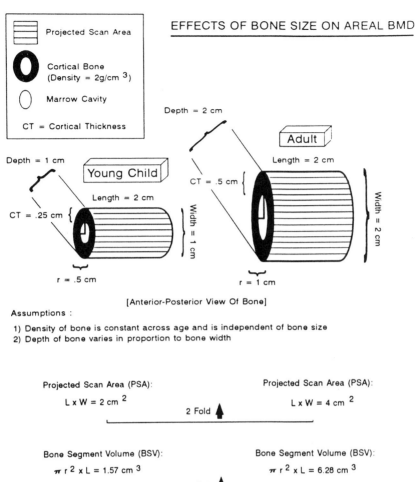

EFFECTS OF BONE SIZE ON AREAL BMD

Projected Scan Area

Cortical Bone
(Density = 2g/cm^3)

Marrow Cavity

CT = Cortical Thickness

Depth = 2 cm

Adult

Depth = 1 cm

Length = 2 cm

Young Child

CT = .5 cm

Length = 2 cm

Width = 1 cm

CT = .25 cm

Width = 2 cm

r = .5 cm

r = 1 cm

[Anterior-Posterior View Of Bone]

Assumptions :

1) Density of bone is constant across age and is independent of bone size
2) Depth of bone varies in proportion to bone width

Projected Scan Area (PSA):

L x W = 2 cm^2

2 Fold

Projected Scan Area (PSA):

L x W = 4 cm^2

Bone Segment Volume (BSV):

π r^2 x L = 1.57 cm^3

4 Fold

Bone Segment Volume (BSV):

π r^2 x L = 6.28 cm^3

Cortical Bone Volume (CBV):

BSV - Marrow Cavity Volume = 1.17 cm^3

Cortical Bone Volume (CBV):

BSV - Marrow Cavity Volume = 4.71 cm^3

Bone Mineral Content (BMC) :

CBV x Cortical Bone Density = 2.35 g

Bone Mineral Content (BMC) :

CBV x Cortical Bone Density = 9.42 g

Areal BMD :

BMC / PSA = 1.17 g/cm^2

Areal BMD :

BMC / PSA = 2.35 g/cm^2

FIGURE 4-3. *Effects of bone size on areal bone mineral density (BMD).* A schematic representation of the effect of bone size on areal BMD measures derived from absorptiometric techniques.

and may limit gender comparisons of mineralization trends with aging because absorptiometry will not accurately detect changes in bone volume consequent to continued periosteal bone accretion that accompanies increases in bone diameter in males. Additionally, because bone volume will change proportionally more than projected scan area, areal BMD measures will probably underestimate the loss in true volumetric BMD with aging in both sexes (Kanis & Adami, 1994). Computed tomography, on the other hand, adequately adjusts for bone size effects by providing equitable comparisons on a per unit volume basis, regardless of age, gender, or skeletal size.

Various normalization approaches have been used to overcome the inability of absorptiometry to determine bone volume (Katzman et al. 1991; Kroger et al. 1992, 1993). With these approaches, absorptiometric measures of bone mineral content (BMC) are normalized for estimates of bone volume derived from the product of site-specific projected scan area and either bone width or height (for the femoral neck and lumbar spine, respectively), or stature (for the total body). The derived measure is bone-mineral-apparent-density ($g \cdot cm^{-3}$). Whether the interpretation of developmental changes in bone mineralization is improved with these normalization approaches, compared to the interpretation derived from the actual and highly precise unadjusted measure of areal bone density itself, remains to be determined.

Scanning Technique Limitations And Bone Composition

The absorptiometric techniques cannot distinguish between cortical and trabecular bone compartments, and the resultant measure of bone density represents the integral densities of both tissue types at a particular region. Interpretation of the developmental patterns for cortical and trabecular bone derived from absorptiometric measurements must, therefore, take into consideration the proportional distributions of the two bone types at specific scan sites (Mazess & Wahner, 1988). The measure of total body bone mineral is considered to reflect predominantly (80%) cortical bone. The distal region of the radius is composed mostly of trabecular bone (90–95%), whereas the mid-shaft is composed mostly of cortical bone (90–95%). The femoral neck and Ward's triangle are composed of slightly more trabecular (55–65%) than cortical bone, with Ward's triangle having a slightly higher proportion of trabecular bone than the femoral neck region. Absorptiometric measures of the whole vertebrae are generally considered to reflect predominantly trabecular bone (65–75%), although a morphological study by Nottestad et al. (1987) suggested that the thoraco-lumbar vertebrae have a higher proportion of cortical than trabecular bone.

Measurements derived from computed tomography provide a more straightforward interpretation of cortical and trabecular mineralization patterns. This technique is capable of isolating the two bone types at specific regions, but at the expense of greater radiation exposure when compared to the absorptiometric techniques.

Micro And Macro Bone Density Distinction

Both the absorptiometric and computed tomography techniques provide measures of macro bone density, that is, the mineral mass of the whole skeleton or skeletal segment divided by the volume of osseous material substance (bone cells and matrix) and the non-osseous space (pores, canals, and vascular and intertrabecular space) included in the scan. In healthy individuals, the macro bone density measures will always be less than the true (micro) density of isolated bone tissue because of the dilution of the mineral mass by the non-osseous space. The micro or true density of bone osseous material alone, determined by gravimetric analysis, ranges between 1.4 $g \cdot cm^{-3}$ during the initial stages of mineralization to 2.2 $g \cdot cm^{-3}$ when fully mature (Grynpas, 1993; Parfitt, 1988).

DEVELOPMENTAL AND AGING CONSIDERATIONS

Emphasis in the following section is placed on developmental and aging changes in bone mineral for the total body, the radius, the lumbar spine, and the proximal femur. To minimize the effects of changes in bone size across the life span, we have presented mineralization patterns only in terms of areal and volumetric BMD. The relative merits of expressing mineral measures as bone content or density have been eloquently argued in several reviews (Compston, 1995; Genant et al., 1994; Prentice et al., 1994). Additional rationale for selecting BMD as the measurement unit in the following section are summarized in Table 4-2.

Changes Before Puberty

Areal BMD $(g \cdot cm^{-2})$ increases between infancy and the onset of puberty in both sexes for the total body (Faulkner et al., 1993a; Geusens et al., 1991; Gordon & Webber, 1993; Katzman et al., 1991; Lu et al., 1994; Rico et al., 1992), radial (Bell et al., 1991; Geusens et al., 1991; Li et al., 1989; Rubin et al., 1993; Sugimoto et al., 1994), femoral neck (Lu et al., 1994;

TABLE 4-2. *Reasons for choosing bone mineral density (BMD) as the primary measure of bone mineral*

- **BMD is a useful predictor of fracture risk for adults**
- **BMD discriminates between osteoporotic and normal bone**
- **BMD measurements are more reproducible than those for bone mineral content (BMC)**
- **BMD standardizes in whole (tomography: QCT) or in part (absorptiometry: DPA, DXA) for differences in bone size**
  Absorptiometric measures of BMD reflect elements of both size and density of bone. This facilitates comparisons of individuals of different size and comparisons to reference populations.

Thomas et al., 1991), and lumbar spine (Bell et al., 1991; Del Rio et al., 1994; DeSchepper et al., 1991; Geusens et al., 1991; Glastre et al., 1990; Henderson & Hayes, 1994; Kroger et al., 1992, 1993; Lu et al., 1994; McCormick et al., 1991; Ponder et al., 1990; Rubin et al., 1993; Southard et al., 1991; Thomas et al., 1991) (Figure 4-4). The rates of gain in BMD during this period vary from 1.2%–3.9% per year for females, to slightly greater values of 1.5%–7.7% per year for males (Kroger et al., 1993; Lu et al., 1994; Thomas et al., 1991). Some studies have reported slightly greater BMD values for males (Bonjour et al., 1991; Gunnes 1994; Kroger et al., 1992, 1993; Li et al., 1989; Miller et al., 1991), whereas others have reported similar or slightly higher values for females (Del rio et al., 1994; DeSchepper et al., 1991; Glastre et al., 1990; Grimston et al., 1992; Henderson & Hayes, 1994; Kroger et al., 1993; McCormick et al., 1991; Miller et al., 1991; Rubin et al., 1993), and yet others (Bonjour et al., 1991; Faulkner et al., 1993a; Geusens et al., 1991; Grimston et al., 1992; Lu et al., 1994; Thomas et al., 1991) have failed to find a gender difference at comparable ages or when collapsed across wide age ranges during this prepubertal period.

Available data on racial differences in BMD during the prepubertal period are limited. Several studies suggest that African-American boys and girls may have greater areal BMD at the radial, femoral neck, and lumbar spine sites than do Caucasian children (Bell et al., 1991; Li et al., 1989), whereas another study failed to find any difference in lumbar spine BMD between African-American and Caucasian children during the prepubertal years (Southard et al., 1991).

Changes During Puberty And Adolescence

Areal BMD for the total body (Faulkner et al., 1993a; Geusens et al., 1991; Katzman et al., 1991; Lu et al., 1994), radial (Geusens et al., 1991; Gunnes, 1994; Katzman et al., 1991; Matkovic et al., 1990; Rubin et al., 1993; Slemenda et al., 1994), femoral neck (Bonjour et al., 1991; Grimston et al., 1992; Henderson, 1991; Katzman et al., 1991; Kroger et al., 1992; Miller et al., 1991; Slemenda et al., 1994; Theintz et al., 1992; Thomas et al., 1991), and lumbar spine sites (Bonjour et al., 1991; Del Rio et al., 1994; DeSchepper et al., 1991; Grimston et al., 1992; Katzman et al., 1991; Kroger et al., 1993; Rubin et al., 1993; Sentipal et al., 1991; Slemenda et al., 1994; Southard et al., 1991) increases more rapidly during the circum-pubertal years (10–16 y) than at times prior to or following this period for both girls (Figure 4-5) and boys.

In relation to pubertal status, most (Geusens et al., 1991; Katzman et al., 1991; Matkovic et al., 1990), but not all (Rubin et al., 1993), studies indicate substantial increases in total body (Lu et al., 1994), radial, femoral neck (Bonjour et al., 1991; Grimston et al., 1992; Katzman et al., 1991;

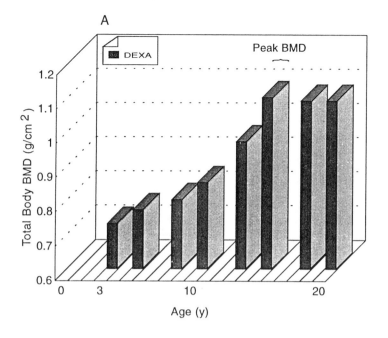

A

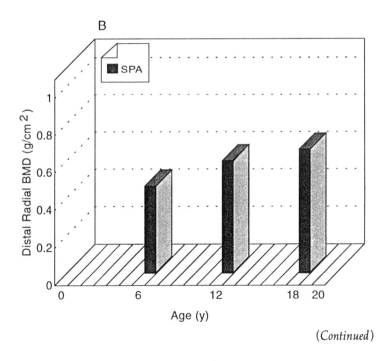

B

(*Continued*)

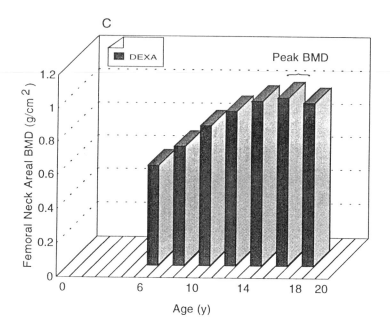

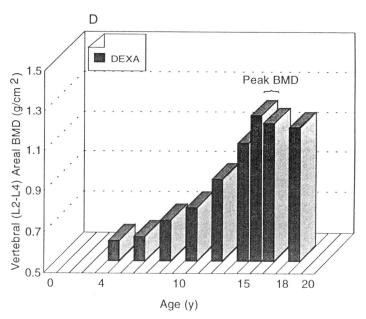

FIGURE 4-4. *Age-related changes in areal bone mineral density (BMD) during childhood—females.* Panel A was adapted from Lu et al. (1994), panel B from Geusens et al. (1986), panel C from Kroger et al. (1992), and panel D from Lu et al. (1994). DEXA = dual-energy x-ray absorptiometry; SPA = single-photon absorptiometry.

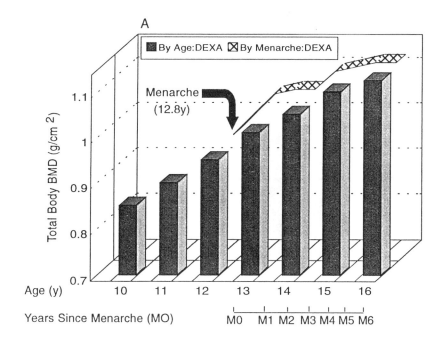

A

By Age:DEXA ⊠ By Menarche:DEXA

Total Body BMD (g/cm ^{2})

Menarche
(12.8y)

Age (y) 10 11 12 13 14 15 16

Years Since Menarche (MO) M0 M1 M2 M3 M4 M5 M6

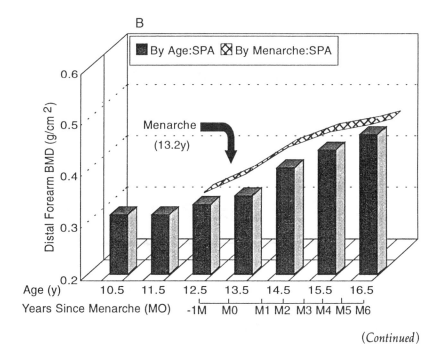

B

By Age:SPA ⊠ By Menarche:SPA

Distal Forearm BMD (g/cm ^{2})

Menarche
(13.2y)

Age (y) 10.5 11.5 12.5 13.5 14.5 15.5 16.5

Years Since Menarche (MO) -1M M0 M1 M2 M3 M4 M5 M6

(Continued)

BONE MINERALIZATION PATTERNS   **85**

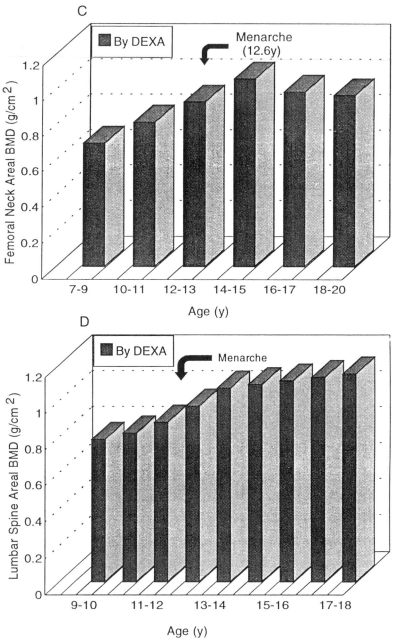

FIGURE 4-5. *Pubertal and adolescent changes in areal bone mineral density (BMD) in females.* Panel A was adapted from Lu et al. (1994), panel B from Gunnes et al. (1994), panel C from Kroger et al. (1993), and panel D from Del Rio et al. (1994). DEXA = dual-energy x-ray absorptiometry; SPA = single-photon absorptiometry.

Kroger et al., 1992; Theintz et al., 1992), and lumbar spine areal BMD (Bonjour et al., 1991; Del Rio et al., 1994; Grimston et al., 1992; Katzman et al., 1991; Kroger et al., 1993), with advancing levels of sexual maturity in both genders during this period.

For females, the largest gains occur during the first 2 y following the onset of menarche (Gunnes et al., 1994) for radial BMD, during the year prior to menarche for femoral neck BMD (Kroger et al., 1993), and between Tanner pubertal stages 3 and 5 (commencing about 13.5 y for girls) for lumbar spine BMD (Bonjour et al., 1991; Del Rio et al., 1994; DeSchepper et al., 1991; Glastre et al., 1990; Grimston et al., 1992; Katzman et al., 1991; Kroger et al., 1993; Rubin et al., 1993; Southard et al., 1991; Theintz et al., 1992). The rates of gain in radial, femoral neck and lumbar spine BMD abate substantially in females during the later stages of puberty and adolescence (Bonjour et al., 1991; Geusens et al., 1991; Katzman et al., 1991; Kroger et al., 1993; Matkovic et al., 1990; Theintz et al., 1992). In males, however, radial (Geusens et al., 1991; Rubin et al., 1993) and lumbar spine BMD (Bell et al., 1991; Del Rio et al., 1994; Henderson & Hayes, 1994; Lu et al., 1994; McCormick et al., 1991; Ponder et al., 1990; Southard et al., 1991; Thomas et al., 1991) continue to increase from late puberty until the late teens and early adulthood.

There is no clear gender difference in the maximal rate of gain or the magnitude of change in radial, femoral neck, or lumbar spine BMD during this period (Bonjour et al., 1991; Del Rio et al., 1994; DeSchepper et al., 1991; Glastre et al., 1990; Grimston et al., 1992; Kroger et al., 1993; McCormick et al., 1991; Rubin et al., 1993; Southard et al., 1991; Theintz et al., 1992) and no evident gender difference in BMD at comparable stages of maturity (Bonjour et al., 1991; Del Rio et al., 1994; DeSchepper et al., 1991; Geusens et al., 1991; Grimston et al., 1992; Katzman et al., 1991; Miller et al., 1991; Sugimoto et al., 1994). Males, however, appear to have slightly higher radial (Geusens et al., 1991; Rubin et al., 1993), femoral neck (Bonjour et al., 1991; Grimston et al., 1992; Kroger et al., 1992; Kroger et al., 1993; Lu et al., 1994; Thomas et al., 1991), and lumbar spine areal BMD (Bonjour et al., 1991; Del Rio et al., 1994; Lu et al., 1994) than do females by full sexual maturity during the later years of adolescence.

Total body BMD does not appear to be correlated with age of onset of menarche in normally active, healthy, adolescent females (Lu et al., 1994; Rice et al., 1993), although it is positively related to years after menarche during the first 2 y following the onset of menstruation (Lu et al., 1994). By contrast, a recent study (Robinson et al., 1995) reported a negative correlation between age at menarche and total body, femoral neck, and lumbar spine areal BMD in competitive female gymnasts. The negative correlations for the gymnasts may have been influenced by restriction of dietary energy and nutrients and/or by delayed menarche. We are unaware of any published data on areal BMD differences between African-American and Caucasian children during the pubertal and adolescent period.

Normalization For Growth-Related Changes In Bone Size

After adjusting for bone size effects, there was no evident change in total body bone-mineral-apparent-density (BMAD) in females 9-20 y of age (Katzman et al., 1991), a substantial (but smaller percentage change compared to areal BMD) increase in femoral neck BMAD for females but not for males 7-15 y of age (Kroger et al., 1993), and a 20-25 % increase in lumbar spine BMAD (Figure 4-6A) in both sexes 7-18 y of age (Katzman et al., 1991; Kroger et al., 1992, 1993). These studies suggest that areal BMD values unadjusted for bone size (Figure 4-6B) overestimate apparent volumetric bone density changes during the growth years. Age-related increases and gender differences in areal BMD reported in the preceding section appear highly influenced by changes in bone size that occur during childhood and adolescence.

Areal BMD values have also been normalized for body mass. With this approach, African-American children of both genders had higher relative (per body mass) lumbar spine BMD than did Caucasian children (McCormick et al., 1991) during the pubertal years, and females had higher values than males at comparable ages and stages of sexual maturity (McCormick et al., 1991; Rubin et al., 1993).

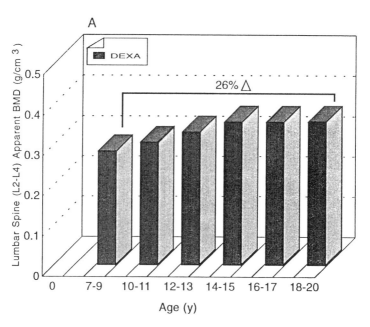

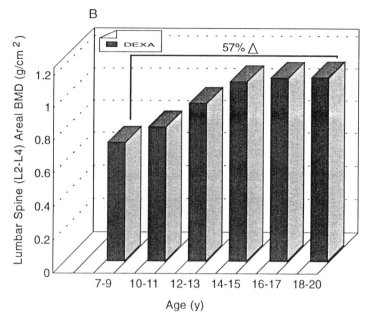

B

(Y-axis: Lumbar Spine (L2-L4) Areal BMD (g/cm²), values 0, 0.2, 0.4, 0.6, 0.8, 1, 1.2)

DEXA   57% △

7-9   10-11   12-13   14-15   16-17   18-20

Age (y)

FIGURE 4-6. *Lumbar spine apparent and areal bone mineral density (BMD) changes in females.* Panels A and B were adapted from Kroger et al. (1993). DEXA = dual-energy x-ray absorptiometry.

Recently, peripheral computed tomography (pQCT) has also been used to determine true volumetric radial BMD in children. Shonau et al., (1993) found no differences in distal radial total or trabecular BMD among a small sample (N = 8) of prepubescent children and adults of varying ages, suggesting that there is no age-related change in radial volumetric BMD from childhood to adulthood. However, unpublished data on larger samples from our own laboratory suggest that distal radial BMD does increase with age in females from before puberty to mid-adulthood, but the increase is smaller than the reported changes in absorptiometrically determined areal BMD at the distal radius over the same period (Blimkie, unpublished).

Quantitative computed tomography (QCT) has also been used to study age- and gender-related changes in true volumetric lumbar spine BMD (mg·cm⁻³) during the growth years. Based on limited data, lumbar spine trabecular BMD appears to increase only slightly and insignificantly in both sexes during the prepubertal and early pubertal years (Figure 4-7A) (Gilsanz et al., 1988a, 1988b, 1991, 1994b). These same studies show that lumbar spine volumetric BMD increases rather dramatically, however, in females (Figure 4-7B) and males around mid-puberty (puberty stage III), and appears to plateau during late adolescence.

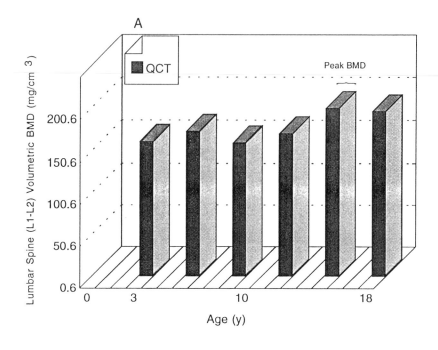

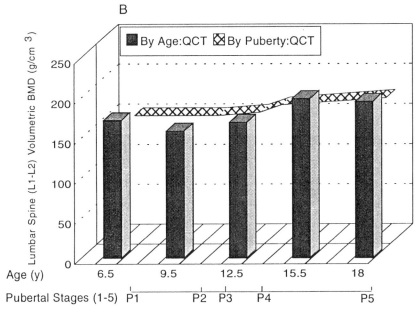

FIGURE 4-7. *Lumbar spine volumetric bone mineral density (BMD) changes during childhood in females.* Panel A was adapted from Gilsanz et al. (1988) and panel B from Gilsanz et al. (1991). QCT = quantitative computed tomography.

Lumbar spine volumetric density increases from 12–22% in Caucasian males and females (40% in African-American females) from early childhood to adulthood (Gilsanz et al., 1988a, 1988b, 1991). About 83–90% of the growth-related increase in lumbar spine volumetric BMD in Caucasian children, and 75% of the increase in African-American girls occurs after mid-puberty (Gilsanz et al., 1988b, 1991, 1994b).

Information about racial differences in BMD during the pubertal and adolescent period is scant. Nevertheless, one study (Gilsanz et al., 1991) reported no difference in lumbar spine volumetric BMD between African-American and Caucasian females prior to mid-puberty (stage 3) but greater lumbar spine BMD in the African-American girls during the later stages of puberty.

Changes During Early Adulthood

Total body areal BMD peaks and plateaus in females (Figure 4-8A) during the last half of the 2nd or first half of the 3rd decade (Gallagher et al., 1987; Gotfredsen et al., 1987; Lu et al., 1994; Rico et al., 1991) and then remains stable or decreases slightly from its peak until the onset of menopause around 50 y of age (Gallagher et al., 1987; Gotfredsen et al., 1987; Nilas & Christiansen, 1988; Rico et al., 1991). Peak total body BMD in males is achieved during the latter part of the 2nd or 3rd decades, or the early part of the 4th decade, and is higher than in females (Gotfredsen et al., 1987; Lu et al., 1994).

Radial areal BMD appears to reach a plateau in females between the 3rd to 5th decades (Figure 4-8B) and peaks in the 4th or early part of the 5th decades (Buchanan et al., 1988b; Luisetto et al., 1993; Mazess & Barden, 1991; Nordin et al., 1986, 1987; Prentice et al., 1991; Sowers et al., 1992). For males, radial BMD increases slightly from the 2nd to 3rd decades and then plateaus during the later part of the 3rd or early part of the 4th decades (Blunt et al., 1994; Compston et al., 1988; Geusens et al., 1986; Meier et al., 1984).

Femoral neck areal BMD peaks between late adolescence and the 4th decade (Figure 4-8C) in females, and density does not vary across ages during this interval (Bonjour et al., 1991; Casez et al., 1994; Laitinen et al., 1991; Mazess & Barden, 1991; Mazess et al., 1987; Rodin et al., 1990). Femoral neck BMD is lost at a rate of between 0.25–5.0% per year from its peak to the onset of menopause (Mazess et al., 1987; Pocock et al., 1987), and this premenopausal loss represents about one-third of the lifetime reduction in femoral neck BMD (Rodin et al., 1990). There is no apparent gender difference in femoral neck BMD between premenopausal females and their male twins (Kelly et al., 1990).

Vertebral areal BMD was reported in one study (Buchanan et al., 1988b) to peak in females in the late teens, whereas others (Casez et al.,

A

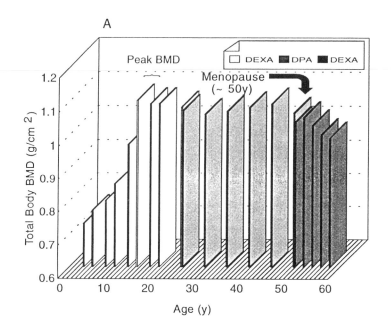

B

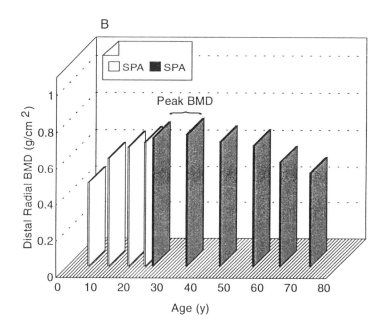

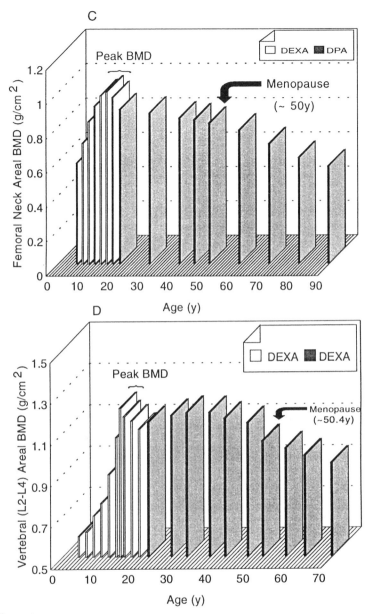

FIGURE 4-8. *Life span changes in areal bone mineral density (BMD) in females.* Panel A was adapted from Lu et al. (1994, white bars); Gallagher et al. (1987, medium-gray bars); and Wang et al. (1994, dark-gray bars). Panel B was adapted from Geusens et al. (1986, white bars, and 1991, gray bars). Panel C was adapted from Kroger et al. (1992, white bars) and Beck et al. (1993, gray bars). Panel D was adapted from Lu et al. (1994, white bars) and Laitinen et al. (1991, gray bars). DEXA = dual-energy x-ray absorptiometry; SPA = single-photon absorptiometry; DPA = dual-photon absorptiometry. Note: The DPA technique usually provides greater BMD values than does the DEXA technique.

1994; Hagiwara et al., 1989; Laitinen et al., 1991; Luckey et al., 1989; Mazess et al., 1987; Nilas & Christiansen, 1988; Pocock et al., 1987; Recker, 1993; Ribot et al., 1988) suggest that it increases beyond the teen years, reaching its peak between the 3rd and 4th decades (Figure 4-8d). In most studies (Casez et al., 1994; Gallagher et al., 1987; Laitinen et al., 1991; Mazess & Barden, 1991; Mazess et al., 1987; Ribot et al., 1988), there is little difference in vertebral areal BMD across ages during the adult premenopausal years (Figure 4-8d). About one-third to one-fourth of the lifetime loss in vertebral areal BMD (from its peak) occurs during the premenopausal years (Gallagher et al., 1987; Hansson & Roos, 1986; Hagiwara et al., 1989).

Vertebral true volumetric BMD (determined by computed tomography) peaks in females during the latter part of the 2nd or early part of the 3rd decades (Figure 4-7) (Gilsanz et al., 1988a). Volumetric density remains fairly stable during most of the premenopausal period (Compston et al., 1988; Gilsanz et al., 1988a), begins to decrease during the immediate premenopausal period, and continues to decrease with increasing age throughout the postmenopausal years (Gilsanz et al., 1988a).

Peak lumbar spine areal BMD occurs for males during the 3rd decade (Cann et al., 1985; Geusens et al., 1986; Hagiwara et al., 1989) and may be slightly higher than, or not statistically different from, values for females 20–30 y of age (Cann et al., 1985; Compston et al., 1988; Geusens et al., 1986; Hagiwara et al., 1989). Several studies indicate that lumbar spine areal BMD diminishes linearly with age for males from the 2nd or 3rd through the 9th decades (Cann et al., 1985; Compston et al., 1988; Meier et al., 1984), whereas others indicate a linear reduction between the 3rd and 5th decades, with a plateau beyond the 6th decade (Blunt et al., 1994; Geusens et al., 1986; Nguyen et al., 1994). There is no apparent difference in vertebral trabecular true volumetric BMD (determined by computed tomography) between young adult males and premenopausal females of comparable age (Gilsanz et al., 1994a).

Premenopausal African-American females have higher total (Adams et al., 1992), radial (Nelson et al., 1988a; Prentice et al., 1991), femoral neck (Marcus et al., 1994), and lumbar spine (Liel et al., 1988; Luckey et al., 1989; Marcus et al., 1994) areal BMD than do Caucasian females of comparable ages. From its peak, the pattern of bone loss (at least for the radius) during the adult premenopausal period is similar for African-American and Caucasian females (Nelson et al., 1988a; Prentice et al., 1991). We are unaware of any published information on differences in BMD between African-American and Caucasian males.

Changes During Menopause

Numerous studies indicate an accelerated (compared to the premenopausal period) diminution in total body (Gallagher et al., 1987;

Gotfredsen et al., 1987; Wang et al., 1994), radial (Blunt et al., 1994; Genant et al., 1982; Luisetto et al., 1993; Ross et al., 1994; Sowers et al., 1991; Steiger et al., 1992; Talmage et al., 1986), femoral neck (Beck et al., 1993; Greenspan et al., 1994; Mazess et al., 1987; Nguyen et al., 1994; Ravn et al., 1994), and lumbar spine BMD (Buchanan et al., 1988a; Casez et al., 1994; Elders et al., 1989; Ettinger et al., 1987; Gallagher et al., 1987; Gilsanz et al., 1991; Hagiwara et al., 1989; Harris & Dawson-Hughes, 1992; Laitinen et al., 1991; Nilas & Christiansen, 1988; Pocock et al., 1987; Ribot et al., 1988) with the onset of menopause (Figure 4-9). However, some studies have failed to show an acceleration in bone loss in the transition from premenopause to menopause or during the first 10 y of menopause for radial (Harris & Dawson-Hughes, 1992; Prentice et al., 1991), femoral neck (Harris & Dawson-Hughes, 1992; Hreschyshyn et al., 1988; Marcus et al., 1994), and lumbar spine BMD (Lindquist et al., 1983).

Controversy exists regarding the timing of the onset of vertebral bone loss and the loss rates during the premenopausal and postmenopausal periods. Several studies suggest that vertebral BMD is lost from its peak premenopausal level at a constant linear rate of 0.38–1.2% per year, continuing into old age (Cann et al., 1985; Compston et al., 1988; Dawson-Hughes et al., 1987b; Hansson & Ross, 1986; Isaia et al., 1990; Riggs et al., 1986). Other studies, however, indicate that lumbar spine BMD is diminished at a slow, steady rate of 0.14–1.0% per year during the premenopausal years (Buchanan et al., 1988; Gallagher et al., 1987; Hagiwara et al., 1989; Luckey et al., 1989; Nilas & Christiansen, 1988; Pocock et al., 1987; Ribot et al., 1988; Rodin et al., 1990), with an accelerated rate of loss of 0.3–2.6% per year during menopause (Cann et al., 1985; Ettinger et al., 1987; Gallagher et al., 1987; Hagiwara et al., 1989; Harris & Dawson-Hughes, 1992; Laitinen et al., 1991; Nilas & Christiansen, 1988; Pocock et al., 1987; Ribot et al., 1988).

The relationship between years since menopause and rate of BMD loss has also been investigated. Loss rates for total body areal BMD are higher during the first 5–10 y following menopause than for later intervals (Gallagher et al., 1987; Gotfredsen et al., 1987; Wang et al., 1994), and there is an apparent increased loss rate for vertebral areal BMD during the immediate (first 1–3 y) postmenopausal period (Ettinger et al., 1987; Gallagher et al., 1987; Genant et al., 1982; Luisetto et al., 1993; Nilas & Christiansen, 1988), which is followed with a plateau or deceleration during the later years (Cann et al., 1988; Gallagher et al., 1987; Harris & Dawson-Hughes, 1992; Laitinen et al., 1991; Luisetto et al., 1993; Nilas & Christiansen, 1988; Ribot et al., 1988). The relationship between years since menopause and bone loss rates for radial BMD (Blunt et al., 1994; Genant et al., 1982; Harris & Dawson-Hughes, 1992; Luisetto et al., 1993; Prentice et al., 1991) and femoral neck BMD (Dawson-Hughes et al.,

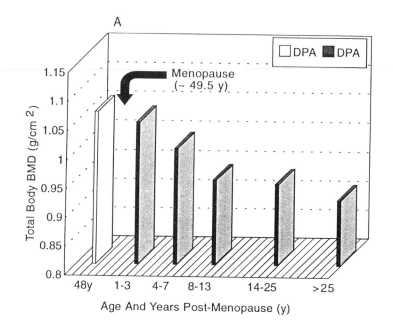

A

Total Body BMD (g/cm^2)

Menopause
(~ 49.5 y)

☐ DPA ■ DPA

48y 1-3 4-7 8-13 14-25 >25

Age And Years Post-Menopause (y)

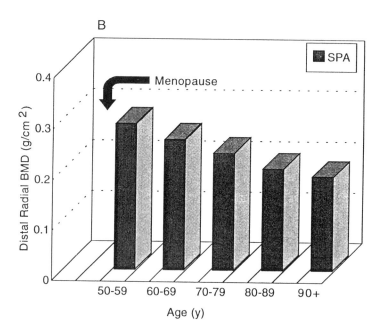

B

Distal Radial BMD (g/cm^2)

Menopause

■ SPA

50-59 60-69 70-79 80-89 90+

Age (y)

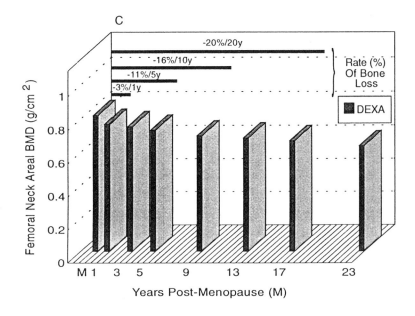

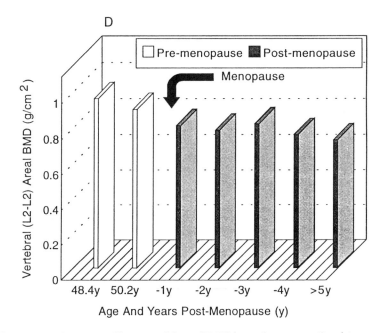

FIGURE 4-9. *Changes in areal bone mineral density (BMD) during the menopause.* Panel A was adapted from Gallagher et al. (1987), panel B from Blunt et al. (1994), panel C from Ravn et al. (1994), and panel D from Elders et al. (1989). DPA = dual-photon absorptiometry; SPA = single-photon absorptiometry; and DEXA = dual-energy x-ray absorptiometry. Note: The DPA technique usually provides greater BMD values than does the DEXA technique.

1987b; Harris & Dawson-Hughes, 1992; Marcus et al., 1994; Nguyen et al., 1994) are less clearly established and remain equivocal.

Postmenopausal radial bone loss trends are similar for African-American and Caucasian women (Nelson et al., 1988a; Prentice et al., 1991), but African-American women have higher radial areal BMD (Nelson et al., 1988a; Prentice et al., 1991), femoral neck areal and volumetric BMD (Marcus et al., 1994), and lumbar spine areal BMD (Luckey et al., 1989; Marcus et al., 1994) than do Caucasian females at comparable ages after menopause.

Lifetime Losses Of Bone Mineral Density

In males, total body and radial areal BMD decrease from their peaks at a constant rate of 0.10–0.35% per year into the 9th and 10th decades (Blunt et al., 1994; Compston et al., 1988; Geusens et al., 1986; Gotfredsen et al., 1987; Meier et al., 1984). Males lose a smaller proportion (5–6%) of their peak total and radial BMD over a comparable time period compared to females: 13–15% and 30% reductions in total body (Gallagher et al., 1987; Gotfredsen et al., 1987) and radial BMD (Prentice et al., 1991), respectively, by the 8th and 9th decades. Males also have higher radial BMD than do females at comparable ages beyond their respective peak levels (Blunt et al., 1994; Compston et al., 1988; Geusens et al., 1986; Kelly et al., 1990).

Femoral neck BMD decreases in males beyond 50 y of age at a constant rate of about 0.5–0.9% per year (Blunt et al., 1994; Hannan et al., 1992; Nguyen et al., 1994). Loss rates for females during the same part of the life span are similar to (Hannan et al., 1992) or greater than those for males (Beck et al., 1993; Dawson-Hughes et al., 1987b; Harris & Dawson-Hughes, 1992; Hreschyshyn et al., 1988; Mazess et al., 1987; Pocock et al., 1987; Ravn et al., 1994; Rodin et al., 1990; Steiger et al., 1992). About 30–35% of femoral neck peak BMD is lost in females by 80 y of age (Mazess et al., 1987; Pocock et al., 1987). There are no comparable data for males.

In males, lumbar spine areal BMD either decreases from its peak in a constant linear fashion (0.16–1.2% per year) into the 9th decade (Cann et al., 1985; Compston et al., 1988; Meier et al., 1984), or decreases only until the 6th decade, and then plateaus (Blunt et al., 1994; Geusens et al., 1986; Nguyen et al., 1994). Although there is considerable variability and overlap in the range of bone loss values between genders, males are generally thought to lose less spinal BMD than females (12–50% vs 16–37%) over the course of the adult life spans (Cann et al., 1985; Compston et al., 1988; Gallagher et al., 1987; Geusens et al., 1986; Hagiwara et al., 1989; Hansson & Roos, 1986). Beyond the 6th decade, males have higher lumbar spine areal BMD than do females (Blunt et al., 1994; Cann et al., 1985;

Compston et al., 1988; Geusens et al., 19886; Hagiwara et al., 1989; Nguyen et al., 1994).

No longitudinal absorptiometry or computed tomography studies of BMD bridge all stages of the life span. The patterns of BMD described in the previous section (Figures 4-4 to 4-9) were derived mostly from composites of cross-sectional or population studies and, in fewer instances, from longitudinal studies that covered abridged periods of the life span. Reliance on these types of data to infer longitudinal (life span) patterns for bone mineralization may be problematic (Kanis & Adami, 1994). Whereas the patterns of bone mineralization derived from cross-sectional and population studies probably provide a fairly accurate reflection of longitudinal trends, inferences regarding the magnitude and rates of change in BMD likely will be less accurate than inferences obtained from purely longitudinal studies.

Peak Bone Density

Peak bone density reflects the maximal lifetime amount of bone mineral accrued in individual bones and the whole skeleton. It is the consequence of net accretion of mineral due to growth during the childhood years and the balance between accretion and resorption rates in the immediate postgrowth period.

Insufficient peak bone mineral during the early adult years is considered an important risk factor for increased susceptibility to fractures and osteoporosis in females in later life (Mazess & Barden, 1991; Recker et al., 1992; Riggs & Melton, 1986). In this regard, a one standard deviation increase (+ 1 S.D.) in peak bone mass is associated with a reduction of more than 50% in fracture risk in old age (Cummings et al., 1993; Slemenda et al., 1994), and premenopausal peak bone mineral status has been estimated to account for two-thirds of the risk for fracture in later life (Horsman & Birchall, 1990; Horsman & Burkinshaw, 1989).

Controversy exists surrounding the precise timing of peak bone mass in females. Individuals and populations differ considerably in their hereditary predispositions and lifestyle behaviors (e.g., physical activity and diet) that are known to influence bone mineral accretion (Christian et al., 1989; Krall & Dawson-Hughes, 1993; Moller et al., 1978; Morrison et al., 1994; Pollitzer & Anderson, 1989; Smith et al., 1973; Teegarden & Weaver, 1994). Most likely, peak bone mass will occur when hereditary and lifestyle factors are temporally synchronized and operating at their optimal levels. The synchronization of these factors may occur at various times for different skeletal sites, individuals, and populations (Table 4-3).

Paradoxical Increase In Bone Density With Aging

Results from studies using single and dual photon absorptiometry, dual-energy x-ray absorptiometry, and computed tomography are all con-

TABLE 4-3. *Site variability in the attainment of peak BMD in females.*

Skeletal Site	Period of the Lifespan
Total BMD	Between the last part of the 2nd, and the mid-part of the 3rd decades
Distal Radial	Between the 4th and early part of the 5th decades
Femoral Neck BMD	Between late adolescence and the early part of the 4th decade
Lumbar Spine BMD	Between late adolescence and the 4th decade

sistent in describing a reduction in BMC and BMD in females at most skeletal sites with increasing age during adulthood. These techniques cannot distinguish qualitative differences between newly formed bone, which is incompletely mineralized, and older bone, which is fully and highly mineralized.

Density fractionation separates new from old bone and permits the determination of the proportions by weight of high- and low-density bone within a given tissue sample. This technique provides a qualitative measure of the micro density of isolated bone which, unlike the macro density measure derived from the other techniques, is not influenced by non-osseous space or changes in bone geometry. Density fractionation indicates that there is a general shift of both cortical and trabecular bone mineralization profiles of the femur toward higher densities with advancing age (Grynpas, 1993; Parfitt, 1993). In other words, femurs from the elderly have a greater proportion (by weight) of highly mineralized matrix compared to younger femurs, and there is shift toward greater proportions of highly mineralized bone with increasing age.

Whether a similar trend occurs at other sites besides the femur in humans, and whether this shift is linear throughout the adult life span remains to be determined. Variable age-related changes in activation frequency of osteonal remodelling may temporarily alter the linear progression of this shift at specific periods during the adult life span (Crofts et al., 1994; Frost, 1963). Nevertheless, it appears that there is a reduction in mineral mass or content of bone with aging, with a concomitant shift in the quality of the extant bone towards higher levels of mineralization.

REPRODUCTIVE ENDOCRINOLOGY, BONE MINERALIZATION, AND EXERCISE

Estrogen and perhaps progesterone appear to play essential roles in the development of bone mineral mass during puberty, in the optimization of peak BMD during late adolescence or early adulthood, and in the maintenance of skeletal integrity in menopausal and postmenopausal females. Estrogen, produced during both the follicular and luteal phases of the normal menstrual cycle, increases the efficiency of intestinal absorption of calcium (Ca^{2+}), decreases urinary Ca^{2+} loss (Heaney et al., 1978b, 1989), and suppresses the rate of bone remodelling (Heaney et al., 1978a). The effects of progesterone, released during the second half (luteal phase) of the normal menstrual cycle, are not as well understood. There is some evidence that progesterone decreases the rate of bone resorption because when administered to estrogen-deficient females, progesterone reduces urinary excretion of hydroxyproline, a marker of bone resorption (Friedman et al., 1993).

The effects of estrogen and progesterone on bone are most evident during puberty and adolescence and at the menopause. However, these reproductive hormones also have important modulating effects on bone metabolism during the premenopausal period when their production is adversely affected by dietary restriction and weight loss associated with extreme exercise (Carbon, 1992; Loucks & Horvath, 1985) and when exogenous hormones are administered for contraception or hormone replacement therapy. A summary of the effects of estrogen (E) and progesterone (P) on BMD at different stages of the life span is presented in Table 4-4.

Influences During Puberty And Adolescence

Puberty represents a crucial period for the development of peak bone mass; about 45–50% of adult peak total body bone mass is accrued during this period of rapid somatic growth and sexual maturation (Sentipal et al., 1991). Reproductive hormone secretion rates also increase dramatically in both genders during this transition period (Winter, 1978), and it is tempting to infer a causal relationship between changes in reproductive hormone status and bone mineral accretion at this time.

TABLE 4-4. *Effects of estrogen (E) and progesterone (P) on BMD.*

- Prepuberty
  —Large increases in BMD in absence of significant E & P
- Puberty
  —Rapid increases in BMD with increases in E & P
  —Greatest rates of increase 1st 2 years after menarche
- Adolescence and Early Adulthood
  —Reduced BMD associated with eating disorders
  —Reduced BMD associated with irregular menses
  —Reduction in BMD associated with age at onset, duration and severity of menstrual dysfunction
  —Equivocal relationship between E and BMD in athletes without eating disorders
  —Positive effect on BMD with exogenous E
- Peri- and Post-Menopause
  —Reduced BMD with reduction in E & P
  —Increased or maintained BMD with exogenous E & P
  —E & P most effective in immediate post-menopause period

Developmental Considerations. Only a few studies have investigated concurrent changes in bone mineral and in reproductive hormone secretion across the circumpubertal period. In boys, increasing serum testosterone is associated with increased forearm BMC (Krabbe et al., 1979; 1984). In girls, urinary estrogen has been reported (Lloyd et al., 1992) to be positively correlated with total body BMC and BMD during the immediate premenarcheal stages of puberty (Tanner stages I-III), and plasma estradiol was a significant contributor to the variance in lumbar spine BMD in adolescent female runners (Baer et al., 1992).

Despite the statistical significance of these associations, the relationship between reproductive hormones and bone mineral status was fairly weak, and other studies (Blimkie et al., 1992; Rice et al., 1993) have failed to detect such relationships in menarcheal adolescent girls. To our knowledge, there are no studies of the association between reproductive hormone status and bone mineral that span the pubertal period. Correlative studies of this kind suggest, but cannot confirm, that bone mass development during puberty is dependent on reproductive hormone status.

Effects Of Menstrual Cycle Dysfunction. Adolescent females with anorexia nervosa and primary or secondary amenorrhea typically exhibit lower BMD (Bachrach et al., 1990; Young et al., 1994) and lower metacarpal cortical thickness (Ayers et al., 1984) than healthy age-matched controls. There is a strong negative relationship between duration of anorexia nervosa and bone density in adolescent females (Bachrach et al., 1990) and a positive relationship between the age at onset of menstrual dysfunction during adolescence and reduced BMD in young anoretic adults (Biller et al., 1989; Seeman et al., 1992). The use of estrogen-containing oral contraceptives during adolescence appears to offer some protection against bone mineral loss in females with anorexia nervosa (Seeman et al., 1992).

Reproductive hormone status was not assessed directly in most studies involving adolescent females; based on prior studies of young oligomenorrheic and amenorrheic adults, this status was assumed to be lower than normal (Baer et al., 1992; Lloyd et al., 1988; Snead et al., 1992). This may not be a valid assumption, however, because a number of studies (Ayers et al., 1984; Biller et al., 1989) failed to find suppressed estradiol levels in adolescent females with anorexia nervosa.

Exercise And Menstrual Cycle Dysfunction. Baer et al. (1992) reported no significant difference in vertebral BMD between amenorrheic athletes with suppressed serum estradiol and eumenorrheic runners with normal estradiol levels. A more recent study (Young et al., 1994) reported normal or slightly higher than normal BMD in weight-bearing regions of the skeleton, but reduced BMD at non-weight-bearing sites in adolescent female ballet dancers who had a high prevalence of menstrual dysfunction. One study failed to find any relationship between level of habitual physical activity and bone mineral in oligomenorrheic and amenorrheic adolescent girls with reduced bone mineral (Bachrach et al., 1990). Although by no means unanimous, these studies suggest that reproductive hormone deficiency during menstrual dysfunction in adolescent girls is associated with reduced bone mineral and that intense training, but perhaps not habitual activity, may provide some protection against bone mineral loss. This is particularly true for weight-bearing sites, even in the presence of lower than normal reproductive hormone levels.

Influences In Premenopausal Adult Females: Exercise, Menstrual Cycle Dysfunction, And Exogenous Hormones

An interruption in menses, a decreased level of estrogen and progesterone production, and decreased bone mass may occur in young adult females in response to extremes of exercise training (Drinkwater et al., 1984). Bone mineral density is reduced at most sites in amenorrheic, compared with eumenorrheic, adult athletes (Drinkwater et al., 1984), and positive correlations have been reported between serum estradiol levels and BMD in young amenorrheic runners (Buchanan et al., 1988; Snead et al., 1992) but not in non-athletic females with anorexia nervosa (Treasure et al., 1987). Additionally, bone density in young collegiate female athletes is also negatively correlated with severity of menstrual dysfunction, measured as the number of missed menses during adolescence (Lloyd et al., 1988).

The positive effects of certain types of weight-bearing exercise may wholly or partially offset the negative effects of amenorrhea on bone, allowing amenorrheic athletes to attain BMD measurements similar to or greater than those of sedentary counterparts. Whole body BMC and BMD were maintained in amenorrheic runners and figure skaters when compared to eumenorrheic sedentary individuals (Myerson et al., 1992; Slemenda & Johnston, 1993). Likewise, young adult female gymnasts with a high prevalence of menstrual dysfunction had higher whole body, lumbar spine, and femoral neck BMD than did controls and age-matched runners (Robinson et al., 1995). However, several studies have reported significant reductions in lumbar spine (Marcus et al., 1985; Snead et al., 1992) and femoral mid-shaft (Myburgh et al., 1993) BMD in amenorrheic runners versus sedentary controls. From these studies, it could be hypothesized that BMD is maintained or increased at weight-bearing appendicular and axial sites, especially when activity is of a high-impact nature, and that general weight-bearing activity, including running, may not be sufficient to protect BMD at axial or appendicular sites.

To date, only two prospective studies have investigated the effects of intense training on menstrual cycle function and reproductive hormone status. Both studies found disturbances in the luteal phase of the menstrual cycle as a result of intense training (Bullen et al., 1985; Prior et al., 1990). In the study of Prior et al. (1990) changes in spinal trabecular BMD seemed to be related to changes in plasma progesterone levels. Luteal phase index (the proportion of the cycle in the luteal phase) accounted for a significant proportion (24%) of the variance in BMD changes. Thus, it seems that adequate levels of progesterone are important for maintenance of BMD, at least in the early stages of training.

The relative effects of exercise-induced changes in estrogen and progesterone on BMD cannot really be separated because there is an interaction between the two hormones; the rise in progesterone during the luteal phase is dependent on the estrogen-stimulated luteinizing hormone surge during the latter part of the follicular phase. From the above studies, however, it appears that decreases in both estrogen and progesterone production with overly intense training may result in reductions in BMD in young adult females.

The effect of exogenous hormones on BMD in premenopausal women has not been extensively studied. Recker et al. (1992) followed BMD changes in 156 females (average age 21.4 y) for up to 5 y and found that total body BMD gain was positively associated with use of oral contraceptives, independent of the effects of physical activity and Ca^{2+} intake. More recently, Haenggi et al. (1994) reported small but significant increases in lumbar spine BMD (0.2-2.9%) in 15 young women with long standing amenorrhea who were on estrogen replacement for 12-24 mo. Thus, it seems that exogenous reproductive hormones may enhance peak BMD in young adult females with a history of menstrual dysfunction.

Influences In Perimenopausal Females: Oral Contraceptive Use

In a cross-sectional study of 939 perimenopausal women (average age of 53.4 y), Tupparainen et al. (1994) found that past oral contraceptive users had a slightly higher (1%) BMD of the lumbar spine than the nonusers. However, when the analysis was restricted to only the 387 premenopausal women or to the 1427 women not receiving hormone replacement therapy, there were no differences between contraceptive users and non-users. This cross-sectional study does not clearly indicate whether contraceptive use during either the premenopausal or perimenopausal period had a beneficial effect on BMD during the perimenopausal years.

A single longitudinal trial has provided stronger proof of the beneficial effects of short-term oral contraceptive use on BMD during the perimenopausal period. Gambacciani et al. (1994) studied 30 eumenorrheic and 60 oligomenorrheic perimenopausal women; the oligomenorrheic women were randomly assigned to receive oral contraceptives or Ca^{2+} supplement. Over 2 y, there were no changes in BMD in the eumenorrheic group, whereas lumbar spine BMD decreased by 2.1% in the oligomenor-rheic subjects receiving Ca^{2+} and increased by 1.3% in the oligomenorrheic group receiving oral contraceptives. It appears from this study that exogenous reproductive hormones increase BMD in perimenopausal women with menstrual dysfunction.

Influences During Menopause And Old Age: Hormone Replacement Therapy And Fracture Rates

To determine the long-term effects of estrogen-replacement therapy on BMD, Felson et al. (1993) compared well-matched groups of estrogen-treated and non-treated postmenopausal women. Lumbar spine, proximal femur, mid-radial, and distal radial BMD were higher by an average of 11.2% in females less than 75 y of age who received estrogen-replacement therapy for $\geq$ 7 y. Females older than 75 y who had a similar duration of estrogen-replacement therapy had an average BMD level that was only 3.2% greater than that for non-treated women. It appears from this study that estrogen-replacement therapy can have a powerful protective effect against bone loss if begun immediately after menopause and continued for at least 7 y.

Longitudinal, double-blind, placebo-controlled trials have convincingly demonstrated the beneficial effects of hormone-replacement therapy on BMD during the postmenopausal period. Bone mineral density of the lumbar spine, proximal femur, radius and whole body increased annually by approximately 5%, 3%, 1.5%, and 4%, respectively, in early postmeno-pausal (Lufkin et al., 1992; Riis et al., 1987) and older osteoporotic women (Christiansen & Riis, 1990; Lindsay & Tohme, 1990) treated with estro-gen or estrogen-progesterone combinations, whereas BMD decreased consistently at most sites in the placebo control group.

The interaction between hormone replacement and exercise on BMD in this population is equivocal. In one study (Heikkinen et al., 1991), bone-loading exercise failed to increase lumbar spine and femoral neck BMD in postmenopausal women beyond the increase due to hormone treatment (combined estrogen and progesterone) alone, over a 1-y period. In another study (Ballard et al., 1988), however, the reduction in radial BMD was more attenuated over a 1-y period by combined exercise and estrogen therapy than by exercise or estrogen intervention separately in postmeno-pausal women.

A cross-sectional study of a large population of postmenopausal women indicated a higher proportion of fractures of the hip and forearm in women not on hormone replacement therapy compared to those on es-trogen therapy (Weiss et al., 1980). Additionally, one long-term prospec-tive trial demonstrated a reduced risk of vertebral fracture over 12 y in women on estrogen replacement therapy compared to placebo-treated, postmenopausal, osteoporotic women who had established vertebral fractures (Riggs et al., 1982). It appears that estrogen replacement therapy reduces both bone loss and risk of osteoporotic fracture at the three most clinically relevant and susceptible bone sites (proximal femur, lumbar spine, and distal radius) in postmenopausal women.

CALCIUM INTAKE AND BONE MINERALIZATION

Nutrition is one of several lifestyle factors that is considered to play an important role in the development and retention of bone mineral throughout the life span. The role of general nutrition on bone mineralization in both health and disease has been extensively reviewed (Angus et al., 1988; Avioli & Heaney, 1991; Bronner, 1994; Clarkson & Haymes, 1995; Cumming, 1990; Heaney, 1988, 1991; Kanis, 1991b; McCulloch & Bailey, 1990). This section will focus solely on the influence of calcium intake on BMD across the life span in otherwise healthy women.

Calcium Intake During Childhood

The importance of nutrition during childhood on bone mineral development has been derived from several different research approaches, e.g., retrospective studies of bone mineral in young adults with different nutritional histories during their childhood years; comparative studies of bone mineral between adequately nourished and malnourished groups of children; correlative studies of nutritional status and bone mineral at different stages during childhood; and controlled intervention studies in which the effects of nutritional supplementation on bone mineral are examined prospectively at different stages of development during childhood.

Retrospective, Group Comparison, And Correlative Studies.

Results from retrospective studies of childhood calcium intake and bone mineral status during adulthood are equivocal. Several of these studies have reported positive correlations between childhood intake of calcium in milk and adult bone density (Garn, 1970; Odland et al., 1972; Sandler et al., 1985), whereas a more recent study found no correlation between calcium intake during adolescence and bone mass or density in adult females (Welten et al., 1994). In the latter study, however, there was a nonsignificant trend towards higher lumbar spine bone density in the female group with relatively high calcium intakes during the adolescent years, compared to the low intake group (Welten et al., 1994).

Studies of children and adolescents (Henderson & Hayes, 1994; Lee et al., 1993) with varying dietary calcium intakes and normal reproductive hormone status provide strong support for the hypothesis that nutritional status may have an independent effect on bone mineral development during the formative growth years. Radial BMC was reported to be greater in Chinese children aged 5 y who were raised in a region with relatively high calcium intake, compared to children from a low-intake region (Lee et al., 1993), and higher in North American children (2–16 y) whose calcium intake exceeded 1000 mg daily, compared to those with a lower intake (Chan, 1991). In a more recent study of children (5–14 y) (Henderson & Hayes, 1994), femoral neck and lumbar spine bone density increased serially across calcium intake quartile groups. Another study of Finnish children (6–19 y), however, failed to find any difference in femoral neck or lumbar spine BMD across quartiles of daily calcium intake (Kroger et al., 1992).

Results of cross-sectional correlative studies are generally equivocal. Positive correlations have been reported between dietary calcium and BMD at the spine (Grimston et al., 1992; Sentipal et al., 1991), femur (Grimston et al., 1991b; Henderson & Hayes, 1994; Turner et al., 1992), and the radius (Chan, 1991; Rubin et al., 1993). An equally large number of studies, however, failed to demonstrate significant correlations between calcium intake and BMD at the spine (Bachrach et al., 1990; Glastre et al., 1990; Katzman et al., 1991; Kroger et al., 1992, 1993; Rubin et al., 1993; Turner et al., 1992), femur (Katzman et al., 1991; Kroger et al., 1992, 1993), radius (Bachrach et al., 1990; Katzman et al., 1991), or whole body sites (Bachrach et al., 1990; Katzman et al., 1991) in young females.

Supplementation Studies. The strongest evidence in support of the importance of calcium for bone mineral development during childhood comes from prospective studies of calcium supplementation and bone mineral. The effects of calcium supplementation on BMD at various stages of the life span, including childhood, are summarized in Table 4-5.

Supplementation (718 mg daily of calcium malate) over the course of 3 y resulted in significant increases in mid-shaft radial (5.1%) and lumbar

TABLE 4-5. *Calcium supplementation and BMD in females.*

- Prepuberty
  —Significant increases in BMD at most sites
  —Positive effects with calcium malate and carbonate
- Early Puberty
  —Significant increases in BMD at most sites
  —Positive effect with calcium citrate
- Mid-Puberty—Adolescence
  —No significant effect on BMD, but a positive trend
  —Unsuccessful with calcium malate, carbonate and milk
- Early-Mid-Adulthood
  —Equivocal effects: no effect, maintenance effect, or small increase
  —Dairy products, natural foods, or calcium citrate tablets
- Peri- & Post-Menopausal
  —Equivocal effects on BMD: small increases or attenuation of losses
  —Effectiveness may be dependent on estrogen status

spine BMD (2.8%), as well as a trend toward significant increases in Ward's triangle (2.9%) and the greater trochanter (3.5%) in prepubescent identical twin boys and girls (Johnston et al., 1992). The effects of supplementation, however, were impermanent because BMD at all sites was not different from placebo controls 3 y after discontinuation of the supplementation protocol (Slemenda et al., 1993; Slemenda, personal communication).

Calcium supplementation of 300 mg daily of calcium carbonate for a period of 18 mo increased radial BMC (2.5%) and density (3.14%) in 7-year-old Chinese children with habitually low (280 mg daily) calcium intakes (Warren et al., 1994). Another study of initially premenarcheal girls reported greater increases in lumbar spine BMC (4.7%), lumbar spine BMD (2.9%), and total body BMD (1.3 %) in subjects taking calcium supplements (354 mg daily of calcium citrate malate) compared to a placebo control group over a period of 18 mo (Lloyd et al., 1993).

The effects of calcium supplementation on bone mineral during adolescence are less clear. In the study of Johnston et al. (1992), supplementation of 718 mg daily of calcium malate for 3 y had no significant effect on any of the measures of bone mineral in subjects who went through puberty or were postpubertal during the course of the study. Similarly, 2 y of calcium supplementation (an additional 890 mg daily) from milk or calcium carbonate tablets failed to result in any significant increase in radial or lumbar spine BMD in postmenarcheal adolescent females, compared to controls with a low calcium intake (Matkovic et al., 1990). Although the differences between supplemented and control groups in this study were not significant, there was a trend toward a more pronounced increase in bone mineral in the supplemented compared to the control group (Matkovic et al., 1990).

The lack of a significant effect of calcium supplementation in postmenarcheal girls in the studies of Johnston et al., (1992) and Matkovic et al. (1990) suggest that higher levels of supplementation might be required to alter bone mineral during this stage of development. In this regard, Matkovic et al. (1990) demonstrated that calcium accretion had not been saturated in adolescent girls even with a high intake of 1600 mg daily. Based on recent information about calcium absorption efficiencies, calcium retention requirements, and daily obligatory calcium losses, Heaney (1991) has proposed recommended daily allowances (RDA) for calcium of 800 mg and 1400–1600 mg, respectively, for children (up to 10–12 y of age) and adolescents.

Calcium Intake During Adulthood

Calcium balance studies (Heaney et al., 1977, 1978b) indicate that the majority of both pre-and postmenopausal women are in a negative Ca^{2+} balance (Ca^{2+} excretion is greater than dietary intake). The Ca^{2+} intake required to produce a balance of zero was estimated to be 990 mg/d in premenopausal and 1500 mg/d in postmenopausal women, values that exceed the current Recommended Nutrient Intakes. This implies that over a lifetime, Ca^{2+} deficiency may lead to a gradual decrease in BMD, with an accelerated loss at menopause.

Young And Middle-Aged Premenopausal Women. Multiple regression analyses indicate that current Ca^{2+} intake has either relatively small or nonsignificant effects on BMD in young to middle-aged women. Intake of Ca^{2+} accounts for small amounts (5–20%) of the variation in BMD of the radius (Metz et al., 1993), lumbar spine (Krall & Dawson-Hughes, 1993; Ramsdale et al., 1994), and proximal femur (Ramsdale et al., 1994) in some studies, but has failed to predict BMD at these sites in others (Krall & Dawson-Hughes, 1993; Mazess & Barden, 1991).

Cross-sectional studies have been more successful at demonstrating differences in BMD among groups with varied dietary Ca^{2+} intakes; groups with high Ca^{2+} intakes have greater BMD at the femoral neck (Mazess & Barden, 1991), radius, and lumbar spine (Kanders et al., 1988) than do groups with low intake. Additionally, there appears to be a threshold level of Ca^{2+} intake of about 800–1000 mg/d, above which there are no increases in BMD. This corresponds nicely to the value which Heaney et al. (1977) estimated to be required to produce a Ca^{2+} balance of zero. Thus, while results from multiple regression analyses suggest that Ca^{2+} intake contributes little to BMD of premenopausal women with adequate dietary calcium intake, women with very low intake may have a deficit in BMD.

In contrast to cross-sectional and regression studies, longitudinal studies of young to middle-aged females have found beneficial effects of increased Ca^{2+} intake on BMD, even in those with average initial intakes close to the recommended levels. Recker et al. (1992) followed 156 young women (average age of 21.4 y) for a period of 3.4 y, measuring dietary habits by 7-d food intake diaries, repeated over approximately 7 visits. Average Ca^{2+} intake was 781 mg/d, close to the Recommended Nutrient Intake. Bivariate and multiple regression analyses, using age, activity level, and Ca^{2+} intake as independent variables, showed that changes in Ca^{2+} intake accounted for a significant, although small, proportion of the change in lumbar spine BMD. With activity level held constant, BMD increased with increased Ca^{2+} intake up to 2100 mg/d. In contrast to the cross-sectional studies described earlier, there was no apparent Ca^{2+} intake threshold at which bone mass ceased to increase.

Likewise, Baran et al. (1989) found beneficial effects of 3 y of calcium supplementation on BMD in a group of slightly older women (aged 30–42 y). Twenty women who had an initial Ca^{2+} intake of about 900 mg/d were randomized to a treatment group and increased their Ca^{2+} intake by ~610 mg/d through increased consumption of dairy products, or to a nonsupplemented control group. The control group had a greater loss of lumbar spine BMD than did the supplemented group over the 3-y period (−2.9% vs 0.4%).

Not all intervention studies have demonstrated positive effects of calcium supplementation in this age group. In a recent study (Friedlander et al., 1995), there was no difference in BMD after 2 y of follow-up between groups of young (20–35 y), relatively inactive females who were on a combined stretching and calcium supplementation program (400–1200 mg/d from calcium-citrate tablets in combination with dietary calcium to bring individual levels up to 1500 mg/d), compared to controls who received a placebo and participated in an identical stretching program. As indicated earlier, skeletal mass reaches its peak in the latter part of the 2nd or during the 3rd decade. Additional randomized, placebo-controlled, calcium intervention studies are required to determine whether supplementation during this period is effective at increasing peak bone mass and density of young adult females.

Few studies have examined the relative effectiveness of calcium supplementation, compared to exercise, on BMD in healthy adult premenopausal women. In a recent randomized, double blind study (Friedlander et al., 1995), daily calcium supplementation alone (up to 1500 mg/d from calcium citrate tablets and dietary intake) or in combination with exercise did not add any significant benefit to BMD beyond that achieved solely by an exercise program of combined aerobics and weight training, in women 20–35 y of age. Additional studies incorporating diverse types and intensities of exercise in combination with different calcium supplementation regimens are required before the relative effectiveness of calcium supplementation and exercise intervention on BMD in this population is clearly established.

Perimenopausal Women. The effects of calcium supplementation on BMD of perimenopausal women are equivocal. Elders et al. (1991) conducted a 2-y longitudinal study of a large group (n = 300) of women 46–55 y of age, with an average Ca^{2+} intake of 1150 mg/d. Subjects were randomized to a control group, a group receiving a 1000 mg Ca^{2+} supplement daily, and a group receiving a 2000 mg Ca^{2+} supplement daily. After 2 y, lumbar spine BMD was diminished in all groups; however, the losses were smaller in the treatment groups (1.3% and 0.7% decreases in the 1000 and 2000 mg Ca^{2+}/d groups, respectively) compared to the control group (loss of 3.5%). Differences between the treatment groups were not significant. The results from this study suggest that Ca^{2+} supplementation can reduce BMD loss during the perimenopausal period, even in women with a relatively high initial calcium intake.

Several other studies suggest that calcium supplementation alone may not be effective in increasing BMD in perimenopausal women. Heaney et al. (1978b) demonstrated that estrogen replacement was required before postmenopausal women could achieve improved Ca^{2+} balance with increased Ca^{2+} intake. Likewise, Gambacciani et al. (1994) found that oligomenorrheic perimenopausal women randomized to treatment with estrogen (as an oral contraceptive) increased lumbar spine BMD by 1.3% over 2 y, whereas a group receiving a Ca^{2+} supplement (500 mg/d) had a 2.1% loss. Thus, although Ca^{2+} supplementation alone may be effective in some cases, estrogen replacement seems to be the preferred therapy for arresting bone loss in perimenopausal women.

Postmenopausal Women. Life-time Ca^{2+} intake, rather than current Ca^{2+} intake, seems to be important in influencing the BMD of postmenopausal women. Sandler et al. (1985) studied 255 postmenopausal women (aged 49–66 y) and found that those who reported drinking milk with every meal during childhood had a 2% greater radial BMD than those who drank milk less frequently; current Ca^{2+} intake did not correlate with BMD in this study. A similar association appears to exist between lifetime calcium intake and fracture rate. Cooper et al. (1988) found that current Ca^{2+} intake failed to predict fracture rate of the proximal femur, whereas Matkovic et al. (1979) found that fracture rate was reduced in regions of Yugoslavia with a high childhood and lifetime Ca^{2+} intake.

In one study (Riggs et al., 1982), long-term (12 y) Ca^{2+} supplementation in postmenopausal osteoporotic women reduced fracture rate by one half, compared to a placebo group. Contrary to the previous studies, the latter study suggests that long-term calcium supplementation during the postmenopausal period may be effective at reducing fracture rates in postmenopausal women.

Longitudinal, randomized Ca^{2+} intervention trials, in which treatment and control groups were matched and not taking exogenous estrogen, have shown small positive effects of supplementation on BMD at the whole body, proximal femur (Aloia et al., 1994), lumbar spine (Reid et al., 1993), and distal radius (Dawson-Hughes et al., 1990). Dawson-Hughes et al. (1990) found that supplementation was of greatest benefit during late menopause in women with low initial Ca^{2+} intake. The negative effects of rapid decreases in estrogen production early in menopause most likely obscured the effects of the relatively small dose of Ca^{2+} supplementation (500 mg/d) given to the early postmenopausal subjects. With a higher supplementation dose, Aloia et al. (1994) demonstrated positive effects in their early postmenopausal women. From these results, it may be recommended that supplemental doses of at least 1200 mg/d are needed for BMD maintenance during early menopause.

Combined estrogen replacement therapy and calcium supplementation seem to provide the best protection against bone loss during the postmenopausal period. Riis et al. (1987) compared the two modes of therapy and found that early postmenopausal women randomized to estrogen-replacement therapy maintained BMD at the forearm, lumbar spine, and whole body, whereas Ca^{2+} supplementation (2000 mg/d) prevented loss of BMD only at the forearm. Lumbar spine and whole body BMD diminished by 4–8% in the Ca^{2+} supplemented and control groups. These results suggest that regions of high cortical bone composition, such as the forearm, may be most sensitive to calcium supplementation (Seeman, 1994) in this age group and that estrogen replacement therapy provides a stronger and more general bone mineral sparing effect in postmenopausal women than does Ca^{2+} supplementation.

Old Age. The effects of Ca^{2+} supplementation on BMD during old age are equivocal. Andon et al. (1991) reported that older women (aged 64.7 y) with low Ca^{2+} intake (402 mg/d) had lower lumbar spine BMD than did those with a higher intake (878 mg/d). The Ca^{2+} intake was a significant predictor of BMD, although it accounted for only 3.6% of the variance. Positive effects of calcium were found in several prospective studies. In one study (Smith et al., 1981), calcium supplementation increased radial BMD in a group of elderly women (mean of 81 y) over a 36-mo period. In another study (Dawson-Hughes et al., 1987a), women (40–70 y old) were separated into groups with low (<405 mg/d) and high (>777 mg/d) Ca^{2+} intake and followed for 7 mo. The low-intake group lost lumbar spine BMD at a rate of 4.8% per year, while BMD increased in the high intake group by 2.5% per year (Dawson-Hughes et al., 1987a). In contrast to these studies, Riggs et al. (1987) found no relationship between Ca^{2+} intake and changes in lumbar spine or radial BMD in 106 women (aged 73–84 y) followed over 4 y. There are few studies of the relative effectiveness of calcium supplementation versus exercise on BMD in this population. In the study of Smith et al. (1981), elderly postmenopausal women who took part in an exercise program demonstrated larger increases in radial BMD than did a calcium-supplemented group (2.29% vs 1.58%) over a period of 36 mo. A combination of exercise and calcium was less effective than either exercise or calcium alone and failed to prevent a loss in BMD in this study.

Considerations in Interpreting Correlational and Supplementation Studies

As is evident from the preceding section, there is considerable controversy regarding the importance of dietary calcium for bone mineral accretion. There are numerous possible explanations for these apparent discrepant results, and several of these have been eloquently presented in a recent editorial (Avioli & Heaney, 1991). Because dietary calcium is only one of a number of factors that might influence bone mineral development, it is likely that correlations will be constrained and of a low order of magnitude. With small sample sizes, statistical power may be inadequate to detect these weak correlations. Nutrient intakes, including calcium, also vary widely from one population to another, and it is possible that the importance of calcium will vary accordingly with the degree of current and historical nutritional adequacy. Moreover, the relative importance of dietary calcium may vary during different stages of the life span in relation to the adequacy and level of other determinants of bone mineral, such as physical activity and levels of circulating reproductive hormones.

There also appears to be a threshold effect between calcium intake and calcium balance (Matkovic & Heaney, 1992), both during childhood and adolescence, so associations between calcium intake and bone mineral during childhood may only be detectable in studies in which calcium intake is below this threshold level. Additionally, current levels of calcium intake are poorly correlated with past dietary history, so generalizations about prior calcium intakes and BMD based on current dietary status are tenuous at best.

Furthermore, calcium balance is influenced not only by intake but also by absorption efficiency and excretory loss. There may be higher absorption efficiencies for the same calcium intake in males compared to females and lower urinary calcium loss in black compared to white children (Bell et al., 1993). The results from the study by Bell and colleagues suggest that differences in calcium absorption efficiency and urinary loss, rather than differences in calcium intake, are responsible for gender and racial differences in bone mineral that are evident during childhood. Clearly, conclusions about the importance of calcium for bone mineral development based solely on studies that measured calcium intakes must be made cautiously.

Lastly, there is considerable variability in the absolute amount, elemental composition (proportion by weight), and bioavailability (absorption efficiency) of calcium in various foods and supplements (Aloia, 1989). These differences must also be considered when comparing and interpreting results of correlative and supplementation studies involving calcium.

PHYSICAL ACTIVITY AND BONE MINERALIZATION

Immobilization imposed by long-term bed rest causes a marked loss of bone (LeBlanc et al., 1990). Frost (1987a, 1987b, 1988) proposed that in the absence of weight-bearing activity, bone resorption is favored over formation in the remodelling cycle. With mechanical stimulation, remodelling is uncoupled, and bone formation is stimulated, resulting in an increase in bone mass until it has adjusted to the increased loads.

In response to mechanically induced strain, osteocytes located throughout the bone matrix may synthesize proliferation or differentiation factors, which, when released, could directly affect osteoblasts responsible for bone formation (El Haj et al., 1990). Thus, lack of exercise increases bone resorption, and increased exercise supposedly increases bone formation (Frost, 1991).

Physical Activity During Childhood

Until recently, the effect of physical activity on BMD was studied mostly in adults. There are several excellent reviews of this topic (Bailey & McCulloch, 1990; Chilibeck et al., 1995; Drinkwater, 1990; Forwood & Burr, 1993; Gutin & Kasper, 1992; Marcus et al., 1992; Snow-Harter and Marcus, 1991; Wolman, 1990). With the realization that peak bone mass and density may occur sometime during late adolescence or early adulthood, attention has recently been directed towards investigating the importance of physical activity on BMD during the childhood and adolescent years. This topic has also been thoroughly reviewed (Bailey, 1995; Bailey & Martin, 1994; Loucks, 1988).

General Physical Activity. Turner et al. (1992) found that physical activity was associated with increased BMD of the hip in high school girls (16.4 y). Physical activity measured as a continuous variable of energy expenditure (kcal/d) was a significant contributor to variance in axial (lumbar spine), but not appendicular (radius), BMD in white children (6–18 y), after correcting for the influence of weight and pubertal status (Rubin et al., 1993). Femoral neck BMD was also greater in the most-active compared to the moderate- and least-active Finnish children (6–19 y), after adjusting for differences in age, height, and body weight (Kroger et al., 1992). Lumbar spine BMD followed the same trend, but failed to reach significance. Authors of this latter study concluded that children with higher BMD were more likely to be physically active, owing partially to their more robust body sizes.

Another study reported higher radial, femoral, and spinal BMD in active compared to inactive monozygotic twins (5–14 y), after adjusting for age and gender influences (Slemenda et al., 1991b). Authors of this study concluded that, depending on the specific skeletal site, an active child could emerge from adolescence with 5–10% higher BMD than an inactive child. In a follow-up study, weight-bearing physical activity was a significant predictor of bone mineral in prepubertal, but not pubertal, children (Slemenda et al., 1994).

Not all studies have demonstrated positive effects of physical activity on BMD during childhood. Southard et al., (1991) failed to find any effect of physical activity on bone mineral in healthy young children after making adjustments for pubertal status and body weight, and physical activity was not a significant predictor of total body or lumbar spine BMD in healthy postmenarcheal adolescent girls (Rice et al., 1993). After adjusting for the effects of bone size, Kroger et al. (1993) failed to find any significant relationships between physical activity and apparent BMD of the lumbar spine and femoral neck in children and adolescents 13–17 y old. Physical activity was not correlated with lumbar spine, radial, or femoral BMD in prepubertal and pubertal girls (Katzman et al., 1991), and weight-bearing physical activity between 13 and 27 y of age was not a significant predictor of lumbar spine BMD in Dutch females, although it was significant for males (Welten et al., 1994).

Weight-Bearing Activity. Children with recent (within the past 2.3 y) uncomplicated fractures of either the femur or tibia had lower BMD at the hip on the affected compared to non-affected side (Henderson et al., 1992). The larger the BMD deficit, the longer the period of immobilization. Additionally, Bailey et al. (1995) found lower BMD at the affected compared to the contralateral unaffected hip in children with Legg-Calve-Perthes disease. Results from these studies demonstrate the importance of continued weight-bearing activity for the maintenance of normal skeletal mineralization during childhood.

Several studies have concluded that weight-bearing activity during childhood and adolescence will lead to greater than normal bone densities. McCulloch et al. (1992) compared the BMD of adolescent (13–17 y) soccer players (weight-bearing activity) with age- and weight-matched swimmers (weight-supported activity) and sedentary controls. There was a trend towards greater BMD in the os calcis, a weight-supporting bone in the foot, in soccer players, compared to the controls and swimmers. There were no group differences in BMD of the distal radius, a non-weight-bearing bone. Calcaneal BMD (measured by computed tomography) was also higher in varsity volleyball and basketball players who had participated in their sports throughout high school, compared to varsity swimmers (Risser et al., 1990).

The effects of intense weight-bearing activity on BMD of elite, late adolescent (17 y), female ballet dancers was recently studied by Young et al. (1994). Dancers practiced more than 32 h/wk, and many had irregular menses. It was concluded that BMD at weight-bearing sites was positively affected by training, despite the occurrence of oligomenorrhea and reduced body weight; also, the higher density in the lower limbs of the dancers may have resulted from several years of practice and increased accumulation of bone during the prepubertal years. Results from this study suggest that cortical bone may be more responsive to weight-bearing mechanical loads than is more centrally located (within the medullary cavity) trabecular bone because muscle tendons insert into cortical bone.

Slemenda and Johnston (1993) studied the site-specific effects of weight-bearing activity on bone mineral in female figure skaters aged 10–23 y. Skaters (40% with menstrual dysfunction) trained 25–40 h/wk and were compared to sedentary, eumenorrheic girls of the same age. There were no differences in age- and weight-adjusted upper-body bone densities between groups, but mean densities of the skaters' leg and pelvic bones were greater by 5.5% and 11%, respectively, suggesting a site-specific effect of training. The authors concluded that the powerful jumping actions in figure skating served as a potent-mechanical stimulus to enhance lower-body BMD. Differences in BMD between skaters and controls in this study were not evident until the mid-teens. The apparent ineffectiveness of this specific type of weight-bearing activity on BMD for the pre-teens, however, must be interpreted cautiously because there were only two skaters in this age category. The increased BMD in the adolescent skaters may have been due to their longer sport-specific training history, a greater genetic potential for increased BMD that may not be manifest until after puberty, or a combination of these factors. Limited evidence suggests that the full effects of genetics on BMD may not be evident until after puberty (Smith et al., 1973). Alternatively, these findings may indicate a selection bias, whereby adolescent girls with high BMD may be more tolerant of heavy training demands, more resistant to injury, and more likely to sustain their participation in the sport.

Risser et al. (1990) found that swimmers had lower lumbar spine BMD than did controls, basketball players, and volleyball players after adjusting for height and weight. Swimmers appear consistently to have lower bone densities than do children in weight-bearing sports; quite often, swimmers exhibit lower densities than do sedentary children (Cassell et al., 1993; Grimston et al., 1993; McCulloch et al., 1992; Slemenda et al., 1991b). Self-selection into swimming may explain some of these apparent effects of swimming, i.e., children who have lower BMD at certain sites may be more buoyant and thus more likely to achieve success in swimming. Alternatively, the relative weightlessness while in the water may facilitate diminution in BMD similar to the zero-gravity effect in astronauts. For young females, it seems that the pulling actions of muscles on the skeleton during swimming do not provide any additional stimulus for bone mineral accrual beyond that provided by normal habitual physical activity.

High-Impact Activity. High-impact activities impart large compressive strains to bones that may stimulate bone accretion. Grimston et al. (1993) compared BMD of youths (13.2 y) who participated in competitive high-impact or weight-bearing sports (running, gymnastics, tumbling, and dance) with elite swimmers. All athletes trained for 60 min at least three times weekly. For the females, there was a trend toward higher femoral neck BMD measures for the high-impact and weight-bearing groups compared to those for the swimmers. There was no difference in lumbar spine BMD among groups. The lack of a positive effect at the lumbar region and the trend for higher densities in the proximal femur suggest that the femur may be under greater mechanical strain than the spine during high-impact and weight-bearing activities. Interestingly, there was no significant correlation between BMD of the femoral neck or lumbar spine and total weight-bearing hours, which is in contrast to the findings of Slemenda et al. (1991b).

Other studies have also investigated the effects of high-impact gymnastics training on BMD in children. For example, Robinson et al. (1993) found higher lumbar spine and femoral neck BMD in gymnasts and controls, compared to long-distance runners. Total body, lumbar spine, and femoral neck BMD have also been shown to be consistently higher in young gymnasts compared to age- and weight-matched controls and swimmers (Cassell et al., 1993; Nichols et al., 1994). Significantly increased distal radial total, cortical, and trabecular volumetric BMD has also been reported in elite (> 15 h training per week), prepubescent (8–10 y) female gymnasts compared to age-matched controls (Dyson et al., 1995). These findings suggest that high site-specific mechanical strains on the skeleton during gymnastics induce positive effects on bone mineral accretion during childhood.

Gymnasts generally have higher bone densities than young athletes from most other sports (e.g., basketball, volleyball, swimming, running, and soccer). The femur, hip, and wrist seem to be the skeletal regions most sensitive to the high-impact loads imparted during gymnastics. These findings are consistent with the results of animal research reported by Rubin and Lanyon (1985), indicating that the absolute magnitude of the mechanical load is an important stimulus for new bone formation.

Preferred Limb Studies. The effect of increased mechanical usage on BMD in children has also been inferred from comparisons of preferred or dominant to nondominant limbs. These studies provide a unique model because extraneous variables such as genetic, endocrine, and nutritional influences are shared by both limbs, and differences in BMD can be attributed solely to mechanical usage. Faulkner et al. (1993b) compared BMC and BMD for dominant and nondominant limbs in children 8–16 y old. Both BMC and BMD were higher in the dominant compared to the nondominant arms, but there was no difference between dominant and nondominant legs. The greater bone mineral in the dominant arm was attributed to its greater habitual usage, whereas the lack of difference in the lower limbs was explained by equal use of both legs in daily weight-bearing activity.

Increased bone mineral has also been reported in the dominant arms of elite young adult (18–28 y) female tennis players (Jacobson et al., 1984) and squash players (Haapasalo et al., 1994). In the latter study, both the years of training and the strength of the arm were correlated with bone mass. Interestingly, athletes who began playing before or during menarche had higher BMD (22% higher) than athletes who began at least 1 y after menarche (Haapasalo et al., 1994).

Retrospective Studies. Talmage and Anderson (1992) found that 25-y-old women who participated in secondary school sports or performed heavy farm chores as children had higher BMD than did women who were less active during their childhood. Tylavsky et al. (1992) reported a significant positive relationship between the amount of activity during adolescence and present BMD levels in college-age females. Distal radial bone dimensions in postmenopausal women were also positively related to physical activity history during childhood, with the strongest association occurring between 14 and 21 y of age (Kriska et al., 1988).

Physical activity during childhood was positively associated with os calcis bone density in young (20–35 y) healthy females (McCulloch et al., 1990), and time spent in sports activity during the first year of high school was positively associated with radial BMC in young women (25 y) who were initially recruited for a 14-y follow-up study of milk supplementation on bone mineral (Fehily et al., 1992). Interestingly, in the latter study, the association with past activity level was stronger than for current sports involvement, suggesting that the greatest effect of activity may be during the adolescent years while the bones are still growing.

Longitudinal Training Studies. There are few controlled longitudinal studies of the effects of exercise training on BMD in children and adolescents. Nichols et al. (1994) studied the effects of 27 wk of high-impact gymnastics training on bone mass and density in eumenorrheic college-age females. Gymnasts had greater BMD at the femoral neck (7.8%) and lumbar spine (7.8%) compared to eumenorrheic controls at the beginning of the study, suggesting that prior training during childhood and adolescence had a positive effect on bone accretion. Training resulted in a significant increase in lumbar spine BMD (+1.3%), and there were no changes in BMD in the controls. The veteran gymnasts increased their lumbar densities by 0.9%, whereas BMD of the freshman gymnasts increased by 1.5%. These findings suggest that the veteran gymnasts were closer to their potential peak bone densities than were the freshman gymnasts; the freshmen had greater potential physiological reserves for increased bone accretion.

The effects of progressive resistance training on BMD of young females have also been investigated. Blimkie et al. (1993b) trained postmenarcheal adolescent girls (14–18 y) for 26 wk with 13 different resistance exercises designed to provide high-level generalized as well as site-specific (lumbar spine) skeletal mechanical strains. Strength increased over the training period, but there was only a transient insignificant increase in lumbar spine BMD and no significant increases in bone mineral at any of the other measured sites. In the only other resistance training study of young women (19 y), 8 mo of training had no effect on BMD of the proximal femur, but it did cause a small significant increase (+1.2%) in lumbar spine BMD (Snow-Harter et al., 1992). The lack of change in femoral BMD in this study was attributed to the lower sensitivity of cortical bone to the mechanically induced strains of training and to the slower turnover of bone at this site.

These longitudinal training studies suggest that training may have a small positive effect on BMD in adolescent and young adult females. The magnitude of the effect is much smaller, however, than would be predicted from the differences between trained and untrained women in cross-sectional and comparative studies.

Physical Activity During Adulthood

With osteoporotic fractures increasing at a faster rate than the increase in age of the population, Martin et al. (1991) hypothesized that an increase in sedentary living is responsible for increased skeletal fragility. Multiple regression analysis has indicated that physical activity level has a small but significant effect on BMD of the radius, lumbar spine, femoral neck, or whole body in young (Krall & Dawson-Hughes, 1993; Metz et al., 1993; Recker et al., 1992; Takeshita et al., 1992), middle-aged (Aloia et al., 1988), perimenopausal (Zhang et al., 1992) and older (Krall & Dawson-Hughes, 1993) women. Others, however, have failed to find an association between physical activity level and average BMD of the total body, radius, spine (Krall & Dawson-Hughes, 1993), and proximal femur (Stevenson et al., 1989) in young women. In studies in which physical activity was positively associated with BMD, activity level alone accounted for only 5–10% of the variability in BMD.

The association between active living and greater BMD is more obvious from cross-sectional comparisons among groups differing in activity level. For example, Talmage et al. (1986) compared 1105 nonathletic and 124 athletic women aged 18–98 y. They performed a segmental regression analysis of age versus BMD to determine the break point at which the loss of radial BMD was accelerated. In the nonathletic group, this breakpoint corresponded to an age between 47 y and 52 y, approximately the time of menopause. In contrast, a break point could not be detected for the athletic group, and they had a greater BMD through menopause. Cross-sectional studies have also shown that active older individuals are less susceptible to osteoporotic fractures. Current and lifetime physical activity estimates are greater in age-matched healthy controls, compared to patients with hip fracture (Astrom et al., 1987; Cooper et al., 1988).

Aerobic Exercise. Aerobic exercise is a common and popular form of activity for many adults. Results generally are equivocal for premenopausal women but indicate a positive effect of aerobic exercise on BMD in postmenopausal women.

Premenopausal Women. Cross-sectional, comparative studies generally show that the average BMD of endurance-trained eumenorrheic runners aged 18–35 y is similar to that of sedentary eumenorrheic controls at the spine, proximal femur, distal radius, and whole body sites (Davee et al., 1990; Heinonen et al., 1993; Heinrich et al., 1990; Myerson et al., 1992, Snead et al., 1992). One study, however, (Kirk et al., 1989) reported a positive correlation in runners between maximal oxygen uptake ($\dot{V}O_2$max) and BMD of the lumbar spine, whereas another (Pocock et al., 1986) failed to confirm this association in a larger group of subjects.

There may be a site-specific effect of endurance training on BMD. Runners may have increased BMD at appendicular weight-bearing sites. Orienteers (Heinonen et al., 1993) had 5% greater BMD at the distal femur and proximal tibia, and runners had 8% greater BMD of the distal femur, compared to sedentary controls (Wolman et al., 1991).

Other endurance-type sports, including lacrosse, basketball, field hockey, cycling, and cross-country skiing, also fail to elicit greater than normal BMD at most bone sites (Baker & Demers, 1988; Buchanan et al., 1988b; Heinonen et al., 1993). In one study (Risser et al., 1990) female swimmers whose average age was 18.4 y had lower lumbar spine BMD than did controls; the authors suggested that the weightlessness of swimming may have been a contributing factor to the lower BMD. Heinrich et al. (1990), however, failed to confirm this finding. The mean BMD of swimmers in this study (aged 21.7 y) was similar to that of controls. Subjects in this study were heavier than in those in the study of Risser et al. (1990), and this may have contributed to the difference in BMD outcomes.

Results from these cross-sectional, comparative studies suggest that areal BMD in young endurance-trained athletes is not different from that in nonathletic controls, with the possible exception of weight-bearing appendicular sites. The effects of weight-supported activity such as swimming on BMD of premenopausal women remains equivocal. Results from these cross-sectional and comparative studies must be interpreted cautiously, however, because the effects of skeletal size on bone density have not been adequately controlled in most studies. In contrast, longitudinal studies generally indicate a positive effect of endurance training alone (Bassey & Ramsdale, 1994; Snow-Harter et al., 1992) or in combination with resistance training (Friedlander et al., 1995) on BMD of the trochanter and lumbar spine in premenopausal females.

Early Postmenopausal Women. Cross-sectional, comparative studies indicate that postmenopausal women who engage in aerobic activities tend to have greater BMD than their sedentary counterparts. Postmenopausal women (aged 50–65 y) who ran on a regular basis had 15–35% and 12–17% greater BMD at the lumbar spine and distal radius, respectively, than did sedentary controls (Jonsson et al., 1992; Lane et al., 1986; Nelson et al., 1988b). One study, however, (Kirk et al., 1989) failed to find a greater lumbar spine BMD in runners compared to controls, and another failed to find differences at the proximal femur (Nelson et al., 1988b).

Several explanations have been put forth to explain the discrepancy between the generally positive effects of endurance training in postmenopausal women in these comparative studies and the negative findings in similar studies of younger premenopausal women: 1) postmenopausal subjects usually have longer training histories than premenopausal women; 2) bone may adapt slowly to exercise, and it may take 10–20 y of endurance training before increases in BMD are evident; and 3) with decreased estrogen secretion and diminished BMD, postmenopausal women may be more "trainable" than younger women, whose initial BMD is greater.

Correlative studies in postmenopausal women also indicate positive effects of endurance exercise on BMD. A positive association was reported by Michel et al. (1989) between minutes of exercise per week and lumbar spine BMD in women (aged 57.3 y) who varied widely in amount of participation in aerobic exercise. The five subjects who trained the most (> 300 min/wk), however, had substantially lower BMD. In this study the relationship between weight-bearing exercise and BMD was best described by a quadratic model; maximal BMD was reached at 217 min of exercise per week and decreased thereafter. The authors hypothesized that body fat is reduced with excessive exercise to a level where peripheral conversion of adrenal steroids to estrogen is negatively affected; the resultant hypoestrogenemia is thought to contribute to diminished BMD. This hypothesis remains to be verified.

Most longitudinal studies (Hatori et al., 1993; Martin & Notelovitz, 1993; Nelson et al., 1991) indicate that moderate-intensity walking may slow the rate of BMD loss in early postmenopausal women. In two of the studies showing positive gains, subjects walked with weighted belts (Nelson et al., 1991) or walked at intensities above their anaerobic thresholds (Hatori et al., 1993). This suggests that walking has to be done at a brisk pace or with the addition of loads (i.e., hand-held weights) to have positive effects on bone. In the study of Martin and Notelovitz (1993), early postmenopausal women also walked at a fairly high intensity and had a substantially smaller reduction in BMD than did the controls. There was no positive effect of training, however, in women who were more than 6 y postmenopausal. This implies that walking may only be effective in the early stages of menopause, when the rate of bone turnover is greatest and probably more sensitive to changes in external factors such as increased exercise.

The only study (Cavanaugh & Cann, 1988) that failed to demonstrate a positive effect of walking on BMD can be criticized on the basis of its small samples, poorer compliance, and unsupervised training. This was the only study in which diet was not monitored and Ca^{2+} supplements were not given. Additionally, upon entry into the study, the exercise group was involved in a greater amount of weight-bearing activity than was the control group; therefore, it is possible that they were already relatively well trained and had little to gain from a training program of moderate intensity.

One other study (Grove & Londeree, 1992) demonstrated positive effects of moderate-intensity aerobic exercise on BMD in early postmenopausal women. Women were randomly assigned to high-impact aerobic (n = 5), low-impact aerobic (n = 10), or control (n = 5) groups. Groups were well matched in all aspects, including diet, and all women were on estrogen replacement therapy. The exercise groups attended aerobics classes for 20 min/d, 3 d/wk for 12 mo and maintained BMD of the lumbar spine; there were no differences in BMD outcome between high- and low-impact exercise groups, but BMD was diminished (6.1%) in the control group. It is difficult with this design to isolate the effects of training from a possible interactive effect with estrogen-replacement therapy.

Older Postmenopausal Women. Aerobic exercise also seems to have positive effects on BMD in older postmenopausal women (> 10 y postmenopausal). Lumbar spine BMD was positively correlated with $\dot{V}O_2$max in a group of postmenopausal women (Bevier et al., 1989). Also, $\dot{V}O_2$max contributed 5.6% of the variance in whole body BMC in 69 women aged 59–84 y (Webber et al, 1993).

Three longitudinal studies (Bloomfield et al., 1993; Dalsky et al., 1988; Krolner et al., 1983) have shown that endurance training can have beneficial effects on BMD of older women. These studies were not randomized, and all included subjects who were either currently or previously on estrogen replacement therapy. The results from one study (Bloomfield et al., 1993) are particularly encouraging because they indicate that stationary cycling, a relatively safe, nonweight-bearing exercise can be beneficial to BMD in elderly women.

Resistance Exercise. Resistance exercise is a less common exercise for adults but is gaining in popularity. Studies of resistance training have generally shown positive effects on BMD.

Premenopausal Women. Body builders or weightlifters exceed endurance athletes or controls in BMD at the lumbar spine, femoral neck, proximal and distal radius, distal femur, patella, and proximal tibia by 8–26% (Davee et al., 1990; Heinonen et al., 1993; Heinrich et al; 1990). Greater BMD is also found in other groups of athletes who incorporate resistance-type exercise into their training programs. For example, volleyball players, rowers, and gymnasts have 4–14% greater BMD at the lumbar spine and femoral neck (Nichols et al., 1994; Risser et al., 1990; Taaffe et al., 1995; Wolman et al., 1990) compared to endurance athletes or sedentary controls. The results of these studies should also be interpreted cautiously, however, because the BMD values are rarely adjusted for possible differences in bone size between groups.

There is also some indication that tension created by muscle contraction stimulates bone formation locally at its site of attachment. Hip adductor strength independently predicts hip BMD, grip strength independently predicts radius BMD (Snow-Harter et al., 1990), and trunk extensor strength independently predicts lumbar spine BMD (Eickhoff et al., 1993). Additional evidence that muscle has a direct local effect on the bone is provided by the unique study of Doyle & Brown (1970). In this study, a positive correlation of 0.72 was reported between the third lumbar vertebrae and the psoas muscle mass in 47 female and male cadavers aged 26–83 y. Additional site-specific studies are required to unequivocally describe the relationship between muscle mass and BMD at local bone attachment sites.

It also has been suggested that the strength of some muscle groups best predicts mineral density of bones other than those to which they attach. Biceps strength was found to best predict hip BMD, whereas grip strength was the best predictor of spine BMD (Pocock et al., 1989; Snow-Harter et al., 1990). Researchers have hypothesized that trunk muscle groups are recruited as stabilizers when upper body muscles are involved in lifting; the resultant large forces on the spine and hip are thought to stimulate bone formation in these distal sites. The association between muscle strength or mass and BMD at sites distant from muscle attachments requires further study.

Longitudinal investigations of resistance training have resulted in relatively smaller changes in BMD than would be expected from cross-sectional, comparative studies of resistance-trained athletes and sedentary controls. Most of these studies (Gleeson et al., 1990; Lohman et al., 1995; Nichols et al., 1994; Snow-Harter et al., 1992) reported small increases in BMD with training, whereas one (Rockwell et al., 1990) reported negative effects. Of those reporting positive effects, only the studies of Lohman et al. (1995) and Snow-Harter et al. (1992) were randomized and, therefore, not subject to a self-selection bias.

The negative results of Rockwell et al. (1990) are difficult to explain. This study can be criticized for its small samples and differences in exercise histories between trained and control groups. Excessive training in the exercise group may have altered endocrine status and negatively affected BMD in this study.

Resistance and endurance training had equally small positive effects on BMD in the study of Snow-Harter et al. (1992), and Friedlander et al. (1995) reported improvements in most measures of BMD in young adult females following 2 y of combined strength, endurance, and stretching training. These findings suggest that resistance and endurance training, whether done separately or together, elicit small increases in BMD in premenopausal women. Despite positive group effects, however, it is interesting to note that 2–3 subjects in both the weight training and running groups in the study by Snow-Harter et al. (1992) demonstrated losses in lumbar spine BMD, despite their participation in moderate-intensity training.

Prospective resistance training studies in this population have elicited smaller increases in BMD than might have been expected based on cross-sectional comparative studies. This discrepancy may be explained in part by the influence of subject selection bias in comparative studies. Elite athletes may have genetically greater BMD before they start training for their sports. The strength-trained athletes in the studies of Heinrich et al. (1990) and Davee et al. (1990) had an average of only 2.5 y of participation in resistance training, yet they had greater BMD than did controls, far greater than those demonstrated in even the most successful longitudinal studies.

Postmenopausal And Older Women. Muscle strength also appears to be positively correlated with BMD at local and distal sites of muscle attachment in older women. Back extensor strength and flexor strength were correlated with lumbar spine BMD in the study of Halle et al. (1990), and grip strength was correlated with BMD at radial (Bevier et al., 1989; Kritz-Silverstein & Barrett-Connor, 1994), lumbar spine (Bevier et al., 1989; Kritz-Silverstein & Barrett-Connor, 1994), and hip sites (Kritz-Silverstein & Barrett-Connor, 1994) in elderly postmenopausal females.

Longitudinal studies (Nelson et al., 1994; Pruitt et al., 1992; Smith et al., 1989) indicate that resistance training has small beneficial effects on BMD in older females. In the study of Nelson et al. (1994), femoral neck (0.9%) and lumbar spine (1.0%) BMD increased in the experimental group after 1 y of strength training. Training was not universally effective, however, because BMD actually decreased in nine subjects in the training group at the femoral neck and in six at the lumbar spine. These, and similar findings in the study by Snow-Harter et al. (1992) for premenopausal women, indicate substantial individual variability in responsiveness to training, and suggest that conclusions about trainability drawn from group data may not be wholly generalizable at the individual level.

Of the prospective studies above, only the study of Nelson et al. (1994) was randomized; in the other studies, however, both the control and exercise subjects were well matched. The bias of a desire for self-improvement, which may occur with self-selection into treatment groups, is evident from results of the study of Smith et al. (1989). Exercise subjects who were self-selected consumed greater amounts of Ca^{2+} and magnesium throughout this study than did controls. It is difficult with this type of bias in nonrandomized studies to separate the effects of exercise training from the effects of dietary changes on the BMD outcome observed in the experimental group.

Impact Loading Exercise. Few comparative studies of the effects of different types of mechanical loading on BMD in adult females have controlled for variability in menstrual or reproductive status. However, in a recent study of eumenorrheic college-age females (Taaffe et al., 1995), gymnasts had greater BMD at the femoral neck and trochanter than did controls, who for the most part had greater BMD than did varsity swimmers. These results suggest that high-intensity impact activity, such as that experienced during gymnastics training, may be a potent osteogenic stimulus and that long-term weight-supported activity such as swimming may not confer any skeletal benefit for young premenopausal females with normal menstrual status.

Impact loading (heel drops) had no effect on BMD after 1 y, in a prospective study of healthy postmenopausal women (Bassey & Ramsdale, 1995). The impact loads in this study, however, were generally less than three times body weight, which is lower than the purported impact loads (up to 18 times body weight) experienced by elite gymnasts (Panzer et al., 1988), and may not have been of sufficient magnitude to elicit changes in BMD in this population. Clearly, the effects of impact loading on BMD in pre-and postmenopausal women require further investigation. A summary of the effects of different types of exercise on BMD at various stages of the life span is provided in Table 4-6.

MEDICAL AND SAFETY CONCERNS

Bone mineral mass and density account for about 80–90% of the variance in bone compressive strength (Mazess & Wahner, 1988). Bone mineral status, therefore, is an important risk factor for skeletal fractures, regardless of age (Seeman, 1994). Fracture rates of all types increase dramatically during the circumpubertal years, and the peak rate of fracture during childhood occurs coincidentally with the growth spurt in stature in both boys and girls (Bailey et al., 1989; Blimkie et al., 1993a; Kleerekoper et al., 1981). Most of these fractures occur at the relatively under-mineralized metaphyseal region of long bones (Davis & Green, 1976; Hagino et al., 1990), and, unlike osteoporotic fractures, they are often associated with significant trauma (Melton, 1988).

Paradoxically, this is also the period of largest lifetime gains in bone mineral mass and density. These observations suggest an uncoupling of

TABLE 4-6.   The effects of different types of exercise on BMD in females.

Activity Type	Childhood	Adolescence	Young-Middle Age	Post-Menopausal & Old Age
Weight-Bearing (WB)	↑	↑	=	↑
Impact Loading (IL)	↑	↑	↑	NE
Weight-Supported (WS)	↓	↓	=	?
Endurance Training (ET)	?	?	↑	↑
Resistance Training (RT)	?	↑	↑	↑

The size and direction of the arrows indicates the relative magnitude of the effects of different types of activity on BMD based on the author's interpretation of the literature.

? unknown effect; = equivocal effect; NE no effect; ↑ large + effect; ↓ small – or + effect the normal relationship between bone mineral mass and fracture risk during the circumpubertal period. An alternative hypothesis, however, proposes a developmental lag between changes in skeletal dimensions (bone length and width) and bone mineralization during this period. A relative lag in the rate of bone mineralization in relation to dimensional growth would temporarily render bones more fragile, predisposing them to fracture.

No study has prospectively assessed the interrelationship between rates of bone mineralization, long bone growth, and skeletal fractures at this stage of the life span. However, a study of adolescent boys reported a 6-mo lag in the timing of peak growth rates for metacarpal cortical thickness relative to the timing of peak growth rates for stature and metacarpal length (Blimkie et al., 1993a). This observation lends support to the concept that a developmental delay in bone mineralization relative to linear skeletal growth may contribute to the increased fracture rates observed during this period.

High activation frequency of osteonal remodelling during puberty may temporarily uncouple bone accretion and resorption rates (Frost, 1963), thereby predisposing children to increased fracture risk and rates during the growth spurt. Parfitt (1994) suggests that the increased fracture incidence during the growth spurt is due to an increase in cortical porosity as a consequence of increased intracortical bone turnover. Increased intracortical turnover would provide additional calcium in support of the rapid growth in bone length at the metaphysis but at the expense of temporarily incomplete or delayed cortical bone mineralization and increased bone fragility. In this sense, normal growth dynamics may place children at increased risk for fracture during the circumpubertal years. Although speculative, fracture risk at this stage of the life span might be more accurately predicted by measuring BMD at the shafts of long bones, which are composed predominantly of cortical bone, rather than at the sites typically used to assess osteoporotic fracture risk in adults.

Young amenorrheic athletes in many (Lloyd et al., 1986; Marcus et al., 1985) but not all (Grimston et al., 1991a) cross-sectional reports seem to be more susceptible to tibial, metatarsal, and even femoral stress fractures than are eumenorrheic athletes and controls. The rate of stress fracture is greater in athletes with eating disorders and low body mass (Frusztajer et al., 1990) and is twice as high in athletes who have never used oral contraceptives compared to those using oral contraceptives for at least 1 y (Barrow & Saha, 1988). To minimize risk of fracture, BMD screening and dietary monitoring may be recommended for the amenorrheic athlete. Treatment may include a reduction in training, improved nutrition, and prescription of hormone replacement, perhaps with oral contraceptives.

For osteoporotic postmenopausal women, screening for low BMD should be performed before initiating an exercise program. Although vigorous exercise may prove beneficial for BMD, individuals with low initial BMD should proceed cautiously with exercise because of their increased susceptibility to stress fractures. Because most recent studies have indicated a positive effect of walking on BMD, a low-impact exercise program of brisk walking may be prescribed.

Only one longitudinal study to date has compared the effects of different types of exercises on fracture rate. Sinaki and Mikkelsen (1984) compared back flexion and extension exercises and their relative effects on fracture rate in 59 postmenopausal women who suffered from osteoporosis and back pain. After 1–6 y, a smaller number of additional vertebral fractures had occurred in the group that performed back extensions, compared to those who did flexion exercises and those in a nonexercise control group. The authors concluded that back extension exercises are beneficial for strengthening musculature and bone and for decreasing fracture incidence; back flexion exercises should be avoided. More research is needed to determine if other types of exercises are beneficial or detrimental with regard to fracture rate.

Fractures at any stage of the life span impose restrictions on physical activity and increase health care costs. The effects of fractures on independent living capability and health care costs in the elderly have been adequately documented and described (Bloomfield, 1995; Snow-Harter & Marcus, 1991). Less attention has been given to the economic costs associated with the increased fracture incidence during the circumpubertal years and to the effects of ensuing restricted activity on peak BMD and subsequent risk of fracture in old age. Achieving and maintaining the highest possible BMD at all stages of the life span is a necessary prerequisite to insure adequate bone strength, but high bone density itself may not be sufficient to protect against risk of fractures. As indicated in the previous sections, optimal BMD may be realized by ensuring adequate physical activity, calcium intake, and a supportive endocrine environment.

DIRECTIONS FOR FUTURE RESEARCH

Better controlled correlative studies are required to determine the absolute and relative importance of physical activity and the effects of different types of physical activity on bone mineral accretion during the different developmental stages of childhood and during adulthood. Such studies should include large samples with discrete maturity or menstrual status groups and evaluate all the known possible determinants of bone mineral, e.g., body mass, muscle strength, $\dot{V}O_2$max, and body fat. These studies also should differentiate among the different types (e.g., weight-bearing versus non-weight-bearing activity) and magnitudes of mechanical loads. Improved methods for the quantification of physical activity are required in these studies to provide the necessary reliability and sensitivity to differentiate the effects of physical activity on bone mineral from other possible determinants.

Much of our understanding of bone mineral development trends for both children and adults has been derived from cross-sectional studies. More longitudinal studies spanning the transitional years between periods of high biological reactivity, e.g., puberty and menopause, in diverse populations are required to provide a clearer description of the normal history of bone mineral development in humans across the life span.

Prospective, controlled, randomized studies incorporating different types and intensities of training within discrete maturity or menstrual status groups are required to determine the trainability of bone mineral at different periods of the life span. More studies of the interaction of different types of training with nutritional and hormonal interventions at the various stages of the life span are also required. These studies must be implemented over several years to differentiate the effects of growth and aging from the effects of training and to counteract both the relatively slow turnover of bone compared to other biological tissues and the bone-remodelling transient (Heaney, 1993; Parfitt, 1988). Additionally, subjects must be more closely screened at entry into these studies to control for confounding influences such as use of oral contraceptives, hormone replacement, and nutritional deficiencies.

Greater effort must also be directed towards understanding the complex interplay among physical activity or training, menstrual dysfunction, and bone mineralization in adolescent and young adult females. Research should be directed towards identifying the upper limits and types of exercises that evoke menstrual dysfunction, the degree to which exercise must be reduced to reinstate normal function, and the interaction among exercise, nutrition, and endocrine (e.g., hormone replacement) interventions in the prevention and management of these conditions.

Absorptiometry is a widely used and precise method for quantitative assessment of BMD (Chilibeck et al., 1994). However, studies have rarely used measurement techniques that provide qualitative assessments of bone geometry and structural architecture, which also influence bone strength. Newer techniques, including ultrasonography, mechanical accelerometry, and computed tomography, have been used to characterize mechanical and geometric properties as well as architectural features of bone and should be incorporated in future physical activity and training studies.

The technique used to measure bone mineral biases the conclusions we make concerning the pattern of bone mineral development during the life span and the effects of physical activity and training at various stages of the life span. Although absorptiometric techniques have been used extensively in recent years with children and adults, these techniques do not fully account for changes in bone size that occur with growth and aging, and they provide measures of areal rather than volumetric bone density. If these techniques continue to be used as extensively as they have in recent years, improvements must be made in the normalization approaches used in the conversion of BMC to measures of BMD. The limitations of the current normalization approaches are clearly recognized (Compston, 1995; Prentice et al., 1994).

Lastly, Morrison et al. (1994) identified the gene for the vitamin D receptor that apparently accounts for up to 75% of the variation in bone density in healthy Caucasian women. Studies should now be undertaken to investigate the complex interactions among physical activity, nutrition, and hormone replacement therapy on BMD at different stages of the life span, while strictly controlling or accounting for this particular genetic influence. This discovery may also prove enlightening in explaining racial differences in bone density and the interaction of race with physical activity, nutrition, and endocrine status in determining bone mineral status.

SUMMARY

Several techniques have been used to assess bone density, but the most current and common are absorptiometry and computed tomography. The absorptiometric techniques generally do not account for bone depth or thickness, cannot distinguish between cortical and trabecular bone, and, unlike computed tomography, are incapable of measuring bone volume. Although computed tomography provides a more straightforward interpretation of cortical and trabecular mineralization patterns, it involves greater radiation exposure compared to the absorptiometric techniques. Bone mineralization patterns are influenced by measurement technique, and caution is warranted when interpreting developmental and aging trends in bone density derived from these different approaches.

Generally bone mineral density (BMD) increases between infancy and the onset of puberty in both sexes. Bone mineral density increases more rapidly during the circumpubertal years than at any other time. Most but not all studies have found an increase in BMD with advancing level of sexual maturity in both genders. The lifetime peak bone density occurs at various times for different bone sites. For example, radial areal BMD plateaus in females between the 3rd to 5th decade, whereas femoral neck areal BMD peaks between late adolescence and the 4th decade. Most studies have found an acceleration in bone loss in the transition from premenopause to menopause. However, controversy exists regarding the timing of the onset of vertebral bone loss and the loss rate during the premenopausal and postmenopausal periods.

Bone mineral density is determined largely by genetics, but it is also influenced by reproductive hormone status, nutrition, and physical activity. Estrogen and perhaps progesterone appear to play essential roles in bone mineralization during puberty, in the optimization of peak BMD during late adolescence or early adulthood, and for the maintenance of skeletal integrity in menopausal and postmenopausal females. Estrogen increases the efficiency of intestinal absorption of calcium (Ca^{2+}), decreases urinary (Ca^{2+}) loss, and suppresses the rate of bone remodelling.

These reproductive hormones are also important modulators of mineralization during the adult premenopausal years when their production may be adversely affected by dietary restriction and weight loss associated with extreme exercise and when exogenous hormone is administered for contraception or hormone replacement therapy. A decline in production of estrogen and progesterone may occur with intense training in young athletic women. This may result in a decrease in BMD and an increased risk of fracture. For the amenorrheic younger woman, menses may return, and BMD may be recovered (at least partially) when training is decreased and calcium and energy intake are increased. The use of oral contraceptives may slightly increase BMD. Estrogen replacement therapy may benefit young amenorrheic women, but it has not been used extensively in this population. Therapy with estrogen plus progesterone is established as the best treatment for postmenopausal osteoporosis, increasing both trabecular and cortical BMD and reducing fracture rate.

Recent studies of children and adolescents with normal reproductive hormone status strongly suggest that dietary calcium may have an independent positive effect on bone mineral development during the formative growth years. The strongest evidence comes from prospective studies of calcium supplementation and bone mineral. Adequate calcium is needed during the early and middle years of adulthood for achievement of greater peak bone mass and prevention of osteoporosis as one enters menopause.

Calcium balance studies indicate that the majority of both pre- and postmenopausal women are in a negative Ca^{2+} balance. The Ca^{2+} intake required to produce a balance of zero was estimated to be 990 mg/d in premenopausal and 1500 mg/d in postmenopausal women, values that exceed the current Recommended Nutrient Intake. This implies that over a lifetime, Ca^{2+} deficiency may lead to a gradual decrease in BMD, with an accelerated loss at menopause. The effects of calcium supplementation on BMD in premenopausal and perimenopausal women are equivocal. Lifetime Ca^{2+} intake, rather than current Ca^{2+} intake, seems to be important in influencing the BMD of postmenopausal women. Estrogen replacement therapy combined with calcium supplementation appears to provide the best protection against bone loss during the postmenopausal period.

Weight-bearing (e.g., walking) and high-impact exercise (gymnastics) appear to be beneficial, whereas weight-supported activity (e.g., swimming) does not appear to have any beneficial effect on bone mineral acquisition during childhood and adolescence. High-magnitude loads are more effective than lower-magnitude loads applied more frequently, even when the absolute volume of loading or total external work is similar. There is evidence of a beneficial effect of high levels of physical activity during the prepubertal years, but excessive physical activity during the pubertal and postpubertal years is often associated with late-onset menses and reduced bone density. Trabecular bone appears to be metabolically more active, more sensitive to hormonal influences, and more rapidly turned over than cortical bone in response to exercise. Lastly, as in adults, BMD in youths is diminished with a reduction in weight-bearing activity or with immobilization.

Cross-sectional studies indicate that active individuals on average have a greater BMD and lower incidence of osteoporotic fracture than do inactive persons. Most studies suggest that moderate exercise, such as walking, can be beneficial for increasing BMD of less fit women who cannot perform heavier exercise due to bone fragility. Young endurance-trained athletes may achieve a greater BMD at weight-bearing appendicular sites compared to sedentary controls. Older endurance-trained athletes have a greater BMD at most sites compared to inactive individuals, indicating that a lifetime of endurance exercise may increase BMD. Longitudinal studies indicate that both endurance and resistance training are similarly effective in increasing BMD in younger and older adult females. Resistance-trained athletes tend to have greater BMD than do endurance-trained athletes and sedentary controls. This may be the result of a bias of studying highly selected groups of elite athletes, whose greater BMD may have genetic roots, or from failure to correct bone mineral measures for differences in bone size. Longitudinal studies of resistance-trained women show gains in BMD, but the gains are much smaller than the apparent effects of resistance training seen in cross-sectional studies. Exercise that incorporates high-impact loading such as gymnastics training may be a potent osteogenic stimulus for girls and young adult females, but impact loading at relatively low intensities may not be sufficient to elicit changes in BMD in older females.

ACKNOWLEDGEMENTS

The authors thank Don Bailey, Angela Smith, and Mitch Kanter for their expert reviews of this chapter and Priscilla Clarkson for her editorial direction and assistance. Special thanks to Colin Webber, J.D. (Rick) Adachi, and Chris Gordon for their continued collaboration and support. Appreciation is also extended to the Ontario Ministry of Tourism and Recreation, Fitness Branch, and Sport Canada for their financial support of the authors' work in this area.

BIBLIOGRAPHY

Adams, W.C., K. Deck-Cote, and K.M. Winters (1992). Anthropometric estimation of bone mineral content in young adult females. *Am. J. Hum. Biol.* 4:767-774.

Aloia, J.F. (1989). *Osteoporosis. A Guide To Prevention & Treatment.* Champaign, IL: Leisure Press.

Aloia, J.F., N.A. Vaswani, J.K. Yeh, and S.H. Cohn (1988). Premenopausal bone mass is related to physical activity. *Arch. Intern. Med.* 148:121-123.

Aloia, J.F., A. Vaswani, J.K. Yeh, P.L. Ross, E. Flaster, and F.A. Dilmanian (1994). Calcium supplementation with and without hormone replacement therapy to prevent postmenopausal bone loss. *Ann. Intern. Med.* 120:97-103.

Andon, M.B., K.T. Smith, M. Bracker, D. Sartoris, P. Saltman, and L. Strause (1991). Spinal bone density and calcium intake in healthy postmenopausal women. *Am. J. Clin. Nutr.* 54:927-929.

Angus, R.M., P.N. Sambrook, N.A. Pocock, and J.A. Eisman (1988). Dietary intake and bone mineral density. *Bone Miner.* 4:265-277.

Arnold, J.S., M.H. Bartley, S.A. Tont, and D.P. Jenkins (1966). Skeletal changes in aging and disease. *Clin. Orthop. Rel. Res.* 49:17-38.

Astrom, J., S. Ahnqvist, J. Beertema, and B. Jonsson (1987). Physical activity in women sustaining fracture of the neck of the femur. *J. Bone Joint Surg.* 69B:381-383.

Avioli, L.V., and R.P. Heaney (1991). Calcium intake and bone health. *Calcif. Tissue Int.* 48:221-223.

Ayers, J.W.T., G.P. Gidwani, I.M.V. Schmidt, and M. Gross (1984). Osteopenia in hypoestrogenic young women with anorexia nervosa. *Fertil. Steril.* 41:224-228.

Bachrach, L.K., D. Guido, D. Katzman, I.F. Litt, and R. Marcus (1990). Decreased bone density in adolescent girls with anorexia nervosa. *Pediatrics* 86:440-447.

Baer, J.T., L.J. Taper, F.G. Gwazdauskas, J.L. Walberg, M.-A. Novascone, S.J. Ritchey, and F.W. Thye (1992). Diet, hormonal, and metabolic factors affecting bone mineral density in adolescent amenorrheic and eumenorrheic female runners. *J. Sport Med. Phys. Fitness* 32:51-58.

Bailey, D.A. (1995). The role of mechanical loading in the regulation of skeletal development during growth. In: C.J.R. Blimkie and O. Bar-Or (eds.) *New Horizons In Pediatric Exercise Science.* Champaign: Human Kinetics, pp. 97-108.

Bailey, D.A., and A.D. Martin (1994). Physical activity and skeletal health in adolescents. *Ped. Exerc. Sci.* 6:330-347.

Bailey, D.A., and R.G. McCulloch (1990). Bone tissue and physical activity. *Can. J. Spt. Sci.* 15:229-239.

Bailey, D., K. Daniels, A. Dzus, K. Yong-Hing, D. Drinkwater, A. Wilkinson, and S. Houston (1992). Bone mineral density in the proximal femur of children with Legg-Calve-Perthes disease. *J. Bone Miner. Res.* 7 (Suppl.): S287.

Bailey, D.A., R.A. Faulkner, and H. McKay (1996). Growth, physical activity and bone mineral acquisition. In: J. Holloszy (ed.) *Exercise and Sport Sciences Reviews.* Vol. 24. Baltimore: Williams and Wilkins. In Press.

Bailey, D.A., J.H. Wedge, R.G. McCulloch, A.D. Martin, and S.C. Bernhardson (1989). Epidemiology of fractures of the distal end of the radius in children as associated with growth. *J. Bone Joint Surg.* 71-A:1225-1231.

Baker, E., and L. Demers (1988). Menstrual status in female athletes: correlation with reproductive hormones and bone density. *Obstet. Gynecol.* 72:683-687.

Ballard, J., J. Holtz, B. McKeown, and S. Zinkgraf (1988). Effect of exercise and estrogen upon postmenopausal bone mass. *Med. Sci. Sports Exerc.* 20 (Suppl.): S51, #304.

Baran, D., A. Sorensen, J. Grimes, R. Lew, A. Karellas, B. Johnson, and J. Roche (1989). Dietary modification with dairy products for preventing vertebral bone loss in premenopausal women: a three-year prospective study. *J. Clin. Endocrinol. Metab.* 70:264-270.

Barrow, G.W., and S. Saha (1988). Menstrual irregularity and stress fractures in collegiate female distance runners. *Am. J. Sports Med.* 16:209-216.

Bassey, E.J., and S.J. Ramsdale (1994). Increase in femoral bone density in young women following high-impact exercise. *Osteoporosis Int.* 4:72-75.

Bassey, E.J., and S.J. Ramsdale (1995). Weight-bearing exercise and ground reaction forces: a 12-month randomized controlled trial of effects on bone mineral density in healthy postmenopausal women. *Bone* 16:469-476.

Beck, T.J., C.B. Ruff, and K. Bissessur (1993). Age-related changes in female femoral neck geometry: implications for bone strength. *Calcif. Tissue Int.* 53 (Suppl): S41-S46.

Bell, N.H., J. Shary, J. Stevens, M. Garza, L. Gordon, and J. Edwards (1991). Demonstration that bone mass is greater in black than in white children. *J. Bone Miner. Res.* 6:719-723.

Bell, N.H., A.L. Yergey, N.E. Vieira, M.J. Oexmann, and J.R. Sharay (1993). Demonstration of a difference in urinary calcium, not calcium absorption, in black and white adolescents. *J. Bone Miner. Res.* 8:1111-1115.

Bevier, W.C., R.A. Wiswell, G. Pyka, K. Kozak, K. Newhall, and R. Marcus (1989). Relationship of body composition, muscle strength, and aerobic capacity to bone mineral density in older men and women. *J. Bone Miner. Res.* 4:421-432.

Biller, B.M.K., V. Saxe, D.B. Herzog, D.I. Rosenthal, S. Holzman, and A. Klibanski (1989). Mechanisms of osteoporosis in adult and adolescent women with anorexia nervosa. *J. Clin. Endocrinol. Metab.*, 68:548–554.

Blimkie, C.J.R., J. Lefevre, G.P. Beunen, R. Renson, J. Dequeker, and P. Van Damme (1993a). Fractures, physical activity, and growth velocity in adolescent Belgian boys. *Med. Sci. Sports Exerc.* 25:801–808.

Blimkie, C.J.R., S. Rice, C.E. Webber, J. Martin, D. Levy, and C.L. Gordon (1993b). Effects of resistance training on bone mass and density in adolescent females. *Med.Sci. Sports Exerc.* 25:S48.

Blimkie, C.J., S. Rice, C. Webber, J. Martin, D. Levy, and D. Parker (1992). Bone density, physical activity, fitness, anthropometry, gynecologic, endocrine and nutritional status in adolescent girls. In: J. Coudert and E. Van Praagh (eds.) *Children and Exercise XVI: Pediatric Work Physiology.* Paris: Masson, pp. 201–203.

Bloomfield, S.A. (1995). Bone, ligament, and tendon. In: D.R. Lamb, C.V. Gisolfi, and E. Nadel (eds.) *Perspectives in Exercise Science and Sports Medicine* Vol. 8. Exercise in Older Adults. Carmel, IN: Cooper Publishing Group, pp. 175–235.

Bloomfield, S.A., N.I. Williams, D.R. Lamb, and R.D. Jackson (1993). Non-weightbearing exercise may increase lumbar-spine bone mineral density in healthy postmenopausal women. *Am. J. Phys. Med. Rehabil.* 72:204–209.

Blunt, B.A., M.R. Klauber, E.L. Barrett-Connor, and S.L. Edelstein (1994). Sex differences in bone mineral density in 1653 men and women in the sixth through tenth decades of life: the Rancho Bernardo study. *J. Bone Miner. Res.* 9:1333–1338.

Bonjour, J.-P., G. Theintz, B. Buchs, D. Slosman, and R. Rizzoli (1991). Critical years and stages of puberty for spinal and femoral bone mass accumulation during adolescence. *J. Clin. Endocrin. Metab.* 73:555–563.

Borders, J., E. Kerr, D.J. Sartoris, J.A. Stein, E. Ramos, A.A. Moscona, and D. Resnick (1989). Quantitative dual-energy radiographic absorptiometry of the lumbar spine: in vivo comparison with dual-photon absorptiometry. *Radiology* 170:129–131.

Bronner, F. (1994). Calcium and osteoporosis. *Am. J. Clin. Nutr.* 60:831–836.

Buchanan, J.R., C. Myers, T. Lloyd, and R.B. Greer III (1988a). Early vertebral trabecular bone loss in normal premenopausal women. *J. Bone Miner. Res.* 3:583–587.

Buchanan, J.R., C. Myers, T. Lloyd, P. Leunenberger, and L.M. Demers (1988b). Determinants of peak trabecular bone density in women: the role of androgens, estrogen, and exercise. *J. Bone Miner. Res.* 3:673–680.

Bullen, B.A., G.S. Skrinar, I.Z. Beitins, G. von Merig, B.A. Turnbull, and J.W. Arthur (1985). Induction of menstrual disorders by strenuous exercise in untrained women. *N. Engl. J. Med.* 312:1349–1353.

Cann, C.E., H.K. Genant, F.O. Kolb, and B. Ettinger (1985). Quantitative computed tomography for prediction of vertebral fracture risk. *Bone* 6:1–7.

Carbon, R.J. (1992). Exercise, amenorrhoea and the skeleton. *Br. Med. Bull.* 48:546–560.

Casez, J.-P., A. Troendle, K. Lippuner, and P. Jaeger (1994). Bone mineral density at distal tibia using dual-energy x-ray absorptiometry in normal women and in patients with vertebral osteoporosis or primary hyperparathyroidism. *J. Bone Miner. Res.* 9:1851–1857.

Cassell, C., M. Benedict, G. Uetrect, J. Ranz, M. Ho, and B. Specker (1993). Bone mineral density in young gymnasts and swimmers. *Med. Sci. Sports Exerc.* 25:S49.

Cavanaugh D.J., and C.E. Cann (1988). Brisk walking does not stop bone loss in postmenopausal women. *Bone* 9:201–204.

Chan, G.M. (1991). Dietary calcium and bone mineral status of children and adolescents. *A.J.D.C.* 145:631–634.

Chilibeck, P., A. Calder, D. Sale, and C. Webber (1994). Reproducibility of bone and body composition by dual energy x-ray absorptiometry. *Can. J. Assoc. Radiol.* 45:297–302.

Chilibeck, P.D., D.G. Sale, and C.E. Webber (1995). Exercise and bone mineral density. *Sports Med.* 19:103–122.

Christian, J.C., P.-L. Yu, C.W. Slemenda, and C.C. Johnston Jr. (1989). Heritability of bone mass: a longitudinal study in aging male twins. *Am. J. Hum. Genet.* 44:429–433.

Christiansen C., and B.J. Riis (1990). 17β-estradiol and continuous norethisterone: A unique treatment for established osteoporosis in elderly women. *J. Clin. Endocrinol. Metab.* 71:836–841.

Clarkson, P.M., and E.M. Haymes (1995). Exercise and mineral status of athletes: calcium, magnesium, phosphorus, and iron. *Med. Sci. Sports Exerc.* 27:831–843.

Compston, J.E. (1995). Bone density: BMC, BMD, or corrected BMD? *Bone* 16:5–7.

Compston, J.E., W.D. Evans, E.O. Crawley, and C. Evans (1988). Bone mineral content in normal UK subjects. *Br. J. Radiol.* 61:631–636.

Cooper, C., D.J.P. Barker, and C. Wickham (1988). Physical activity, muscle strength, and calcium intake in fracture of the proximal femur in Britain. *B.M.J.* 297:1443–1446.

Crofts, R.D., T.M. Boyce, and R.D. Bloebaum (1994). Aging changes in osteon mineralization in the human femoral neck. *Bone* 15:147–152.

Cumming, R.G. (1990). Calcium intake and bone mass: a quantitative review of the evidence. *Calcif. Tissue Int.* 47:194–201.

Cummings, S.R., D.M. Black, M.C. Nevith, W. Browner, J. Cauley, K. Ensrud, H.K. Genant, L. Palmerno, J. Scott, and T.M. Vogt (1993). Bone density at various sites for prediction of hip fractures. *Lancet* 341:72–75.

Dalsky, G.P., K.S. Stocke, A.A. Ehsoni, E. Slatopolsky, W.C. Lee, and S.J. Birge (1988). Weight-bearing exercise training and lumbar-spine bone mineral content in postmenopausal women. *Ann. Intern. Med.* 108:824–828.

Davee, A.M., C.J. Rosen, and R.A. Adler (1990). Exercise patterns and trabecular bone density in college women. *J. Bone. Miner. Res.* 5:245–250.

Davis, D.R., and D.P. Green (1976). Forearm fractures in children. Pitfalls and complications. *Clin. Orthop.* 120:172–184.

Dawson-Hughes, B., G.E. Dallal, E.A. Krall, L. Sadowski, N. Sahyoun, and S. Tannenbaum (1990). A controlled trial of the effect of calcium supplementation on bone density in postmenopausal women. *N. Engl. J. Med.* 323:878–883.

Dawson-Hughes, B., P. Jaques, and C. Shipp (1987a). Dietary calcium intake and bone loss from the spine in healthy postmenopausal women. *Am. J. Clin. Nutr.* 46:685–687.

Dawson-Hughes, B., C. Shipp, L. Sadowski, and G. Dallal (1987b). Bone density of the radius, spine, and hip in relation to percent of ideal body weight in postmenopausal women. *Calc. Tissue Int.* 40:310–314.

Del Rio, L., A. Carrascosa, F. Pons, M. Gusinye, D. Yeste, and F.M. Domenech (1994). Bone mineral density of the lumbar spine in white mediterranean Spanish children and adolescents: changes related to age, sex, and puberty. *Pediatr. Res.* 35:362–366.

DeSchepper, J., M.P. Derde, M. Van Den Broeck, A. Piepsz, and M.H. Jonckheer (1991). Normative data for lumbar-spine bone mineral content in children: influence of age, height, weight, and pubertal stage. *J. Nucl. Med.* 32:216–220.

Doyle, F., and J. Brown (1970). Relation between bone mass and muscle weight. *Lancet* 2:391–393.

Drinkwater, B.L. (1990). Physical exercise and bone health. *J. Am. Med. Women's Assoc.* 45:91–97.

Drinkwater, B.L., K. Nilson, C.H. Chesnut, W.J. Bremner, S. Shainholtz, and M.B. Southworth (1984). Bone mineral content of amenorrheic and eumenorrheic athletes. *N. Engl. J. Med.* 311:277–281.

Dyson, K., C.J.R. Blimkie, E.C. Webber, and J.D. Adachi (1995). Bone density in prepubescent female gymnasts. *Med. Sci. Sports Exerc.* 27 (Suppl.): S68, # 381.

Eickhoff, J., L. Molczyk, J.C. Gallagher, and S. De Jong (1993). Influence of isotonic, isometric and isokinetic muscle strength on bone mineral density of the spine and femur in young women. *Bone Miner.* 20:201–209.

Elders, P.J.M., J.C. Netelenbos, P.Lips, E. Khoe, F.C. van Ginkel, K.F.A.M. Hulshof, and P.F. van der Stelt (1989). Perimenopausal bone mass and risk factors. *Bone Miner.* 7:289–299.

Elders, P.J.M., J.C. Netelenbos, P. Lips, F.C. van Ginkel, E. Khoe, O.R. Leeuwenkamp, W.H.L. Hackeng, and P.F. van der Stelt (1991). Calcium supplementation reduces vertebral bone loss in perimenopausal women: a controlled trial in 248 women between 46 and 55 years of age. *J. Clin. Endocrin. Metab.* 73:533–540.

El Haj, A.J., S.L. Minter, C.F. Rawlinson, R. Suswillo, and L.E. Lanyon (1990). Cellular responses to mechanical loading in vitro. *J. Bone Miner. Res.* 5:923–932.

Ettinger, B., H.K. Genant, and C.E. Cann (1987). Postmenopausal bone loss is prevented by treatment with low-dosage estrogen with calcium. *Ann. Intern. Med.* 106:40–45.

Faulkner, R.A., D.A. Bailey, D.T. Drinkwater, A.A. Wilkinson, C.S. Houston, and H.A. McKay (1993a). Regional and total body bone mineral content, bone mineral density, and total body tissue composition in children 8–16 years of age. *Calcif. Tissue Int.* 53:7–12.

Faulkner, R.A., C.S. Houston, D.A. Bailey, D.T. Drinkwater, H.A. McKay, and A.A. Wilkinson (1993b). Comparison of bone mineral content and bone mineral density between dominant and nondominant limbs in children 8–16 years of age. *Am. J. Hum. Biol.* 5:491–499.

Fehily, A.M., R.J. Coles, W.D. Evans, and P.C. Elwood (1992). Factors affecting bone density in young adults. *Am. J. Clin. Nutr.* 56:579–586.

Felson, D.T., Y. Zhang, M.T. Hannan, D.P. Kriel, P.W.F. Wilson, and J.J. Anderson (1993). The effect of postmenopausal estrogen therapy on bone density in elderly women. *N. Engl. J. Med.* 329:1141–1146.

Forwood, M.R., and D.B. Burr (1993). Physical activity and bone mass: exercises in futility? *Bone Miner.* 21:89–112.

Friedlander, A.L., H.R. Genant, S. Sandowsky, N.N. Byl, and C.-C. Gluer (1995). A two-year program of aerobics and weight training enhances bone mineral density of young women. *J. Bone Miner. Res.* 10:574–585.

Friedman, A.J., M. Daly, M. Juneau-Norcross, M.S. Rein, C. Fine, R. Gleason, and M. Leboff (1993). A prospective, randomized trial of gonadotropin-releasing hormone agonist plus estrogen-progestin or progestin "add back" regimens for women with Leiomyomata Uteri. *J. Clin. Endocrin. Metab.* 76:1439–1445.

Frost, H.M. (1987a). Bone mass and the mechanostat: a proposal. *Anat. Rec.* 219:1–9.

Frost, H.M. (1963). Dynamics of bone remodelling. In: H.M. Frost (ed.) *Bone Dynamics.* Springfield: Charles C. Thomas, pp. 320.

Frost, H.M. (1987b). The mechanostat: a proposed pathogenic mechanism of osteoporoses and the bone mass effects of mechanical and nonmechanical agents. *Bone Miner.* 2:73–85.

Frost, H.M. (1991). Some ABC's of skeletal pathophysiology. 7. Tissue mechanisms controlling bone mass. *Calcif. Tissue Int.* 49:303–304.

Frost, H.M. (1988). Vital biomechanics: Proposed general concepts for skeletal adaptations to mechanical usage. *Calcif. Tissue Int.* 42:145–156.

Frusztajer, N.T., S. Dhuper, M.P. Warren, J. Brooks-Gunn, and R.P. Fox (1990). Nutrition and the incidence of stress fractures in ballet dancers. *Am. J. Clin. Nutr.* 51:779–783.

Gallagher, J.C., D. Goldgar, and A. Moy (1987). Total bone calcium in normal women: effect of age and menopause status. *Bone Miner. Res.* 2:491–496.

Gambacciani, M., A. Spinetti, F. Taponeco, B. Cappagli, L. Piaggesi, and P. Fioretti (1994). Longitudinal evaluation of perimenopausal vertebral bone loss: effects of a low-dose oral contraceptive preparation on bone mineral density and metabolism. *Obstet. Gynecol.* 83:392–396.

Garn, S.M. (1970). *The Earlier Gain and the Later Loss of Cortical Bone.* Springfield: Charles C. Thomas.

Genant, H.K., C.E. Cann, B. Ettinger, and G.S. Gordan (1982). Quantitative computed tomography of vertebral spongiosa: a sensitive method for detecting early bone loss after oophorectomy. *Ann. Intern. Med.* 97:699–705.

Genant, H.K., C.-C. Gluer, and J.C. Lotz (1994). Gender differences in bone density, skeletal geometry, and fracture biomechanics. *Radiology* 190:636–640.

Geusens, P., F. Cantatore, J. Nijs, W. Proesmans, F. Emma, and J. Dequeker (1991). Heterogeneity of growth of bone in children at the spine, radius and total skeleton. *Growth Dev. Aging* 55:249–256.

Geusens, P., J. Dequeker, A. Verstraeten, and J. Nijs (1986). Age-, sex-, and menopause-related changes of vertebral and peripheral bone: population study using dual and single photon absorptiometry and radiogrammetry. *J. Nuc. Med.* 27:1540–1549.

Gilsanz, V., M.I. Boechat, R. Gilsanz, M.L. Loro, T.F. Roe, and W.G. Goodman (1994a). Gender differences in vertebral sizes in adults: biomechanical implications. *Radiology* 190:678–682.

Gilsanz, V., M.I. Boechat, T.F. Roe, M.L. Loro, J.W. Sayre, and W.G. Goodman (1994b). Gender differences in vertebral body sizes in children and adolescents. *Radiology* 190:673–677.

Gilsanz, V., D.T. Gibbens, M. Carlson, M.I. Boechat, C.E. Cann, and E.E. Schulz (1988a). Peak trabecular vertebral density: a comparison of adolescent and adult females. *Calcif. Tissue Int.* 43:260–262.

Gilsanz, V., D.T. Gibbens, T.F. Roe, M. Carlson, M.O. Senac, M.I. Boechat, H.K. Huang, E.E. Schulz, C.R. Libanati, and C.C. Cann (1988b). Vertebral bone density in children: effect of puberty. *Radiol.* 166:847–850.

Gilsanz, V., T.F. Roe, S. Mora, G. Costin, and W.G. Goodman (1991). Changes in vertebral bone density in black and white girls during childhood and puberty. *N. Engl. J. Med.* 325:1597–1600.

Glastre, C., P. Braillon, L. David, P. Cochat, P.J. Meunier, and P.D. Delmas (1990). Measurement of bone mineral content of the lumbar spine by dual energy x-ray absorptiometry in normal children: correlations with growth parameters. *J. Clin. Endocrin. Metab.* 70:1330–1333.

Gleeson, P.B., E.J. Protas, A.D. LeBlanc, V.S. Schneider, and H.J. Evans (1990). Effects of weight lifting on bone mineral density in premenopausal women. *J. Bone. Miner. Res.* 5:153–158.

Gordon, C.L., and C.E. Webber (1993). Body composition and bone mineral distribution during growth in females. *Can. Assoc. Radiol. J.* 44:112–116.

Gotfredsen A., A. Hadberg, L. Nilas, and C. Christiansen (1987). Total body bone mineral in healthy adults. *J. Lab. Clin. Med.* 110:362–368.

Greenspan, S.L., L.A. Maitland, E.R. Myers, M.B. Krasnow, and T.H. Kido (1994). Femoral bone loss progresses with age: a longitudinal study in women over age 65. *J. Bone Miner. Res.* 9:1959–1965.

Grimston, S.K., J.R. Engsberg, R. Kloiber, and D.A. Hanley (1991a). Bone mass, external loads, and stress fracture in female runners. *Int. J. Sport Biomech.* 7:293–302.

Grimston, S.K., K. Morrison, J.A. Harder, and D.A. Hanley (1991b). Bone mineral density and calcium intake in children during puberty. In: P. Buckhardt and R.P. Healey (eds.) *Nutritional Aspects of Osteoporosis.* Rome: Raven Press, pp. 77–89.

Grimston, S.K., K. Morrison, J.A. Harder, and D.A. Hanley (1992). Bone mineral density during puberty in western Canadian children. *Bone Miner.* 19:85–96.

Grimston, S.K., N.D. Willows, and D.A. Hanley (1993). Mechanical loading regime and its relationship to bone mineral density in children. *Med. Sci. Sports Exerc.* 25:1203–1210.

Grove, K.A., and B.R. Londeree (1992). Bone density in postmenopausal women: high impact vs low impact exercise. *Med. Sci. Sports Exerc.* 24:1190–1194.

Grynpas, M. (1993). Age and disease-related changes in the mineral of bone. *Calcif. Tissue Int.* 53 (Suppl. 1):S57–S64.

Gunnes, M. (1994). Bone mineral density in the cortical and trabecular distal forearm in healthy children and adolescents. *Acta. Paediatr.* 83:463–467.

Gutin, B., and M. Kasper (1992). Can vigorous exercise play a role in osteoporosis prevention? A review. *Osteoporosis Int.* 2:55–69.

Haapasalo, H., P. Kannus, H. Sievanen, A. Heinonen, P. Oja, and I. Vuori (1994). Long-term unilateral loading and bone mineral density and content in female squash players. *Calcif. Tissue Int.* 54:249–255.

Haenggi, A.V., J.P Casez, M.H. Birkhaeuser, K. Lippaner, and P. Jaeger (1994). Bone mineral density in young women with long-standing amenorrhea: limited effect of hormone replacement therapy with ethinylestradiol and desogestrel. *Osteoporosis Int.* 4:99–103.

Hagino, H., K. Yamamoto, R. Teshima, H. Kishimoto, and T. Nakamura (1990). Fracture incidence and bone mineral density of the distal radius in Japanese children. *Arch. Orthop. Trauma Surg.* 109:262–264.

Hagiwara, S., T. Miki, Y. Nishizawa, H. Ochi, Y. Onoyama, and H. Morii (1989). Quantification of bone mineral content using dual-photon absorptiometry in a normal Japanese population. *J. Bone Miner. Res.* 4:217–222.

Halle, J.S., G.L. Smidt, K.D. O'Dwyer, and S.Y. Lin (1990). Relationship between trunk muscle torque and bone mineral content of the lumbar spine and hip in healthy postmenopausal women. *Phys. Ther.* 70:690–699.

Hannan, M.T., D.T. Felson, and J.J. Anderson (1992). Bone mineral density in elderly women: results from the Framingham Osteoporosis study. *J. Bone Miner. Res.* 7:547–553.

Hansson, T., and B. Roos (1986). Age changes in bone mineral of the lumbar spine in normal women. *Calcif. Tissue Int.* 38:249–251.

Harris, S., and B. Dawson-Hughes (1992). Rates of change in bone mineral density of the spine, heel, femoral neck and radius in late postmenopausal women. *Calcif. Tissue Int.* 17:87–95.

Hatori, M., A. Hasgawa, H. Adachi, A. Shinozaki, R. Hayashi, H. Okano, H. Miaumuma, and K. Murata (1993). The effects of walking at the anaerobic threshold level on bone loss in postmenopausal women. *Calcif. Tiss. Int.* 52:411–414.

Heaney, R.P. (1993). Is there a role for bone quality in fragility fractures? *Calcif. Tissue Int.* 53(Suppl.):S3–S6.

Heaney, R.P. (1991). Lifelong calcium intake and prevention of bone fragility in the aged. *Calcif. Tissue Int.* (Suppl.) 49:S42–S45.

Heaney, R.P. (1988). Nutritional factors in bone health. In: B. Lawrence and L.J. Melton, III (eds.) *Osteoporosis: Etiology, Diagnosis, and Management.* New York: Raven Press, pp. 359–372.

Heaney, R.P., R.R. Recker, and P.D. Saville (1977). Calcium balance and calcium requirements in middle-aged women. *Am. J. Clin. Nutr.* 30:1603–1611.

Heaney, R.P., R.R. Recker, and P.D. Saville (1978a). Menopausal changes in bone remodelling. *J. Lab. Clin. Med.* 92:964–970.

Heaney, R.P., R.R. Recker, and P.D. Saville (1978b). Menopausal changes in calcium balance performance. *J. Lab. Clin. Med.* 92:953–963.

Heaney, R.P., R.R. Recker, M.R. Stegman, A.J. Moy (1989). Calcium absorption in women: relationship to calcium intake, estrogen status and age. *J. Bone Miner. Res.* 4:469–475.

Heikkinen, J., E. Kurttila-Matero, E. Kyllonen, J. Vuori, T. Takala, and H.K. Vaananen (1991). Moderate exercise does not enhance the positive effect of estrogen on bone mineral density in postmenopausal women. *Calcif. Tissue Int.* 49 (Suppl.):S83–S84.

Heinonen, A., P. Oja, P. Kannus, H. Sievanen, A. Manttari, and I. Vuori (1993). Bone mineral density of female athletes in different sports. *Bone Miner.* 23:1–14.

Heinrich, C.H., S.B. Going, R.W. Pamenter, C.D. Perry, T.W. Boyden, and T.G. Lohman (1990). Bone mineral content of cyclically menstruating female resistance and endurance trained athletes. *Med. Sci. Sports Exerc.* 22:558–563.

Henderson, R.C. (1991). Assessment of bone mineral content in children. *J. Pediatr. Orthop.* 11:314–317.

Henderson, R.C., and P.R.L. Hayes (1994). Bone mineralization in children and adolescents with a milk allergy. *Bone Miner.* 27:1–12.

Henderson, R., G. Kemp, and H. Campion (1992). Residual bone-mineral density and muscle strength after fractures of the tibia or femur in children. *J. Bone Joint Surg. Am.* 74:211–218.

Holbrook, T.L., E. Barnett-Connor, M. Klauber, and D. Sartoris (1991). A population based comparison of quantitative dual-energy absorptiometry with dual-photon absorptiometry of the spine and legs. *Calcif. Tissue Int.* 49:305–307.

Horsman, A., and M.N. Birchall (1990). Assessment and modification of hip fracture risk predictions of a stochastic model. In: H.H. Deluca and R. Mazess (eds.) *Osteoporosis: Physiological Basis, Assessment, and Treatment.* New York: American Elsevier, pp. 45–54.

Horsman, A., and L. Burkinshaw (1989). Stochastic models of femoral bone loss and hip fracture risk. In: M.J. Kleerkoper and S.M. Krane (eds.) *Clinical Disorders of Bone & Mineral Metabolism.* New York: Mary Ann Liebert, Inc., pp. 253–263.

Hreshchyshyn, M.M., A. Hopkins, S. Zylstra, and M. Anbar (1988). Effects of natural menopause, hysterectomy, and oophorectomy on lumbar-spine and femoral neck bone densities. *Obstet. Gynecol.* 72:631–638.

Isaia, G.C., G. Salamano, M. Musseta, and G.M. Molinatti (1990). Vertebral bone loss in menopause. *Exp. Geront.* 25:303–307.

Jacobson, P.C., W. Beaver, S.A. Grubb, T.N. Taft, and R.V. Talmage (1984). Bone density in women: college athletes and older athletic women. *J. Orthop. Res.* 2:328–332.

Johnston, C.C., Jr., J.Z. Miller, C.W. Slemenda, T.K. Reister, S.Hui, J.C. Christian, and M. Peacock (1992). Calcium supplementation and increases in bone mineral density in children. *N. Engl. J. Med.* 327:82–87.

Jonsson, B., K. Ringsberg, P.O. Josefsson, O. Johnell, and M. Birch-Jensen (1992). Effects of physical activity on bone mineral content and muscle strength in women: a cross-sectional study. *Bone* 13:191–195.

Kanders, B., D.W. Dempster, and R. Lindsay (1988). Interaction of calcium nutrition and physical activity on bone mass in young women. *J. Bone Min. Res.* 3:145–149.

Kanis, J.A. (1991a). Calcium requirements for optimal skeletal health in women. *Calcif. Tissue Int.* 49 (Suppl.):S33–S41.

Kanis, J.A. (1991b). Pathophysiology and histopathology. In: J.A. Kanis (ed.) *Pathophysiology and Treatment of Paget's Disease of Bone.* London: Martin Dunitz, pp. 12–40.

Kanis, J.A., and S. Adami (1994). Bone loss in the elderly. *Osteop. Int.* 1 (Suppl.):S59–65.

Katzman, D.K., L.K. Bachrach, D.R. Carter, and R. Marcus (1991). Clinical and anthropometric correlates of bone mineral acquisition in healthy adolescent girls. *J. Clin. Endocrin. Metab.* 73:1332–1339.

Kelly, P.J., L. Twomey, P.N. Sambrook, and J.A. Eisman (1990). Sex differences in peak adult bone mineral density. *J. Bone Miner. Res.* 5:1169–1175.

Kirk, S., C.F. Sharp, N. Elbaum, D.B. Endres, S.M. Simons, J.G. Mohler, and R.K. Rude (1989). Effect of long-distance running on bone mass in women. *J. Bone Miner. Res.* 4:515–522.

Kleerekoper, M., K. Tolia, and A.M. Parfitt (1981). Nutritional, endocrine, and demographic aspects of osteoporosis. *Orthop. Clin. North Am.* 12:547–558.

Krabbe, S., C. Christiansen, P. Rodbro, and I. Transbol (1979). Effect of puberty on rates of bone growth and mineralization. *Arch. Dis. Child.* 54:950–953.

Krabbe, S., L. Hummer, and C. Christiansen (1984). Longitudinal study of calcium metabolism in male puberty. II. Relationship between mineralization and serum testosterone. *Acta Paediatr. Scand.* 73:750–755.

Krall, E.A., and B. Dawson-Hughes (1993). Heritable and life-style determinants of bone mineral density. *J. Bone Miner. Res.* 8:1–9.

Kriska, A.M., R.B. Sandler, J.A. Cauley, R.E. LaPorte, D.L. Hom, and G. Pambianco (1988). The assessment of historical physical activity and its relation to adult bone parameters. *Am. J. Epidemiol.* 127:1053–1063.

Kritz-Silverstein, D., and E. Barrett-Connor (1994). Grip strength and bone mineral density in older women. *J. Bone Miner. Res.* 9:45–51.

Kroger, H., A. Kotaniemi, L. Kroger, and E. Alhava. (1993). Development of bone mass and bone density of the spine and femoral neck—a prospective study of 65 children and adolescents. *Bone Miner.* 23:171–182.

Kroger, H., A. Kotaniemi, P. Vainio, and E. Alhava (1992). Bone densitometry of the spine and femur in children by dual-energy x-ray absorptiometry. *Bone Miner.* 17:75–85.

Krolner, B., B. Toft, S.P. Nelson, and E. Tonevold (1983). Physical exercise as prophylaxis against involutional vertebral bone loss: a controlled trial. *Clin. Sci.* 64:541–546.

Laitinen, K., M. Valimaki, and P. Keto (1991). Bone mineral density measured by dual-energy x-ray absorptiometry in healthy Finnish women. *Calcif. Tissue Int.* 48:224–231.

Lane, N.E., D.A. Bloch, H.H. Jones, W.H. Marshall, P.D. Wood, and J.F. Fries (1986). Long-distance running, bone density and osteoarthritis. *J.A.M.A.* 255:1147–1151.

LeBlanc, A.D., V.S. Schneider, H.J. Evans, D.A. Engelbretson, and J.M. Krebs (1990). Bone mineral loss and recovery after 17 weeks of bed rest. *J. Bone Miner. Res.* 5:843–850.

Lee, W.T.K., S.S.F. Leung, M.-Y. Ng, S.-F. Wang, Y.-C. Xu, W.-P. Zeng, and J. Lau (1993). Bone mineral content of two populations of Chinese children with different calcium intakes. *Bone Miner.* 23:195–206.

Li, J-Y., B.L. Specker, M.L. Ho, and R.C. Tsang (1989). Bone mineral content in Black and White children 1 to 6 years of age. *A.J.D.C.* 143:1346–1349.

Liel, Y., J. Edwards, J. Shary, K.M. Spicer, L. Gordon, and N.H. Bell (1988). The effects of race and body habitus on bone mineral density of the radius, hip, and spine in premenopausal women. *J. Clin. Endocrin. Metab.* 66:1247–1250.

Lindquist, O., C. Bengtsson, T. Hansson, and E. Jonsson (1983). Changes in bone mineral content of the axial skeleton in relation to aging and the menopause. *Scand. J. Clin. Lab. Invest.* 43:333–338.

Lindsay, R., and J.F. Tohme (1990). Estrogen treatment of patients with established postmenopausal osteoporosis. *Obstet. Gynecol.* 76:290–295.

Lloyd, T., M.B. Andon, N.Rollings, J.K. Martel, J.R. Landis, L.M. Demers, D.F. Eggli, K. Kieselhorst, and H.E. Kulin (1993). Calcium supplementation and bone mineral density in adolescent girls. *J.A.M.A.* 270:841–844.

Lloyd, T., C. Myers, J.R. Buchanan, and L.M. Demers (1988). Collegiate women athletes with irregular menses during adolescence have decreased bone density. *Obstet. Gynecol.* 72:639–642.

Lloyd, T., N. Rollings, M.B. Andon, L.M. Demers, D.F. Eggli, K. Kieselhorst, H. Kulin, J.R. Landis, J.K. Martel, G. Orr, and P. Smith (1992). Determinants of bone density in young women. I. Relationships among pubertal development, total body bone mass, and total body bone density in premenopausal females. *J. Clin. Endocrinol. Metab.* 75:383–387.

Lloyd, T., S.J. Triantafyllou, E.R. Baker, P.S. Houts, J.A. Whiteside, A. Kalenak, and P.G. Stumpf (1986). Women athletes with menstrual irregularity have increased musculoskeletal injuries. *Med. Sci. Sports Exerc.* 18:374–379.

Lohman, T.G., S.B. Going, R.W. Pamenter, T. Boyden, L.B. Houtkooper, C. Ritenbaugh, M. Hall, L.A. Bare, A. Hill, and M. Aickin (1992). Effects of weight training on lumbar-spine and femur bone mineral density in premenopaucal females. *Med. Sci. Sports Exerc.* 24 (Suppl.):S188, #1123.

Loucks, A. (1988). Osteoporosis prevention begins in childhood. In: E.W. Brown & C.F. Branta (eds.) *Competitive Sports For Children and Youth. An Overview of Research Issues.* Champaign: Human Kinetics, pp. 213-223.

Loucks, A., and S. Horvath (1985). Athletic amenorrhea—a review. *Med. Sci. Sports Exerc.* 17:56-72.

Lu, P.W., J.N. Briody, G.D. Ogle, K. Morley, I.R.J. Humphries, J. Allen, R. Howman-Giles, D. Sillence, and C.T. Cowell (1994). Bone mineral density of total body, spine, and femoral neck in children and young adults: a cross-sectional and longitudinal study. *J. Bone Miner. Res.* 9:1451-1458.

Luckey, M.M., D.E. Meier, J.P. Mandeli, M.C. DaCosta, M.L. Hubbard, and S.J. Goldsmith (1989). Radial and vertebral bone density in white and black women: evidence for racial differences in premenopausal bone homeostasis. *J. Clin. Endocrin. Metab.* 69:762-770.

Lufkin, E.G., H.W. Wahner, W.M. O'Fallon, S.F. Hodgson, M.A. Kotoqicz, A.W. Lane, H.L. Judd, R.H. Caplan, and B.L. Riggs (1992). Treatment of postmenopausal osteoporosis with transdermal estrogen. *Ann. Intern. Med.* 117:1-9.

Luisetto, G., M. Zangari, L. Tizian, A. Nardi, E. Ramazzina, S. Adami, and P. Galuppo (1993). Influence of aging and menopause in determining vertebral and distal forearm bone loss in adult healthy women. *Bone Miner.* 22:9-25.

Marcus, R., C. Cann, P. Mudvig, J. Minkoff, M. Goddard, M. Bayer, M. Martin, L. Gaudiani, W. Haskell, and H. Genant (1985). Menstrual function and bone mass in elite woman distance runners. *Ann. Intern. Med.* 102:158-163.

Marcus, R., B. Drinkwater, G. Dalsky, J. Dufek, D. Raab, C. Slemenda, and C. Snow-Harter (1992). Osteoporosis and exercise in women. *Med. Sci. Sports Exerc.* 24:S301-S307.

Marcus, R., G. Greendale, B.A. Blunt, T.L. Bush, S. Sherman, R. Sherwin, H. Wahner, and B. Wells (1994). Correlates of bone mineral density in the postmenopausal estrogen/progestin interventions trial. *J. Bone Miner. Res.* 9:1467-1476.

Martin, D., and M. Notelovitz (1993). Effects of aerobic training on bone mineral density of postmenopausal women. *J. Bone Miner. Res.* 8:931-936.

Martin, A.D., K.G. Silverthorn, C.S. Houstyon, S. Bernhordson, A. Wajda, and L.L. Roos (1991). Trends in fracture of the proximal femur in two million Canadians: 1972 to 1984. *Clin. Orthop. Rel. Res.* 266:111-118.

Matkovic V., and R.P. Heaney (1992). Calcium balance during human growth: evidence for threshold behavior. *Am. J. Clin. Nutr.* 55:992-996.

Matkovic, V., D. Fontana, C. Tominac, P. Goel, and C.H. Chestnut III (1990). Factors that influence peak bone mass formation: a study of calcium balance and the inheritance of bone mass in adolescent females. *Am. J. Clin. Nutr.* 52:878-888.

Matkovic, V., K. Kostial, I. Simonovic, R. Buziua, A. Brodarec, and B.E.C. Nordin (1979). Bone status and fracture rates in two regions of Yugoslavia. *Am. J. Clin. Nutr.* 32:540-549.

Mazess, R.B. (1982). On aging bone loss. *Clin. Orthop. Rel. Res.* 165:239-252.

Mazess, R.B., and H.S. Barden (1991). Bone density in premenopausal women: effects of age, dietary intake, physical activity, smoking and birth-control pills. *Am. J. Clin. Nutr.* 53:132-142.

Mazess, R.B., and H.M. Wahner (1988). Nuclear medicine and densitometry. In: B. L. Riggs and L.J. Melton, III (eds.) *Osteoporosis: Etiology, Diagnosis, and Management.* New York: Raven Press, pp. 251-295.

Mazess, R.B., H.S. Barden, M. Ettinger, C. Johnston, B. Dawson-Hughes, D. Baran, M. Powell, and M. Notelovitz (1987). Spine and femur density using dual-photon absorptiometry in US white women. *Bone Miner.* 2:211-219.

McCormick, D.P., S.W. Ponder, H.D. Fawcett, and J.L. Palmer (1991). Spinal bone mineral density in 335 normal and obese children and adolescents: evidence for ethnic and sex differences. *J. Bone Miner. Res.* 6:507-513.

McCulloch, R.G., and D.A. Bailey (1990). Calcium intake and bone density: a review. *Can. J. Aging* 9:167-176.

McCulloch, R.G., D.A. Bailey, C.S. Houston, and B.L. Dodd (1990). Effects of physical activity, dietary calcium intake and selected lifestyle factors on bone density in young women. *Can. Med. Assoc. J.* 142:221-227.

McCulloch, R.G., D.A. Bailey, R.L. Whalen, C.S. Houston, R.A. Faulkner, and B.R. Craven (1992). Bone density and bone mineral content of adolescent soccer athletes and competitive swimmers. *Ped. Exerc. Sci.* 4:319-330.

Meier, D.E., E.S. Orwoll, and J.M. Jones (1984). Marked disparity between trabecular and cortical bone loss with age in healthy men. Measurement by vertebral computed tomography and radial photon absorptiometry. *Ann. Intern. Med.* 101:605-612.

Melton, L.J. (1988). Epidemiology of fractures. In: B.L. Riggs & L.J. Melton, III (eds.) *Osteoporosis: Etiology, Diagnosis, and Management.* New York: Raven Press, pp. 133-154.

Metz, J.A., J.J.B. Anderson, and P.N. Gallagher (1993). Intakes of calcium, phosphorous, and protein, and physical activity level are related to radial bone mass in young adult women. *Am. J. Clin. Nutr.* 58:537–542.

Michel, B.A., D.A. Bloch, and J.F. Fries (1989). Weight-bearing exercise, overexercise, and lumbar bone density over age 50 years. *Arch. Intern. Med.* 149:2325–2329.

Miller, J.Z., C.W. Slemenda, F.J. Meaney, T. K. Reister, S. Hui, and C.C. Johnston (1991). The relationship of bone mineral density and anthropometric variables in healthy male and female children. *Bone Miner.* 14:137–152.

Moller. M., A. Horsman, B. Hervald, M. Hauge, M. Henninsden, and B.E.C. Nordin (1978). Metacarpal morphometry in monozygotic elderly twins. *Calcif. Tissue Res.* 25:197–201.

Montoye, H.J. (1987). Better bones and biodynamics. The 1987 C.H. McCloy Research Lecture. *Res. Quart.* 58:334–348.

Morrison, N.A., J.C. Qui, A. Tokita, P.J. Kelly, L. Crofts, T.V. Nguyen, P.N. Sambrook, and J.A. Eisman (1994). Prediction of bone density from vitamin D receptor alleles. *Nature* 367:284–287.

Mueller, K.H., A. Trias, and R.D. Ray (1966). Bone density and composition. Age-related and pathological changes in water and mineral content. *J. Bone Joint Surg.* 48A:140–148.

Myburgh, K.H., L.K. Bachrach, B. Lewis, K. Kent, and R. Marcus (1993). Low bone mineral density at axial and appendicular sites in amenorrheic athletes. *Med. Sci. Sports Exerc.* 25:1197–1202.

Myerson, M., B. Gutin, M.P. Warren, J. Wang, S. Lichtman, and R.N. Pierson (1992). Total body bone density in amenorrheic runners. *Obstet. Gynecol.* 79:973–978.

Nelson, M.E., M.A. Fiatarone, C.M. Morganti, I. Trice, R.A. Greenberg, and W.J. Evans (1994). Effects of high-intensity strength training on multiple risk factors for osteoporotic fractures. A randomized controlled trial. *J.A.M.A.* 272:1909–1914.

Nelson, M.E., E.C. Fisher, F.A. Dilmanian, G.E. Dallal, and W.J. Evans (1991). A 1-year walking program and increase dietary calcium in postmenopausal women: effects on bone. *Am. J. Clin. Nutr.* 53:1304–1311.

Nelson, D.A., M. Kleerekoper, and A.M. Parfitt (1988a). Bone mass, skin color and body size among black and white women. *Bone Miner.* 4:257–264.

Nelson, M.E., C.N. Meredith, B. Dawson-Hughes, and W.J. Evans (1988b). Hormone and bone mineral status in endurance-trained and sedentary postmenopausal women. *J. Clin. Endocrinol. Metab.* 66:927–933.

Newton-John, H.F., and D.B. Morgan (1970). The loss of bone with age, osteoporosis, and fractures. *Clin. Orthop.* 71:229–252.

Nguyen, T.V., P.J. Kelly, P.N. Sambrook, C. Gilbert, N.A. Pocock, and J.A. Eisman (1994). Lifestyle factors and bone density in the elderly: implications for osteoporosis prevention. *J. Bone Miner. Res.* 9:1339–1346.

Nichols, D.L., C.F. Sanborn, S.L. Bonnick, V. Ben-Ezra, B. Gench, and N.M. DiMarco (1994). The effects of gymnastics training on bone mineral density. *Med. Sci. Sports Exerc.* 26:1220–1225.

Nilas, L., C. Christiansen (1988). Rates of bone loss in normal women: evidence of accelerated trabecular bone loss after the menopause. *Eur. J. Clin. Invest.* 18:529–534.

Nordin, B.E.C., B.E. Chatterton, T.A. Steurer, and C.J. Walker (1986). Forearm bone mineral content does not decline with age in premenopausal women. *Clin. Orthop. Rel. Res.* 211:252–256.

Nordin, B.E., B.E. Chatterton, C.J. Walker, and J. Wishart (1987). The relation of forearm density to peripheral fractures in postmenopausal women. *Med. J. Aust.* 146:300–304.

Nottestad, S.Y., J.J. Baumel, D.B. Kimmel, R.R. Recker, and R.P. Heaney (1987). The proportion of trabecular bone in human vertebrae. *J. Bone Miner. Res.* 2:221–229.

Odland, L.M., R.L. Mason, and A.I. Alexff (1972). Bone density and dietary findings of 409 Tennessee subjects. 1. Bone density considerations. *Am. J. Clin. Nutr.* 25:905–907.

Pacifici, R., R. Rupich, I. Vered, K.C. Fisher, M. Griffin, N. Susman, and L.V. Avioli (1988). Dual energy radiography (DER): a preliminary comparative study. *Calcif. Tissue Int.* 43:189–191.

Panzer, V.P., G.A. Wood, B.T. Bates, and B.R. Mason (1988). Lower extremity loads in landings of elite gymnasts. In: G. deGroot, A. Hollander, P. Huijing, and G. van Ingen Schenau (eds.) *Biomechanics XI.* Amsterdam: Free University Press, pp. 727–735.

Parfitt, A.M. (1993). Bone age, mineral density, and fatigue damage. *Calif. Tissue Int.* 53 (Suppl. 1):S82–S86.

Parfitt, A.M. (1988). Bone remodelling: relationship to the amount and structure of bone, and the pathogenesis and prevention of fractures. In: R.L. Riggs and L.J. Melton, III (eds.) *Osteoporosis: Etiology, Diagnosis, and Management.* New York: Raven Press, pp. 45–93.

Parfitt, A.M. (1994). The two faces of growth: benefits and risks to bone integrity. *Osteop. Int.* 4:382–398.

Pocock, N.A., S. Eberl, J.A. Eisman, M.G. Yeates, P.N. Sambrook, J. Freund, and A. Duncan (1987). Dual-photon bone densitometry in normal Australian women: a cross-sectional study. *Med. J. Aust.* 293–297.

Pocock, N.A., J. Eisman, T. Gwinn, P. Sambrook, P. Kelly, J. Freund, and M. Yeates (1989). Muscle strength, physical fitness, and weight but not age predict femoral neck bone mass. *J. Bone Miner. Res.* 4:441–447.

Pocock, N.A., J.A. Eisman, M.G. Yeates, P.N. Sambrook, and S. Eberl (1986). Physical fitness is a major determinant of femoral neck and lumbar-spine BMD. *J. Clin. Invest.* 78:618–621.

Pollitzer, W.S., and J.J.B. Anderson (1989). Ethnic and genetic differences in bone mass: a review with a hereditary vs environmental perspective. *Am. J. Clin. Nutr.* 50:1244–1259.

Ponder, S.W., D.P. McCormick, D. Fawcett, J.L. Palmer, M.G. McKernan, and B.H. Brouhard (1990). Spinal bone mineral density in children aged 5.00 through 11.99 years. *A.J.D.C.* 144:1346–1348.

Prentice, A., T.J. Parsons, and T.J. Cole (1994). Uncritical use of bone mineral density in absorptiometry may lead to size-related artifacts in the identification of bone mineral determinants. *Am. J. Clin. Nutr.* 60:837–842.

Prentice, A., J. Shaw, M.A. Laskey, T.J. Cole, and D.R. Fraser (1991). Bone mineral content of British and rural Gambian women aged 18–80+ years. *Bone Miner.* 12:201–214.

Prior, J.C., Y.M. Vigna, M.T. Schechter, and A.E. Burgess (1990). Spinal bone loss and ovulatory disturbances. *N. Engl. J. Med.* 323:1221–1227.

Pruitt, L.A., R.D. Jackson, R.L. Bartels, and H.J. Lehnhard (1992). Weight-training effects on bone mineral density in early postmenopausal women. *J. Bone Miner. Res.* 7:179–185.

Ramsdale, S.J., E.J. Bassey, and D.W. Pye (1994). Dietary calcium intake relates to bone mineral density in premenopausal women. *Br. J. Nutr.* 71:77–84.

Ravn, P., M.L. Hetland, K. Overgaard, and C. Christiansen (1994). Premenopausal and postmenopausal changes in bone mineral density of the proximal femur measured by dual-energy x-ray absorptiometry. *J. Bone Miner. Res.* 9:1975–1980.

Recker, R.R. (1993). Current therapy for osteoporosis. Clinical review 41. *J. Clin. Endocrin. Metab.* 76:14–16.

Recker, R.R., K.M. Davies, S.M. Hinders, R.P. Heaney, M.R. Stegman, and D.B. Kimmel (1992). Bone gain in young adult women. *J.A.M.A.* 268:2403–2408.

Reid, I.R., R.W. Ames, M.C. Evans, G.D. Gamble, and S.J. Sharpe (1993). Effect of calcium supplementation on bone loss in postmenopausal women. *N. Engl. J. Med.* 328:460–464.

Ribot, C., F. Tremollieres, J.M. Pouilles, J.P. Louvet, and R. Guiraud (1988). Influence of the menopause and aging on spinal density in French women. *Bone Miner.* 5:89–97.

Rice, S., C.J.R. Blimkie, C.E. Webber, D. Levy, J. Martin, D. Parker, and C.L. Gordon (1993). Correlates and determinants of bone mineral content and density in healthy adolescent girls. *Can. J. Physiol. Pharmacol.* 71:923–930.

Rico, H., M. Revilla, E.R. Hernandez, L.F. Villa, and M. Alvarez del Buergo (1992). Sex differences in the acquisition of total bone mineral mass peak assessed through dual-energy x-ray absorptiometry. *Calcif. Tissue Int.* 51:251–254.

Rico, H., M. Revilla, E.R. Hernandez, L.F. Villa, and A. Lopez-Alonso (1991). Total and regional bone mineral content in normal premenopausal women. *Clin. Rheum.* 10:423–425.

Riggs, L.B., and L.J. Melton III (1986). Involutional osteoporosis. *N. Engl. J. Med.* 314:1676–1684.

Riggs, B.L., E. Seeman, S.F. Hodgson, D.R. Taves, and W.M. O'Fallon (1982). Effect of the fluoride/calcium regimen on vertebral fracture occurrence in postmenopausal osteoporosis. *N. Engl. J. Med.* 306:446–450.

Riggs, B.L., H.W. Wahner, L.J. Melton, L.S. Richelson, H.L. Judd, and W.M. O'Fallon (1987). Dietary calcium intake and rates of bone loss in women. *J. Clin. Invest.* 80:979–982.

Riggs, B.L., H.W. Wahner, L.J. Melton III, L.S. Richelson, H.L. Judd, and K.P. Offord (1986). Rate of bone loss in the appendicular and axial skeletons of women. Evidence of substantial vertebral bone loss before menopause. *J. Clin. Invest.* 77:1487–1491.

Riis, B., K. Thomson, and C. Christiansen (1987). Does calcium supplementation prevent postmenopausal bone loss? *N. Engl. J. Med.* 316:173–177.

Risser, W.L., E.J. Lee, A. LeBlanc, H.B.W. Poindexter, J.M.H. Risser, and V. Schneider (1990). Bone density in eumenorrheic female college athletes. *Med. Sci. Sports Exerc.* 22:570–574.

Robinson, T., C. Snow-Harter, D. Gillis, and J. Shaw (1993). Bone mineral density and menstrual cycle status in competitive female runners and gymnasts. *Med. Sci. Sports Exerc.* 25:S49

Robinson, T.L., C. Snow-Harter, D.R. Taaffe, D. Gillis, J. Shaw, and R. Marcus (1995). Gymnasts exhibit higher bone mass than runners despite similar prevalence of amenorrhea and oligomenorrhea. *J. Bone Miner. Res.* 10:26–35.

Rockwell, J.C., A.M. Sorensen, S. Baker, D. Leahey, J.L. Stock, J. Michaels, and D.T. Baran (1990). Weight training decreases vertebral bone density in premenopausal women: a prospective study. *J. Clin. Endocrin. Metab.* 71:988–993.

Rodin, A., B. Murby, M.A. Smith, M. Caleffi, I. Fentiman, M.G. Chapman, and I. Fogelman (1990). Premenopausal bone loss in the lumbar spine and neck of femur: a study of 225 caucasian women. *Bone* 11:1–5.

Ross. P.D., Y.-F. He, J.W. Davis, R.S. Epstein, and R.D. Wasnich (1994). Normal ranges for bone loss rates. *Bone Miner.* 26:169–180.

Rubin, C.T., and L.E. Lanyon (1985). Regulation of bone mass by mechanical strain magnitude. *Calcif. Tissue Int.* 37:411–417.

Rubin, K., V. Schirduan, P. Gendreau, M. Sarfarazi, R. Mendola, and G. Dalsky (1993). Predictors of axial and peripheral bone mineral density in healthy children and adolescents, with special attention to the role of puberty. *J. Pediatr.* 123:863–870.

Sandler, R.B., C.W. Slemenda, R.E. Laporte, J.A. Cauley, M.W. Schramm, M.L. Barresi, and A.M. Kriska (1985). Post-menopausal bone density and milk consumption in childhood and adolescence. *Am. J. Clin. Nutr.* 42:270–274.

Seeman E. (1994). Reduced bone density in women with fractures: Contribution of low peak bone density and rapid bone loss. *Osteop. Int.* 1 Suppl.:S15–25.

Seeman, E., G.I. Szmukler, C. Formica, C. Tsalamandris, and R. Mestrovic (1992). Osteoporosis in anorexia nervosa: the influence of peak bone density, bone loss, oral contraceptive use, and exercise. *J. Bone Miner. Res.* 7:1467–1474.

Sentipal, J., G.M. Wardlaw, J. Mahan, and V. Matkovic (1991). Influence of calcium intake and growth indexes on vertebral bone mineral density in young females. *Am. J. Clin. Nutr.* 54:425–428.

Shipp, C.C., P.S. Berger, M.S. Dechr, and B. Dawson-Hughes (1988). Precision of dual-photon absorptiometry. *Calcif. Tissue Int.* 42:287–292.

Sinaki, M., and B.A. Mikkelsen (1984). Postmenopausal spinal osteoporosis: flexion versus extension exercises. *Arch. Phys. Med. Rehabil.* 65:593–596.

Sledge, C.B., and C.L.T. Rubin (1989). Formation and resorption of bone. In: W.N. Kelley, E.D. Harris, Jr., S. Ruddy, and C.B. Sledge (eds.) *Textbook of Rheumatology*, 3rd Ed. Philadelphia: W.B. Saunders Co., pp. 54–75.

Slemenda, C.W., and C.C. Johnston (1993). High intensity activities in young women: site specific bone mass effects among female figure skaters. *Bone Miner.* 20:125–132.

Slemenda, C.W., J.C. Christian, C.J. Williams, J.A. Norton, and C.C. Johnston (1991a). Genetic determinants of bone mass in adult women: a reevaluation of the twin model and the potential importance of gene interaction on heritability estimates. *J. Bone Miner. Res.* 6:561–567.

Slemenda, C.W., J.Z. Miller, S.L. Hui, T.K. Reister, and C.C. Johnston (1991b). Role of physical activity in the development of skeletal mass in children. *J. Bone Miner. Res.* 6:1227–1233.

Slemenda, C.W., T.K. Reister, J.Z. Miller, J.C. Christian, and C.C. Johnston Jr.(1994). Influences on skeletal mineralization in children and adolescents: evidence for varying effects of sexual maturation and physical activity. *J. Pediatr.* 125:201–207.

Slemenda, C.W., T.K. Reister, M. Peacock, and C.C. Johnston (1993). Bone growth in children following the cessation of calcium supplementation. *J. Bone Miner. Res.* 8 (Suppl.):S154.

Smith, D.M., W.E. Nance, K.W. Kang, J.C. Christian, and C.C. Johnston Jr. (1973). Genetic factors in determining bone mass. *J. Clin. Invest.* 52:2800–2808.

Smith, E.L. C. Gilligan, M. McAdam, C.P. Ensign, and P. Smith (1989). Deterring bone loss by exercise intervention in premenopausal and postmenopausal women. *Calcif. Tiss. Int.* 44:312–321.

Smith, E.L., W. Reddan, and P.E. Smith (1981). Physical activity and calcium modalities for bone mineral increase in aged women. *Med. Sci. Sports Exerc.* 13:60–64.

Snead, D.B., A. Weltman, J.Y. Weltman, W.S. Evans, J.D. Veldhuis, M.M. Varma, C.D. Teates, E.A. Dowling, and A.D. Rogol (1992). Reproductive hormones and bone mineral density in women runners. *J. Appl. Physiol.* 72:2149–2156.

Snow-Harter, C., and R. Marcus (1991). Exercise, bone mineral density, and osteoporosis. In: J. Holloszy (ed.) *Exercise and Sport Sciences Reviews*. Philadelphia: Williams and Wilkins, Vol. 19, pp. 351–388.

Snow-Harter, C., M.L. Bouxsein, B.T. Lewis, D.R. Carter, and R. Marcus (1992). Effects of resistance and endurance exercise on bone mineral status of young women: a randomized exercise intervention trial. *J. Bone Miner. Res.* 7:761–769.

Snow-Harter, C., M. Bouxsein, B. Lewis, S. Charette, P. Weinstein, and R. Marcus (1990). Muscle strength as a predictor of bone mineral density in young women. *J. Bone Miner. Res.* 5:589–595.

Southard, R.N., J.D. Morris, J.D. Mahan, J.R. Hayes, M.A. Torch, A. Sommer, and W.B. Zipf (1991). Bone mass in healthy children: measurement with quantitative DXA. *Radiology* 179:735–738.

Sowers, M.R., M.K. Clarke, B. Hollis, R.B. Wallace, and M. Jannausch (1992). Radial bone mineral density in pre-and perimenopausal women: a prospective study of rates and risk factors for loss. *J. Bone Miner. Res.* 7:647–657.

Sowers, M.F., K. Clark, R. Wallace, M. Jannausch, and J. Lemke (1991). Prospective study of radial bone mineral density in a geographically defined population of postmenopausal Caucasian women. *Calcif. Tissue Int.* 48:232–239.

Steiger, P., S.R. Cummings, D.M. Black, N.E. Spencer, and H.K. Genant (1992). Age-related decrements in bone mineral density in women over 65. *J. Bone Miner. Res.* 7:625–632.

Stevenson, J.C., B. Lees, M. Devenport, M.P. Cust, and K.F. Ganger (1989). Determinants of bone density in normal women: risk factors for future osteoporosis. *B.M.J.* 298:924–927.

Sugimoto, T., M. Nishino, T. Tsunenari, M. Kawakatsu, K. Shimogaki, Y. Fujii, H. Negishi, M. Tsutsumi, M. Fukase, and K. Chihara (1994). Radial bone mineral content of normal Japanese infants and prepubertal children: influence of age, sex, and body size. *Bone Miner.* 24:189–200.

Taaffe, D.R., C. Snow-Harter, D.A. Connolly, T.L. Robinson, M.D. Brown, and R. Marcus (1995). Differential effects of swimming versus weight-bearing activity on bone mineral status of eumenorrheic athletes. *J. Bone Miner. Res.* 10:586–593.

BONE MINERALIZATION PATTERNS **141**

Takeshita, T., Z. Yamagata, S. Lijima, T. Nakamura, Y. Ouchi, H. Orimo, and A. Asaka (1992). Genetic and environmental factors of bone mineral density indicated in Japanese twins. *Gerontol.* 39(suppl 1):43–49.

Talmage, R.V., and J.J.B. Anderson (1984). Bone density loss in women: effects of childhood activity, exercise, calcium intake and estrogen theory. *Calcif. Tissue Int.* 36:S52.

Talmage, R.V., S.S. Stinnett, J.T. Landwehr, L.M. Vincent, and W.H. McCartner (1986). Age-related loss of bone mineral density in non-athletic and athletic women. *Bone Miner.* 1:115–125.

Teegarden, D., and C.M. Weaver (1994). Calcium supplementation increases bone density in adolescent girls. *Nutr. Rev.* 52:171–173.

Teitelbaum, S.L. (1993). Skeletal growth and development. In: M.J. Favus (ed.) *Primer on the Metabolic Bone Diseases and Disorders of Mineral Metabolism.* Second Ed. New York: Raven Press, pp. 7–11.

Theintz, G., B. Buchs, R. Rizzoli, D. Slosman, H. Clavien, P.C. Sizonenko, and J.-PH Bonjour (1992). Longitudinal monitoring of bone mass accumulation in healthy adolescents: Evidence for a marked reduction after 16 years of age at the levels of lumbar spine and femoral neck in female subjects. *J. Clin. Endocrin. Metab.* 75:1060–1065.

Thomas K.A., S.D. Cook, J.T. Bennett, T.S. Whitecloud III, and J.C. Rice (1991). Femoral neck and lumbar-spine bone mineral densities in a normal population 3–20 years of age. *J. Pediatr. Orthop.* 11:48–58.

Tothill, P. (1989). Methods of bone mineral measurement. *Phys. Med. Biol.* 34:543–572.

Treasure, J.L., G.F.M. Russell, I. Fogelman, and B. Murby (1987). Reversible bone loss in anorexia nervosa. *Brit. Med. J.* 295:474–475.

Trotter, M., and B.B. Hixon (1974). Sequential changes in weight, density, and percentage ash weight of human skeletons from an early fetal period through old age. *Anat. Rec.* 179:1–18.

Tupparainen, M., H. Kroger, S. Saarikoski, R. Honkanen, and E. Alhava (1994). The effect of previous oral contraceptive use on bone mineral density in perimenopausal women. *Osteoporosis Int.* 4:93–98.

Turner, J.G., N.L. Gilchrist, E.M. Ayling, A.J. Hassall, E.A. Hooke, and W.A. Sadler (1992). Factors affecting bone mineral density in high school girls. *NZ. Med. J.* 105:95–96.

Tylavsky, F., J. Anderson, R. Talmage, and T. Taft (1992). Are calcium intakes and physical activity patterns during adolescence related to radial bone mass of college-aged females? *Osteoporosis Int.* 2:232–240.

Wang, Q., C. Hassager, P. Ravn, S. Wang, and C. Christiansen (1994). Total and regional body-composition changes in early postmenopausal women: age-related or menopause-related? *Am. J. Clin. Nutr.* 60:843–848.

Warren, T.K., S.S.F. Leung, S.-H. Wang, Y.-C. Xu, W.-P. Zeng, J. Lau, S.J. Oppenheimer, and J.C.Y. Cheng (1994). Double-blind, controlled calcium supplementation and bone mineral accretion in children accustomed to a low-calcium diet. *Am. J. Clin. Nutr.* 60:744–750.

Webber, C.E., C.L. Gordon, L.F. Chambers, J. Martin, C.J.R. Blimkie, and N. McCartney (1993). Body composition and bone mass in female adolescents and elderly subjects entering exercise programs. *Basic Life Sci.* 60:259–262.

Weiss, N.S., C.L. Ure, J.H. Ballard, A.R. Williams, and J.R. Daling (1980). Decreased risk of fractures of the hip and lower forearm with postmenopausal use of estrogen. *N. Engl. J. Med.* 303:1195–1198.

Welten, D.C., H.C.G. Kemper, G.B. Post, W.van Mechelen, J. Twisk, P. Lips, and G.J. Teule (1994). Weight-bearing activity during youth is a more important factor for peak bone mass than calcium intake. *J. Bone Miner. Res.* 9:1089–1096.

Winter, J.S.D. (1978). Prepubertal and pubertal endocrinology. In: F. Falkner and J.M. Tanner (eds.) *Human Growth. 2. Postnatal Growth.* New York: Plenum Press, pp. 183–213.

Wolman, R.L. (1990). Bone mineral density in elite female athletes. *Ann. Rheum. Dis.* 49:1013–1016.

Wolman, R.L., P. Clark, E. McNally, M. Harries, and J. Reeve (1990). Menstrual state and exercise as determinants of spinal trabecular bone density in female athletes. *B.M.J.* 301:516–518.

Wolman, R.L., L. Faulmann, P. Clark, R. Hesp, and M.G. Harries (1991). Different training patterns and bone mineral density of the femoral shaft in elite, female athletes. *Am. Rheum. Dis.* 50:487–489.

Young, N., C. Formica, G. Szmukler, and E. Seeman (1994). Bone density at weight-bearing and non-weight-bearing sites in ballet dancers: the effects of exercise, hypogonadism, and body weight. *J. Clin. Endocrinol. Metab.* 78:449–454.

Zhang, J., P.J. Feldblum, and J.A. Fortney (1992). Moderate physical activity and bone density among perimenopausal women. *Am. J. Public Health* 82:736–738.

DISCUSSION

WILMORE: The methodological problems you discussed make me less confident that we know very much about exercise and bone development across the life span.

BLIMKIE: It is becoming more confusing because of the interpretation problems associated with these techniques. This whole research area has been heavily driven by the availability of new machines, and as soon as a new one is introduced, a plethora of studies are undertaken without a lot of consideration as to the interpretation of data. In a nutshell, the density of osseous, mineralized tissue *per se* either does not change or it increases somewhat over the life span. The mineral composition of bone based on studies of ash weight changes very little with age and remains around 60–67%. On the other hand, the density of whole bones as "organs" decreases progressively with advancing age, according to results obtained with the dual-photon and the dual-energy techniques. This is due in part to a reduction in bone mass but also to an increased volume of some bones with increasing age.

BAILEY: I don't see why we should continue to perpetuate clearly erroneous information suggesting that BMD doubles from childhood to the mid-teens. Everyone knows this is ridiculous, so why do we keep reporting this? Bob Marcus's group at Stanford estimates that across adolescence 99% of the change in total body and femoral neck bone mineral and 50% of the change in lumbar spine bone mineral can be attributed to an increase in size of the bone rather than to an increase in bone mineral density. I wouldn't use BMD at all, I would use bone mineral content (BMC)and leave it at that, because clearly BMD as measured by DXA does not adequately control for size change in the skeleton that accompanies growth. People will be misled by studies that report tremendous increases in BMD values that are not representative of what is really happening during the growing years.

BLIMKIE: When I started this chapter, it was over 200 pages long and included BMC changes as well as BMD. Bone mineral content will be largely influenced by changes in skeletal size over the life span, so to reduce the size of the chapter, I used the BMD measure, which is less influenced by changes in bone size and is a better variable to use when comparing bone mineral changes across the life span. It is not perfect, but it allows us to make comparisons among children, young adults and older individuals.

BAILEY: I agree partially. Bone mineral density as measured by DXA is appropriate for measuring bone mineral status in adults, because adults don't change in size. But, for evaluating growing children over time, expressing BMD per unit area scanned provides an inappropriate correction for size because it fails to account for changes in bone depth; therefore, it shouldn't be used in developmental studies.

BLIMKIE: This is a bit contentious, too, because bone size will increase at some sites with aging, and this will accentuate the true reduction in bone mineral when assessed by dual-photon and DXA techniques.

BAILEY: To a minimal extent; this is not really an issue in the elderly.

BLIMKIE: I have consolidated these technical issues into a separate section at the beginning of the chapter to alert the reader to their importance when interpreting the literature.

GISOLFI: Depending on where you look, what method you use, and what the effect of the physical activity is, it seems to me that you can get any result you want. What is the best methodology? Should we be using a whole body scan to measure BMD?

BLIMKIE: There is no evidence to indicate that physical activity has a preferential effect on improving cortical vs. trabecular bone when both of those compartments are considered together at the same site, but you can get very different results depending on the site that you select. The best advice that we can give here is that we know that physical activity has a site-specific effect. There may also be some generalized effect, but by and large the site-specific effect is much more predominant than the general effect. For instance, if I isolated my wrist flexors in a weight-training program and chose total body BMD as my outcome measure, I would see no change at all. The total body is predominantly 80% cortical bone, whereas the distal site at the wrist is predominantly trabecular. So you have to be very selective in choosing your technique to minimize bias in your results.

GISOLFI: If I were interested in athletic amenorrhea, for example, could I not bias my results depending on which site I chose?

BLIMKIE: Yes, you could. Most reviewers are aware of these problems, and you would have a hard time getting your results published if, for example, you studied female runners and chose single-photon absorptiometry to study BMD at the wrist. You need to look at the bony site that is being exercised, i.e., the leg and hip region in this example.

BAR-OR: Weight-supported activity such as swimming may even decrease bone density. Which site should be used in this case, i.e., when the whole body is supported?

BLIMKIE: Most of those studies have looked at total body BMD. You can look at the appendicular sites of the arms and the legs as well because you use the legs and the arms in swimming.

HASKELL: It seems to me that the clinically important issue is bone strength.

BLIMKIE: Areal BMD is highly correlated with the compressive strength of certain bony segments. It doesn't totally account for the variation in bone strength, however. Other factors such as the geometry of bone also influence bone strength.

LAMB: In an older person, if the mineral density of a "biopsy plug" of cortical bone is the same as in a younger person or maybe a little greater, but the volume is also greater, is the bone weaker?

BLIMKIE: The expansion in volume partially strengthens the bone. Increases in bone size tend to compensate for any reduction in bone density that might occur.

GREGG: While at Berkeley we were involved in a study of fitness-matched groups of male water-polo players, swimmers, and runners. We found that BMD was actually highest in swimmers and water-polo players. Can these results be explained by the fact that these athletes were involved in other kinds of training activities, especially weight training?

BLIMKIE: Many of the studies I have reviewed don't describe the total activity profiles of their subjects. Most of that data on swimmers comes from cross-sectional studies, and we need to interpret those results very cautiously.

BAR-OR: Is the discrepancy between the outcomes of cross-sectional studies, which usually give more optimistic results about exercise benefits, and longitudinal intervention studies explained simply by the typically brief length of the intervention, or are there other important factors?

BLIMKIE: Most of the training studies have only lasted 1–2 y at the most, and the bone is a very slow-adapting tissue. I suspect that the brief duration of the intervention studies is the best explanation of the more modest results that usually are found with such experiments.

EICHNER: There are epidemiologic studies showing that walking protects against hip fracture. On the other hand, there are epidemiologic studies suggesting that obesity also protects. So it seems that if you want to ward off hip fractures, you should be either a power walker or a couch potato.

BLIMKIE: You may be correct.

GISOLFI: Is there any published information on gender differences in bone loss during space flight? It might be worthwhile to know what happens to BMD in female astronauts.

BLIMKIE: I'm not aware of any data on bone mineral changes in these women, but I'm sure they will be forthcoming.

5

Body Composition and Weight Control: A Perspective on Females

PRISCILLA M. CLARKSON, Ph.D.

SCOTT GOING, Ph.D.

INTRODUCTION

Women's weight-control practices and their concerns over body weight can have a profound impact on their health. Advertisements for weight-loss products clearly demonstrate that women are the primary targets. Despite the limited data to support long-term effectiveness of weight-loss programs, the weight-loss industries, valued at more that 30 billion dollars per year, abound and flourish. Over most of the life span, from prepubescence to adulthood, females are sporadically restricting energy intake. In attempts to lose weight, women risk inadequate energy intake, malnutrition, loss in lean tissue, reduced peak bone mass, increased bone fractures, and the development of eating disorders.

Female athletes not only deal with societal pressure to achieve low body weights, but they also may experience additional pressures from sport participation. For example, gymnastics and dance emphasize leanness for aesthetic reasons, whereas sports such as distance running advocate low body weights for optimal performance. Although athletes exercise regularly and strenuously, many find that the added energy expenditures are not sufficient to maintain the low body weights that they believe are necessary for optimal performance or aesthetics. Thus, weight control is a serious problem for many female athletes.

This chapter begins with a discussion of gender differences in body composition, energy balance, and changes in body composition in response to exercise. Developmental changes and training adaptations in both fat and fat-free masses are discussed since both compartments are significant determinants of health, disease risk, and functional capacity. The information presented in these sections is not specific to athletes, so comparisons between males and females and age-related changes occurring in the general population are addressed. To explain how body weight is controlled, information is presented on energy and nutrient balance and on the responses to aerobic and resistance exercise. Finally, body composition, sport performance, and nutritional concerns for weight control are addressed specifically in female athletes.

GENDER DIFFERENCES IN FAT AND FAT-FREE BODY MASS THROUGHOUT THE LIFE CYCLE

Population-based normative data describing total body fat and fat-free mass (FFM) for different ages of males and females are unavailable. Although various components of the FFM have been measured in some large-scale studies in some segments of the population, few attempts have been made to systematically describe whole-body fat and FFM across the age span. Consequently, descriptions of developmental and aging trends are usually based on composites of data from a variety of smaller scale studies. Despite this limitation, qualitative changes are well described, although the accuracy of absolute values at different ages may be limited.

This situation has occurred in part because of the difficulty in obtaining accurate estimates of body composition in living humans. Direct estimation is not possible. Consequently, indirect methods based on a variety of models with different assumptions have been developed (Wang et al., 1992). The accuracy of any method depends on the validity of the underlying assumptions in the group in which it is applied. More complex multicompartment models are more generalizable and more accurate across groups; however, they require more measurements and are generally not feasible for large groups. As a result, methods based on two compartment models (e.g., fat and fat-free masses) with an underlying assumption of chemical constancy of the fat-free mass are most commonly used in all groups.

It is now well recognized that there is substantial variation in the chemical composition of the FFM, both within and among different populations, and the very developmental, exercise-, and age-related changes that we wish to detect can introduce substantial errors when methods based on the two-compartment model are applied across groups of males and females who vary in age, maturational status, ethnicity, health, and level of physical conditioning. Several reviews of the limitations of various methods and models of body composition and the potential errors in different populations have been published (Baumgartner et al., 1991; Deurenberg et al., 1989; Going et al., 1995; Heymsfield et al., 1989; Lohman, 1986). These errors must be considered when interpreting the available data describing typical age-related changes in body composition and the effects of various interventions.

Fat-Free Body Mass

Malina and Bouchard (1991a) have derived growth curves showing the changes in fat-free body mass (FFM) during childhood and adolescence. Fat-free mass was estimated from measurements of body water and measurements of body density. Although subject to the methodological limitations described above, qualitatively, both methods give similar results.

In both genders, FFM increased fairly linearly during childhood following a growth pattern like those of height and weight (Figure 5-1). There were only minor differences between boys and girls during childhood, whereas gender differences were clearly established during the adolescent growth spurt. Young adult values of FFM are reached earlier in females (15–16 y of age) compared to males (19–20 y). In late adolescence and young adulthood, males have, on average, 1.5 times greater FFM than females. The difference predominately reflects the male adolescent spurt in muscle mass and the sex difference in adult stature, although smaller differences in other components of the FFM also contribute. The sex difference in FFM per unit stature is small in childhood and early adolescence, but after age 14 y, the sex difference increases so that young adult

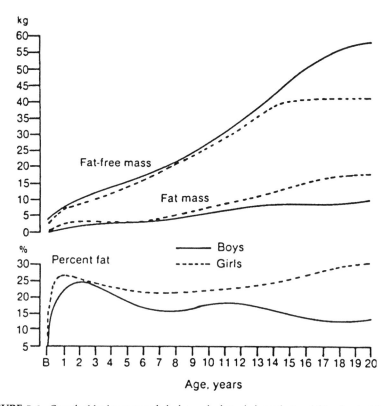

FIGURE 5-1. *Growth of fat-free mass and absolute and relative body fat during childhood and adolescence.* Reprinted from Malina and Bouchard (1991), with permission.

males have about 0.36 kg of FFM/cm height, whereas females have about 0.26 kg/cm (Malina & Bouchard, 1991).

Changes in FFM with aging have been most often estimated from measurements of body potassium (K) at different ages. Forbes (1987a), using cross-sectional data from several studies, estimated that males lose 45 g K (a decline from 155 g to 110 g) from young adulthood to 80 y of age, whereas females lose 20 g K over the same period (a decline from 100 g to 80 g). Assuming that the K/FFM ratio is constant throughout life, this magnitude of loss of K suggests a 30% decline in FFM in men and a 20% decline in women. The average rate of loss is estimated to be 5% per decade for men and 3.5% for women (Forbes & Reina, 1970).

Available longitudinal data (Flynn et al., 1989; Forbes, 1987a; Forbes & Reina, 1970) suggest a somewhat slower rate of loss of approximately 3% per decade or about 3.0 kg per decade in men. In women, Flynn et al. (1989) found no significant loss of body potassium in women until after 50 y of age, although only a small number of women was studied. Estimates of FFM loss per decade (based on cross-sectional measurements of body density, body water, and nitrogen) agree reasonably well with estimates based on longitudinal potassium data, suggesting a 3% decline per decade in FFM for men and a 2% decline for women (Ellis, 1990). Because potassium is found mainly in muscle tissue, the loss of potassium with aging reflects muscle loss, which may occur at a faster rate in men than in women. Significant losses of body water and bone mineral (more so in women than in men) also contribute to the loss of FFM with aging as described below.

Changes In Subcomponents of FFM. Gender- and age-related differences in FFM represent the net effects of differential changes in the subcomponents of the FFM as a result of growth, maturation, and aging. Comprehensive reviews of the changes in water, protein (muscle), and mineral content during childhood and adolescence (Lohman, 1986) and during adulthood (Going et al., 1994; 1995) are available elsewhere. An overview of these changes is given here.

Water. Body water represents the single largest component of the body in both males and females at all ages. The absolute water mass varies with body size, equaling about 50–60% of body weight, although there is considerable interindividual variation due to both variation in hydration and body fatness. Relative to females, adult males at all ages have both higher absolute amounts of body water on average (because of their larger size and muscle mass) and larger fractions of weight as water, primarily due to their lower body fat. In adult males and females water comprises approximately 72–74% of the FFM (Schoeller, 1989).

The hydration of the FFM in children is considerably higher than that in adults, i.e., about 76–77% at age 7–8 y (Boileau et al., 1984), and declines steadily with growth and maturation until the adult value is reached at approximately 18 y of age. Small gender differences (~0.5–1.0%) that seem to persist into adulthood appear during childhood. Absolute volumes of body water increase in both boys and girls with increasing age and size while at the same time the proportion of water in the FFM declines. Although the volume of extracellular water (ECW) is greater than intracellular water (ICW) at birth, ECW increases more slowly than ICW, and by 3 mo of postnatal age ICW volume is greater than that of ECW (Bell, 1985; Friis-Hansen, 1957).

The volume of body water remains relatively constant after ~18 y of age and into middle age. Water as a fraction of body weight declines in men and more so in women beginning as early as the 4th decade, an observation that reflects more the increase in body fat that begins in middle-age than actual decreases in body water. A decline in body water, correlated with loss of muscle mass (Ellis, 1990; Pierson et al.,1982), may begin at approximately age 40–50 y and continue into old age, reaching a loss of ~5–6 L of water (Going et al., 1995) and possibly more (Schoeller, 1989). Intracellular water volume declines at a faster rate than ECW (Pierson et al., 1982). Thus, the ECW:ICW ratio increases in old age. Nevertheless, the proportion of water in the FFM seems to remain relatively constant throughout adult life (Schoeller, 1989).

Mineral Content. Changes in the mineral content of the body with growth, maturation, and aging are typically estimated from changes in bone mineral, which accounts for ~80% of total mineral in adults (Brozek et al., 1963). Information is also available from the analysis of a limited number of skeletons of young individuals (Malina & Bouchard, 1991). The dry defatted skeleton weighs, on average, about 95 g in infant boys (3% of body weight) and slightly less in infant girls, and it increases to about 4 kg in young men and about 2.8 kg in young women, or about 6–7% of body weight. Bone mineral comprises about 63% (females) to 66% (males) of the dry defatted skeleton, or about 2% of body weight at birth and during childhood and 4–5% of body weight in adults. In children, mineral accounts for about 5% of the FFM, and in adults the mineral fraction of FFM is about 6–7%.

With aging, there is significant bone loss in men and women (Going et al., 1995). In both sexes, little if any bone loss occurs until after age 40 y. Thereafter, a consistent decrease in bone mineral occurs. The results of cross-sectional studies suggest that appendicular bone loss in males begins at about 50–60 y and proceeds at a rate of about 0.3% per year (Mazess & Cameron, 1974). Females may begin their decline slightly earlier and lose about 1% of bone mass per year between ages 45–75 y, after which the rate is similar to that in males (Mazess & Cameron, 1974).

There is some evidence that the loss of trabecular bone in the axial skeleton may begin earlier than the loss of compact bone, and several studies suggest that trabecular bone loss in the spine in females accelerates for about 5 y at menopause, followed by a slower decline (Aloia et al., 1990; Riggs et al., 1986). Data from Mazess and colleagues (1987) suggest that apparently healthy women by age 70 y experience about a 20% decrease in vertebral bone mineral density (BMD) and a 25–40% decrease in BMD at the femoral neck and trochanteric regions. In healthy men (Mazess et al., 1990), the decrease in spine (~3%) and femur (~20–30%) BMD by age 70 is less than in women, a fact which helps to explain the lower prevalence of osteoporosis in men.

Protein And Muscle Mass. Because it is the most difficult component of FFM to estimate, especially in children and adolescents, whole body protein in boys and girls is typically calculated from the differences in estimates of total body water, mineral, and FFM. Using this approach, Lohman and colleagues (Lohman, 1986) reported that the protein fraction was approximately 16–18% of FFM in boys and girls. Prior to puberty, gender differences are minor. In contrast, adolescent males experience a slightly greater increase in protein than do same-aged females. Thus, by ~18 y of age, the protein mass reaches its adult values—19–20% of FFM in males and 18–19% in females.

The muscle fraction of FFM is of particular interest because it is more strongly related to functional capacity and possibly to metabolic rate than is FFM, which includes the extracellular fluids and solids in addition to the body cell mass. Estimates of total muscle mass derived from dissection studies suggest that muscle comprises about 22–25% of body weight at birth and 40–45% of body weight in adults (Malina & Bouchard, 1991). Dissection data for children and adolescents are not available.

The growth of muscle mass in children and adolescents has been estimated from anthropometric measurements, soft-tissue x-rays, whole-body potassium, and urinary creatinine excretion (Falkner & Tanner, 1986; Malina, 1969; Tanner et al.,1981). The findings from each of these methods present similar patterns of muscle growth (Figure 5-2).

Both boys and girls experience a gradual increase in muscle growth from birth to puberty. A small (~2% body weight) but consistent sex difference that is evident by age 5 y increases during and after the adolescent growth spurt. Muscle mass (estimated from creatinine excretion) relative to body weight increases from about 42% to 54% in boys between 5 and 17 y of age. In girls it increases from about 40% to 45% of body weight between 5 and 13 y and then declines somewhat after age 13 y. The decline is due to fat accumulation during female adolescence, resulting in increased body fat percentage, rather than to a decline in absolute muscle mass.

Estimates of protein mass for representative samples of adult males and females at different ages have been derived from estimates of whole-body nitrogen content by neutron activation analysis, and muscle mass has been estimated from whole-body potassium content (Cohn et al.,

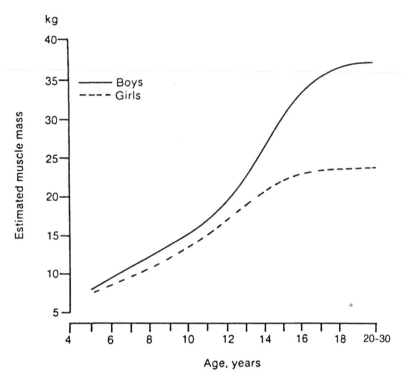

FIGURE 5-2. *Growth of muscle mass during childhood and adolescence.* Reprinted from Malina and Bouchard (1991), with permission.

1980; Ellis, 1990; Flynn et al., 1989). Based on these cross-sectional data, protein mass appears to decline by about 13% in men (13.1 kg to 11.4 kg) and 20% in women (9.3 to 7.4 kg) from the third to the eighth decade of life. In men, a slower loss of nitrogen than of potassium was observed, suggesting that muscle protein was lost at a faster rate than nonmuscle protein. In contrast, in women the declines in nitrogen and potassium were similar. Thus, the loss of muscle mass with aging, estimated from the K/FFM ratio, appears to be substantially larger in males ($\sim$10–15%) than in females ($\sim$3–9%), although it must be noted that most available estimates are based on cross-sectional data, and a considerable range of estimates has been reported (Cohn et al., 1980; Ellis, 1990; Pierson et al., 1982; Womersley et al., 1976).

The age-related loss of muscle mass, sometimes referred to as sarcopenia (Evans & Rosenberg, 1991), and the associated change in metabolic rate (Tzankoff & Norris, 1978) are intimately associated with the age-related increases in total and central body fat described below. Together, these age-related shifts in body composition contribute to an increased risk of developing many chronic disorders, including hypercholesterolemia, atherosclerosis, hyperinsulinemia, insulin resistance, non-insulin-dependent diabetes, and hypertension. Sarcopenia is the major factor in the decline in muscle strength associated with aging and inactivity; it contributes to increased inactivity that, in turn, contributes to further muscle loss and the accumulation of body fat. Thus, interventions aimed at maintaining and increasing muscle mass have an important role in maintaining optimal body composition and reducing disease risk.

Body Fat

Using data from both direct and indirect studies of the chemical composition of individuals between infancy and young adulthood, Malina and Bouchard (1991d) have derived composite growth curves indicating age- and sex-associated variations in body fat. Fat mass at birth equals about 0.5 kg or ~8% of body weight. Fat mass increases during the first 2 or 3 y of life and then is relatively stable until 5 or 6 y of age. The sex difference in fat mass is negligible at these ages. Subsequently, fat mass increases more rapidly in girls than in boys. Fat mass continues to increase in girls during adolescence but reaches a plateau or increases only slightly during adolescence in boys. Consequently, fat mass is about 1.5 times greater, on average, in adolescent and young adult females, compared to same-aged males.

The growth curve for relative fatness (Figure 5-1) is somewhat different than for absolute fatness (Malina & Bouchard, 1991). Relative body fat increases rapidly in both sexes during infancy and then declines during early childhood. Girls tend to have only slightly more relative fat than do boys during infancy and childhood. However, after age 5–6 y through adolescence, girls consistently have greater percentages of body fat, compared to boys. The relative fatness increases during adolescence in girls just as absolute fat does. Relative fatness also increases in boys until the adolescent growth spurt and then gradually declines. Thus, in contrast to absolute fat, relative fatness declines during male adolescence, due to the rapid growth of FFM and much slower accumulation of body fat.

Based on composite data, Vogel and Friedl (1992) derived estimates of 18% and 28% body fat, respectively, for nonathletic, young adult reference man and woman. The greater relative fatness in women reflects a gender difference in essential or obligatory fat more so than in storage fat (Table 5-1).

In men, obligatory fat is considered to be lipid that is required for structural support and protection (e.g., perirenal fat), for nutritional support (e.g., pericardial fat), and for reserves that can be chemically extracted from tissues rather than dissected as adipose tissue. In women, additional sites, most importantly the breasts, hips, and thighs, are also obligatory and may be essential for normal physiological function. Men do

TABLE 5-1. *Reference body composition values for young adult nonathletic women and men (% of total body mass). Values are constructed from a composite of reference sources.*

Variable	Women	Men	Ratio (W/M)
Height (cm)	163	177	0.92
Body mass (kg)	60	75	0.80
Body mass index	22.2	23.6	0.94
Fat mass (kg)	16.8 (28%)	13.5 (18%)	1.24
essential	7.2 (12%)	1.2 (3%)	3.13
storate	9.6 (16%)	11.3 (15%)	0.85
Fat-free mass (kg)	43.2 (72%)	61.5 (82%)	0.70
skeletal muscle	21.6 (36%)	33.8 (45%)	0.64
bone	7.2 (12%)	11.3 (15%)	0.64
other	14.4 (24%)	16.4 (22%)	0.88
Minimal weight (kg)	50.4	63.8	0.79
Waist/hip ratio[a]	0.75	0.83	

[a]Waist = abdominal circumference at the navel; hips = circumference at the greatest projection of the buttocks.

not have this obligatory storage, and they deposit excess fat in the abdominal region that in healthy young women is teleologically "reserved" for the abdominal expansion that accompanies fetal growth (Vogel & Friedl, 1992).

The results of studies examining age-related changes in body fat suggest two somewhat contrasting patterns of change. Cross-sectional skinfold data (sum of triceps and subscapular skinfolds) from the second National Health and Nutrition Examination Survey (NHANES II) show that, within a given percentile, skinfold thickness increases from age 18 to 54 y and that from ages 55 to 74, there is a leveling off or a decline in skinfold thickness (Najjar & Rowland, 1987). Unfortunately, data for persons older than 74 y were not collected in NHANES II, and it is not clear whether the changes in skinfold thicknesses represent a decrease in body fat at older ages or a shift in body fat from subcutaneous to visceral depots. Recent studies of total body fat also suggest an increase in body fat in middle age and early old age followed by a reduction in later old age. Using bioelectric impedance analysis, Silver et al. (1993) observed higher percent body fats in both men and women aged 40–64 y as compared to their older (> 85 y) counterparts. Similarly, higher estimates of percent fat derived from dual-energy x-ray absorptiometry were found in women aged 65 y compared to women 81 y of age (Rico et al.,1993). Finally, Ellis (1990), using a multiple-component model of body composition that minimizes bias from age-related changes in bone mineral, water, and protein, reported mean body fats of 27.1% in women 20–29 y old, 42.1% in women 50–59 y old, and 36.7% in women 70–79 y old. Although these data suggest a decline in body fat in old age, they are limited by their cross-sectional nature and the likelihood of selection bias.

In contrast to the studies noted above, cross-sectional studies of body composition that used hydrostatic weighing (Durnin & Womersley, 1974) and ^{40}K gamma spectroscopy (Flynn et al., 1989; Forbes & Reina, 1970), as well as longitudinal ^{40}K gamma spectroscopy (Flynn et al., 1989; Forbes & Reina, 1970), suggest that body fat increases continuously with advancing age. Durnin and Womersley (1974) estimated body fat percentages from body density and the Siri equation (Siri, 1956) in 209 men and 272 women 16–72 y of age. These data support the qualitative trend of gradually higher body fat percentages at older ages. In men and women the average body fat percentage was higher in each successive age group from age 16 through age 72. However, because the data were stratified by age groups with discrepant interval widths, it is difficult to quantify the differences in body fat with increasing age.

In an effort to replicate the qualitative trends identified by Durnin and Womersley (1974) and to better quantify the relationship between age and body fat percentage, Going and colleagues (1995) analyzed body density data from white men (N = 229) and women (N = 229) 40–81 y of age. The mean ± SD values for body fat percentage (% fat) were 26.4 ± 6.5 in men and 35.8 ± 7.3 in women. Body fat percentage was correlated with age in both men and women. The age-related differences in % fat were roughly +2.2 ± 0.4% fat per decade in men (Figure 5-3) and +3.6 ± 0.4% fat per decade in women (Figure 5-4).

These results compare favorably with longitudinal estimates of changes in body fat percentage in 564 men and 61 women with initial ages ranging from 28 to 60 y (Flynn et al., 1989). The average rate of increase

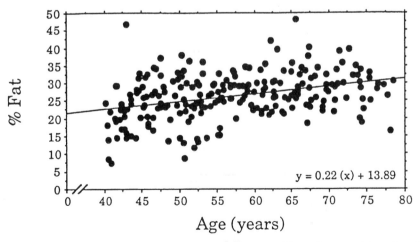

FIGURE 5-3. *Percent body fat in men 40 to 80 years of age.* Reprinted from Going et al.(1995), with permission.

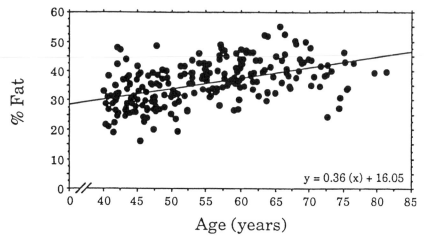

FIGURE 5-4. *Percent body fat in women 40 to 80 years of age.* Reprinted from Going et al. (1995), with permission.

in body fat over the 18 y of follow-up (estimated from ^{40}K gamma spectroscopy) was 3.0% fat per decade in men and 5.2% fat per decade in women. Taken together, the qualitative and quantitative agreement between the cross-sectional densitometric (Going et al., 1995) and longitudinal ^{40}K gamma spectroscopic (Flynn et al., 1989) data suggest that there may be a continuous and relatively linear increase in body fat percentage with advancing age.

Fat Topography and Fat Distribution. Recent studies using computed axial tomography (CT) have shown consistent gender differences in subcutaneous and visceral fat areas (Enzi et al., 1986; Kvist et al., 1986; Weits et al., 1988) and confirmed Garn's (1957) early observation that "women carry more of their fat on and less in their smaller frames" compared to men. Because women tend to be smaller and have less bone and muscle mass, absolute skinfold thicknesses for a given percent body fat are smaller than for men, despite the greater distribution of fat near the surface (Durnin & Womersley, 1974). Women also tend to distribute more subcutaneous fat on the extremities compared to men, as reflected in greater skinfold thicknesses at the triceps and thigh than on the trunk.

The predominant region for fat storage in men is in the abdominal region, whereas women typically deposit fat in the hips and buttocks (Krotkiewski et al., 1983). Vague (1956) first described these patterns as the android (or central and upper body) fat pattern typical of men and the gynoid (or peripheral and lower body) fat patterning of women. The android pattern has been associated with greater visceral fat storage (Enzi et al., 1986; Kvist et al., 1986; Weits et al., 1988). This upper-body fatness typically is described by a high waist-to-hip circumference ratio (WHR), although the results of some studies suggest that waist circumference may be a better predictor of visceral fat (Pouliot et al., 1994). In men, WHR is correlated with increasing fatness because of the trend to store excess fat in the abdominal region. The correlation with fatness in women is not as marked; nevertheless, the WHR or waist circumference may be useful for identifying women with android versus gynoid patterns of fat distribution (Vogel & Friedl, 1992).

The tendency for a central or truncal distribution of fat versus a more peripheral distribution of fat toward the arms and legs has also been associated with a greater ratio of subscapular-to-triceps skinfold thicknesses, which tends to be greater in males than in females (Baumgartner et al., 1986; Haffner et al., 1986). As Vogel and Friedl (1992) have noted, this expression reflects only subcutaneous fat, whereas the waist circumference in the WHR reflects both visceral and subcutaneous fat; the two measures thus may have different physiological meanings. Mueller and colleagues (1987) have suggested using the waist-to-thigh circumference ratio, which distinguishes central and upper-body fat from extremity and lower-body fat and which Seidell et al. (1987) found to be more highly correlated with intraabdominal fat than with WHR in women.

Changes in the distribution of fat with growth have been studied using measurements of skinfold thicknesses (Malina & Bouchard, 1988) and, in some cases, fat widths from standardized radiographs (Malina & Roche, 1983) rather than from CT because the relatively high radiation exposure limits CT use in children. Radiographic data demonstrate that girls have more subcutaneous fat than do boys at all ages from early infancy through young adulthood. After an early rapid increase in subcutaneous fat from birth to 6 mo, both boys and girls experience a reduction in subcutaneous fat through age 6–7 y. Girls then show a reasonably linear increase in subcutaneous fat with age through adolescence. In contrast, boys show a slight increase in fat thickness between 7 and 12–13 y of age, followed by a decrease in subcutaneous fat during adolescence (Figure 5-5). For girls, skinfold data, as compared to radiographic data, suggest an almost identical pattern of subcutaneous fat accumulation in girls.

Radiographic data and skinfold data also correspond quite well in boys between 4 and 13 y of age, whereas after 13 y of age, radiographic data suggest a more dramatic decline in subcutaneous fat than is demonstrated by skinfold data. The discrepancy is methodological because radiographs are usually taken at a few sites on the extremities, whereas skinfolds are measured at multiple sites on the extremities and trunk.

The ratio of the sum of skinfold thicknesses measured on the trunk versus on the extremities has been used to indicate changes in the relative distribution of subcutaneous fat during growth (Malina & Bouchard, 1988). During childhood, the ratio is similar and rather stable in both sexes

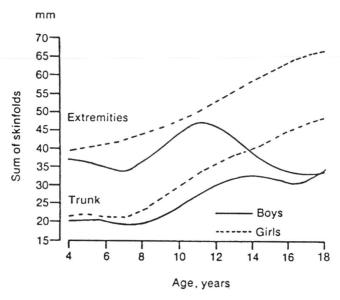

mm

Sum of skinfolds

Extremities

Trunk

——— Boys

------ Girls

Age, years

FIGURE 5-5. *Sum of trunk and extremity skinfolds during childhood and adolescence.* Reprinted from Malina and Bouchard (1991), with permission.

(Figure 5-6). The ratio then increases after age 8 to 9 in girls and age 9 to 10 in boys. It continues to increase with age through male adolescence but changes only slightly after age 12 to 13 y in girls. The increasing ratio in boys reflects the tendency to gain more fat on the trunk than on the extremities between about 10 and 13 y. Subsequently, extremity fat declines while truncal fat continues to slowly increase. In girls, increases in trunk fat are greater than in extremity fat between 8 and 12 y; thereafter, both trunk and extremity fat appear to accumulate at a reasonably similar rate. Hence, the increase in this ratio is not as marked in girls as in boys, resulting in a gender difference in the distribution of subcutaneous fat.

A gender difference in internal fat may also develop during adolescence, as inferred from the ratio of subcutaneous fat to total fat mass (Malina & Bouchard, 1988). The ratio decreases in girls from age 9 to 18 y, suggesting that internal fat accumulates at a faster rate than subcutaneous fat. In contrast, in boys, the ratio tends to increase after puberty, reflecting the differential changes in extremity and trunk subcutaneous fat noted above as well as a shift in the relationship between subcutaneous and total fat.

In women, regional fat changes also occur during pregnancy and lactation, and with menopause. Using skinfold measurements, several investigators have demonstrated that fat is added predominately to the trunk during pregnancy, although fat is also added to the mid-thigh (Forsum et

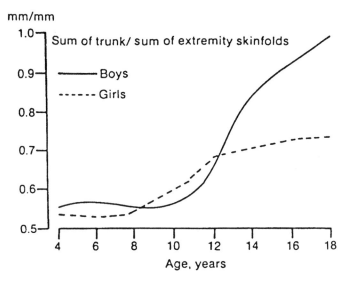

FIGURE 5-6. *Trunk-to extremity skinfold ratio during childhood and adolescence.* Reprinted from Malina and Bouchard (1991), with permission.

al., 1989; Taggart et al., 1967). With lactation the reverse occurs, and under the influence of prolactin (Steingrimsdottir et al., 1980; Zinder et al., 1974) thigh fat mobilization is enhanced as lipase activity decreases while abdominal wall lipase remains unchanged (Rebuffe-Scrive et al., 1985). Several investigators have reported increases in upper-arm and subscapular skinfolds in postpartum women during lactation, even as body weight declines (Brewer et al., 1989; Forsum et al., 1989; Quandt, 1983). Thus, while fat is mobilized from the thigh, there is a redistribution of fat to the arms, breasts, and upper trunk. Fat distributions appear to return to prepregnancy measurements 6 mo or more after delivery.

Fat redistribution also occurs with aging in middle-aged and older men and women. Increasing truncal skinfold thicknesses (Chien et al., 1975; Chumlea et al., 1984a, 1984b) and increased abdominal fat measured by dual-energy x-ray absorptiometry (Ley et al., 1992) suggest a redistribution of subcutaneous fat from the limbs to the trunk, and circumference measurements (Heitmann, 1992; Shimokata et al., 1988; Stevens et al., 1991) indicate that distribution of fat from the upper to the lower body also increases with age. The results of studies using computed tomography to differentiate subcutaneous from visceral fat are suggestive of an age-related internalization of body fat (Baumgartner et al., 1988; Borkan & Norris, 1977; Borkan et al., 1985; Enzi et al., 1986; Schwartz et al., 1990). Although longitudinal changes in waist and abdominal circumferences indicate that the accumulation of abdominal fat with advancing age is greater in males than in females, there are some cross-sectional CT data implying that men and women may have similar age-related changes in visceral fat (Baumgartner et al., 1988, 1993; Enzi et al., 1986).

The regional fat changes with aging in middle-aged women may be caused by the hormonal events associated with menopause. Several studies have shown that postmenopausal women undergo a shift in fat distribution to a pattern typically associated with males, and estrogen replacement therapy for postmenopausal women preserves the premenopausal fat distribution pattern (Den Tonkelaar et al., 1989; Lindberg et al., 1989). Increased truncal fat may be independently related to both increasing androgenicity and obesity in women (Dunaif & Graf, 1989; Evans et al., 1983), although given the difficulties associated with accurate assessment of total body fat, it is difficult to make this conclusion with certainty. Indeed, in one study of nearly 60,000 overweight women, age and weight but not menstrual status were significant determinants of an increased WHR (Lanska et al., 1985).

By any assessment, the net result of increasing upper body fatness in women and men is an increased risk of cardiovascular disease (Despres et al., 1989; Lapidus et al., 1984, 1989) and diabetes (Lundgren et al., 1989; Pasquali et al., 1990), possibly as a result of a series of consequences associated with increased portal delivery of fatty acids to the liver (Rebuffe-Scrive et al., 1990). Whether metabolic complications are caused by increased visceral fat or whether visceral fat is simply a marker of a maladaptive response to stress is not known (Bjorntorp, 1991).

There is some evidence that women may increase body fat considerably more than do men before they express the same metabolic derangements as men (Krotkiewski et al., 1983). Regional variations in fat distribution have been related to differences in lipoprotein lipase activity and to adipocyte sensitivity to insulin (Arner et al., 1981, 1991; Evans et al., 1983), although whether or not the relationship is causal is not clear. In women, compared to men, enzyme activity is greater in femoral fat regions (Fried & Kral, 1987), and before menopause the activity is greater in femoral fat than in breast or abdominal fat (Rebuffe-Scrive et al., 1986). In addition, regional differences in the regulation of lipase activity may account for shifts in the fat distribution of females during different phases of maturation and reproductive life (Rebuffe-Scrive et al., 1985). It is likely that variations in lipase activity also contribute to differential responses of various fat depots to conditions of energy deficit and surfeit as well as to exercise (Forbes, 1990).

Male-pattern obesity in women is also associated with increased muscle and bone mass, possibly caused by androgen action (Krotkiewski & Bjorntorp, 1986; Mueller et al., 1982). The reduction in bone mass that has been reported in amenorrhoeic women, for example, is not observed in women with hirsutism and amenorrhoea, and this has been suggested to be a benefit of elevated androgens (Dixon et al., 1989). Moreover,

Baumgartner et al. (1986) demonstrated that truncal fat distribution was associated with greater internal fat as well as with greater muscle and bone mass, regardless of age, gender, and ethnicity.

ENERGY BALANCE, NUTRIENT BALANCE, AND WEIGHT CONTROL: EFFECTS OF ENERGY INTAKE AND EXPENDITURE

The principle of energy conservation is the underlying basis of energy balance in humans. Thus, the expected change in body energy stores with a change in energy intake or expenditure is usually estimated from the classic energy balance equation:

Change In Energy Balance = Energy Intake — Energy Expenditure.

When energy intake exceeds expenditure, energy stores and body mass are expected to increase, and when expenditure exceeds intake, they decrease. However, the actual weight gain or loss is often less than predicted from the classic equation (Miller et al., 1967; Ravussin & Swinburn, 1993; Ravussin et al., 1985b); in early studies, this discrepancy led to the notion of heat wasting (Neumann, 1902). A more likely explanation, proposed by Alpert (1990) and reviewed by Ravussin and Swinburn (1992, 1993), is that the traditional "static" model cannot account for the dynamics of energy balance. As shown by Alpert, under conditions of semistarvation (1988) and hyperphagia (1990), not only does the composition of the tissue lost or gained play a critical role in predicting weight gain or loss, but also small changes in body weight can offset the imbalance.

The use of a dynamic equation that introduces time dependency ("rates"), i.e., *Rate Of Change Of Energy Stores = Rate Of Energy Intake — Rate Of Energy Expenditure*, allows the effect of changing energy stores (fat-free mass, fat mass, and weight) to enter into the prediction of weight change (Alpert, 1990; Ravussin & Swinburn, 1993). Thus, a small initial energy surfeit does not lead to large weight gains over many years as would be predicted from the static equation. Rather, after a short period of positive energy balance, the energy stores (fat and FFM) increase and cause an automatic increase in energy expenditure that then balances the increased energy intake. The person will then once again be in energy balance, albeit with a higher energy intake, higher energy expenditure, and higher body energy stores.

Nutrient Balance

Dynamic nutrient balance equations, in a fashion analogous to energy balance equations, can be examined to determine the contribution of chronic imbalance between nutrient intake and oxidation to overall energy balance, assuming that each nutrient is regulated separately and is not converted into another nutrient compartment for storage. Although not true in the strict sense, this assumption is reasonable under the dietary conditions of industrialized countries (Ravussin & Swinburn, 1993). Based on this approach, work by Flatt (1988) and others suggests that oxidation rates of carbohydrate (Acheson et al., 1987, 1988) and protein (Abbott et al., 1988) are largely determined by carbohydrate and protein intakes. In contrast, fat oxidation is not determined by fat intake but by the difference between the total intake of protein and carbohydrate and the total rate of oxidation of protein and carbohydrate (Flatt et al., 1985; Schutz et al., 1989). Thus, chronic imbalances of carbohydrate and protein are unlikely to be direct causes of significant weight gain, although by contributing to overall energy balance, they indirectly affect fat balance.

An important prediction of this model is that the oxidation rates of protein and carbohydrate are rapidly affected by changes in the intakes of protein and carbohydrate, whereas fat oxidation is not immediately influenced by changes in fat intake. Work by Bennett et al. (1992), Flatt (1987), Flatt et al. (1985), and Schutz et al. (1989) suggests that this indeed is true. Excess fat intake, even in conditions of spontaneous overfeeding (Rising et al., 1992), is stored as body fat. Based on these observations, Ravussin and Swinburn (1992) suggested that energy balance is virtually equivalent to fat balance, and for body weight to change (largely dependent on adipose tissue) there must be an imbalance between fat intake and fat oxidation.

The energy balance equation offers two possible alternatives for weight reduction—increasing energy expenditure through exercise or consciously limiting total energy intake, i.e., dieting. In contrast, the fat balance equation—*Rate Of Change Of Fat Stores = Rate Of Fat Intake — Rate Of Fat Oxidation*—offers three alternatives for weight reduction. The first two, increased exercise and decreased energy intake, act by increasing fat oxidation. The third alternative is to decrease fat intake, i.e., alter the quality of the diet. This concept implies that a high-fat, *ad libitum* diet will cause weight gain, whereas a low-fat, *ad libitum* diet will result in weight loss (Kendall et al., 1991; Ravussin & Swinburn, 1992).

According to Flatt's model (1988), a high-fat, low-carbohydrate diet would lead to early depletion of glycogen stores, a greater food intake, and a positive energy balance. The imbalance would persist until the adipose tissue mass was enlarged sufficiently to provide a greater supply of fat for oxidation. When the higher rate of fat oxidation matches the higher rate of fat intake, the individual can then be in fat balance but at a higher percent body fat. Conversely, if an overweight person changed to a low-fat, *ad libitum* diet, fat mass would diminish, and fat would be oxidized at an increasingly slower rate until a new equilibrium with lower fat stores, lower rate of fat oxidation, and lower fat intake was reached. Studies that support this concept include those reporting higher fat intakes in obese persons compared to lean persons (Dreon et al., 1988; Prentice et al.,

1986; Tremblay et al., 1989); greater energy intakes and weight gains in persons eating *ad libitum*, high-fat versus low-fat diets (Kendall et al., 1991; Lissner & Levitsky, 1987); greater weight losses on low-fat diets (Wood et al., 1988, 1991); and an association between higher percents body fat and greater fat oxidation (Zurlo et al., 1990).

Response To Restricted Dietary Energy

Based on the equations for energy balance and nutrient balance, a hypoenergy diet is expected to decrease body weight, particularly if fat intake is also reduced. Indeed, energy restriction is more effective for inducing weight loss than is increased energy expenditure through increased physical activity, although the composition of weight loss may be affected by activity (Stefanick, 1993).

The common features of hypoenergy diets are a rapid initial weight loss, followed by a diminished and eventually flattened rate of weight loss unless further restriction is imposed (Forbes, 1987b; Ravussin & Swinburn, 1992). The amount and composition of weight loss depend on the degree and duration of energy restriction (Forbes, 1987b; 1992), diet composition (Flatt, 1988), and the initial body weight and body composition (Forbes, 1987b). Generally, the proportion of weight loss that is fat increases with increasing duration of energy restriction until a critical level of body fat is reached (Forbes, 1987b). The degree to which the FFM is eroded depends on the severity of energy restriction. Starvation and semi-starvation diets result in large losses of water, electrolytes, protein, and probably bone (Buskirk et al., 1963; Grande, 1968; Grande et al., 1958; Keys et al., 1950; Krotkiewski et al., 1981; Passmore et al., 1958; Yang & Van Itallie, 1976). Even mild energy restriction, when used alone to induce weight loss, results in the loss of moderate amounts of water and other fat-free tissue, particularly if initial levels of body fat are already low (Forbes, 1987b; Goldman et al., 1963; Weltman et al., 1980; Zuti & Golding, 1976). Although a diet low in energy but relatively high in protein may minimize the loss of fat-free mass (Wadden et al., 1983), even high protein intakes may not offset the effects of low levels of body fat on increasing the loss of lean tissue.

Eventually, most subjects regain some or all of the lost weight (Johnson & Drenick, 1977). Although the decrease in the rate of weight loss and the subsequent weight gain may be caused by poor diet adherence, a reduction in metabolic rate leading to lower daily energy expenditure in response to energy restriction may also contribute (Ravussin & Swinburn, 1992).

Components of Daily Energy Expenditure. In assessing the impact of energy restriction on metabolism, it is important to consider separately the components of energy expenditure. Daily energy expenditure can be divided into three components: the resting metabolic rate (RMR), the thermic effect of food, and the thermic effect of activity (Figure 5-7). The RMR represents the largest portion of total energy expenditure in an inactive person, accounting for 60–75% of total energy expenditure. It includes the cost of maintaining the integrated systems of the body and body temperature at rest and constitutes the energy needed to maintain electrolyte gradients, to sustain cardiovascular and pulmonary work, and to provide energy used by the central nervous system and other chemical reactions. Dietary-induced thermogenesis, i.e., the thermic effect of a meal, which accounts for the increased energy expenditure above RMR after a meal, accounts for another 10% of daily energy expenditure. Lastly, physical activity, the most variable component, accounts for about 15–30% of total energy expenditure in relatively inactive adults, whereas in very active individuals it can account for significantly more energy expenditure.

Energy Restriction And Daily Energy Expenditure. Observations of less weight loss than predicted as a consequence of energy restriction have led to the suggestion that a metabolic adaptation expressed as a lowering of metabolic rate occurs in response to energy restriction to protect energy stores and minimize weight loss. Although several studies have clearly demonstrated decreased energy expenditure with energy restric-

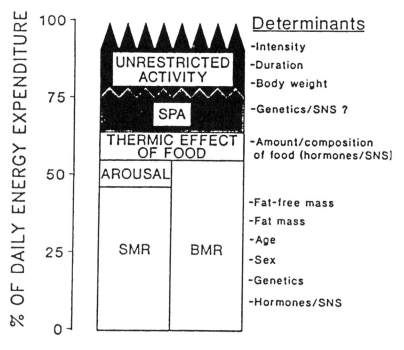

FIGURE 5-7. *Components and determinants of daily energy expenditure.* Modified from Ravussin and Swinburn (1993), with permission.

tion, it does not necessarily follow that a metabolic adaptation has occurred. As Ravussin and Swinburn (1992) explained, when a hypoenergy diet is imposed, some or all of the components of energy expenditure must decrease to match the lower energy intake. If the energy balance is reached at an energy expenditure that is about what would be expected for the body size and composition, then the metabolic changes are predictable, and a metabolic adaptation has not occurred. In contrast, if the decrease in metabolic rate is greater than can be explained from its known determinants, then an adaptation has occurred.

Predictable decreases in the components of daily energy expenditure do indeed happen. In response to lower energy intake, the thermic effect of food can be expected to decline in proportion (10%) to its contribution to total energy expenditure. In response to weight loss, the RMR will also decline, mainly as a function of the loss of FFM and, to a lesser degree, the loss of fat mass. The energy cost of activity is also proportional to body weight, so this component will decrease even when physical activity is constant.

Whether or not a metabolic adaptation to restricted energy intake occurs remains controversial (Ravussin & Swinburn, 1992). While most studies have shown a decrease in 24-h energy expenditure, the measured decline has not always exceeded the expected decline based on changes in body size and composition (Apfelbaum et al., 1971; Bessard et al., 1983; de Boer et al., 1986; de Groot et al., 1990; Garby et al., 1988; Ravussin et al., 1985a; Webb & Abrams, 1983). Also, it is not clear which component of daily energy expenditure may account for the adaptation if one does indeed occur. Several studies have found a decrease in RMR but have not reported the RMR normalized to FFM (Apfelbaum et al., 1977; Bray, 1969; Garrow & Webster, 1989; Morgan, 1984; Welle et al., 1984). In studies of changes in RMR relative to FFM, many, but not all, have shown no significant decline in the RMR-to-FFM ratio (Belko et al., 1987; Davies et al., 1989; de Boer et al., 1986; Elliot et al., 1989; Foster et al., 1990; Henson et al., 1987; Heshka et al., 1990; Wadden et al., 1990; Weigle, 1988; Weigle et al., 1988). The conflicting evidence may be due to differences in diet, initial body composition, and the rate of weight loss because all of these factors have been shown to influence the decrease in RMR (Garrow & Webster, 1989; Hendler & Bonde, 1988, 1990; Hendler et al., 1986). In addition, individual variability in response and technical error in RMR measurement must be considered. The timing of measurements is also important and may explain the conflicting results because RMR has often been measured during active weight loss rather than after the new equilibrium is reached.

Based on their comprehensive review, Ravussin and Swinburn (1992) concluded that an adaptation of RMR to weight loss does not occur, except possibly under certain circumstances, because the fall in RMR may be greater in lean than in obese persons and greater with severe energy restriction and a rapid weight loss than with a more gradual loss (Garrow & Webster, 1989).

Assuming that an adaptation in RMR does not occur, then an adaptation in a component of the nonresting metabolic rate would be required for an adaptation in 24-h energy expenditure to occur. Although reports of a greater than predicted decline in the thermic effect of food suggest an adaptation to low-energy diets (Davies et al., 1989; Schutz et al., 1984, 1987), even a large adaptation would likely have only a small effect on the final body weight (Ravussin & Swinburn, 1992). Thus, it appears that an adaptation in physical activity may be the most plausible explanation of an adaptation in 24-h energy expenditure.

Indeed, some limited evidence suggests that an adaptation in physical activity does occur. In a weight loss study of 12 obese men (Weigle, 1988), the weight lost by six of the men was replaced by lead weights worn in a vest. The added, artificial weight had no effect on the RMR, but it did attenuate the reduction in nonresting energy expenditure observed at the lower body weight. Thus, the reduction in total energy expenditure could be attributed to a lower energy cost of physical activity. Adjustment for this effect and the lower RMR relative to FFM suggested that 100–200 kcal of the lower energy expenditure might be considered "adaptive." Weigle (1988) also showed a lower level of activity, and other investigators have shown a decline in spontaneous activity (de Groot et al., 1989). It would be valuable if additional studies were conducted on the effects of energy restriction and weight loss on planned and spontaneous physical activity, with gender as an independent variable.

Response To Dietary Energy Surfeit

The results of deliberate overfeeding experiments have clearly shown that excess energy intake in men and women results in weight gain (Bouchard et al., 1990; Forbes et al., 1986). The magnitude of the increase is proportional to the daily energy surfeit and the duration of overfeeding, which together determine the total amount of excess energy consumed. The rate of weight gain is proportional to the daily excess. Because maintenance energy requirement is a function of body weight (Jequier & Schultz, 1983), overfed subjects kept on a given level of intake gain less weight as body weight increases up to a new level for which the diet represents a maintenance requirement. Thus, for long periods of overfeeding, the rate of weight gain is expected to decline over time in a curvilinear fashion.

A significant increase in FFM in addition to fat mass is induced by energy surfeit. Although there is considerable individual variation, FFM accounts for approximately 40% of weight gain, on average, in overfeeding experiments lasting up to 100 d (Bouchard et al., 1990; Forbes et al., 1986). Spontaneous weight gain is also accompanied by an increase in FFM of about 40%, although this is somewhat higher than the percentage (~25–30%) of excess weight contributed by FFM in persons with established obesity, suggesting that in the initial phase of overfeeding a somewhat higher proportion of weight gain is FFM than is the proportion after prolonged overfeeding (Forbes et al., 1986). Based on data from a number of studies in the literature, Forbes and colleagues (1986) concluded that individual variation in the composition of weight gain (FFM versus fat) was unaffected by the type of excess food (carbohydrate, fat, or mixed), although it is clear from other sources that adequate protein intake is required for FFM to increase (Barac-Nieto et al., 1978; Miller & Mumford, 1967). In the study by Forbes et al. (1986), gender, initial body weight, and initial body fat were not significant determinants of FFM gain. In contrast, in a more recent analysis, Forbes (1987b) has described a curvilinear relationship between FFM and body fat in females and showed that leaner persons gain relatively larger amounts of FFM with excess energy intake, whereas fatter persons gain proportionately more body fat.

Early observations of less weight gain than predicted during deliberate overfeeding lead to the notion that the body adapts and "wastes" energy in response to overfeeding (Gulick, 1922; Neumann, 1902). More recent work, however, suggests that energy wasting does not occur (Garrow, 1978) and demonstrates the potential for confusion when the static energy balance equation is applied. For example, in an experiment by Ravussin and colleagues (1985a), only 25% of excess energy was dissipated as increased energy expenditure after 9 d of overfeeding; the rest was stored. One-third of the increase in energy expenditure was accounted for by an increase in RMR, mostly related to an increase in FFM. Another one-third was accounted for by an increase in the thermic effect of food in response to the increased energy intake, and the remainder by an increase in energy cost of activity at the heavier body weight. Thus, all the excess energy expenditure could be explained without the need to invoke an adaptive response. Similarly, Roberts et al. (1990) found all the excess energy intake in their subjects was explained by increases in body weight and energy expenditure.

The importance of genetic background to the response to overfeeding has been demonstrated by Bouchard et al. (1990). These investigators overfed 12 pairs of monozygotic twins for 100 d, inducing an average weight gain of 8.1 kg (range = 4.3–13.3 kg). The similarity within each pair in response to overfeeding was significant with respect to body weight, percent fat, fat mass, and subcutaneous fat, with about three times more variance among pairs than between pairs. Moreover, after adjustment for gains in fat mass, the within-pair similarity was particularly impressive with respect to changes in regional fat distribution and amount of abdominal visceral fat. These results clearly demonstrate the different susceptibilities to excess energy intake and the role of genetic factors in governing the determinants of resting energy expenditure and the tendency to store energy as FFM or fat.

ADAPTATION OF BODY WEIGHT AND COMPOSITION TO AEROBIC OR RESISTANCE TRAINING

Comprehensive reviews of the effects of exercise on body weight and composition in athletes and in obese and nonobese nonathletes have been published by Oscai (1973), Epstein and Wing (1980), Wilmore (1983), Stefanick (1993), Ballor and Keesey (1991), Hill et al. (1994) and Atkinson and Walberg-Rankin (1994). The majority of data suggests that increased energy expenditure through exercise results in a decrease in body fat, maintenance of and possibly an increase in fat-free mass, and a decline in body weight that depends on both the direction and magnitude of the change in fat and fat-free mass. Interestingly, the decrease in body fat does not always equal the decrement expected from the calculated energy deficit. One possible explanation for this finding is that exercise may stimulate an increase in appetite, but there is conflicting evidence on this point (Anderson et al., 1991; Oscai, 1973; Thompson et al., 1982; Wilmore, 1983). Moreover, there may be gender differences in the compensation of energy intake to a change in exercise participation, but this point is also controversial (Stefanick, 1993). The application of the static rather than the dynamic energy balance equation to estimate expected loss may have contributed to the uncertainty.

In a recent meta-analysis, Ballor and Keesey (1991) assessed the effects of exercise type and the frequency, intensity, and duration of exercise on changes in total, fat, and fat-free masses, and in percent fat in adults males and females. Studies that included at least five previously sedentary subjects per group and did not combine sexes were included in the analysis. Other inclusionary criteria included adequate reports of pre- and post-intervention body mass and percent fat, exercise energy expenditure (or sufficient information to calculate EE), and exercise type (no mixing of exercise types). Studies that involved exercise sessions longer than 60 min duration or programs of greater than 36 wk were excluded from the analysis. In the 53 studies (41 of males and 12 of females) that met these criteria (of 500 studies reviewed), weight loss after aerobic-type training was shown to be modest in both sexes, although greater in males. All exercise was associated with a reduction in fat mass, whereas an increase in fat-free mass was seen with cycling and resistance exercise in males, such that the actual fat mass loss was greater than total weight loss. No studies of weight training in females were included in the analysis. In males, only slightly more weight loss was associated with aerobic-type exercise compared to resistance exercise, and the rate of change in fat mass (kg/wk) was similar for these two classes of activity. The energy expended during exercise and the initial levels of body fat and total mass accounted for most of the variance associated with changes in body composition; in females, weeks of training and duration of exercise sessions were also significant factors.

The role of the initial body weight and composition on the change in composition with exercise is important to note. Based on a model of two energy reservoirs, Forbes (1987b) has examined the relationship between FFM and fat mass and has shown that the former is a curvilinear function of the latter. Thus, in persons losing or gaining weight as a result of restricted or excess energy intake, the change in FFM is inversely related to . body fat content. In more recent work, Forbes (1991) has shown that a similar relationship exists in exercising persons. Based on a variety of data from the literature, Forbes estimates that individuals with small or modest amounts of body fat tend to lose or gain ~0.5 kg of FFM for every kilogram change in body weight with exercise, and those persons who maintain their weight tend to gain an average of 0.67 kg of FFM and lose an equal amount of fat. If these same persons lose more than ~1.5 kg of weight, they tend to lose FFM, despite engaging in an exercise program. It is important to emphasize these estimates of compositional change represent average values, and individuals may show substantial variations from these average figures.

In contrast, having larger fat stores serves to protect the individual somewhat from loss of FFM as weight is lost and hence favors the loss of body fat during exercise. Individuals with larger fat stores lose or gain only ~0.25 kg of FFM for every kilogram of body weight change, and those whose weight is maintained during exercise gain almost twice as much FFM as do leaner individuals and so lose more fat (Forbes, 1991).

Metabolic Adaptation To Exercise

Aerobic Training. Aerobic-type exercise training has been recommended for programs of weight loss based on the rationale that most individuals can accumulate greater energy expenditures during sustained low- to moderate-intensity aerobic activities than during more anaerobic activities such as resistance training (ACSM, 1983). However, as Ballor and Keesey (1991) have shown, to the degree that energy expenditure is equivalent, both types of exercise can be expected to contribute similarly to energy deficit and loss of fat mass, but the reduction in body mass may be greater with aerobic exercise because the increased FFM with resistance training offsets the decline in total body mass.

In keeping with the notion that energy balance is essentially equal to fat balance (Ravussin & Swinburn, 1992), activities that promote the greatest increase in fat oxidation should be most useful in programs designed to maximize weight loss. Aerobic exercise may be particularly beneficial in this regard. With acute aerobic exercise, sympathoadrenal activity increases and insulin decreases, thereby stimulating hormone-sensitive lipase (HSL) activity, hydrolysis of triglycerides in adipose tissue, and free-fatty acid (FFA) release.

Intramuscular triglycerides are also hydrolyzed during exercise (Walker et al., 1991), depending on intensity (Oscai & Palmer, 1988), whereas circulating triglycerides are not a major lipid source during exercise after fasting (Stefanick, 1993). In contrast, circulating triglycerides represent a significant source of lipid substrate for oxidation during moderate-intensity exercise after a fat-containing meal (Nikkila & Konttinen, 1962); however, this reduces oxidation of FFA released from adipose tissue. Therefore, a high-fat diet would reduce exercise-induced loss of fat weight.

After a transition period of anaerobic metabolism and glucose oxidation, lipids account for a significant portion (up to 65%) of the oxidative metabolism during moderate intensity exercise (less than 50% $\dot{V}O_2$max). Furthermore, there is evidence that the proportion of energy derived from FFA steadily increases with increasing duration of exercise at a fixed work rate (Wolfe et al., 1990), suggesting that a single bout of long duration may be more beneficial in terms of FFA consumption than the same amount of exercise accumulated through several bouts of shorter duration.

Bjorntorp (1990), Despres (1994), and Stefanick (1993) have reviewed the metabolic effects of chronic aerobic exercise in muscle and adipose tissue in relation to lipid utilization and weight control. There is some evidence that regular aerobic exercise may increase the proportion of oxidative versus glycolytic fibers in skeletal muscle, thereby increasing the oxidative capacity of the tissue (Saltin & Gollnick, 1983).

Endurance exercise training also induces important changes in the oxidative potential of muscle fibers, irrespective of their contractile characteristics. For example, training increases mitochondrial number and size, particularly in slow oxidative fibers, resulting in greater concentrations of enzymes for the citric acid cycle and electron transfer (Saltin & Gollnick, 1983), as well as for fatty acid oxidation (Kiens & Saltin, 1985). Increases in skeletal muscle and adipose tissue LPL activity (Kiens & Lithell, 1989; Svedenhag et al., 1983) together serve to decrease circulating plasma triglycerides, and epinephrine-stimulated lipolysis also increases (Despres et al., 1984), resulting in increased fatty acid release from adipose tissue. Thus, trained persons are capable of greater reliance on FFA oxidation during submaximal exercise than are untrained persons (Henriksson, 1977). Moreover, the intensity at which muscles switch from fatty acid oxidation to anaerobic metabolism of glucose also increases with training (Andrews, 1991). The increased endurance that results from training permits longer exercise bouts, which further promotes fat utilization.

There is evidence that regional adipose tissue depots respond differently to exercise designed to induce weight loss, probably because of differential regulation among subcutaneous and visceral fat depots (Arner et al., 1981; Efendic, 1970; Ostman et al., 1979). Regulatory differences may also explain gender differences in the response of regional fat depots to exercise. Arner and colleagues (1991) demonstrated that aerobic exercise mobilized fatty acid release from adipose tissue in the abdominal region more readily than in the gluteal area, and that the differences were more pronounced in women than men. In men, changes in skinfolds suggest that weight loss through exercise results in greater mobilization of trunk fat than extremity fat (Despres et al., 1985), and changes in CT scans in obese premenopausal women who trained for 14 mo indicated a greater loss of deep abdominal fat compared to midthigh fat (Despres et al., 1991). Thus, it is possible that women with a male distribution of fat may benefit more from exercise for weight reduction than do women who deposit fat in the more resistant gluteal and thigh areas, possibly because of preferential lipolysis of visceral fat with stimulation of the sympathetic nervous system during exercise (Krotkiewski & Bjorntorp, 1986). Variation in fat distribution may also explain why in some studies changes in fatness with exercise are correlated with initial fatness in men but not in women (Tremblay et al., 1984).

In addition to the direct energy cost, acute and chronic aerobic exercise may also contribute to increased 24-h energy expenditure by increasing RMR. Available data on this point suggest that RMR may remain elevated for a period of at least 12 h after exercise, and possibly longer, dependent on the duration and intensity of exercise (Bahr et al., 1987; Devlin & Horton, 1986; Poehlman, 1989) relative to the individual's level of fitness. Acute exercise may also potentiate postprandial thermogenesis (Segal & Pi-Sunyer, 1989), but this point remains controversial (Stefanick, 1993). The results of some studies suggest that the sequence of a meal and exercise may interact with body composition (lean versus obese)to affect RMR in men (Segal & Pi-Sunyer, 1989); the effects in women are uncertain.

The degree to which chronic exercise affects RMR remains controversial (Poehlman, 1989; Stefanick, 1993). Cross-sectional studies of RMR and aerobic capacity have shown that trained individuals with high levels of maximal oxygen consumption (> 60 mL $O_2 \cdot kg$ FFM$^{-1} \cdot min^{-1}$) have higher RMRs than individuals with lower aerobic capacity (Poehlman, 1989); however, the influence of factors other than training cannot be discounted. Similarly, the results of training studies are inconclusive due to a variety of methodological differences that have contributed to discrepant results (Poehlman, 1989). Nevertheless, some data suggest that an increase in RMR occurs with training in men and women (Poehlman, 1989). For example, Tremblay et al. (1986) reported an 8% increase in RMR per kg FFM after an 8-wk training program in moderately obese women. Lawson et al. (1987) and Lennon et al. (1985) also observed a higher average RMR after an exercise program in females, but high-intensity exercise may be necessary to achieve the effect (Lennon et al., 1985).

Observations of an increased RMR/kg FFM suggest an adaptation (as defined above) to chronic exercise, but not all investigators reported such a response (Broeder et al., 1992a; Segal & Pi-Sunyer, 1989). Any increase in RMR, if indeed it occurs, suggests that physical conditioning may increase resting energy expenditure, which may be useful in long-term weight control. On this point some evidence indicates that including exercise may be more important in women than in men for preventing a decline in RMR during energy restriction for weight loss (Lennon et al., 1985), although additional research on this issue is certainly needed.

Resistance Training. Fat-free mass, and in particular the muscle component of that mass, are significant predictors of RMR and major determinants of 24-h energy expenditure. Moreover, adequate muscle mass and muscle strength are required for participation in moderate to vigorous physical activity, and low levels of muscle mass and strength undoubtedly contribute to low levels of physical activity and decreased energy expenditure. Thus, any intervention that can maintain or increase fat-free mass, especially muscle mass, would be expected to have a significant role in weight control (Ballor & Keesey, 1991).

The muscle-building effects of resistance training are well known. Although the exact exercise prescription to elicit maximal results remains controversial, muscle hypertrophy accompanies chronic resistance exercise such as weightlifting in postpubescent males and in young adult and middle-aged men (Frontera et al., 1988; Sale, 1989; Tesch, 1988). However, the muscular adaptation to such training in children and women is somewhat different from that of men, due to their different endocrine profiles. Prior to puberty, boys and girls respond similarly to weight training, with increases in muscle strength and little or no increase in muscle mass (Ramsay et al., 1990; Sale, 1989). Adolescent girls and especially young women may experience more muscle hypertrophy than prepubescent girls, but the degree of hypertrophy is less than that of same-aged males. Interestingly, females experience similar relative gains in muscle strength as do males, which has lead to speculation that strength gains in females result more from neural adaptation than from changes in body composition (Pollock & Wilmore, 1990). It seems quite likely that an increase in functional capacity as a result of improved muscle strength may encourage more physical activity and thereby cause greater 24-h energy expenditure and improved body weight control.

In a series of studies, Frontera et al. (1988) and Fiatarone and colleagues (1990) have examined the muscular adaptation to resistance exercise in old and very old men and women. In contrast to the notion that muscle trainability is impaired in old age, significant increases in muscle strength and muscle hypertrophy were demonstrated in men and women in the ninth and tenth decades of life. The results suggested that physical inactivity is a major cause of muscle atrophy and weakness in older people. An important finding in these investigations was that older men and women were capable of resistance exercise at relative loads (> 75% maximum strength) similar to those often employed with younger subjects. Thus, with an appropriate stimulus, older men and women are capable of increasing muscle mass and muscle strength, both of which may contribute to increased 24-h energy expenditure and better weight control.

The effects of resistance exercise on resting metabolic rate have been largely uninvestigated. In what may be the only study of its type, Broeder et al. (1992b) compared the effects of high-intensity resistance exercise versus aerobic exercise on RMR in nondieting men aged 18–35 y. A significant decline in relative body fat was observed in both exercise groups, due either to a reduction in fat weight and maintenance of FFM (aerobic exercise) or to a reduction in fat weight and an increase in FFM (resistance exercise). However, in agreement with some other studies in which exercise was the primary determinant of a negative energy balance (Bingham et al., 1989; Tremblay et al., 1990), RMR in absolute terms or relative to FFM was unchanged in both groups. These results suggest that exercise may help maintain RMR during periods of negative energy balance by either preserving or increasing FFM.

The metabolic consequences of resistance exercise have been reviewed by Dudley (1988). In comparison to aerobic exercise, the effects of resistance exercise on lipid metabolism have received relatively little attention. Nevertheless, observations of reduced intramuscular triglyceride content and increased free-fatty-acid content of blood during high–intensity resistance exercise (Tesch, 1987; Tesch et al., 1986) suggest that β-oxidation is a meaningful source of energy during this type of resistance exercise (Saltin & Gollnick, 1983). There is a need for resistance-exercise training studies in men and women of all ages, with accurate measurements of energy intake and expenditure, to assess the associations among increased muscle mass, energy expenditure, and risk factors for cardiovascular disease (CVD).

Exercise Plus Restricted Energy

Exercise plus energy restriction is generally regarded as the best strategy for inducing optimal changes in body composition (Stefanik, 1993). The addition of exercise to a weight loss program involving energy restriction results in greater weight loss and fat loss (Weltman et al., 1980; Zuti

& Golding, 1976), as well as maintenance of and possibly an increase in FFM (Franklin et al., 1979; Pollock, 1973), especially if a portion of the energy restriction is replaced by increased energy expenditure via exercise. In contrast, if exercise is added to a constant dietary restriction such that it results in a greater loss of body mass, the sparing effect of exercise on FFM may be lost (Hagan et al., 1986).

Programs conducted for at least 20 min per exercise session at least 3 d/wk and of sufficient intensity and duration to expend 300 kcal per session have been suggested as a threshold level for total body weight and fat weight reduction (ACSM, 1983). Increasing energy expenditure above 300 kcal/session and increasing frequency of exercise sessions will further enhance fat loss while possibly sparing FFM. However, the composition of weight change is strongly affected by both the magnitude of body mass loss and the initial body fat stores (Forbes, 1991, 1992; Hagan et al., 1986). As Forbes (1991, 1992) has shown, individuals with larger body fat stores have a degree of protection against FFM loss as body weight is lost. However, exercise cannot conserve FFM in the face of significant energy deficit, particularly in persons with low levels of body fat.

Diet composition may play a role in the response to energy restriction and exercise (Stefanik, 1993). In the second Stanford Weight Control Project (SWCP-II) (Wood et al., 1991), moderately overweight men and women lost significant amounts of fat weight in response to a low-fat diet or a low-fat diet plus exercise, as compared to controls. In comparison to men in the first Stanford Weight Control Project (Wood et al., 1988), in which diet composition was unchanged, the men in SWCP-II achieved greater fat loss on a low-fat diet, and with the addition of exercise an even greater loss of fat occurred. The macronutrient content of weight-reducing diets may also influence the effect of exercise on FFM (Barac-Nieto et al., 1978; Miller & Mumford, 1967; Walberg, 1989), but even a high-protein diet cannot completely overcome the effects of significant energy deficit (Forbes, 1991, 1992).

Exercise has been reported to be one of the few factors positively correlated with successful long-term maintenance of body weight (Brownell et al., 1986; Pavlou et al., 1989; Technology Assessment Conference Panel, 1992). The results of a survey of 700 women recruited from a large health maintenance organization support this point (Kayman et al., 1990). Fifty women were randomly selected from each of the following self-selected categories: relapsers (obese women who regained weight after successful weight reduction), maintainers (formerly obese, at average weight), or always at average weight (controls). Data obtained on 44 relapsers, 30 maintainers, and 30 controls showed that few relapsers exercised (34%), whereas 90% of maintainers and 82% of controls exercised regularly. Thus, the contribution of exercise to weight maintenance may be its most significant effect.

BODY COMPOSITION AS A LIMITING FACTOR
IN SPORT PERFORMANCE

The previous sections dealt with body composition, nutrient balance, and energy expenditure in relation to weight control, predominantly for the general population. The following sections will consider weight control issues that could have profound effects on the health of female athletes.

Many athletes see low body weight as an important performance factor. Female varsity-level college athletes who used pathogenic forms of weight-control (n = 30) were surveyed as to the reason for their behavior (Rosen et al., 1986). Only 7% used pathogenic methods to improve appearance, whereas 80% did so to improve athletic performance. It should be noted that of the 10 sports represented, only one (gymnastics) emphasized physique.

Although athletes tend to have larger fat-free mass levels than nonathletes, a strong relationship between performance and body fat is not a consistent finding. For activities such as running and jumping, in which body mass must be moved through space, generally the higher the body fat the poorer the performance, probably because body fat adds mass without adding power (Claessens et al., 1994; Malina, 1992). However, the relationship between fatness and performance is difficult to establish because several additional variables (e.g., training status, energy expenditure related to training, and energy intake) could influence the relationship. Also, low levels of body fat could be attributed to genetic predisposition, diet, training, and other factors. As one example of the many apparent exceptions to the rule that "leaner is better" for sport performance, Wilmore (1977) examined the body compositions of female distance runners and reported that one runner who had the highest percent body fat (35.8%) in the group established the best time in the world for the 50-mile run.

The data regarding fatness and performance are mostly descriptive. No experimental studies have shown that changes in fatness can alter performance. Therefore, no cause-and-effect relationship has been established; in fact, several studies (e.g., Watts et al., 1993) have found no significant correlation between performance and fatness.

Female bodybuilders, gymnasts, and dancers generally have low body fat levels (Calabrese et al., 1983; Clarkson et al., 1985; Elliot et al., 1987; Fleck, 1983); these may improve performance but are probably sought by these athletes primarily for esthetic reasons. In sports where body fat is not an essential factor for performance or esthetics, correlations between performance and body fat are low, and the average body fat levels are higher (Fleck, 1983; Malina, 1992).

Unfortunately, the belief that lower percentages of body fat always translate into enhanced performance has led some coaches to set inappropriate weight standards for athletes. These coaches (and some athletes) may have adopted the philosophy that if a small weight loss will enhance performance by a small amount, a large weight loss should improve performance markedly (Wilmore, 1992). Experts in body composition believe there is a desirable range of lean mass/fat ratio for a given sport (Johnson et al., 1989; Roundtable, 1990) and that a minimum weight in certain sports (e.g., gymnastics) should be set (Roundtable, 1990). Oppliger and Cassady (1994) state that assessment of body composition should be related to optimal performance of an individual rather than to arbitrary body fat values.

Alterations in body composition with severe dieting can actually impair performance, especially aerobic capacity (Malina, 1992). Ingjer and Sundgot-Borgen (1991), using a case-control study, found that seven elite endurance-trained female athletes showed a significant decrease in maximal oxygen uptake and running speed relative to controls during a period of weight loss achieved by pathogenic weight control methods.

NUTRITIONAL CONCERNS FOR WEIGHT CONTROL IN ATHLETES

Disordered Eating

Assessment. This section will describe disordered eating and assessment techniques. Based on the current diagnostic criteria from the Diagnostic and Statistical Manual (DSM-IV) of the American Psychiatric Association, there are four classes of eating disorders: anorexia nervosa (AN), bulimia nervosa (BN), binge eating disorder, and eating disorders not otherwise classified (American Psychiatric Association, 1994). These conditions share the criteria of attempting to control body weight to prevent weight gain. For anorexia nervosa, the criteria include refusal to maintain normal body weight, intense fear of gaining weight, disturbance of body image, and absence of three consecutive menstrual cycles. Diagnostic criteria for bulimia nervosa include recurrent episodes of binge eating or inappropriate compensatory behavior (vomiting, laxatives, etc.) occurring at least twice a week for three months.

"Binge eating disorder" and "Eating disorder not otherwise specified" were established as categories in 1994 and provide criteria that are not as restrictive as those for AN and BN (American Psychiatric Association, 1994). This is important to take into account when reviewing the studies cited in this paper because most of these studies have not evaluated many of pathogenic weight control methods and behaviors that now are now considered as clinically significant; therefore, the studies probably underestimate the prevalence of eating disorders. For a full description of eating disorder criteria, see the Diagnostic and Statistical Manual (DSM-IV) of the American Psychiatric Association (American Psychiatric Association, 1994).

While the term "eating disorder" typically refers to labels and criteria set forth by the American Psychiatric Association, it must be recognized that disordered eating could also include restrained eating, insufficient energy intake, or inappropriate behaviors such as bingeing and purging only once a week, which do not meet the DSM-IV criteria but may have serious implications for athletes. Because of this problem with the DSM-IV classification, Sundgot-Borgen (1994a) recommended a classification of disordered eating of athletes called "anorexia athletica" (Table 5-2). Athletes with anorexia usually indicate that a coach has suggested that they lose weight. For these athletes, the restricted energy intake is below that needed to sustain the amount of training. They frequently report binge eating, vomiting, use of laxatives, and/or use of diuretics. However, athletes who binge usually do not consume an amount of food greater than what would be ingested by an unaffected athlete.

The Eating Aptitude test (EAT) and the Eating Disorder Inventory (EDI) commonly are used to assess the presence of an eating disorder (Garner & Garfinkel, 1979; Garner et al., 1983). The most recent EAT test (EAT-26) requires an individual to respond to 26 statements concerning abnormal weight and eating conditions and emotional disturbances of anorexia nervosa (Garner & Garfinkel, 1979). For each statement, such as "I feel that food controls my life," "I give too much time and thought to food," "I vomit after I have eaten," a responder must select a number on a 6-point scale that ranges from "never" to "always." A score of 20 or higher in this test is typical of the scores for patients with anorexia nervosa.

The EDI tests for psychological characteristics of anorexia and bulimia nervosa and indicates disturbed attitudes towards eating and body image (Garner et al., 1983). The EDI is composed of a series of 64 statements that are grouped into eight categories: Drive for thinness, Bulimia, Body Dissatisfaction, Ineffectiveness, Perfectionism, Interpersonal distrust, Interoceptive awareness, and Maturity fears (Sundgot-Borgen & Corbin, 1987). The first four are the attitude/behavior subscales, and the latter

TABLE 5-2. *Diagnostic criteria for anorexia athletica.* Proposed by Sundgot-Borgen (1994a).

Weight loss (> 5% of expected body weight)	+
Delayed puberty [no menstrual bleeding at age 16 (primary amenorrhea)]	(+)
Menstrual dysfunction (primary amenorrhoea, secondary amenorrhea, and oligomenorrhea)	(+)
Gastrointestinal complaints	(+)
Absence of medical illness or affective disorder explaining the weight reduction	+
Distorted body image	(+)
Excessive fear of becoming obese	+
Restriction of food (<1200 kcal/d)	+
Use of purging methods (self-induced vomiting, use of laxatives and diuretics)	(+)
Binge eating	(+)
Compulsive exercise	(+)

Symbols: + denotes absolute criteria; (+) denotes relative criteria.

four are psychological trait subscales. In addition to one total score, subscores for each category are obtained.

Another test of disordered eating is the Michigan State University (MSU) Weight Control Survey (Dummer et al., 1987; Rosen et al., 1986). This survey is not primarily concerned with diagnosing anorexia and bulimia, but it attempts to identify pathogenic weight control methods (Rosen & Hough, 1988). Also, the EAT and EDI tests are often modified or abbreviated (Sundgot-Borgen, 1994a).

The EAT and EDI are reliable and valid for the general public (Garner et al., 1983; Garner & Garfinkel, 1979). However, there has been some question regarding their validity for athletes. Wilmore (1991) reported that 110 elite women athletes were administered the EAT, and of the 87 who returned the questionnaire, no athlete scored in the disordered eating range. Yet, in the 2-y period that followed, 18 of these athletes were treated for eating disorders. In a second study, Wilmore (1991) administered the EDI to 14 nationally ranked women distance runners—nine amenorrheic and five eumenorrheic. Results of the EDI showed that three of these athletes had "possible" problems but no frank eating disorder. However, of the nine amenorrheic athletes, four were subsequently diagnosed as having anorexia, two as having bulimia, and one as having both conditions.

Why the validity of these tests would be lower for athletes is uncertain. It is clear from the questions on these tests that the objective is to assess disordered eating. To respond accurately, an individual must have the assurance of anonymity. Wilmore (1991) suggests that athletes may try to cover up their problems, fearing that their coaches, despite anonymity assurance, would discover which athletes have disordered eating. An athlete suspected of having disordered eating behavior could be dropped from a team or not allowed to compete. Based on use of these questionnaires or inventories, there appears to be a significant under-identification of disordered eating in athletes.

Sundgot-Borgen (1993b) used a combination of a questionnaire, interview, and clinical exam. Athletes tended to underreport the use of some pathogenic methods (e.g., vomiting) and overreport the use of other methods (e.g., bingeing) in the screening study using the questionnaires compared to the interviews. The authors recommended that questionnaires should be used only as screening tools and should be followed up by personal interviews and clinical evaluations.

Prevalence in the General Population. Weight control is a concern for many, and especially for girls and women. This has led to an increased frequency of eating disorders such as anorexia nervosa, bulimia, and other abnormal eating behaviors. It has been estimated that when rigid diagnostic criteria are used, 1–5% of the population has anorexia and 2–18% has bulimia nervosa, and of these, 10% or less are males (Brown, 1993; Zerbe,

1993). It has been estimated that 8–12% of college-age women have disordered eating patterns (Raciti & Norcross, 1987). However, these statistics do not account for subclinical eating disorders or the number of females who have exaggerated concerns with body weight. For example, it has been estimated that 79% of female college students have bulimic episodes (Brown, 1993).

Prevalence rates for anorexia nervosa based on hospitalized patients and psychiatric case registers from 1935–1984 were reported to be highest for females aged 15–19 y, followed by females aged 20–24 y (Lucas & Huse, 1994). There was a linear increase in the incidence of anorexia nervosa over the years of the reporting period for the females aged 15–24 y. For example, from 1935–1939 the incidence rate was 13.4/100,000, and from 1980–1984 the rate had grown to 76.1/100,000.

An examination of black and white college students showed that white females had the highest rate of pathogenic eating behaviors (16%) and scored higher on the eating disorder questionnaires compared with the black women (8%) (Chandler et al., 1994). The lower values for black women were related to more positive body images, despite the fact that they weighed more than the white college-age women. Nevertheless, many black females display disordered eating behavior, and they may present this behavior differently than do white women. A survey (Pumariega et al., 1994) of 600 black women showed that their rates of abnormal eating behaviors were similar to those of whites when comparing their responses to a 1983–1984 *Glamour* survey.

The percentage of children scoring in the anorectic range has been estimated at 7%, with anorexia being more frequent than bulimia (Zerbe, 1993). Concerns about body weight are frequent in young girls (11–13 y); although only 4% were actually overweight, more than 40% considered themselves overweight. By age 18, 80% of females have dieted to lose weight, and this practice started early. By age 13, 60% had begun dieting practices (Brown, 1993). Females as young as 5 y reported that they restricted food intake to prevent weight gain (Ciliska, 1993). Black female adolescents appear to diet to lose weight less than white female adolescents, but they are more likely to use fasting, laxatives, and diuretics (Melnyk & Weinstein, 1994).

Prevalence in Athletes. Female athletes generally tend to have a greater frequency of disordered eating compared either to males or to female non-athletes (Brownell & Rodin, 1992; Brownell & Steen, 1992; Leon, 1991; Nattiv et al., 1994, Putukian, 1994; Wilmore, 1991). This section will provide information on the frequency of disordered eating in various groups of athletes and will examine possible mechanisms responsible for these disorders. Comparison among studies is difficult because not all investigators used the same measurement instruments and because the validity of these instruments for athletes is somewhat questionable. However, general patterns emerge, and, while the exact prevalence of disordered eating is not completely known, the data do suggest that significant numbers of female athletes are at risk.

Adolescent Athletes. There are few studies of disordered eating behavior in adolescent athletes. Using the MSU Weight-Control Survey, Dummer et al. (1987) studied 487 girls and 468 boys aged 9–18 y who were attending a competitive swimming camp. Unfortunately, swimmers were not separated by age groups. The percentage of girls and boys who used pathogenic weight control methods was 15.4% and 3.6%, respectively.

Little difference in the risk for developing an eating disorder was found among groups of high school girls, 100 athletes and 112 non-athletes (Taub & Blinde, 1992). The athletes mostly represented sports such as volleyball, basketball, tennis, and softball, none of which emphasizes leanness, although athletes in track and cross-country running were also included. In another study, Benson et al. (1990) administered the EDI to 30 Swiss adolescent athletes (12 gymnasts, and 18 swimmers) and to 34 non-athletes. They found a small but significant risk for eating disorders in these adolescents, but there appeared to be no greater risk among the athletes. There was no significant difference between the groups in preoccupation with weight, but significantly more swimmers (38%) scored high on body dissatisfaction than did controls (9%) or gymnasts (1%). Although swimmers are thought to represent a sport where leanness is not emphasized, their distress over body weight may be due to concern with personal appearance because they must train and compete in swim suits. It is also possible that swimmers in this group were relatively fat, perhaps giving them more reason to be concerned.

Adolescent ballet dancers (11–14 y) were followed for 2–4 y to determine the persistence of eating disorders and to identify factors that could predict an eating disorder (Garner et al., 1987). Inventories of eating disorders (EDI) were administered, and it was found at follow-up that 25.7% met the criteria for anorexia nervosa and 14.2% had bulimia nervosa or a "partial syndrome." On the EDI scales, "drive for thinness" and "body dissatisfaction" predicted the development of eating disorders at follow-up.

College and Young Adult Athletes. Black and Burckes-Miller (1988) administered a self-developed questionnaire to assess inappropriate weight loss methods of 695 college athletes, of whom 55% were women representing eight unspecified sports, and found that as many as 14.7% of the women and 8.6% of the men reported that they had previously fasted for at least 24 h on one or more occasions. Values were lower for other disordered eating behaviors, i.e., fad dieting, vomiting, and use of laxatives, diuretics, and enemas. In another large study, 18.5% of 227 college females from six sports who completed an EAT apparently had disordered eating behaviors (Gustafson, 1989). Rosen et al. (1986) found that of 182 female varsity-level collegiate athletes, 32% practiced at least one pathogenic weight control behavior. Sykora et al. (1993) administered the EAT test to 162 collegiate rowers during the racing season and found that the women had significantly higher EAT scores than did the men.

Sixty-two percent of 42 college gymnasts used at least one pathogenic form of weight control based on the MSU Weight Control Survey (Rosen & Hough, 1988). A study of 218 collegiate gymnasts found that 78% reported eating behaviors that could be classified as disordered, but only a small percentage were actually diagnosed as having bulimia (Petrie, 1993; Petrie & Stoever, 1993). Davis and Cowles (1989) administered the EDI to 64 athletes in "thin-build" sports and to 62 in "normal-build" sports. The females from the thin-build sports tended to have a greater drive for thinness, more body dissatisfaction, more aberrant eating behavior, and generally more abnormal scores on the EDI subscales than did the other athletes and the controls. The "Drive for Thinness" category of the EDI inventory was found to be useful in identifying females at risk for problems associated with eating disorders (O'Connor et al., 1995).

Sundgot-Borgen and Corbin (1987) examined EDI scores of 101 non-athletes, 35 athletes in activities emphasizing leanness (ballet, cheerleading, bodybuilding, gymnastics), and 32 athletes in activities not emphasizing leanness. Results showed that about 4% of non-athletes, 11% of athletes in activities emphasizing leanness, and 0% of athletes with no emphasis on leanness were exceptionally preoccupied with their body weights. Also, approximately 4% of non-athletes, 5% of athletes in activities emphasizing leanness, and 0% of athletes with no emphasis on leanness demonstrated a tendency toward eating disorders. Those reporting EDI subscale scores similar to or higher than those of known anorectics were more commonly among the athletes in "lean" sports. It was interesting to note that when examining only the preoccupation with weight, athletes in sports not emphasizing leanness actually had a bit lower index than did non-athletes (Figure 5-8).

Based on the EDI, a significantly larger percentage (15.5%) of women who participated in weightlifting and body building had elevated scores on the subscale of "drive for thinness" compared with controls (8.7%). Similar percentages of weightlifters and controls (23.3% and 27.2%, respectively) showed high scores on the body-dissatisfaction subscale. Based on a questionnaire developed by the investigators, more weightlifters than controls were classified as "weight preoccupied."

Elite Athletes. Sundgot-Borgen (1993b) obtained EDI test data from 522 elite Norwegian female athletes and 448 controls. Twenty-two percent of the athletes and 26% of the controls were classified as being at risk for an eating disorder. Four categories were determined from the EDI results: 1) those athletes who scored in the abnormal range, 2) those athletes who scored in the normal range, 3) those non-athletic controls who scored in the abnormal ("at risk") range, and 4) those non-athletic controls

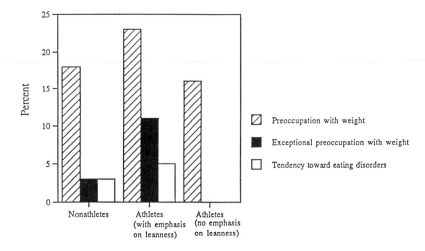

FIGURE 5-8. *Percentage of 168 subjects with preoccupation with weight (hatched bar), exceptional preoccupation with weight (solid bar) and tendencies toward eating disorders (open bar).* Data from Sundgot-Borgen and Corbin (1987), with permission.

who scored in the normal range. Members of these groups were chosen at random to continue with the second part of the study, which contained an interview and clinical exam. Results of the interview showed that 89% of the "at risk" athletes and only 20% of the "at risk" non-athletes met the criteria for anorexia nervosa or bulimia nervosa. Thus, when calculating these numbers for the whole group, there was a significantly greater number of athletes (18%) than non-athletes (5%) suffering from disordered eating. These values were based on the anorexia athletica criteria (see Table 5-2).

The reason for the underreporting of disordered eating in these elite athletes is unclear. It is not known if the athletes actually realize they have a problem and hide it or if they believe they are answering the question truthfully. Sundgot-Borgen (1993b) suggested that athletes may underreport because they do not realize they have disordered eating behavior because their body weights are within accepted ranges. However, fear of discovery by a coach could result in losing a place on the national team, and this could be perceived as more important for elite than for nonelite athletes. The extent to which coaches may perpetuate this problem by giving athletes the impression that disordered eating behavior is acceptable as long as they "don't get caught" is not known.

Generally, sports that have an esthetic component, such as gymnastics, appear to have a greater frequency of disordered eating. In the Sundgot-Borgen study (1993b), the data were also examined for various sport groups. In Figure 5-9, it can be seen that athletes in sports classified

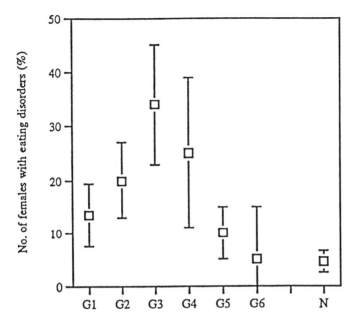

FIGURE 5-9. *Prevalence of eating disorders in female elite athletes in various sport groups:* technical (G1), endurance (G2), aesthetic (G3), weight-dependent (G4), ball games (G5), power sports (G6), and for nonathletes (N). Data from Sundgot-Borgen (1994a), with permission.

as esthetic (34%), weight dependent (27%), or endurance (20%) had greater prevalences of disordered eating.

Figure skaters and professional ballet dancers represent sports in which body weight is emphasized for esthetic reasons. In nationally competitive figure skaters (17 males and 23 females), EAT assessment showed that 48% of women but no men were within the anorectic range (Rucinski, 1989). Also, Brooks-Gunn and colleagues (1987) studied 55 dancers from national and regional classical ballet companies in America and Western Europe and found that 33% reported either having anorexia, bulimia, or both.

Hamilton and colleagues (1985) reported that of 11 black and 34 white professional ballet dancers, none of the black dancers and 33% of the white dancers self-reported anorexia and/or bulimia (Hamilton et al., 1985). Furthermore, the white dancers exhibited more behavior linked to anorexia nervosa than did the black dancers, and the black dancers had more positive body images and were less concerned about dieting. The authors suggest that these results could be due to black dancers being less likely to report eating disorders because one-third of the black dancers' body weights were 20% below ideal (Hamilton et al., 1985). The paucity of data on racial differences in the prevalence of disordered eating in athletes underscores the need for further studies in this area.

Weight and Noakes (1987) studied the top 15 finishers in two major South African ultra-marathon races in addition to 85 female marathon runners, 25 college cross-country runners who participated in the cross-country championships, and 25 non-runner controls. Of the entire group, 18 runners had EAT scores > 20, and of these, five had low body masses and histories of amenorrhea. Three of the five were in the elite category. (Patients with anorexia nervosa have typical scores of 20 or higher on the EAT.) The greatest percentage of abnormal EAT scores (> 30) was found for the elite runners (about 20%), followed by the cross-country runners (about 13%), suggesting that the more skilled runners had a greater incidence of disordered eating.

Dancers from companies that choose their dancers from the company's school (a more select and skilled group) had a lower incidence of disordered eating (11%) compared with companies who chose their dancers from general auditions (46%) (Hamilton et al., 1988). The esthetics of having a very slim body is an essential component of classical ballet, which puts pressure on young dancers to achieve this image. Young dancers can only fight against their natural body types for so long before giving up or settling for a less select company in which fluctuations in body weight or higher percentages of body fat may be tolerated. Only those individuals who naturally have an ectomorphic body type will "survive" a company school and make it into the company. On the other hand, based on the results of Wilmore (1991) and Sundgot-Borgen (1993b), there may be a greater incidence of underreporting of eating disturbances in the most skilled dancers. It is possible that an artistic director could reduce performances and even drop a dancer from a company because of an eating disorder. While the stakes are high for elite athletes whose coaches may discover an eating disorder, the stakes are even greater for professional dancers whose livelihoods depend on being able to perform.

Older Athletes. There is virtually no information available on the incidence of disordered eating behaviors in older or masters athletes. Although poor social networks, low physical activity, high alcohol consumption, and high body-mass index are independent risk indicators of inadequate dietary habits in the elderly (Steen, 1990), it would be quite unlikely to find these characteristics in older athletes. Moreover, mature adults may be less susceptible to social pressures to achieve a certain body shape and would not be under undue influence of a coach. Nevertheless, research is needed to evaluate disordered eating in this population.

Development of Disordered Eating

Females have a greater incidence of disordered eating than do males, and females in sports where body weight is emphasized appear to have the greatest incidence (Johnson et al., 1989). Sundgot-Borgen (1994a) developed a schematic of the factors that contribute to disordered eating in athletes (Figure 5-10). It should be noted in Figure 5-10 that there are predisposing factors that make some athletes more vulnerable. The risk to those vulnerable athletes can be increased or decreased by other circumstances, such as injury, age at onset of training, age at onset of dieting, acceptance of puberty, and changes in training conditions. Societal pressure for girls and women to be thin contribute to the

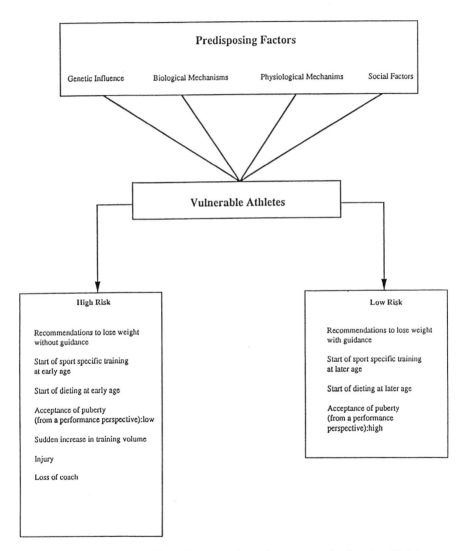

FIGURE 5-10. *Model proposed by Sundgot-Borgen (1994a) on how general and sport specific factors can contribute to the development of eating disorders in athletes.* Model used with permission.

risk of eating disorders. Psychological factors such as the stress of athletics or a predisposition that allows some young women who begin strict diets to let the behavior "get out of hand" may be involved (Sundgot-Borgen, 1994a). Koff and Rierdan (1993) examined whether or not advanced pubertal development was associated with increased risk of an eating disorder in early adolescent girls. They found that girls with more advanced pubertal development generally had elevated levels of eating disturbances, weight preoccupation, increased body fatness, and more negative body images. The authors concluded that the psychological response of a negative body image was an important factor in promoting an eating disturbance.

The "attraction to sport" hypothesis suggests that individuals with a predisposition for disordered eating are attracted to sport (Sundgot-Borgen, 1994a). It is possible that the same personality traits, such as concentration, focus, and discipline, that allow young girls to be successful at a given sport are also factors that predispose them to disordered eating behavior. For example, although ballet does emphasize thinness, it also stresses discipline, keeping the hair in a tight bun, wearing a certain color leotard to class, not allowing runs in tights, and repeating the same fine movements time and time again. Davis and Cowles (1989) reported that athletes in sports that require a thin build were more emotionally labile and dissatisfied. Whether more emotionally labile individuals gravitate toward these kinds of activities or whether the pressure of the activity leads to more emotional reactivity is not known.

Skowron and Friedlander (1994) examined psychological distress and weight preoccupation in a group of 55 highly ranked collegiate swimmers. They found that, like non-athletic college women, athletes most at risk for an eating disorder experience distress in trying to achieve a separate and adequate sense of self, are conflictually dependent upon parents, and engage in punitive, destructive forms of self-control. Mallick and colleagues (1987) suggested that those who appear to be at risk for an eating disorder based on menstrual and dieting patterns are not likely to be at risk unless their mental states and social functioning have deteriorated to a low level.

College runners did not score sufficiently high on the EDI to be categorized as eating disordered, but the psychological inventories showed that the eating-disturbed runners (29 out of 60 runners) appeared to be more concerned with food and dieting than were other runners (Parker et al., 1994). However, unlike athletes with frank eating disorders, these runners did not show disturbances in psychopathology, such as problems in self-esteem or interpersonal relationships, or in psychological disturbances of a more general nature. Athletes predisposed to acquiring an eating disorder may have underlying psychiatric factors such as low self-esteem and depression.

Hormonal and neurotransmitter imbalances may play a role in eating disorders. Kaye and Weltzin (1991) presented some data from animal and human studies relating imbalances in serotonin and norepinephrine with bulimic or bingeing behaviors. Also, persons with bulimia have a lower secretion of cholecystokinin (Kaye & Weltzin, 1991), a peptide secreted by the small intestine during digestion that appears to suppress hunger (Strubbe, 1994). However, Hirschberg et al. (1994) found that cholecystokinin response to a meal could not explain the insufficient food intake in amenorrheic and oligomenorrheic female long-distance runners.

Sundgot-Borgen (1994a) examined trigger factors associated with the onset of an eating disorder. Athletes who were identified with an eating disorder (n = 85) were asked in an interview: "Do you have any suggestion as to why you developed an eating disorder?" Their responses indicated that three factors were most important: 1) prolonged periods of dieting or weight fluctuations; 2) traumatic events such as illness, injury to oneself or a family member, new coach, failure at school, problems at home, etc.; and 3) significant increases in training volume.

Coaches may play an important role in increasing the incidence of eating disorders. A study of 247 college athletes (44% women) representing 27 varsity teams (Selby et al., 1990) showed that 14% of the men and 63% of the women considered themselves overweight. A third of these women believed that their coaches also saw them as overweight, whereas only 9% of the men believed this. In contrast to their high estimates of coaches' perceptions of their overweight status, only 14% and 21% of the women believed their peers and parents, respectively, saw them as overweight. In the study of college gymnasts by Rosen and Hough (1988), 75% of the gymnasts who were told by their coaches that they were too heavy resorted to pathological eating behaviors.

In the past few decades some alarming changes in the physical characteristics of gymnasts have occurred. Figure 5-11 presents the dramatic

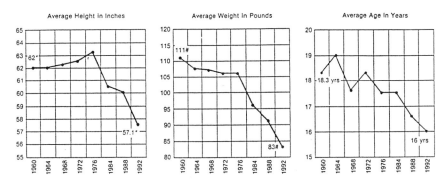

FIGURE 5-11. *Height, weight, and age trend of U.S. Olympic women gymnasts from 1960 to 1992.* Data from Nattiv et al. (1994), with permission.

decreases in height, weight, and age of elite women gymnasts since 1960. In 1960, the height and weight of the 18-y-old gymnasts was in the region of the 20th and 25th percentile, respectively, of the growth charts of the National Center for Health Statistics (NCHS) (Hamill et al., 1979). In 1992, the 16-y-old gymnasts fell below the 5th percentiles for both height and weight. There is virtually no information on how changes in body composition during growth and puberty affect performance; however, it is clear that selection of physical characteristics by coaches or trainers occurs early.

Diet Adequacy of Female Athletes at Risk of Disordered Eating

Before presenting data on dietary patterns in athletes, it is important to address the inadequacies of the techniques used to assess dietary intake in populations. For a detailed review of the strengths and weaknesses of diet-assessment techniques see Pao and Cypel (1990). Factors that contribute to measurement errors of nutrient intake are: 1) respondent biases, 2) interviewer biases, 3) respondent memory lapses, 4) incorrect estimation of portion sizes and tendencies to overestimate low intake and underestimate high intakes, 5) inattention to supplement use, 6) coding and computation errors, and 7) errors associated with computer programs and associated data bases (Garry & Koehler, 1990; Gibson, 1993).

Diet surveys tend to underestimate dietary intake, because subjects underreport what they have eaten (Gibson, 1993; Schoeller, 1990). The results of food frequency questionnaires completed by parents to determine food intake in their children showed that the questionnaires overestimated energy intake by about 810 kcal when compared to the more accurate doubly-labeled water method to determine total energy expenditure (Kaskoun et al., 1994). Schoeller (1990) reviewed eight studies of adults and one of adolescents in which doubly-labeled water assessment and self-reported energy intake were compared in subjects who maintained stable body weights. It was found that reported intakes tended to be lower than expenditures and thus underestimated true energy intakes. Because of the errors described above, deviations of 25% or less from the RDA may not be meaningful.

An excellent review of the energy intake of female athletes is presented by Ruud and Grandjean (1994). Studies have shown a wide range of energy intakes among various sports and even within a sport. However, women and girls in those sports in which body weight or shape is an important factor generally have low energy intakes. A comprehensive survey of athletes' dietary intakes that also addresses the problem with diet surveys can be found in a review paper by Short (1994). Thus, this section will highlight only a few studies of dietary intake of athletes representing various age groups, with specific attention to those athletic groups who may be at risk for disordered eating.

Adolescent Athletes. The average daily energy intakes of adolescent gymnasts and ballet dancers have been reported as 1,838 kcal (Loosli et al., 1986) and 1,890 kcal (Benson et al., 1985), respectively. It is important to notice that these results were published in 1985, and, according to Figure 5-11, the body weights of gymnasts have dropped. In a more recent study, Swiss gymnasts were ingesting 1,544 kcal daily (Benson et al., 1990).

More than 30% of adolescent gymnasts and ballet dancers consumed less than 2/3 of the RDA for vitamin B_6, folic acid, and vitamin E; 7–20% consumed less than 2/3 of the RDA for thiamin, niacin, vitamin B_{12}, vitamin C, and vitamin A (Benson et al., 1985; Loosli et al., 1986). Low calcium intakes have been reported for adolescent female gymnasts (Moffatt, 1984), ballet dancers (Benson et al., 1985), and distance runners (Moen et al. 1992). Forty-one percent of adolescent gymnasts (Loosli et al., 1986) and 43.4% of adolescent ballet dancers (Benson et al., 1985) did not meet 2/3 of the RDA for magnesium. Among female adolescent athletes, gymnasts, ballet dancers, and runners consumed considerably less iron than the RDA (Benson et al., 1991; Loosli et al., 1986; Moen et al., 1992; Moffatt, 1984). More than 70% of adolescent ballet dancers and gymnasts ingested less than 2/3 the RDA for zinc (Benson et al., 1985; Loosli et al., 1986). Although mean values for adolescent female swimmers showed that they were ingesting more than the RDA for vitamins A, C, B_1, and B_2; niacin; calcium; and iron, many individual swimmers reported values substantially lower than the means (Berning et al., 1991). An examination of the dietary intakes of the Swiss national gymnastics team and 18 highly trained swimmers showed that both groups had mean intakes of folic acid and iron that were < 75% of the RDA (Benson et al., 1990). For swimmers, the mean micronutrient intake was < 75% of the RDA for calcium and vitamin B_6.

It appears that the energy intake are low in female adolescents in sports that emphasize leanness. This leads to an insufficient consumption of many micronutrients that could have serious implications for growth and health in later years. It is important, however, to know to what extent these data are due to underreporting of dietary intakes before firm conclusions can be drawn regarding the inadequacy of the diets.

Young Adult Athletes. Economos et al. (1993) reviewed studies concerning the energy needs of athletes and recommended that elite female athletes should ingest 45–50 $kcal \cdot kg^{-1} \cdot d^{-1}$. The studies that were reviewed showed that 88% of "aerobic" athletes and 100% of "anaerobic" athletes consumed less than this recommendation, yet the majority of athletes fell within the normal range for body weight and percent body fat in females. This may indicate an underreporting of energy intake. Long-distance running and bodybuilding were two sports in which energy intake, body weight, and body fat were low.

Women who consumed < 2000 kcal or < 45 kcal/kg had lower dietary intakes of iron, calcium, magnesium, zinc, and vitamin B_{12}. However, 80% of women in aerobic sports and 100% of women in anaerobic sports reported that they regularly used vitamin supplements. Provided that the supplements represented micronutrients for which they were deficient, most adult female athletes could be ingesting sufficient micronutrients, assuming that the supplements contained micronutrients that are active and usable, a concern with this unregulated industry. For example, Bazzarre et al. (1993) found that 15 female athletes who took supplements were ingesting more than 75% of the RDA for all vitamins and minerals. However, those who did not take supplements failed to consume more than 75% of the RDA for iron and magnesium.

Many young adult women in the general population have lower iron, zinc, and calcium intakes than the RDA, and this pattern is generally true for female athletes (Clarkson & Haymes, 1994; 1995). Similar to the adolescent athletes, adult athletes in sports that emphasize leanness appear to have low energy intakes and less than adequate intake of several micronutrients (Applegate, 1989; Grandjean, 1989; Kaiserauer et al., 1989; Rucinski, 1989; Sundgot-Borgen, 1993a). Although many adult athletes take vitamin and mineral supplements and may be meeting their micronutrient requirements, a low energy intake may result an increased risk of malnutrition. Also, some athletes may be taking supplements containing only one or two micronutrients that could be unrelated to those in which they may be deficient. The long-term implications of poor diets is not known, although those who do not ingest sufficient micronutrients can be vulnerable to an increased risk of stress fractures (Frusztajer et al., 1990). As with the adolescent athletes, the data here should be viewed with caution because the extent to which these athletes may underreport dietary intake is not known.

Older Athletes. Data for older athletes are scant. Blair and colleagues (1981) examined dietary intakes of 34 male and 27 female long-distance runners aged 35–59 y. The mean energy intake for the women was 2386 kcal or 42 kcal/kg, which appears to be on the low side of the recommendation for young adult athletes but may be adequate for older women with less muscle mass. Dietary intakes were assessed for 103 adult women runners and compared with those for inactive controls (Pate et al., 1990). The mean energy intake for the runners was 1603.2 kcal (27.5 kcal/kg), not different from that of the controls. Both the runners and controls ingested < 75% of the RDA for magnesium, vitamin D, vitamin B_6, zinc, and iron. The low energy intakes for both the runners and controls may indicate underreporting or undereating on the day of recording intake.

Lloyd and colleagues (1992) examined dietary intakes of 108 premenopausal recreational women runners. The runners aged 36 y or older had an average energy intake of 32.4 kcal·kg^{-1}·d^{-1} (about 1824 kcal/d), which probably did not meet the recommended energy intake for most of the runners. However, the older runners had greater intakes of iron, magnesium, calcium, and vitamin B₆ compared with the younger adult runners. Whether this was associated with vitamin and mineral supplementation was not reported.

MEDICAL AND SAFETY CONCERNS

In the general population, there is an age-related loss in muscle mass, a decline in resting metabolic rate, and an increase in total and central body fat. These changes are associated with other risk factors, including dyslipidemia, hypertension, hypersinsulinemia, insulin resistance, and hyperglycemia, all of which appear to precede the development of non-insulin-dependent diabetes and coronary artery disease. The loss of muscle mass may be a precursor to osteoporosis and also affects the ability to produce force so that performance declines. Decreases in performance cause individuals to be less active, which promotes greater losses in functional capacity. Therefore, interventions aimed at maintaining and increasing muscle mass should be strongly advised. These interventions can play an important role in maintaining optimal body composition and reducing disease risk.

During aging there is an increase in upper body fatness in women that has been associated with an increased risk of cardiovascular disease (Despres et al., 1989; Lapidus et al., 1984, 1989) and diabetes (Lundgren et al.,1989; Pasquali et al., 1990). Although the effects of hormone replacement therapy (HRT) on the risk-factor profile in postmenopausal women have been described, few studies have directly compared either the effects of HRT versus exercise or the interaction of HRT and exercise on body composition and CVD risk in women at different ages. Exercise studies with measurements of dietary energy intake and expenditure in premenopausal women with and without estrogen replacement are sorely needed. This is an especially important area given the increasing numbers of older women and the reluctance of many women to begin HRT or continue it for long periods.

Most of the medical concerns of the older female athlete stem from undernutrition and amenorrhea as an adolescent or young adult. Inadequate estrogen levels and low calcium intakes in young girls compromise bone mass accretion so that peak bone mass is not attained. This has negative consequences later in life (Constantini & Warren, 1994; Nelson et al., 1986).

Women participating in sports such as track and field seek to achieve a large muscle mass. To this end, some women athletes take anabolic steroids. Yesalis et al. (1990) surveyed five National Collegiate Athletic Association Division 1 universities and estimated that 14.7% of men and 5.9% of women athletes used steroids. Although steroid use is greater in men, this should still be considered a significant medical concern for women athletes in sports demanding large musculature. Steroid use in women can result in side effects such as masculinization, menstrual irregularities, increases in secondary sex characteristics, irritability, and aggressiveness (Catlin et al., 1993; Nevole Jr. & Prentice, 1987).

Sports that demand low body weights are associated with delayed menarche (Bale, 1994; Malina, 1992; Malina et al., 1994; Merzenich et al., 1993; Warren, 1992). The long-term consequences of delayed menarche are not known. However, the lack of estrogen may compromise bone mass accretion that occurs in adolescents and thus affect peak bone mass (Constantini & Warren, 1994). The risk of breast cancer is decreased as age at menarche increases (Merzinich et al., 1993). This might lead to the conclusion that a delayed menarche is beneficial. However, if delayed menarche is due to undernutrition and/or if a girl remains amenorrheic, the negative consequences would far outweigh any benefits.

Theintz and colleagues (1993) assessed whether or not intense physical activity during puberty could alter the growth potential of females and found that gymnasts showed a delayed menarche and a reduced stature that could be attributed to a marked stunting of lower limb growth. In an earlier study, Theintz et al. (1989) reported that fathers and mothers of gymnasts were significantly shorter and lighter than those of other athletes. Peltenburg et al. (1984) performed a retrospective study of Dutch female athletes and schoolgirls aged 1–11 y. The results showed that the gymnasts were smaller than the other groups from 1 year of age, and their heights appeared to be related to their mothers' heights. The authors suggested that the short stature of gymnasts is to some extent selected and not due to increased physical activity during growth. Once selected into gymnastics, inadequate diets could affect growth potential.

Many females with eating disorders are also amenorrheic (Brooks-Gunn et al., 1987; Gadpaille et al. 1987). The reduction in circulating estrogen associated with amenorrhea has a profound effect on the loss of bone, and studies have found an increased incidence of stress fractures in amenorrheic athletes and in athletes with restricted diets (Frusztajer et al., 1990; Karpakka et al., 1994; Olson, 1989). A study of ballet dancers with irregular menstrual cycles showed bone density deficits in non-weight-bearing sites that were similar to deficits found for girls with anorexia nervosa (Young et al., 1994).

Females with eating disorders can have other serious medical problems (Pomeroy & Mitchell, 1992). Mortality of patients with anorexia is as high as 19%. Pomeroy and Mitchell (1992) have presented a detailed list of complications associated with anorexia and bulimia nervosa. Nearly every system in the body can be affected. A particularly dangerous complication is a disturbance in fluid balance and electrolytes, especially hypokalemia, which can result in cardiac arrhythmias, inadequate cardiac output, and death.

DIRECTIONS FOR FUTURE RESEARCH

Although qualitative trends have been described, the need to rely on indirect methods in human beings has limited the accuracy of estimates of various body constituents at most ages. Thus, there is a need to apply more complex models of body composition, especially in children and elderly men and women, to better quantify growth patterns and aging-related changes in fat mass, FFM, and FFM subcomponents.

Longitudinal studies combining traditional laboratory methods, anthropometry, and state-of-the-art imaging techniques to describe changes in internal (visceral) and external (subcutaneous) fat depots are especially needed to better understand the relationship between developmental and aging-related changes in simple, external measurements and total body compartments. In this way, more valid field techniques for estimating total fat, FFM, and indices of fat distribution could be derived. Better indices of fat distribution are needed if screening programs are to be undertaken. This is especially true for women, in whom body composition has often been measured using inappropriate models designed for use in men. Also, the persistence (tracking) of fat distribution patterns from adolescence into adulthood and the sensitivity and specificity of measures of adolescent and young adult fat distribution for predicting incidence of various CVD risk factors and NIDDM later in life need to be better established

There is also a need for comprehensive analyses of body composition in studies of weight loss and weight gain and of the metabolic responses to changes in energy intake and expenditure. Traditional two-component criterion methods are confounded by the changes in FFM subcomponents (especially changes in hydration and, to a lesser degree, protein and bone mineral) that accompany changes in body weight as a result of changes in energy balance. The application of more complex approaches would allow a more accurate assessment of the changes in body composition that accompany changes in energy balance and make it possible to determine whether the metabolic changes that occur with weight loss or gain represent true metabolic adaptations or predictable consequences of changes in fat and FFM. If CVD risk factors were also measured, it would be possible to determine the relationship between changes in body composition and risk factor profile. While the cross-sectional associations between total and regional fat masses and CVD risk factors are well established, there have been considerably fewer longitudinal studies, and typically body composition has been estimated from anthropometric indices such as the body mass index rather than by direct measurements.

Intervention studies are also needed. While the relative merits of diet, exercise, and diet plus exercise for modifying body composition have been described, there is a continued need for systematic studies to define the best prescription of diet and exercise for achieving optimal body composition in women. Recent work has defined the interrelationship between fat and FFM and shown that initial fatness is an important determinant of the change in composition in response to both diet and exercise. The notion that exercise spares FFM during weight loss is not supported by all studies, and the conflicting results may well be due to initial differences in body fat and variability in the magnitude of the total energy deficit. The type of exercise is also an important determinant, and there is a need to further investigate the effects of different types of exercise on body composition at various levels of energy intake across the typical range of body fatness. There is some evidence that aerobic and resistance exercise may be equally effective for inducing fat loss in men if energy expenditure is equated. Whether or not similar effects occur in women is not clear. The relative effects of aerobic and resistance exercise on fat distribution is not known, and this is an especially important area for future investigation given the strong association between fat distribution and the risk of metabolic aberrations.

There have been few studies of the metabolic responses to diet and especially exercise, in part, due to the effects of hormonal fluctuations throughout the menstrual cycle. Well-designed intervention studies in women are needed to separate the effects of diet and different types exercise on changes in composition and metabolism at different ages. It would be advantageous to study premenopausal and postmenopausal women undergoing the same intervention to facilitate comparisons among women with different menstrual statuses.

While there is much to learn in general about the body composition of females throughout the life span, there is also a need for information on body composition as related to the health of female athletes. Some female athletes participating in sports in which large muscle mass is desirable may be using anabolic steroids (Yesalis et al., 1990). However, there is a paucity of data on the number of women athletes who take steroids, the amount of muscle mass achievable, and the side effects or risks. Although anabolic steroid use can alter menstrual function, the long-term effects in women are not known.

Many female athletes restrict their energy intakes because they believe that low body weights are necessary for optimal performance. To date, the studies have been descriptive in nature; no experimental research studies have been performed. More information is needed to identify those sports in which low body fat provides an advantage and to determine how low the body fat should be before it becomes a disadvantage for either performance or health. There is a need for further research on the negative impact of excessive weight loss on performance, or the possible positive impact of a small/moderate weight loss on performance. It is important to demonstrate to athletes, coaches, and trainers that there could be a threshold for body weight and/or energy intake below which performance and health will deteriorate.

The validity of techniques to assess the prevalence of disordered eating in athletes is questionable. There is not sufficient, accurate information regarding prevalence rates of disordered eating in athletes. There may be a significant underreporting in various athlete groups, and this should be addressed. Furthermore, there is a paucity of data for preadolescent and adolescent girls involved in sport. The development of behaviors associated with disordered eating may start as early as prepubescence. Also, there is no information regarding prevalence rates of disordered eating in older athletes.

Why some athletes develop disordered eating while others do not is not well understood. More information on the causes of disordered eating and on why some athletes are more predisposed to these disorders than others should be gathered.

Based on self-reported food intakes, many female athletes ingest less than optimal amounts of energy and micronutrients. Better tools are needed to assess qualitative and quantitative aspects of energy intake in female athletes. Well-designed and controlled studies conducted in metabolic wards are needed. Several studies have suggested that energy restriction and poor nutrient intakes are associated with an increased incidence of injury, particularly stress fractures. More data are needed to determine injury risks associated with energy restriction in all age groups of female athletes.

The term "Female Athlete Triad" was established to describe the conditions of amenorrhea, osteoporosis, and disordered eating that are frequently found in female athletes. More research is needed to fully understand each of these processes, how they are linked to exercise and energy intake, and how these conditions may be linked to each other.

SUMMARY

Gender-related differences in body composition, first evident in childhood, become more apparent during adolescence. Males experience a rapid gain in FFM and a reduction in relative fat, whereas females experience a more modest increase in FFM and an increase in percent body fat. The greater body water, muscle, and bone masses that develop during adolescence persist throughout life and are significant determinants of differences in functional capacity, athletic performance, and some aspects of disease risk. The characteristic male (truncal or android pattern) and fe-male (gluteofemoral or gynoid pattern) patterns of fat distribution also develop during adolescence. It is now well established that both men and women with the android pattern have a greater risk of developing meta-bolic disorders and CVD than age- and sex-matched individuals with the gynoid pattern.

With aging, both men and women experience a loss of FFM and a gradual increase in body fat. Women also experience significant changes in body composition during pregnancy and lactation, and with menopause. The long-term metabolic consequences of repeated weight gain and loss, and the redistribution of body fat that accompanies multiple pregnancies and lactation, are not clear. Redistribution of body fat, associated with es-trogen withdrawal and increasing androgenicity, also occurs with meno-pause. The increased truncal fat and visceral fat in postmenopausal women contributes to a more adverse CVD risk factor profile in middle-aged and older women who forego hormone replacement therapy.

Many women at all ages, dissatisfied with their appearances or for health reasons, attempt to control their body weights and change body compositions through dieting, exercise, or both. While it is clear that energy restriction can result in more rapid loss of body weight than can exercise, the loss of FFM and the reduction in energy expenditure that can accompany energy restriction may make weight maintenance and subse-quent attempts to lose weight more difficult. In contrast, exercise usually acts to conserve and possibly increase FFM and metabolic rate and, in combination with moderate energy restriction, may increase fat loss, al-though the overall weight loss may be less. Individual responses to energy restriction, energy surfeit, and increased energy expenditure vary widely and have a significant genetic component, although other factors such as initial body composition, severity and duration of energy restriction and energy expenditure, diet composition, age, and menopausal status must be considered when predicting the outcome of a change in energy balance.

Energy restriction is a common practice for many female athletes who are disturbed about their body weights. While some athletes, such as those involved in dance and gymnastics, are concerned for esthetic rea-sons, others believe that low body weights translate into improved per-formance. There are limited data supporting the latter belief, and there is concern that too low a body weight may jeopardize sport performance.

Female athletes have an increased risk for disordered eating. A signif-icant number of adolescent female athletes, especially those participating in sports emphasizing leanness, were found to use pathogenic weight control methods and were negatively preoccupied with body weight. An increased prevalence of disordered eating or body dissatisfaction has been found in college and elite female athletes. However, there appears to be a serious underreporting of disordered eating in these athletes, which may be due to fear of discovery by a coach. Why some athletes are more predisposed than others to eating disorders is not well understood.

Female athletes who restrict energy intakes in attempt to reduce their body weights risk inadequate energy intakes and nutritional deficiencies. Adolescents who diet could consume inadequate levels of nutrients and micronutrients that could affect growth and increase the risk of stress fractures.

Low body weights in athletes are associated with delayed menarche, eating disorders, and amenorrhea. These conditions have profound implications for the health of female athletes of all ages. In certain situations, encouraging weight loss in female athletes could border on malpractice. Coaches, trainers, and other professionals who deal with athletes need to understand the consequences and implications of low body weights before recommending that any female athlete lose weight.

Overall, weight control is a serious issue for females in the general population as well as for female athletes. Increased body fat and the loss of muscle and bone mass with age affect women's health and quality of life in later years. The concern over body fat in many young women and girls has led to deficits in energy intake, compromised micronutrient status, and disordered eating. These problems are particularly striking in female athletes. More research is needed to fully understand the relationships among weight control, body composition, and health risks so that we can safeguard the health of women for a life time.

ACKNOWLEDGEMENTS

The authors thank Jack Wilmore, Craig Horswill, Jean-Pierre Despres, Robin Levine, and Stella Volpe for their expert and comprehensive reviews of this manuscript.

BIBLIOGRAPHY

Abbott, W.G.H., B.V. Howard, L. Christin, D. Freymond, S. Lillioja, V.L. Boyce, T.E. Anderson, C. Bogardus and E. Ravussin (1988). Short-sterm energy balance: relationship with protein, carbohydrate, and fat balances. *Am. J. Physiol.* 255:E332–E337.

Acheson, K.J., Y. Schutz, T. Bessard, K. Anantharaman, J.P. Flatt, and E. Jéquier (1988). Glycogen storage capacity and de novo lipogenesis during massive carbohydrate overfeeding in man. *Am. J. Clin. Nutr.* 48:240–247.

Acheson, K.J., Y. Schutz, T. Bessard, J.P. Flatt, and E. Jéquier (1987). Carbohydrate metabolism and de novo lipogenesis in human obesity. *Am. J. Clin. Nutr* 45:78–85.

Aloia, J.F., A. Vaswani, P. Ross, and S.H. Cohn (1990). Aging bone loss from the femur, spine, radius, and total skeleton. *Metabolism* 39:1144–50.

Alpert, S. (1988). The energy density of weight loss in semistarvation. *Int. J. Obes.* 12:533–542.

Alpert, S. (1990). Growth, thermogenesis, and hyperphagia. *Am. J. Clin. Nutr.* 52:784–792.

American College of Sports Medicine (1983). Proper and improper weight loss programs. *Med. Sci. Sports Exerc.* 15:1, pp. ix–xiii.

American Psychiatric Association (1994). *Diagnostic and Statistical Manual of Mental Disorders*, 4th ed. (DSM-IV). Washington, D.C.: American Psychiatric Association, pp. 539–550, 731.

Anderson, B., X. Xu, M. Rebuffe-Scrive, K. Terning, M. Krotkiewski, and P. Bjorntorp (1991). The effects of exercise training on body composition and metabolism in men and women. *Int. J. Obes.* 15:75–81.

Andrews, J.F. (1991). Exercise for slimming. *Proc. Nutr. Soc.* 50:459–471.

Apfelbaum, M., J. Bostsarron, and D. Lacatis (1971). Effect of caloric restriction and excessive caloric intake on energy expenditure. *Am. J. Clin. Nutr.* 24:1404–1409.

Apfelbaum, M., L. Brigant, and M. Joliff (1977). Effects of severe diet restriction on the oxygen consumption of obese women during exercise. *Int. J. Obes.* 1:387-393.

Applegate, E. (1989). Nutritional concerns of the ultraendurance athlete. *Med. Sci. Sports Exerc.* 21: S205-S208.

Arner, P., P. Engfeldt, and H. Lithel (1981). Site differences in the basal metabolism of subcutaneous fat in obese women. *J. Clin. Endocrinol. Metab.* 53:948-952.

Arner, P., H. Lithell, H. Wahrenberg, and M. Bronnegard (1991). Expression of lipoprotein lipase in different human subcutaneous adipose tissue regions. *J. Lipid Res.* 32:423-429.

Atkinson, R.L., and J. Walberg-Rankin (1994). Physical activity, fitness and severe obesity. In: C. Bouchard, R.J. Shephard, and T. Stephens (eds.) *Physical Activity, Fitness and Health. International Proceedings and Consensus Statement.* Champaign, IL: Human Kinetics, pp. 696-711.

Bahr, R., I. Ingnes, O. Vaage, O.M. Sejersted, and E. Newsholm (1987). Effect of duration of exercise on postexercise O_2 consumption. *J. Appl. Physiol.* 62:485-490.

Bale, P. (1994). Body composition and menstrual irregularities of female athletes. Are they precursors of anorexia? *Sports Med.* 17:347-352.

Ballor, D.L., and R.E. Keesey (1991). A meta-analysis of the factors affecting exercise-induced changes in body mass, fat mass and fat-free mass in males and females. *Int. J. Obes.* 15:717-726.

Barac-Nieto, M., G.B. Spurr, H. Lotero, and M.G. Maksud (1978). Body composition in chronic undernutrition. *Am. J. Clin. Nutr.* 31:23-40.

Baumgartner, R.N., S.B. Heymsfield, S. Lichtman, J. Wang, and R.N. Pierson (1991). Body composition in elderly people: The effect of criterion estimates on predictive equations. *Am. J. Clin. Nutr.* 53:1345-1353.

Baumgartner, R.N., S.B. Heymsfield, A.F. Roche, and M. Bernardino (1988). Abdominal composition quantified by computed tomography. *Am. J. Clin. Nutr.* 48:936-945.

Baumgartner, R.N., R.L. Rhyne, P.J. Garry, and S.B. Heymsfield (1993). Imaging techniques and anatomical body composition in aging. *J. Nutr.* 123:444-448.

Baumgartner, R.N., A.F. Roche, S. Guo, T. Lohman, R.A. Boileau, and M.H. Slaughter (1986). Adipose tissue distribution: the stability of principal components by sex, ethnicity and maturation stage. *Hum. Biol.* 58:719-735.

Bazzarre, T.L., A. Scarpino, R. Sigmon, L.F. Marquart, S.L. Wu, and M. Izurieta (1993). Vitamin-mineral supplement use and nutritional status of athletes. *J. Am. Col. Nutr.* 12:162-169.

Belko, A.Z., M. Van Loan, T.F. Barbieri, and P. Mayclin (1987). Diet, exercise, weight loss, and energy expenditure in moderately overweight women. *Int. J. Obes.* 11:93-104.

Bell, E.F. (1985). Body water in infancy. In: A.F. Roche (ed.) *Body Composition Assessments in Youth and Adults.* Report of the Sixth Ross Conference on Medical Research. Columbus, Ohio: Ross Laboratories, pp. 30-33.

Bennett, C., G.W. Reed, J.C. Peters, N.N. Abumrod, M. Sun, and J.O. Hill (1992). Short-term effects of dietary-fat ingestion on energy expenditure and nutrient balance. *Am. J. Clin. Nutr.* 55:1071-1077.

Benson, J., Y. Allemann, G.E. Theintz, and H. Howald (1990). Eating problems and calorie intake levels in Swiss adolescent athletes. *Int. J. Sports Med.* 11:249-252.

Benson, J., D.M. Gillien, K. Bourdet, and A.R. Loosli (1985). Inadequate nutrition and chronic calorie restriction in adolescent ballerinas. *Phys. Sportsmed.* 13:79-90.

Berning, J.R., J.P. Troup, P.J. VanHandel, J. Daniels, and N. Daniels (1991). The nutrition habits of young adolescent swimmers. *Int. J. Sport Nutr.* 1:240-248.

Bessard, T., Y. Schutz, and E. Jéquier (1983). Energy expenditure and postprandial thermogenesis in obese women before and after weight loss. *Am. J. Clin. Nutr.* 38:680-693.

Bingham, S.A., G.R. Goldberg, W.A. Coward, A.M. Prentice, and J. H. Cummings (1989). The effect of exercise and improved physical fitness on basal metabolic rate. *Br. J. Nutr.* 61:155-173.

Bjorntorp, P. (1990). Adipose tissue adaptation to exercise. In: C. Bouchard, R.J. Shephard, T. Stephens, J.R. Sutton, and B.D. McPherson (eds.) *Exercise, Fitness and Health: A Consensus of Current Knowledge.* Champaign, IL: Human Kinetics, pp. 315-323.

Bjorntorp, P.J. (1991). Visceral fat accumulation: The missing link between psychosocial factors and cardiovascular disease? *J. Intern. Med.* 230:195-201.

Black, D.R., and M.E. Burckes-Miller (1988). Male and female college athletes: Use of anorexia nervosa and bulimia nervosa weigh loss methods. *Res. Q. Exerc. Sport* 59:252-256.

Blair, S.N., N.M. Ellsworth, W.L. Haskell, M.P. Stern, J.W. Farquhar, and P.D. Wood (1981). Comparison of nutrient intake in middle-aged men and women runners and controls. *Med. Sci. Sports Exerc.* 13:310-315.

Boileau, R.A., T.G. Lohman, M.H. Slaughter, T.E. Ball, S.B. Going, and M.K. Hendrix (1984). Hydration of the fat-free body in children during maturation. *Hum. Biol.* 56:651-666.

Borkan, G.A., D.E. Hults, S.G. Gerzof, and A.H. Robbins (1985). Comparison of body composition in middle-aged and elderly males using computed tomography. *Am. J. Phys. Anthropol.* 66:289-295.

Borkan, G.A., and A.H. Norris (1977). Fat redistribution and the changing body dimensions of the adult male. *Hum. Biol.* 49:494-514.

Bouchard, C., A. Tremblay, J.P. Després, A. Nadeau, P.J. Lupier, G. Theriault, J. Dussault, S. Moorjani, S. Pinault, and G. Fournier (1990). The response to long-term overfeeding in identical twins. *N. Engl. J. Med.* 322:1477–1482.

Bray, G.A. (1969). Effect of caloric restriction on energy expenditure in obese patients. *Lancet*, ii, 397–398.

Brewer, M.M., M.R. Bates, and L.P. Vannoy (1989). Postpartum changes in maternal weight and body fat depots in lactating vs. nonlactating women. *Am. J. Clin. Nutr.* 49:259–265.

Broeder C.E., K.A. Burrhus, L.S. Svanevik, and J.H. Wilmore (1992a). The effects of aerobic fitness on resting metabolic rate. *Am. J. Clin. Nutr.* 55:795–801.

Broeder, C.E., K.A. Burrhus, L.S. Svanevik, and J.H. Wilmore (1992b). The effects of either high-intensity resistance or endurance training on resting metabolic rate. *Am. J. Clin. Nutr.* 55:802–810.

Brooks-Gunn, J., M.P. Warren, and L.H. Hamilton (1987). The relation of eating problems and amenorrhea in ballet dancers. *Med. Sci. Sports Exerc.* 19:41–44.

Brown, C. (1993). The continuum: anorexia, bulimia, and weight preoccupation. In: C. Brown and K. Jasper (eds.) *Consuming Passions*. Toronto: Second Story Press, pp. 53–68.

Brownell, K.D., and J. Rodin (1992). Prevalence of eating disorders in athletes. In: K.D. Brownell, J. Rodin, and J.H. Wilmore (eds.) *Eating, Body Weight and Performance in Athletes. Disorders of Modern Society*. Philadelphia: Lea & Febiger, pp. 128–145.

Brownell, K.D., and S.N. Steen (1992). Weight cycling in athletes: Effects on behavior, physiology, and health. In: K.D. Brownell, J. Rodin, and J.H. Wilmore (eds.) *Eating, Body Weight and Performance in Athletes. Disorders of Modern Society*. Philadelphia: Lea & Febiger, pp. 159–171.

Brownell, K.D., G.A. Marlat, E. Lichtenstein, and G.T. Wilson (1986). Understanding and preventing relapse. *Am. J. Psychol* 41:765–782.

Brozek, J., F. Grande, J.T. Anderson, and A. Keys (1963). Densitometric analysis of body composition: Revision of some quantitative assumptions. *Ann. N.Y. Acad. Sci.* 110:113–140.

Buskirk, E.R., R.H. Thompson, L. Lutwak, and G.D. Whedon (1963). Energy balance of obese patients during weight reduction: influence of diet restriction and exercise. *Ann. N.Y. Acad. Sci.* 110:918–940.

Calabrese, L.H., D.T. Kirkendall, M. Floyd, S. Rapoport, G.W. Williams, G.G. Weiker, and J.A. Bergfeld (1983). Menstrual abnormalities, nutritional patterns, and body composition in female classical ballet dancers. *Phys. Sportsmed.* 11:86–98.

Catlin, D., J. Wright, H. Pope, Jr., M. Liggett (1993). Assessing the threat of anabolic steroids. *Phys. Sportsmed.* 21:36–44.

Chandler, S.B., D.A. Abood, D.T. Lee, M.Z. Cleveland, and J.A. Daly (1994). Pathogenic eating attitudes and behaviors and body dissatisfaction difference among black and white college students. *Eat. Disord.* 2:319–328.

Chien, S., M.T. Peng, K.P. Chen, T.F. Huang, C. Chang, and H.S. Fang (1975). Longitudinal studies on adipose tissue and its distribution in human subjects. *J. Appl. Physiol.* 39:825–830.

Chumlea, W.C., A.F. Roche, and E. Rogers (1984a). Replicability for anthropometry in the elderly. *Hum. Biol.* 56:329–337.

Chumlea, W.C., A.F. Roche, and P. Webb (1984b). Body size, subcutaneous fatness and total body fat in older adults. *Int. J. Obes.* 8:311–317.

Ciliska, D. (1993). Why diets fail. In: C. Brown and K. Jasper (eds.) *Consuming Passions*. Toronto: Second Story Press, pp. 80–90.

Claessens, A.L., S. Hlatky, J. Lefevre, and H. Holdhaus (1994). The role of anthropometric characteristics in modern pentathlon performance in female athletes. *J. Sports Sci.* 12:391–401.

Clarkson, P.M., and E.M. Haymes (1995). Exercise and mineral status of athletes: calcium, magnesium, phosphorus, and iron. *Med. Sci. Sports Exerc.* 27:831–843.

Clarkson, P.M., and E.M. Haymes (1994). Trace mineral requirements for athletes. *Int. J. Sport Nutr.* 4:104–119.

Clarkson, P.M., P.S. Freedson, B. Keller, D. Carney, and M. Skrinar (1985). Maximal oxygen uptake, nutritional patterns, and body composition of adolescent female ballet dancers. *Res. Q Exerc. Sport* 56:180–184.

Cohn, S.F., D. Vartsky, and S. Yasumura (1980). Compartmental body composition based on total-body nitrogen, potassium, and calcium. *Am. J. Physiol.* 239:E524–E530.

Constantini, N.W., and M.P. Warren (1994). Special problems of the female athlete. *Bailliers's Clin. Rheumatol.* 8:199–219.

Davies, A.H., I. Baird, J. Fowler, I.H. Mills, J.E. Baillie, S. Rattan, and A.N. Howard (1989). Metabolic response to low- and very-low-calorie diets. *Am. J. Clin. Nutr.* 49:745–751.

Davis C., and M. Cowles (1989). A comparison of weight and diet concerns and personality factor among female athletes and non-athletes. *J. Psychosom. Res.* 33:527–536.

de Boer, J.O., A.J.H. van Es, L.C.A. Roovers, J.M.A. van Raaij, and J.G.A.J. Hautvast (1986). Adaptation of energy metabolism of overweight women to low-energy intake, studied with whole-body calorimeters. *Am. J. Clin. Nutr.* 44:585–595.

de Groot, C.P.G.M., A.J.H. van Es, J.M.A. van Raaij, J.E. Vogt, and J.G.A.J. Hautvast (1989). Adaptation of energy metabolism of overweight women to alternating and continuous low energy intake. *Am. J. Clin. Nutr.* 50:1314–1323.

de Groot, C.P.G.M., A.J.H. van Es, J.M.A. van Raaij, J.E. Vogt, and J.G.A.J. Hautvast (1990). Energy metabolism of overweight women 1 mo and 1 yr after an 8-wk slimming period. *Am. J. Clin. Nutr.* 51:578–583.

Den Tonkelaar, I., J.C. Seidell, P.A.H. Van Noord, E.A. Baanders-van Halewijn, J.H. Jacobus, and P.F. Bruning (1989). Factors influencing waist/hip ratio in randomly selected pre- and post-menopausal women in the DOM-project. *Int. J. Obes.* 13:817–824.

Despres, J.P. (1994). Physical activity and adipose tissue. In C. Bouchard, R.J. Shephard, and T. Stephens (eds.) *Physical Activity, Fitness and Health. International Proceedings and Consensus Statement.* Champaign, IL: Human Kinetics, pp. 358–368.

Despres, J.P., C. Bouchard, A. Tremblay, R. Savard, and M. Marcotte (1984). The effect of a 20-week endurance training program on adipose-tissue morphology and lipolysis in men and women. *Metabolism* 33:235–239.

Despres, J.P., C. Bouchard, A. Tremblay, R. Savard, and M. Marcotte (1985). Effects of aerobic training on fat distribution in male subjects. *Med. Sci. Sports Exerc.* 17:113–118.

Despres, J.P., S. Moorjani, A. Tremblay, M. Ferland, P.J. Lupien, A. Nadeau, and C. Bouchard (1989). Relation of high plasma triglyceride levels associated with obesity and regional adipose tissue distribution to plasma lipo-protein-lipid composition in premenopausal women. *Clin. Invest. Med.* 12:374–380.

Despres, J.P., M.C. Pouliot, S. Moorjani, A. Nadeau, A. Tremblay, P.J. Lupien, G. Theriault, and C. Bouchard (1991). Loss of abdominal fat and metabolic response to exercise training in obese women. *Am. J. Physiol.* 261:E159–E167.

Deurenberg, P., J.A. Weststrate, and K. van der Kooy (1989). Is an adaptation of Siri's formula for the calculation of body fat percentage from body density in the elderly necessary? *Eur. J. Clin. Nutr.* 43:559–568.

Devlin, J.T., and E.S. Horton (1986). Potentiation of the thermic effect of insulin by exercise: differences between lean, obese, and noninsulin-dependent diabetic men. *Am. J. Clin. Nutr.* 43:884–890.

Dixon, J.E., A. Rodin, B. Murby, M.G. Chapman, and I. Fogelman (1989). Bone mass in hirsute women with androgen excess. *Clin. Endocrinol.* 30:271–277.

Dreon, D.M., B. Frey-Hewitt, N. Ellsworth, P.T. Williams, R.B. Terry, and P.D. Wood (1988). Dietary fat: carbohydrate ratio and obesity in middle-aged men. *Am. J. Clin. Nutr.* 47:995–1000.

Dudley, G.A. (1988). Metabolic consequences of resistive-type exercise. *Med. Sci. Sports Exerc.* 20(Suppl):- S158–S161.

Dummer, G.M., L.W. Rosen, W.W. Heusner, P.J. Roberts, and J.E. Counsilman (1987). Pathogenic weight-control behaviors of young competitive swimmers. *Phys. Sportsmed.* 15:75–86.

Dunaif A., and M. Graf (1989). Insulin administration alters gonadal steroid metabolism independent of changes in gonadotropin secretion in insulin-resistant women with the polycystic ovary syndrome. *J. Clin. Invest.* 83:23–29.

Durnin, J.V.G.A., and J. Womersley (1974). Body fat assessed from total body density and its estimation from skinfold thickness: measurements on 481 men and women aged from 16 to 72 years. *Br. J. Nutr.* 32:77–97.

Economos, C.D., S.S. Bortz, and M.E. Nelson (1993). Nutritional practices of elite athletes. Practical recommendations. *Sports Med.* 16:381–399.

Efendic, S. (1970). Catecholamine and metabolism of human adipose tissue. III. Comparison between the regulation of lipolysis in omental and subcutaneous adipose tissue. *Acta Med. Scand.* 187:477–483.

Elliot, D.L., L. Goldberg, K.S. Kuehl, and W.M. Bennett (1989). Sustained depression of the resting metabolic rate after massive weight loss. *Am. J. Clin. Nutr.* 49:93–96.

Elliot, D.L., L. Goldberg, K.S. Kuehl, and D.H. Catlin (1987). Characteristics of anabolic-androgenic steroid-free competitive male and female bodybuilders. *Phys. Sportsmed.* 15:169–179.

Ellis, K.J. (1990). Reference man and woman more fully characterized: Variations on the basis of body size, age, sex, and race. *Biol. Trace Elem. Res.* 26–27:385–400.

Enzi, G, M. Gasparo, P.R. Biondetti, D. Fiore, M. Semisa, F. Zurlo (1986). Subcutaneous and visceral fat distribution according to sex, age, and overweight, evaluated by computed tomography. *Am. J. Clin. Nutr.* 44:739–746.

Epstein, L.H., and R.R. Wing (1980). Aerobic exercise and weight. *Addict. Behav.* 5:371–388.

Evans, D.J., R.G. Hoffman, R.G. Kalkhoff, and A.H. Kissebah (1983). Relationship of androgenic activity to body fat topography, fat cell morphology and metabolic aberrations in premenopausal women. *J. Clin. Endocrinol. Metab.* 57:304–310.

Evans, W.J., and I.R. Rosenberg (1991). *Biomarkers: The Ten Determinants of Aging You Can Control.* New York: Simon & Schuster.

Falkner, F., and J.M. Tanner (eds.) (1986). *Human Growth: A Comprehensive Treatise: Vol 2. Postnatal Growth; Neurobiology* (2nd ed.) New York: Plenum.

Fiatarone, M.A., E.C. Marks, N.D. Ryan, C.N. Meredith, L.A. Lipsitz, and W.J. Evans (1990). High-intensity strength training in nonagenarians. Effects on skeletal muscle. *J.A.M.A.* 263:3029–3034.

Flatt, J.P. (1988). Importance of nutrient balance in body weight regulation. *Diabetes. Metab. Rev.* 6:571–581.

Flatt, J.P. (1987). Dietary fat, carbohydrate balance, and weight maintenance: effects of exercise. *Am. J. Clin. Nutr.* 45:296–306.

Flatt, J.P., E. Ravussin, K.J. Acheson, and E. Jequier (1985). Effects of dietary fat on postprandial substrate oxidation and on carbohydrate and fat balance. *J. Clin. Invest.* 76:1019–1024.

Fleck, S.J. (1983). Body composition of elite American athletes. *Am. J. Sports Med.* 11:398–403.

Flynn, M.A., G.B. Nolph, A.S. Baker, W.M. Martin, and G. Krause (1989). Total body potassium in aging humans: A longitudinal study. *Am. J. Clin. Nutr.* 50:713–717.

Forbes, G.B. (1990). The abdomen: hip ratio—normative data and observations on selected patients. *Int. J. Obes.* 14:149–157.

Forbes, G.B. (1991). Exercise and body composition. *J. Appl. Physiol.* 70:994–997.

Forbes, G.B. (1992). Exercise and lean weight: The influence of body weight. *Nutr. Rev.* 50:157–161.

Forbes, G.B. (1987a). *Human Body Composition: Growth, Aging, Nutrtion, and Activity.* New York: Springer-Verlag, pp. 179–181.

Forbes, G.B. (1987b). Lean body mass-body fat interrelationships in humans. *Nutr. Rev.* 45:225–231.

Forbes, G.B., and J.C. Reina (1970). Adult lean body mass declines with age: Some longitudinal observations. *Metabolism* 9:653–663.

Forbes, G.B. M.R. Brown, S.L. Welle, and B.A. Lipinski (1986). Deliberate over feeding in women and men: energy cost and composition of weight gain. *Br. J. Nutr.* 56:1–9.

Forsum, E., A. Sadurskis, and J. Wager (1989). Estimation of body fat in healthy Swedish women during pregnancy and lactation. *Am. J. Clin. Nutr.* 50:465–473.

Foster, G.D., T.A. Wadden, I.D. Feurer, A.S. Jennings, A.J. Stunkard, L.O. Crosby, J. Ship, and J.L. Mullen (1990). Controlled trial of the metabolic effects of a very-low-calorie diet: Short- and long-term effects. *Am. J. Clin. Nutr.* 51:167–172.

Franklin, B., E. Buskirk, J. Hodgson, H. Gahagan, J. Kollias, and J. Mendez (1979). Effects of physical conditioning on cardiorespiratory function, body composition and serum lipids in relatively normal-weight and obese middle-aged women. *Int. J. Obes.* 3:97–109.

Fried, S.K., and J.G. Kral (1987). Sex differences in regional distribution of fat cell size and lipoprotein lipase activity in morbidly obese patients. *Int. J. Obes.* 11:129–140.

Friis-Hansen, B. (1957). Changes in body water compartments during growth. *Acta Paediatr.* (Suppl.) 110:1.

Frontera, W.R., C.N. Meredith, K.P. O'Reilly, H.G. Knuttgen, and W.J. Evans (1988). Strength conditioning in older men: skeletal muscle hypertrophy and improved function. *J. Appl. Physiol.* 64: 1038–1044.

Frusztajer, N.T., S. Dhuper, M.P. Warren, J. Brooks-Gunn, and R.P. Fox (1990). Nutrition and the incidence of stress fractures in ballet dancers. *Am. J. Clin. Nutr.* 51:779–783.

Gadpaille, W.J., C.F. Sanborn, and W.W. Wagner, Jr. (1987). Athletic amenorrhea, major affective disorders, and eating disorders. *Am. J. Psychiatry* 144:939–942.

Garby, L., M.S. Kurzer, O. Lammert, and E. Nielsen (1988). Effect of 12 weeks' light-moderate underfeeding on 24-hour energy expenditure in normal male and female subjects. *Eur. J. Clin. Nutr.* 42:295–300.

Garn, S.M. (1957). Fat weight and fat placement in the female. *Science* 125:1091–1092.

Garner, D.M., and P.E. Garfinkel (1979). The eating attitudes test: and index of the symptoms of anorexia nervosa. *Psychol. Med.* 9:273–279.

Garner, D.M., P.E. Garkinkel, W. Rockert, and M.P. Olmsted (1987). A prospective study of eating disturbances in the ballet. *Psychother. Psychosom.* 48:170–175.

Garner, D.M., M.P. Olmsted, and J. Polivy (1983). The eating disorder inventory: a measure of cognitive-behavioral dimensions of anorexia nervosa and bulimia. In: *Anorexia Nervosa: Recent Developments in Research.* New York: Alan R. Liss, pp. 173–184.

Garrow, J.S. (1978). The regulation of energy expenditure in man. In: G.A. Bray (ed.) *Recent Advances in Obesity Research*, Vol. 2. London: Newman, pp. 200–210.

Garrow, J.S., and J.D. Webster (1989). Effects on weight and metabolic rate of obese women of a 3–4 mJ (800 kcal) diet. *Lancet*, i:1429–1431.

Garry, P.J., and K.M. Koehler (1990). Problems in interpretation of dietary and biochemical data from population studies. In: M.L. Brown (ed.) *Present Knowledge in Nutrition.* Washington, D.C.: International Life Sciences Institute, pp. 407–414.

Gibson, R.S. (1993). *Principles of Nutritional Assessment.* New York: Oxford University Press, pp. 37–136.

Going, S., D. Williams, and T. Lohman (1995). Aging and body composition: biological changes and methodological issues. In: J.O. Holloszy (ed.) *Exercise and Sport Sciences Reviews*, Vol. 23. Baltimore: Williams and Wilkins, pp. 411–458.

Going, S.B., D.P. Williams, T.G. Lohman, and M.J. Hewitt (1994). Aging, body composition, and physical activity: A review. *J. Aging Phys. Activ.* 2:38–66.

Goldman, R.F., B. Bullen, and C. Seltzer (1963). Changes in specific gravity and body fat in overweight female adolescent as a result of weight reduction. *Ann. N.Y. Acad. Sci.* 110:913–917.

Grande, F. (1968). Energy balance and body composition changes. *Ann. Intern. Med.* 68:467–480.

Grande, F., H.L. Taylor, J.T. Anderson, E. Buskirk, and A. Keys (1958). Water exchange in men on a restricted water intake and a low calorie carbohydrate diet accompanied by physical work. *J. Appl. Physiol.* 12:202–210.

Grandjean, A.C. (1989). Macronutrient intake of U.S. athletes compared with the general population and recommendations made for athletes. *Am. J. Clin. Nutr.* 49: 1070–1076.

BODY COMPOSITION AND WEIGHT CONTROL **203**

Gulick, A. (1922). A study of weight regulation in the adult human body during over-nutrition. *Am. J. Physiol.* 60:371–395.

Gustafson, D. (1989). Eating behaviors of women college athletes. *Melpomene J.* 8:11–12.

Haffner, S.M., M.P. Stern, H.P. Hazuda, J. Pugh, J.K. Patteson, et al. (1986). Upper body and centralized adiposity in Mexican Americans and non-Hispanic whites: relationship to body mass index and other behavioral and demographic variables. *Int. J. Obes.* 10:493–502.

Hagan, R.D., S.J. Wong, L. Wong, and J. Whittam (1986). The effects of aerobic conditioning and/or caloric restriction in overweight men and women. *Med. Sci. Sports Exerc.* 18:87–94.

Hamill, P.V.V., T.A. Drizd, C.L. Johnson, R.B. Reed, A.F. Roche, and W.M. Moore (1979). Physical growth: national center for health statistics percentiles. *Am. J. Clin. Nutr.* 32:607–629.

Hamilton, L.H., J. Brooks-Gunn, and M.P. Warren (1985). Sociocultural influences on eating disorders in professional female ballet dancers. *Int. J. Eat. Disord.* 4:465–477.

Hamilton, L.H., J. Brooks-Gunn, M.P. Warren, and W.G. Hamilton (1988). The role of selectivity in the pathogenesis of eating problems in ballet dancers. *Med. Sci. Sports Exerc.* 20:560–565.

Heitmann, B.L. (1992). The effects of gender and age on associations between blood lipid levels and obesity in Danish men and women aged 35–65 years. *J. Clin. Epidemiol.* 45:693–702.

Hendler, R.G., and A.A. Bonde (1990). Effects of sucrose on resting metabolic rate, nitrogen balance, leucine turnover and oxidation during weight loss with low calorie diets. *Int. J. Obes.* 14:927–938.

Hendler, R.G., and A.A. Bonde (1988). Very-low-calorie diets with high and low protein content: impact on triiodothyronine, energy expenditure, and nitrogen balance. *Am. J. Clin. Nutr.* 48:1239–1247.

Hendler, R.G., M. Walesky, and R.S. Sherwin (1986). Sucrose substitution in prevention and reversal of the fall in metabolic rate accompanying hypocaloric diets. *Am. J. Med.* 81:280–284.

Henriksson, J. (1977). Training induced adaptation of skeletal muscle and metabolism during submaximal exercise. *J. Physiol.* 270:661–675.

Henson, L.D., D.C. Poole, C.P. Donahoe, and D. Heber (1987). Effects of exercise training on resting energy expenditure during caloric restriction. *Am. J. Clin. Nutr.* 46:893–899.

Heshka, S., M.U. Yang, J. Wang, P. Burt, and F.X. Pi-Sunyer (1990). Weight loss and change in resting metabolic rate. *Am. J. Clin. Nutr.* 52:981–986.

Heymsfield, S.B., J. Wang, S. Lichtman, Y. Kamen, J. Kehayias, and R.N. Pierson (1989). Body composition in elderly subjects: a critical appraisal of clinical methodology. *Am. J. Clin. Nutr.* 50:1167–1175.

Hill, J.O., H.J. Drougas, and J.C. Peters (1994). Physical activity, fitness and moderate obesity. In: C. Bouchard, R.J. Shephard, and T. Stephens (eds.) *Physical Activity, Fitness and Health. International Proceedings and Consensus Statement.* Champaign, IL: Human Kinetics, pp. 684–695.

Hirschberg, A.L., C. Lindholm, K. Carlstrom, and B. Von Schoultz (1994). Reduced serum cholecystokinin response to food intake in female athletes. *Metabolism* 43:217–222.

Ingjer, F., and J. Sundgot-Borgen (1991). Influence of body weight reduction on maximal oxygen uptake in female elite athletes. *Scand. J. Med. Sci. Sports* 1:141–146.

Jéquier, E., and Y. Schultz (1983). Long-term measurements of energy expenditure in humans using a respiratory chamber. *Am. J. Clin. Nutr.* 38:989–998.

Johnson, D., and E.J. Drenick (1977). Therapeutic fasting in morbid obesity: Long-term follow-up. *Arch. Intern. Med.* 137:1381–1382.

Johnson, G.O., L.J. Nebelsick-Gullett, W.G. Thorland, and T.J. Housh (1989). The effect of a competitive season on the body composition of university female athletes. *J. Sports Med. Phys. Fit.* 29:314–320.

Kaiserauer, S., A.C. Snyder, M. Sleeper, and J. Zierath (1989). Nutritional, physiological, and menstrual status of distance runners. *Med. Sci. Sports Exerc.* 21:120–125.

Karpakka, J., J. Leppavuori, S. Orava, and J. Heikkinen (1994). Recurrent stress fractures in a female athlete with primary amenorrhea: a case report. *Clin. J. Sport Med.* 14:136–138.

Kaskoun, M.C., R.K. Johnson, and M.I. Goran (1994). Comparison of energy intake by semiquantitative food-frequency questionnaire with total energy expenditure by the doubly-labeled water method in young children. *Am. J. Clin. Nutr.* 60:43–47.

Kaye, W.H., and T.E. Weltzin (1991). Neurochemistry of bulimia nervosa. *J. Clin. Psychiat.* 52:21–28.

Kayman, S., W. Bruvold, and J.S. Stern (1990). Maintenance and relapse after weight loss in women: behavioral aspects. *Am. J. Clin. Nutr.* 52:800–807.

Kendall, A., D.A. Levitsky, B.J. Strupp, and I. Lissner (1991). Weight loss on a low fat diet: consequence of the imprecision of the control of food intake in humans. *Am. J. Clin. Nutr.* 53:1124–1129.

Keys, A., J. Brozek, A. Henshel, O. Mickelson, and H.L. Taylor (1950). *The Biology of Human Starvation.* Minneapolis: University of Minnesota Press.

Kiens, B., and H. Lithell (1989). Lipoprotein metabolism influenced by training-induced changes in human skeletal muscle. *J. Clin. Invest.* 83:558–564.

Kiens, B., and B. Saltin (1985). Enhanced fat oxidation by exercising skeletal muscle after endurance training. *Clin. Physiol.* 5(Suppl 4):86a (Abstract).

Koff, E., and J. Rierdan (1993). Advanced pubertal development and eating disturbance in early adolescent girls. *J. Adoles. Health* 14:433–439.

Krotkiewski, M., and P. Bjorntorp (1986). Muscle tissue in obesity with different distribution of adipose tissue: effects of physical training. *Int. J. Obes.* 10:331–341.

Krotkiewski, M., P. Bjorntorp, L. Sjostrom, and U. Smith (1983). Impact of obesity on metabolism in men and women. Importance of regional adipose tissue distribution. *J. Clin. Invest.* 72:1150–1162.

Krotkiewski, M., L. Toss, P. Bjorntorp, and G. Holm (1981). The effect of a very low-calorie diet with and without chronic exercise on thyroid and sex hormones, plasma proteins, oxygen uptake, insulin and c peptide concentrations in obese women. *Int. J. Obes.* 5:287–293.

Kvist, H., L. Sjostrom, and U. Tylen (1986). Adipose tissue volume determination in women by computed tomography: technical considerations. *Int. J. Obes.* 10:53–67.

Lanska, D.J., M.J. Lanska, A.J. Hartz, and A.A. Rimm (1985). Factors influencing anatomic location of fat tissue in 52,953 women. *Int. J. Obes.* 9:29–38.

Lapidus, L., C. Bengtsson, T. Hallstrom, and P. Bjorntorp (1989). Adipose tissue distribution and health in women—results from a population study in Gothenburg, Sweden. *Appetite* 12:25–35.

Lapidus, L., C. Bengtsson, B. Larsson, K. Pennert, F. Rybo, and L. Sjostrom (1984) Distribution of adipose tissue and risk of cardiovascular disease and death: 12 year follow-up of participants in the population study of women in Gothenburg, Sweden. *Br. Med. J.* 289:1257–1261.

Lawson, S., J.D. Webster, P.J. Pacy, and J.S. Garrow (1987). Effect of a 10-week aerobic exercise programme on metabolic rate, body composition and fitness in lean sedentary females. *Br. J. Clin. Pract.* 41:684–688.

Lennon, D., F. Nagle, F. Stratman, E. Shrago, and S. Dennis (1985). Diet and exercise training effects on resting metabolic rate. *Int. J. Obes.* 9:39–47.

Leon, G.R. (1991). Eating disorders in female athletes. *Sports Med.* 12:219–227.

Ley, C.J., B. Lees, and J.C. Stevenson (1992). Sex- and menopause-associated changes in body-fat distribution. *Am. J. Clin. Nutr.* 55:950–954.

Lindberg, U.B., N. Crona, G. Silfverstolpe, P. Bjorntrop, and M. Rebuffe-Scrive (1989). Regional adipose tissue metabolism in postmenopausal women after treatment with exogenous sex steroids. *Horm. Metab. Res.* 22:345–351.

Lissner, L., and D.A. Levitsky (1987). Dietary fat and the regulation of energy intake in human subjects. *Am. J. Clin. Nutr.* 46:886–892.

Lloyd, T., L.A. Dolence, and M.J. Bartholomew (1992). Nutritional characteristics of recreational women runners. *Nutr. Res.* 12:359–366.

Lohman, T.G. (1986). Applicability of body composition techniques and constants for children and youths. In: K.B. Pandolf (ed.) *Exercise and Sport Sciences Reviews*, Vol. 14. New York: MacMillan, pp. 325–357.

Loosli, A.R., J. Benson, D.M. Gillien, and K. Bourdet (1986). Nutrition habits and knowledge in competitive adolescent female gymnasts. *Phys. Sportsmed.* 14:118–130.

Lucas, A.R., and D.M. Huse (1994). Behavioral disorders affect food intake: anorexia nervosa and bulimia nervosa. In: M.E. Shils, J.A. Olson, and M. Shike (eds.) *Modern Nutrition in Health and Disease.* 8th edition. Philadelphia: Lea and Febiger, p. 979.

Lundgren H., C. Bengtsson, G. Blohme, L. Lapidus, and L. Sjöstrom (1989). Adiposity and adipose tissue distribution in relation to incidence of diabetes in women: results from a prospective population study in Gothenburg, Sweden. *Int. J. Obes.* 13:413–423.

Malina, R.M. (1992). Physique and body composition: effects on performance and effects of training, semistarvation, and overtraining. In: K.D. Brownell, J. Rodin, and J.H. Wilmore (eds.) *Eating, Body Weight and Performance in Athletes. Disorders of Modern Society.* Philadelphia: Lea & Febiger, pp. 94–111.

Malina, R.M. (1969). Quantification of fat, muscle, and bone in man. *Clin. Orthop.* 65:9–38.

Malina, R.M., and C. Bouchard (1991). *Growth, Maturation, and Physical Activity.* Champaign, IL: Human Kinetics, pp. 68–150.

Malina, R.M., and A.F. Roche (1983). *Manual of physical status and performance in childhood: Vol. 2. Physical Performance.* New York: Plenum.

Malina, R.M., R.C. Ryan, and C.M. Bonci (1994). Age at menarche in athletes and their mothers and sisters. *Ann. Hum. Biol.* 21:417–422.

Mallick, M.J., T.W. Whipple, and E. Huerta (1987). Behavioral and psychological traits of weight-conscious teenagers: a comparison of eating-disordered patients and high- and low-risk groups. *Adolescence* 22:157–168.

Mazess, R.B., and J.R. Cameron (1974). Bone mineral content in normal U.S. whites. In: R.B. Mazess (ed.) *International Conference on Bone Mineral Measurement.* Washington, D.C.: U.S. Government Printing Office, pp. 228–237.

Mazess, R.B., H.S. Barden, P.J. Drinka, S.F. Bauwens, E.S. Orwoll, and N.H. Bell (1990). Influence of age and body weight on spine and femur bone mineral density in U.S. white men. *Bone Miner.* 5:645–652.

Mazess, R.B., H.S. Barden, M. Ettinger, C. Johnston, B. Dawson-Hughes, D. Baran, M. Powell, and M. Notelovitz (1987). Spine and femur density using dual-photon absorptiometry in U.S. white women. *Bone Miner.* 2:211–219.

Melnyk, M.G., and E. Weinstein (1994). Preventing obesity in black woman by targeting adolescents: A literature review. *J. Am. Diet Assoc.* 94:536–540.

Merzenich, H., H. Boeing, and J. Wahrendorf (1993). Dietary fat and sports activity as determinants for age at menarche. *Am. J. Epidemiol.* 138:217–224.

Miller, D.S., and P. Mumford (1967). Gluttony: I. An experimental study of low- or high-protein diets. *Am. J. Clin. Nutr.* 20:1212–1222.

Miller, D.S., P. Mumford, and M.J. Stock (1967). Gluttony. II. Thermogenesis in overeating man. *Am. J. Clin. Nutr.* 20:1223–1229.

Moen, S.M., C.F. Sanborn, and N. DiMarco (1992). Dietary habits and body composition in adolescent female runners. *Women Sport Phys. Activ. J.* 1:85–95.

Moffatt, R.J. (1984). Dietary status of elite female high school gymnasts: inadequacy of vitamin and mineral intake. *J. Am. Diet. Assoc.* 84:1361–1363.

Morgan, J.B. (1984). Weight-reducing diets, the thermic effect of feeding and energy balance in young women. *Int. J. Obes.* 8:629–640.

Mueller, W.H., R.F. Shoup, and R.M. Malina (1982). Fat patterning in athletes in relation to ethnic origin and sport. *Ann. Hum. Biol.* 9:371–376.

Mueller, W.H., M.L. Wear, C.L. Hanis, S.A. Barton, and W. J. Schull (1987). Body circumferences as alternatives to skinfold measurements of body fat distribution in Mexican-Americans. *Int. J. Obes.* 11:309–318.

Najjar, M.F., and M. Rowland (1987). *Anthropometric Reference Data and Prevalence of Overweight.* (DHEW publication [PHS]). Rockville, MD: National Center for Health Statistics, Vital and Health Statistics, Series 11.

Nattiv, A., R. Agostini, B. Drinkwater, and K.K. Yeager (1994). The female athlete triad. The interrelatedness of disordered eating, amenorrhea, and osteoporosis. *Clin. Sports Med.* 13:405–418.

Nelson, M.E., E.C. Fisher, P.D. Catsos, C.N. Meredith, R.N. Turksoy, and W.J. Evans (1986). Diet and bone status in amenorrheic runners. *Am. J. Clin. Nutr.* 43:910–916.

Neumann, R.O. (1902). Experimentelle Beiträge zur Lehre von dem täglichen. Nahrungsbedarf des Menschen unter besonderer Berucksichtigung der notwendigen Eiweissmenge. *Arch. Hygiene* 45:1–87.

Nevole, Jr., G.J., and W.E. Prentice (1987). The effect of anabolic steroids on female athletes. *Athlet. Train.* 22:297–299.

Nikkila, E.A., and A. Konttinen (1962). Effect of physical activity on postprandial levels of fats in serum. *Lancet* I:1151–1154.

O'Connor, P.J., R.D. Lewis, and E.M. Kirchner (1995). Eating disorder symptoms in female college gymnasts. *Med. Sci. Sports Exerc.* 27:550–555.

Olson, B.R. (1989). Exercise-induced amenorrhea. *Am. Fam. Pract.* 39:213–221.

Oppliger, R.A., and S.L. Cassady (1994). Body composition assessment in women. Special considerations for athletes. *Sports Med.* 17:353–357, 1994.

Oscai, L.B. (1973). The role of exercise in weight control. *Exerc. Sports Sci. Rev.* 1:103–123.

Oscai, L.B., and W.K. Palmer (1988). Muscle lipolysis during exercise: an update. *Sports Med.* 6:23–28.

Ostman, J., P. Arner, P. Engfeldt, and L. Kager (1979). Regional differences in the control of lipolysis in human adipose tissue. *Metabolism* 28:1198–1205.

Pao, E.M., and Y.S. Cypel (1990). Estimation of dietary intake. In: M.L. Brown (ed.) *Present Knowledge in Nutrition.* Washington, D.C.: International Life Sciences Institute, pp. 399–406.

Parker, R.M., M.J. Lambert, and G.M. Burlingame (1994). Psychological features of female runners presenting with pathological weight control behaviors. *J. Sport Exerc. Psychol.* 16:119–134.

Pasquali, R., F. Casimirri, L. Plate, and M. Capelli (1990). Characterization of obese women with reduced sex hormone-binding globulin concentrations. *Horm. Metab. Res.* 22:303–306.

Passmore, R., J.A. Strong, and F.J. Ritchie (1958). The chemical composition of the tissue lost by obese patients on a reducing regimen. *Br. J. Nutr.* 12:113–122.

Pate, R.R., R.G. Sargent, C. Baldwin, and M.L. Burgess (1990). Dietary intake of women runners. *Int. J. Sports Med.* 11:461–466.

Pavlou, K.N., S. Krey, and W.P. Steffee (1989). Exercise as an adjunct to weight loss and maintenance in moderately obese subjects. *Am. J. Clin. Nutr.* 49:1115–1123.

Peltenburg, A.L., W.B.M. Erich, M.L. Zonderland, M.J.E. Bernink, J.L. VanDenBrande, and I.A. Huisveld (1984). A retrospective growth study of female gymnasts and girl swimmers. *Int. J. Sports Med.* 5:262–267.

Petrie, T.A. (1993). Disordered eating in female collegiate gymnasts: prevalence and personality/attitudinal correlates. *J. Sport Exerc. Psychol.* 15:424–436.

Petrie T.A., and S. Stoever (1993). The incidence of bulimia nervosa and pathogenic weight control behaviors in female collegiate gymnasts. *Res. Q. Exerc. Sport* 64:238–241.

Pierson, R.N., D.H.Y. Lin, and R.A. Phillips (1982). Body composition measurements in normal man: the potassium, sodium, sulfate and tritium spaces in 58 adults. *J. Chron. Dis.* 35:419–428.

Poehlman, E.T. (1989). A review: exercise and its influence on resting energy metabolism in man. *Med. Sci. Sports Exerc.* 21:515–525.

Pollock, M.L. (1973). The quantification of endurance training programs. In: J. Wilmore (ed.) *Exercise and Sport Sciences Reviews,* Vol. 1. New York: Academic Press, pp. 155–188.

Pollock, M.L., and J.H. Wilmore (1990). *Exercise in Health and Disease: Evaluation and Prescription for Prevention and Rehabilitation* (2nd ed.) Philadelphia: W.B. Saunders Company, pp. 202–236.

Pomeroy, C. and J.E. Mitchell (1992). Medical issue in the eating disordered. In: K. Brownell, J. Rodin, and J.H. Wilmore (eds.) *Eating, Body Weight and Performance in Athletes. Disorders of Modern Society.* Philadelphia: Lea & Febiger, pp. 202-221.

Pouliot, M.C., J.P. Despres, S. Lemieux, S. Moorjani, C. Bouchard, A. Tremblay, A. Nadeau, and P.J. Lupien (1994). Waist circumference and abdominal sagittal diameter: best simple anthropometric indexes of abdominal visceral adipose tissue accumulation and related cardiovascular risk in men and women. *Am. J. Cardiol.* 73:460-468.

Prentice, A.M., A.E. Black, W.A. Coward, H.L. Davies, G.R. Goldberg, P.R. Murgatroyd, J. Ashford, M. Sawyer, and R.G. Whitehead (1986). High levels of energy expenditure in obese women. *Br. Med. J.* 292:983-987.

Pumariega, A.J., C.R. Gustavson, J.C. Gustavson, P.S. Motes, and S. Ayers (1994). Eating attitudes in African-American women: the "essence" eating disorders survey. *Eat. Disord.* 2:5-15.

Putukian, M. (1994). The female triad. Eating disorders, amenorrhea, and osteoporosis. *Sports Med.* 78:-345-356.

Quandt, S.A. (1983). Changes in maternal postpartum adiposity and infant feed patterns. *Am. J. Phys. Anthropol.* 60:445-461.

Raciti, M.C., and J.C. Norcross. (1987). The EAT and EDI: Screening, interrelationships, and psychometrics. *Int. J. Eat. Disord.* 6:579-586.

Ramsay J.A., C.J.R. Blimkie, K. Smith, S. Garner, J.D. MacDougall, and D.G. Sale (1990). Strength training effects in prepubescent boys. *Med. Sci. Sports Exerc.* 22:605-614.

Ravussin, E., and B.A. Swinburn (1992). Effect of caloric restriction and weight loss on energy expenditure. In: T.A. Wadden, and T.B. Van Itallie (eds.) *Treatment of the Seriously Obese Patient.* New York: Guilford Press, pp. 163-189.

Ravussin, E., and B.A. Swinburn (1993). Energy metabolism. In: A.J. Stunkard and T.A. Wadden (eds.) *Obesity: Theory and Therapy,* 2nd edition. New York: Raven Press, pp. 97-123.

Ravussin, E., B. Burnand, Y. Schutz, and E. Jéquir (1985a). Energy expenditure before and during energy restriction in obese patients. *Am. J. Clin. Nutr.* 41:753-759.

Ravussin, E., Y. Schutz, K.J. Acheson, M. Dusmet, L. Bourquin, and E. Jéquir (1985b). Short-term, mixed diet overfeeding in man: no evidence for "luxuskonsumption." *Am. J. Physiol.* 249:E470-E477.

Rebuffe-Scrive, M., B. Anderson, L. Olbe, and P. Bjorntorp (1990). Metabolism of adipose tissue in intrabdominal depots in severely obese men and women. *Metabolism* 39:1021-1025.

Rebuffe-Scrive, M., J. Eldh, L.O. Hafstrom, and P. Bjorntorp (1986). Metabolism of mammary, abdominal, and femoral adipocytes in women before and after menopause. *Metabolism* 35:792-797.

Rebuffe-Scrive, M., L. Enk, N. Crona, P. Lonnroth, L. Abrahamsson, U. Smith, and P. Bjorntorp (1985). Fat cell metabolism in different regions in women: effect of menstrual cycle, pregnancy, and lactation. *J. Clin. Invest.* 75:1973-1976.

Rico, H., M. Revilla, R. Hernandez, J.M. Gonzalez-Riola, and L.F. Villa (1993). Four-compartment model of body composition of normal elderly women. *Age Ageing* 22:265-268.

Riggs, B.L., H.W. Wahner, L.J. Melton III, L.S. Richelson, H.L. Judd, and K.P. Offord (1986). Rates of bone loss in the appendicular and axial skeletons of women: evidence of substantial vertebral bone loss before menopause. *J. Clin. Invest.* 7:1487-1491.

Rising, R., S. Alger, V. Boyce, H. Seagle, R. Ferraro, A.M. Fontvieille, and E. Ravussin (1992). Food intake measured by an automated food-selection system: relationship to energy expenditure. *Am. J. Clin. Nutr.* 55:343-349.

Roberts, S.B., V.R. Young, P. Fuss, M.A. Fiatarone, B. Richard, H. Rasmussen, D. Wagner, L. Joseph, E. Holehouse, and W.J. Evans (1990). Energy expenditure and subsequent nutrient intakes in overfed young men. *Am. J. Physiol.* 259:R461-R469.

Rosen, L.W., and D.O. Hough (1988). Pathogenic weight-control behaviors of female college gymnasts. *Phys. Sportsmed.* 16:140-146.

Rosen, L.W., D.B. McKeag, D.O. Hough, and V. Curley (1986). Pathogenic weight-control behavior in female athletes. *Phys. Sportsmed.* 14:79-86.

Roundtable (1990). Body composition for athletes. Participants: P. Clarkson, F. Katch, W. Sinnning, and J. Wilmore. *Sports Sci. Exchange,* Winter. Chicago: The Quaker Oats Company, pp. 1-4.

Rucinski, A. (1989). Relationship of body image and dietary intake of competitive ice skaters. *J. Am. Diet. Assoc.* 89:98-100.

Ruud, J.S., and A.C. Grandjean (1994). Nutritional concerns of female athletes. In: I. Wolinsky and J.F. Hickson, Jr. (eds.) *Nutrition and Sport,* 2nd ed. Boca Raton: CRC Press, pp. 347-365.

Sale, D.G. (1989). Strength training in children. In: C.V. Gisolfi and D.R. Lamb (eds.) *Perspectives in Exercise Science and Sports Medicine,* Vol. 2, Youth, Exercise, and Sport. Indianapolis, IN: Benchmark Press, pp. 165-216.

Saltin, B., and P.D. Gollnick (1983). Skeletal muscle adaptability: significance for metabolism and performance. In: *Handbook of Physiology: Skeletal Muscle* Sec. 10, Chap. 19. Bethesda, MD: American Physiological Society, pp. 555-631.

Schoeller, D.A. (1989). Changes in total body water with age. *Am. J. Clin. Nutr.* 50(Suppl):1176-1181.

Schoeller, D.A. (1990). How accurate is self-reported dietary energy intake? *Nutr. Rev.* 48:373-379.

Schutz, Y., T. Bessard, and E. Jéquier (1987). Exercise and postprandial thermogenesis in obese women before and after weight loss. *Am. J. Clin. Nutr.* 45:1424-1432.

Schutz, Y., J.P. Flatt, and E. Jéquier (1989). Failure of dietary fat intake to promote fat oxidation: a factor favoring the development of obesity. *Am. J. Clin. Nutr.* 50:307-314.

Schutz, Y., A. Golay, J.P. Felber, and E. Jéquier (1984). Decreased glucose-induced thermogenesis after weight loss in obese subjects: a predisposing factor for relapse of obesity? *Am. J. Clin. Nutr.* 39:380-387.

Schwartz, R.S., W.P. Shuman, V.L. Bradbury, K.C. Cain, G.W. Fellingham, J.C. Beard, S.E. Kahn, J.R. Stratton, M.D. Cerqueira, and I.B. Abrass (1990). Body fat distribution in healthy young and older men. *J. Gerontol.* 45:M181-M185.

Segal, K.R., and F.X. Pi-Sunyer (1989). Exercise and obesity. *Med. Clin. North Am.* 73:217-236.

Seidell, J.C., A. Osterlee, M.A.O. Thijssen, J. Burema, P. Deurenberg, J.G.A.J. Hautvast, and J.H.J. Ruijs (1987). Assessment of intraabdominal and subcutaneous abdominal fat: relation between anthropometry and computed tomography. *Am. J. Clin. Nutr.* 45:7-13.

Selby, R., H.M. Weinstein, and T.S. Bird (1990). The health of university athletes: attitudes, behaviors, and stressors. *Coll. Health* 39:11-18.

Shimokata, H., R. Andres, P.J. Coon, D. Elahi, D.C. Muller, and J.D. Tobin (1988). Studies in the distribution of body fat. II. Longitudinal effects of change in weight. *Int. J. Obes.* 13:455-464.

Short, S.H. (1994). Surveys of dietary intake and nutritional knowledge of athletes and their coaches. In: I. Wolinsky and J.F. Hickson, Jr. (eds.) *Nutrition and Sport*, 2nd ed. Boca Raton: CRC Press, pp. 367-416.

Silver, A.J., C.P. Guillen, M.J. Kahl, and J.E. Morley (1993). Effect of aging on body fat. *J. Am. Geriatr. Soc.* 41:211-213.

Siri, W.E. (1956). The gross composition of the body. *Adv. Biol. Med. Phys.* 4:239-280.

Skowron, E.A. and M. L. Friedlander (1994). Psychological separation, self-control, and weight preoccupation among elite women athletes. *J. Counsel. Devel.* 72:310-315.

Steen, B. (1990). Factors affecting the nutritional situation in the elderly outside and inside hospital. In: D.M. Prinsley and H.H. Sandstead (eds.) *Nutrition and Aging.* New York: Alan R. Liss, pp. 345-354.

Stefanick, M.L. (1993). Exercise and weight control. In: J.O. Holloszy (ed.) *Exercise and Sport Sciences Reviews*, Vol. 21. Baltimore: Williams and Wilkins, pp. 363-396.

Steingrimsdottir, L., M.R. Greenwood, and J.A. Brasel (1980). Effect of pregnancy, lactation and a high-fat diet on adipose tissue in Osborne-Mendel rats. *J. Nutr.* 110:600-609.

Stevens, J., R.G. Knapp, J.E. Keil, and R.R. Verdugo (1991). Changes in body weight and girths in black and white adults studied over a 25-year interval. *Int. J. Obes.* 15:803-808.

Strubbe, J.H. (1994). Regulation of food intake. In: M.S. Westerterp-Plantenga, S.W.H.M. Fredrix, and A.B. Steffens (eds.) *Food Intake and Energy Expenditure.* Boca Raton: CRC Press, pp. 141-154.

Sundgot-Borgen, J. (1994a). Eating disorders in female athletes. *Sports Med.* 17:176-188.

Sundgot-Borgen, J. (1993a). Nutrient intake of female elite athletes suffering from eating disorders. *Int. J. Sport Nutr.* 3:431-442.

Sundgot-Borgen, J. (1993b). Prevalence of eating disorders in elite female athletes. *Int. J. Sport Nutr.* 3:29-40.

Sundgot-Borgen, J. (1994b). Risk and trigger factors for the development of eating disorders in female elite athletes. *Med. Sci. Sports Exerc.* 26:414-419.

Sundgot-Borgen, J., and C.B. Corbin (1987). Eating disorders among female athletes. *Phys. Sportsmed.* 15:89-95.

Svedenhag, J., H. Lithell, A. Juhlin-Dannfelt, and J. Henriksson (1983). Increase in skeletal muscle lipoprotein lipase following endurance training in man. *Atherosclerosis* 49:203-207.

Sykora, C., C.M. Grilo, D.E. Wilfley, and K.D. Brownell (1993). Eating, weight, and dieting disturbances in male and female lightweight and heavyweight rowers. *Int. J. Eat. Disord.* 14:203-211.

Taggart, N.R., R.M. Holiday, W.Z. Billewicz, F.E. Hytten, and A.M. Thomson (1967). Changes in skinfolds during pregnancy. *Br. J. Nutr.* 21:439-451.

Tanner, J.M., P.C.R. Hughes, and R.H. Whitehouse (1981). Radiographically determined widths of bone, muscle and fat in the upper arm and calf from age 3-18 years. *Ann. Hum. Biol.* 8:495-517.

Taub, D.E. and E.M. Blinde (1992). Eating disorders among adolescent female athletes: influence of athletic participation and sport team membership. *Adolescence* 27:833-848.

Technology Assessment Conference Panel (1992). Methods for voluntary weight loss and control: Technology assessment conference statement. *Ann. Intern. Med.* 116:942-949.

Tesch, P.A. (1987). Acute and long-term metabolic changes consequent to heavy-resistance exercise. *Med. Sport Sci.* 26:67-89.

Tesch, P.A. (1988). Skeletal muscle adaptations consequent to long-term heavy resistance exercise. *Med. Sci. Sports Exerc.* 20(Suppl):S132-S134.

Tesch, P.A., E.B. Colliander, and P. Kaiser (1986). Muscle metabolism during intense, heavy-resistance exercise. *Eur. J. Appl. Physiol.* 26:67-89.

Theintz, G.E., H. Howald, Y. Allemann, and P.C. Sizonenko (1989). Growth and pubertal development of young female gymnasts and swimmers: a correlation with parental data. *Int. J. Sports Med.* 10:87-91.

Theintz, G.E., H. Howald, U. Weiss, and P.C. Sizonenko (1993). Evidence for a reduction of growth potential in adolescent female gymnasts. *J. Pediatr.* 122:306–313.

Thompson, J.K., G.J. Jarvie, B.B. Lahey, and K.J. Cureton (1982). Exercise and obesity: etiology, physiology, and intervention. *Psychol. Bull.* 91:55–79.

Tremblay, A., J.P. Despres, C. Leblanc, and C. Bouchard (1984). Sex dimorphism in fat loss in response to exercise-training. *J. Obes. Weight Regulat.* 3:193–203.

Tremblay, A., E. Fontaine, E.T. Poehlman, D. Mitchell, L. Perron, and C. Bouchard (1986). The effect of exercise-training on resting metabolic rate in lean and moderately obese individuals. *Int. J. Obes.* 10:511–517.

Tremblay, A., A. Nadeau, J.P. Després, L. St-Jean, G. Thériault, and C. Bouchard (1990). Long-term exercise training with constant energy intake. 2: Effect on glucose metabolism and resting energy metabolism. *Int. J. Obes.* 14:75–84.

Tremblay, A., G. Ploure, J.P. Déspres, and C. Bouchard (1989). Impact of dietary fat content and fat oxidation on energy intake in humans. *Am. J. Clin. Nutr.* 49:799–805.

Tzankoff, S.P., and A.H. Norris (1978). Longitudinal changes in basal metabolic rate in man. *J. Appl. Physiol.* 33:536–539.

Vague, J. (1956). The degree of masculine differentiation of obesities: a factor determining predisposition to diabetes, atherosclerosis, gout and uric calculous disease. *Am. J. Clin. Nutr.* 4:20–34.

Vogel, J.A., and K.E. Friedl (1992). Body fat assessment in women. Special considerations. *Sports Med.* 13(4):245–269.

Wadden, T.A., G.D. Foster, K.A. Letizia, and J.L. Mullen (1990). Long-term effects of dieting on resting metabolic rate in obese outpatients. *J.A.M.A.* 264:707–711.

Wadden, T.A., A.J. Stunkard, and K.D. Brownell (1983). Very low calorie diets: their efficacy, safety, and future. *Ann. Intern. Med.* 99:675–684.

Walberg, J.L. (1989). Aerobic exercise and resistance weight-training during weight reduction: implications for obese persons and athletes. *Sports Med.* 47:343–346.

Walker, M., B.G. Cooper, C. Elliott, J.W. Reed, H. Orskov, and K.G.M.M. Alberti (1991). Role of plasma non-esterified fatty acids during and after exercise. *Clin. Sci.* 81:319–325.

Wang, Z.M., R.N. Pierson, and S.B. Heymsfield (1992). The five-level model: a new approach to organizing body-composition research. *Am. J. Clin. Nutr.* 56:19–28.

Warren, M.P. (1992). Eating, body weight, and menstrual function. In: K.D. Brownell, J. Rodin, and J.H. Wilmore (eds.) *Eating, Body Weight and Performance in Athletes. Disorders of Modern Society.* Philadelphia: Lea & Febiger, pp. 222–234.

Watts, P.B., D.T. Martin, and S. Durtschi (1993). Anthropometric profiles of elite male and female competitive sport rock climbers. *J. Sports Sci.* 11:113–117.

Webb, P., and T. Abrams (1983). Loss of fat stores and reduction in sedentary energy expenditure from undereating. *Hum. Nutr. Clin. Nutr.* 37:271–282.

Weight, L.M., and T.D. Noakes (1987). Is running an analog of anorexia?: a survey of the incidence of eating disorders in female distance runners. *Med. Sci. Sports Exerc.* 19:213–217.

Weigle, D.S. (1988). Contribution of decreased body mass to diminished thermic effect of exercise in reduced-obese men. *Int. J. Obes.* 12:567–578.

Weigle, D.S., K.J. Sande, P.H. Iverius, E.R. Monsen, and J.D. Brunzell (1988). Weight loss leads to a marked decrease in nonresting energy expenditure in ambulatory human subjects. *Metabolism* 37:930–936.

Weits, T., E.J. van der Beek, M. Weden, and B.M. Ter Haar Romeny (1988) Computed tomography measurement of abdominal fat deposition in relation to anthropometry. *Int. J. Obes.* 12:217–225.

Welle, S.L., J.M. Amatruda, G.B. Forbes, and D.H. Lockwood (1984). Resting metabolic rates of obese women after rapid weight loss. *J. Clin. Endocrinol. Metab.* 59:41–44.

Weltman, A., S. Matter, and B.A. Stamford (1980). Caloric restriction and/or mild exercise: effects on serum lipids and body composition. *Am. J. Clin. Nutr.* 33:1002–1009.

Wilmore, J.H. (1983). Body composition in sport and exercise: directions for future research. *Med. Sci. Sports Exerc.* 15:21–31.

Wilmore, J.H. (1977). Body physique and composition of the female distance runner. *Ann. N.Y. Acad. Sci.* 301:764–776.

Wilmore, J.H. (1992). Body weight standards and athletic performance. In: K.D. Brownell, J. Rodin, and J.H. Wilmore (eds.) *Eating, Body Weight and Performance in Athletes. Disorders of Modern Society.* Philadelphia: Lea & Febiger, pp. 315–327.

Wilmore, J.H. (1991). Eating and weight disorders in the female athlete. *Int. J. Sport Nutr.* 1:104–117.

Wolfe, R., R.S. Klein, F. Carraro, and J.M. Weber (1990). Role of triglyceride-fatty acid cycle in controlling fat metabolism in humans during and after exercise. *Am. J. Physiol.* 258:E382–E389.

Womersley, J., J.V.G.A. Durnin, K. Boddy, and M. Mahaffy (1976). Influence of muscular development, obesity and age on the fat-free mass of adults. *J. Appl. Physiol.* 41:223–229.

Wood, P.D., M.L. Stefanick, D.M. Dreon, B. Frey-Hewitt, S.C. Garay, P.T. Williams, H.R. Superko, S.P. Fortmann, J.J. Albers, K.M. Vranizan, N.M. Ellsworth, R.B. Terry, and W.L. Haskell (1988). Changes in plasma lipids and lipoproteins in overweight men during weight loss through dieting as compared with exercise. *N. Engl. J. Med.* 319:1173–1179.

Wood, P.D., M.L. Stefanick, P.T. Williams, and W.L. Haskell (1991). The effects on plasma lipoproteins of a prudent weight-reducing diet, with or without exercise, in overweight men and women. *N. Engl. J. Med.* 325:461–466.

Yang, M., and T.B. Van Itallie (1976). Metabolic responses of obese subjects to starvation and low calorie ketogenic and nonketogenic diets. *J. Clin. Invest.* 58:722–730.

Yesalis, C.E., W.E. Buckley, W.A. Anderson, M.Q. Wang, J.A. Norwig, G. Ott, J.C. Puffer, and R.H. Strauss (1990). Athletes' projections of anabolic steroid use. *Clin. Sports Med.* 2:155–171, 1990.

Young, N., C. Formica, and G. Szmukler (1994). Bone density at weight-bearing and nonweight-bearing sites in ballet dancers: the effects of exercise, hypogonadism, and body weight. *J. Clin. Endocrinol. Metab.* 78:449–454.

Zerbe, K.J. (1993). *The Body Betrayed.* Washington, D.C.: American Psychiatric Press, pp. 15, 125, 130.

Zinder, O., M. Hamosh, T.R. Fleck, and R.O. Scow (1974). Effect of prolactin on lipoprotein in lipase in mammary gland and adipose tissue of rats. *Am. J. Physiol.* 226:744–748.

Zurlo, F., S. Lillioja, A. Esposito-Del Puente, B.L. Nyomba, I. Raz, M.F. Saad, B.A. Swinburn, W.C. Knowler, C. Bogardus, and E. Ravussin (1990). Low ratio of fat to carbohydrate oxidation as a predictor of weight gain: study of 24-h R Q. *Am. J. Physiol.* 259:E650–E657.

Zuti, W.B. and L.A. Golding (1976). Comparing diet and exercise as weight reduction tools. *Phys. Sportsmed.* 4:49–53.

DISCUSSION

DESPRES: How should we define obesity in premenopausal women? There are many women with body mass indices of 26–27 who are very concerned about their body compositions while they are perfectly healthy. We have to stop overemphasizing that they should lose weight and that they should exercise. They are protected because there is a several-fold difference in the risk of developing cardiovascular disease and diabetes in women compared to men. We have to provide a fair judgment regarding the contribution of exercise in premenopausal women. I m not saying that they should not exercise, but we should have a balanced view here.

WILMORE: Studies that have looked at the effects of exercise alone on weight loss show that there are only small changes in both total mass and fat mass. Fat-free mass doesn't change that much either. I think our future research should focus on the role of exercise in preventing weight gain, which I think is the major benefit of exercise in weight control. Exercise does work in combination with diet to help weight loss, but if we look 5–10 y down the road, the results aren't encouraging in terms of people maintaining the weight loss. Compliance of subjects to a training and/or dietary restriction program is a major issue in determining the success or failure of weight loss regimens. We concluded one study 12 y ago in which we had people training for 20 wk while taking beta-blocking drugs. Many of them were firemen and policemen who were getting bonus pay for doing this, and they were excited about all of the positive health changes and the bonus pay. A year later none of them was exercising. We must start early in life to get exercise built in as a fun part of the lifestyle of an individual and not make it "exercise," which has a negative connotation. It is hard to take people who are 30, 40, 50, or 60 years of age and expect them to continue an exercise program habitually.

OLDRIDGE: Our research has suggested that there are major gender differences in adherence to exercise in cardiac patients. There are also major age differences in adherence to an exercise prescription.

GOING: There is certainly some evidence to show that people who begin energy restriction coupled with an exercise program are more likely to maintain their weight loss. Exercise would seem to be very critical in maintenance of weight loss.

OLDRIDGE: People tend to "yo-yo" with regard to weight loss/gain. Is there a real health risk to that?

DESPRES: At this stage it is really premature to raise the issue that losing weight and gaining weight several times during a life span might increase risk. The cause-and-effect association has not been properly addressed, and we have little information on factors involved in weight fluctuations in these studies. I would prefer to see someone who has a dyslipidemic profile, insulin resistance, and hypertension attempting to keep the cardiovascular disease risk profile under control for a few years, even if this person is not quite successful in the long run, i.e., even if the diet and exercise program is interrupted by periods in which the subject would be at a higher body weight. If we consider the fact that atherosclerosis is a progressive process, maybe this process may be slowed down by having a healthier profile a few times during the life span.

EICHNER: It is true that women as compared to men are protected from heart disease, but among women, as shown by the Nurses Health Study, 40% or so of the prediction for early heart attack is governed by obesity. On exercise not being a "major player," when you treat obese people, it can be self-defeating to try to get them to start only by dieting or cutting fat. But if they start an exercise program, begin to feel proud of themselves, then maybe you can broach the diet and get the combined benefit of exercise and a low-fat diet. Isn't it fair to say that oxidation of carbohydrate and protein are fairly tightly regulated on an unrestricted diet, so that if exercise creates an energy deficit, over time the weight loss is essentially fat loss?

DESPRES: Dr. Eichner, you are right about the nurse study, but you have to look at the absolute rate of heart disease. There is no way you can compare those values with those for men.

COYLE: We've heard discussion that exercise should be used as a way to prevent weight gain, especially as people age. Also, you have mentioned in the chapter that there is a large loss of muscle mass with age, but this occurs less in women than in men if they continue to exercise. Do you think that women can potentially prevent this large decline in muscle mass with aging, especially if they are doing aerobic exercise that stresses the lower body where most of the muscle mass in women is located? Can women more effectively prevent a decline in muscle mass with aerobic exercise, whereas men need more resistance training or stimulation of the upper body?

GOING: Whether the loss of muscle can be retarded more in women than in men is unclear. I am not aware of any studies comparing the effects of resistance exercise vs. running or some other lower-body activity in men and women at different ages.

DESPRES: I think we should not overemphasize the maintenance of lean body mass quantity without considerations of the quality of that lean mass during weight loss in overweight women. It would be much more important to increase the oxidative potential of the skeletal muscle component of this fat-free mass while the quantity of lean tissue is being maintained. We know that overweight women have a larger fat-free mass than do normal-weight women, and the obese are bound to lose some fat-free mass eventually if they lose a substantial amount of body fat. Having said that, there is a very nice paper recently published in the *Journal of Clinical Investigation* by Colberg, Kelly, and Simoneau which showed that carnitine-palmitoyl-transferase activity was markedly reduced in viscerally obese women who had low oxidative potentials in their skeletal muscles. In that respect, I see endurance exercise as a very nice way to increase the oxidative potential of the skeletal muscle irrespective of mass considerations. As an approach to reach some sort of balance between this high mobilization of free-fatty acids and utilization by the skeletal muscle, I believe that the oxidative potential of lean tissue should be considered as perhaps at least as important as the mass of the tissue.

COYLE: I think you are right that it is important to maintain the oxidative ability. We have done studies in untrained subjects and found that they can mobilize much more fat than they can oxidize. Fat oxidation is probably limited by their muscle mitochondria and other factors. With endurance training, there is a very close match between mobilization of fatty acids and their oxidation during low-intensity exercise. I think untrained people have no problem mobilizing fat and generating high concentrations of plasma fatty acids, but most of those fatty acids are not oxidized and are simply reesterfied to form triglycerides somewhere in the body.

KRISKA: The health consequences surrounding total obesity and centrally distributed obesity are an especially important issue with many of our minority populations. Compared to their white counterparts, levels of total and central obesity are usually found to be relatively greater in black, Hispanic, and native American women, who by the way, also have more chronic diseases.

Also, you mentioned that there are gender differences in how exercise affects the pattern of fat distribution, but you didn't mention why you think they exist. Is the effect of exercise on central fat distribution in women the same across the life span? Is this effect the same after they become postmenopausal?

GOING: Based on the results of only a few studies, men and women with more visceral fat tend to be more responsive to exercise than those with fat depots in the gluteo-femoral region.

KRISKA: In other words, if you have a man and a woman with the same amount of central fat, you would hypothesize that they would respond equally to exercise?

GOING: I don't know whether they would respond equally, but I believe that women with more visceral fat are more likely to lose fat than are the women with the typical female gynoid pattern, regardless of whether they are premenopausal or postmenopausal women.

KRISKA: Since women become more android through menopause then would they respond better to exercise after menopause?

DESPRES: They have more visceral fat to start with. They are going to show a preferential mobilization of visceral fat, just like men. Before menopause, if they have little visceral fat, there is obviously very little room for mobilization.

WILMORE: The question of what happens to spontaneous activity when people undertake exercise programs is very important and needs to be further studied. If people expend 500 kcal/d during exercise, which is a pretty substantial volume, it would be very difficult for them to decrease their spontaneous activity by that much. Wim Saris's lab addressed this issue using doubly-labeled water and showed no decrease in spontaneous activity. However, there probably are certain groups whose spontaneous activity might decrease if they increase their exercise levels.

NADEL: The relatively small size of the Japanese after World War II was in part due to nutritional deficits following the war. Studies compared Japanese residents of Japan with 1st, 2nd, and 3rd generation Japanese Americans, who attained the size of their American counterparts. The reason I'm bringing this up is that I was very impressed with the report that the current trend in gymnasts demonstrated a very dramatic decrease in height and weight. Is this due to voluntary starvation and, probably more importantly, is this reversible?

CLARKSON: I am not aware of data regarding whether gymnasts who stop training will attain normal growth patterns. In a retrospective study, gymnasts were found to be smaller than normal even at 1 y of age. There seems to be some relationship to the heights of parents as well. However, even taking this into account, gymnasts are still somewhat shorter in stature than the average young person. Several factors probably contribute: genetics, selection, and caloric restriction during the growth process.

BAILEY: Theintz et al. studied elite gymnasts who were training in excess of 30 h/wk. These investigators have reported in the *Journal of Pediat-*

rics a stunting of growth, particularly lower body growth. This paper has certain problems, but animal studies provide incontrovertible evidence that excessive exercise in developing animals can stunt growth, and I think we should not discount this possibility. If you looked at the competitors in the world gymnastic championships last year, you would find 17- and 18-year-old girls 4'10" tall and weighing 80 lb. who hadn't yet reached menarche. This hardly seems normal to me. Excessive, heavy usage may adversely affect somatic growth.

LOUCKS: We don't know the answer whether there is a delay in growth, but I would side with Robert Malina and say that we may have a selection process going on in these gymnasts. Maybe the sport at this elite level is selecting another population of women. I would also side with Malina regarding this concept of delayed menarche. It is not clear that it is delayed. We may have late menarche, and it may be due to self-selection.

BAR-OR: There are data from the Netherlands showing that short gymnasts were short before they became gymnasts.

OLDRIDGE: I was also impressed by these big changes over time in the gymnasts. What role was played by the fact that gymnasts are competing at younger ages?

CLARKSON: Partially it is due to the age decrease. If you compare gymnasts' stature to national surveys of children, gymnasts are smaller than children of the same age. This difference is much more exaggerated for the 16-year-old gymnast in 1992 compared to the 18-year-old gymnast in 1960.

6

Cardiorespiratory Function

HÉLÈNE PERRAULT, Ph.D.

INTRODUCTION

The participation of men in organized sports to test the limits of human performance goes back as far as ancient Greek, Roman, or Egyptian
societies. According to Hult (1986), there was also a female version of
the Olympic Games, the Heraean games, which consisted essentially of a

215

154-m run with entries for three different age groups. Unfortunately, there are no available records of such performances by women. The first "official" recognition of participation in track and swimming events by women was an outcome of the 1916 Amateur Athletic Association convention in which a motion was approved to keep records of female performances in these events (Hult, 1986). The first women's world championships took place in 1922, and the longest running distance was 1000 m (Kuscsik, 1977). Because data on running and swimming endurance events are more readily available than those for other sports, the analysis in this chapter of gender-related differences in cardiorespiratory function and endurance performance will be limited to running and swimming.

FEMALE PERFORMANCE IN ENDURANCE EVENTS

An account of gender differences in Olympic performances between 1960 and 1976 was published by Raine in 1978. A general comparison of track records showed that men performed roughly 10% better than women for running distances between 400 and 1500 m (Raine, 1978). The ratios of running times for men to running times for women have been calculated using current world records (Matthews, 1994) over running distances between 1500 m and 500 km and are illustrated in Figure 6-1. Most record holders were young adult competitors ranging in age between 20 y and 35 y when their records were established. For running distances up to 20 km the best performance by a woman remains within approximately 8–15% of the best record for a man, with the best performance ratio (male run time/female run time) of 92.4% recorded for the 3000 m running distance. These observations are similar to previous accounts of performance ratios for 1984 and 1989 (Wells, 1991) and reflect a marked improvement in both absolute and relative performances by women in the last 30 y.

Performance times recently have been improving faster in women than in men, which lead to the much debated speculation that women will ultimately perform the same as or better than men (Joyner, 1994). In early 1992, Whipp and Ward presented evidence suggesting that male and female marathon running performances would soon converge. This prediction is only valid if selected world records are plotted at set time intervals, e.g., one record per decade as reported by Whipp and Ward, resulting in a linear progression of female running records. Refined analyses of successive marathon world records for both men and women between 1964 and 1981 clearly show a curvilinear progression toward a plateau in world records (Noakes, 1986; Péronnet, 1993). Thus, although it is unlikely that elite women will outrun elite men in the near future, elite women do indeed outrun most men. An exception to this might be performances over

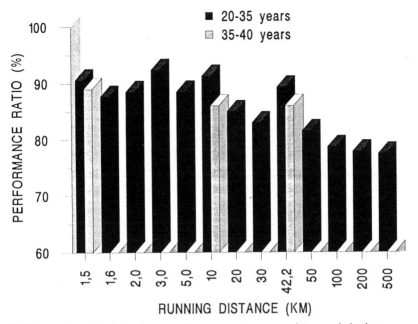

FIGURE 6-1. *Ratios of male/female running times over various running distances calculated using current world records. Age groups of 20–35y and 35–40 y are shown.*

very long distances because, as shown in Figure 6-1, ratios of women's to men's records decline from roughly 90% for the marathon to 77.5% for a 500 km event. However, it must be recognized that for sociocultural reasons the pool of male competitors for ultraendurance events is probably much greater than that of female competitors. Thus, the decline in performance ratios for longer distances does not necessarily reflect differences in aerobic endurance caused by gender *per se.*

The analysis of age-related changes in endurance running performances for 1500 m and marathon events is summarized in Figure 6-2. Gender ratios for performance times of young participants were calculated from "Junior Olympics" comprehensive results and from high school records and are shown for running and swimming in Table 6-1. As can be seen in Figure 6-2, a widening in gender differences develops progressively between the 11–12 y category and the 15–16 y category. It is likely that this coincides with growth, sexual maturation, and muscle mass development in boys that in turn affect running economy, aerobic endurance, or maximal aerobic power.

The increase in performance ratio observed in young world record holders (20–25 y) over those of high school age categories indicates an improvement in women's running performances that may be associated with their intense and specific training regimens. Unlike results for the

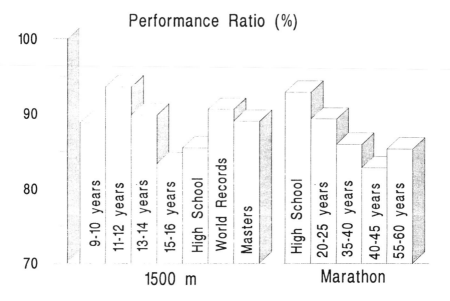

FIGURE 6-2. *Age-related changes in ratios of male/female running times for running 1500 m and marathon distances.*

TABLE 6-1. *Ratios of male/female performance times in children and adolescents*.*

CATEGORY	RUNNING				SWIMMING
	1500 m	3000 m	10 km	42.2 km	400 m Freestyle
Bantam (9–10 y)	88.8	—	—	—	—
Midget (11–12 y)	93.6	90.8	—	—	98.1
Youth (13–14 y)	89.8	93.1	—	—	93.7
Intermediate (15–16 y)	83.4	82.1	—	—	—
High School (17–18 y)	85.5	88.5	86.5	92.9	91.9
World Record (20–25 y)	90.6	92.4	91.3	89.3	92.2

*Data calculated from record times from U.S. High School and Junior Olympics published in the January issue of *Track and Field News*, 1991.

1500-m event, ratios of male/female run times that were calculated for marathon running in high school athletes (93%) are comparable to those found for older Olympic athletes (89%). However, the data suggest a widening of the gender-related performance differences with advancing age. Using notable performance marks reported by Joyner (1994) for male and female runners 35 y of age or older, run-time ratios were calculated for marathon running. As can be seen in Figure 6-2, in older competitors values range between 83% and 86%, i.e., roughly 3–6% lower than those for young competitors. From combined male and female records for popular running events in the United States, a 6–9% decline in running performance could be expected between 30 and 50 y of age, with a more rapid decline thereafter (Joyner, 1994). In accordance with suggestions from Joyner (1994), results from Figure 6-2 suggest that the age-related decline in performance is presumably more rapid in women. It should be recognized, however, that differences in the training states of subjects could perhaps account for such a discrepancy.

Physiological Factors Affecting Running Performance

It is generally accepted that distance running performance depends on the interaction among several physiological factors including maximal aerobic power ($\dot{V}O_2$max), sustained fractional utilization of $\dot{V}O_2$max, and running economy, i.e., the average oxygen cost to run at a given speed (Conley et al., 1981; DiPrampero et al., 1993; Helgerud, 1994; Joyner, 1994; Lacour et al., 1990; Padilla et al., 1992; Péronnet & Thibault, 1989). Although there is much less information on the relationships among these factors and running performance in women than there is in men, the same factors appear to contribute to running performance in both genders. Direct comparisons of running economies at various running speeds are not possible, because the fastest female runners are slower than the fastest males. Rough comparisons of data for women running at 230–248 m/min with those for men at 241–322 m/min generally suggest no gender difference in the oxygen cost of running (Bunc & Heller, 1989; Joyner, 1994; Helgerud, 1994; Padilla et al., 1992; Sparling & Cureton, 1983) except for the data from Daniels and Daniels (1992) that show a higher running economy in elite male runners compared to elite female runners at running speeds between 250 and 330 m/min. Similarly, it appears that the fractional utilization of $\dot{V}O_2$max during running is similar for men and women (Conley et al., 1981; Helgerud, 1994; Helgerud et al. 1990; Wells et al., 1981). Similar to what has been observed in men, running performance in women is closely related to maximal aerobic power (Davies & Thompson, 1979; Padilla et al., 1992; Ramsbottom et al., 1989), and the slower running times of females have mainly been attributed to their lower values for $\dot{V}O_2$max.

MAXIMAL AEROBIC POWER

Theoretically, the gender difference in $\dot{V}O_2$max is predominantly related to differences in body composition and oxygen-carrying capacity. Women typically show a higher fat percentage and a lower fat-free mass than men, and men exhibit, on the average, a hemoglobin concentration that is 20 g/L higher than that of women. Differences in habitual levels of physical activity between men and women may also contribute to the gender differences in $\dot{V}O_2$max.

The Influence Of Body Composition

In an attempt to quantify the gender effect for different expressions of $\dot{V}O_2$max, Sparling (1980) conducted a meta-analysis of $\dot{V}O_2$max data from 13 studies of male and female subjects of various levels of habitual physical activity. The average sex differences were 56% for $\dot{V}O_2$max expressed in L/min, 28% for $\dot{V}O_2$max expressed relative to body weight, and 15% for $\dot{V}O_2$max expressed relative to fat-free mass. Thus, a considerable portion of the gender difference in $\dot{V}O_2$max may be eliminated by considering only fat-free mass (FFM) or muscle mass (Cureton & Sparling, 1980). Recognizing that different levels of physical conditioning may act as a confounding factor, Cureton et al. (1986) compared $\dot{V}O_2$max values of men and women matched for habitual level of physical activity. Although they observed a 47% gender-related difference in $\dot{V}O_2$max expressed in L/min, they found no significant difference between men and women when $\dot{V}O_2$max was expressed relative to fat-free mass. These observations suggest that a large portion of the gender-related difference in $\dot{V}O_2$max can be attributed to the higher relative fat mass and relatively lower fat-free mass of women.

The Influence Of The Oxygen-Carrying Capacity

Because a positive relationship between $\dot{V}O_2$max and total body hemoglobin content has been documented it has been suggested that the lower $\dot{V}O_2$max of women may be related to lower average hemoglobin content. Considering that $\dot{V}O_2$max values relative to fat-free mass of female subjects remained 12–15% lower than those of their male counterparts, Sparling (1980) concluded in his meta-analysis of studies comparing $\dot{V}O_2$max of men and women that a substantial portion of this remaining difference could probably be attributed to a gender-related difference in hemoglobin content. In an attempt to determine the proportion of the gender difference in $\dot{V}O_2$max attributable to differences in hemoglobin concentrations, Cureton et al. (1986) performed blood withdrawal in 10 healthy men to reduce their mean hemoglobin concentration to exactly that of the 11 women participating in the study. Equalizing the hemoglobin concentration reduced the gender-related difference in $\dot{V}O_2$max (L/min) by 7.5%, thus accounting for only a small portion of the initial 47% gender-related difference. However, it must be recognized that there exists a wide variability of hemoglobin concentrations within and across genders that could lead to an overlap of hemoglobin concentrations in men and women. In addition, because venesection or infusion of red blood cells induces changes in blood volume as well as in the hemoglobin concentration, the use of these procedures does not account for the selective influence of the hemoglobin concentration on $\dot{V}O_2$max (Warren & Cureton, 1989). Nevertheless, these observations suggest that the generally lower oxygen-carrying capacity of women is not the predominant factor for their lower $\dot{V}O_2$max, although it may contribute to the gender-related difference.

The Effects Of Growth And Maturation

A classical representation of the effects of growth and maturation on physiological determinants of physical performance is the linear increase in $\dot{V}O_2$max until ages 13 and 16 y for girls and boys, respectively (Bar-Or, 1983; Malina & Bouchard, 1991). Before 12 y of age, average values of $\dot{V}O_2$max for females are typically 85–90% of those for males; this is compatible with a 7% lower relative muscle mass in girls (Figure 6-3). Following adolescent growth and sexual maturation, $\dot{V}O_2$max values for females reach only about 70% of those for male. However, because the growth-related increase in $\dot{V}O_2$max is not linearly related to the resulting increase in total body size (Berg et al., 1991) and because the proportion of fat-free body mass differs between men and women, it is difficult to make valid comparisons of gender-related differences in $\dot{V}O_2$max throughout growth and maturation.

Expressing $\dot{V}O_2$max in relation to body weight somewhat decreases the gap between male and female values, i.e., relative $\dot{V}O_2$max values for prepubescent girls are 90–95% and for late adolescent girls are roughly 80% of male values (Malina & Bouchard, 1991). Average values of $\dot{V}O_2$max/FFM reported in preadolescent and adolescent boys are 10% greater than those found in girls (Malina & Bouchard, 1991), whereas an average 15% difference has been reported in adults (Sparling, 1980).

The Effects Of Aging

In general, data from cross-sectional comparisons of $\dot{V}O_2$max measured using cycle ergometry or treadmill running in healthy sedentary individuals of both sexes ranging in age from 15 to 80 y indicate a 9–10% fall per decade after age 30 y (Åstrand, 1960; Drinkwater et al., 1975; Folkow & Svanborg, 1993; Paterson, 1992; Plowman et al., 1979; Stamford, 1988) (Figure 6-3). The average reported annual loss in $\dot{V}O_2$max between ages 20 y and 85 y may be calculated to be about 0.43 mL·kg^{-1}·min^{-1} for males and 0.41 mL·kg^{-1}·min^{-1} for females (Paterson, 1992; Stamford, 1988; Shvartz & Reibold, 1990). When expressed as percentages of initial $\dot{V}O_2$max values, the average yearly decline among males is 1.05% for cycle ergometry and 0.92% for treadmill running (Paterson, 1992; Stamford, 1988). The corresponding average annual declines in females are 1.27% for cycle ergometry and 0.90% for treadmill running. Thus, although there are considerably fewer investigations of females than of males, there appear to be similar rates of yearly decline in $\dot{V}O_2$max for both genders. Taking exception to this general statement, Wells et al. (1992) recently reported a yearly rate of decline in $\dot{V}O_2$max of 0.47

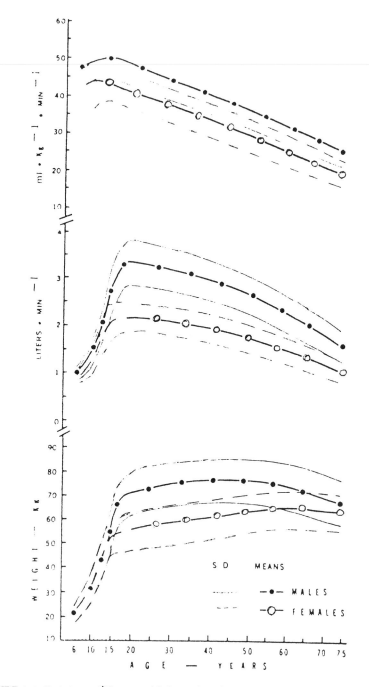

FIGURE 6-3. *Variations in* $\dot{V}O_2max$ *and body weight with maturation and aging.* From: Shvartz & Reibold (1990), with permission.

$mL \cdot kg^{-1} \cdot min^{-1}$ in female masters runners aged between 35 and 70 years of age, suggesting a higher rate of decline in highly trained women compared to sedentary or moderately trained women. A clear explanation for this finding remains to be provided.

Several factors including a decrease in oxygen utilization due to a loss in muscle mass (Plowman et al., 1979) as well as an age-related weight gain or change in physical training habits may account for interindividual differences in the rate of decline of $\dot{V}O_2max$. The higher rate of decline in highly trained women could be related to a selection bias associated with the sociologically less prominent, older female competitive athlete. However, in trained individuals, differences in training status with advancing age may also contribute to the variation in $\dot{V}O_2max$. In a 10-y follow-up of active men who trained 3 h weekly at an intensity of 86% of $\dot{V}O_2max$, Kasch and Wallace (1976) reported no change in $\dot{V}O_2max$. Similarly, the age-related decrement in $\dot{V}O_2max$ was reduced by up to 50% in men who pursued regular endurance training and participated in masters running competitions (Heath et al., 1981; Pollack et al., 1974; Rogers et al., 1990). Similar findings have also been reported in physically active women (Drinkwater, 1984; Drinkwater et al., 1975; Plowman et al., 1979).

Repeated testing of individuals at regular intervals across the life span provides a more accurate assessment of the changes in cardiorespiratory fitness with aging than do ex post facto cross-sectional comparisons. In 1949, Åstrand et al. (1973) studied 31 male and 35 female physical education students using cycle ergometry. Twenty-one years later, as active physical education teachers, the same subjects were retested. Mean $\dot{V}O_2max$ had decreased annually by 0.64 $mL \cdot kg^{-1} \cdot min^{-1}$ for male subjects and by 0.44 $mL \cdot kg^{-1} \cdot min^{-1}$ for female subjects, corresponding to relative decrements in $\dot{V}O_2max$ of 1.09% and 0.92%, respectively. The reported decrement in $\dot{V}O_2max$ for male subjects is much higher than that generally reported from cross-sectional studies, perhaps reflecting a greater age-related loss of muscle mass. In women, however, the calculated decline is comparable to that from cross-sectional comparisons.

The Effects Of Training Status

Can training eliminate the gap between males and females $\dot{V}O_2max$? In humans, values of $\dot{V}O_2max$ as high as 85 $mL \cdot kg^{-1} \cdot min^{-1}$ have been reported in elite male endurance athletes (Pollock, 1977). A subsequent investigation of 16 female elite runners revealed $\dot{V}O_2max$ values ranging between 61 and 73 $mL \cdot kg^{-1} \cdot min^{-1}$ and averaging 67 $mL \cdot kg^{-1} \cdot min^{-1}$ (Pate et al., 1987; Pollack et al., 1987; Sparling et al., 1987). Although lower than that reported for male elite runners (Pollock, 1977), the mean value for the elite women is only 4% lower than the 70.3 $mL \cdot kg^{-1} \cdot min^{-1}$ average reported for male marathon runners (Costill & Winrow, 1970). Despite the relatively low percentages of body fat in elite female distance runners

(Graves et al., 1987), correcting $\dot{V}O_2$max values for FFM further reduces the differences in $\dot{V}O_2$max between men and women. In the group of elite female distance runners studied by Pate et al. (1987), expression of $\dot{V}O_2$max per unit of FFM increased the average relative $\dot{V}O_2$max by 15%, i.e. from 67.1 to 77.8 mL·kg FFM^{-1}·min^{-1}. However, correction for percent body fat may not eliminate differences in $\dot{V}O_2$max between male and female athletes. For example, in recreational runners there was a 5% gender-related difference in $\dot{V}O_2$max expressed relative to FFM (Sparling & Cureton, 1983).

THE OXYGEN TRANSPORT SYSTEM: A FEMALE PERSPECTIVE

Maximal aerobic power reflects the potential for delivery of oxygen to the exercising muscles and their capacity to utilize it in oxidative phosphorylation in the mitochondria. A 5–15% gender-related difference in $\dot{V}O_2$max persists between highly trained men and women despite correction for body weight or muscle mass. Thus, an inherent biological difference seems to exist between men and women in one or more components of the oxygen transport/utilization system. The relationship between these components is best described by the Fick equation (Eq. 1) relating oxygen consumption ($\dot{V}O_2$), cardiac output (Qc), and arteriovenous oxygen difference (a-v O_2):

$$\text{Eq.1: } \dot{V}O_2 = Qc \times (\text{a-v } O_2)$$

By substitution, the equation can be rewritten as follows:

$$\text{Eq. 2: } \dot{V}O_2 = (HR \times Qs) \times (CaO_2\text{-}CvO_2),$$

where HR = heart rate (beats/min); Qs = stroke volume (mL); CaO_2 = arterial oxygen content (mL/L); and CvO_2 = mixed venous oxygen content (mL/L). By another substitution, Eq. 2 can be rewritten as:

$$\text{Eq. 3: } \dot{V}O_2 = HR(LVEDV\text{-}LVESV)(CaO_2\text{-} CvO_2),$$

where LVEDV = left ventricular end-diastolic volume and LVESV = left ventricular end-systolic volume.

In the following sections I will first examine gender-related structural differences in circulatory, pulmonary, and skeletal muscle function that could account for baseline differences in the elements of the equation. Next, I will consider gender-related differences in the responses of these elements during exercise in an attempt to account for the biological difference in $\dot{V}O_2$max between men and women.

The Oxygen Transport System In Female Proportions

From a purely structural point of view the oxygen transport and utilization system of the human female may be seen as a petite version of its male counterpart. As reflected by equations 2 and 3, oxygen transport is determined by ventricular pump function, which in turn is dependent upon filling capacity and ejection potential. Although there is no evidence for differences in the potential for ventricular ejection or systolic function between men and women, ventricular filling capacity may be reduced on account of a smaller left ventricle in females. Heart size is proportional to body size (Feigenbaum, 1986), so it follows that women would exhibit smaller left ventricular dimensions. A contributing factor to the lower end-diastolic ventricular dimensions of female subjects is that, relative to males, they typically have lower blood volumes, which in humans typically represent roughly 8% of total body weight. Furthermore, results from postmortem studies have documented smaller weight-adjusted relative myocardial mass in women compared to men (Grande & Taylor, 1965; Smith, 1928), although these observations did not account for gender-related differences in body composition or lean body mass. Nuclear magnetic resonance imaging in female endurance athletes confirms the earlier postmortem findings and suggests that the lower left ventricular mass of women persists when corrected for lean body mass (Riley-Hagan et al., 1992).

Oxygen-carrying capacity is also lower in women than in men, although there are large intersubject differences. In general, 95% of women exhibit hemoglobin concentrations between 120 and 160 g/L, whereas the corresponding values for men are between 140 and 180 g/L (Freedson, 1981). Considering average hemoglobin concentrations of 160 g/L and 140 g/L in adult males and females, respectively, a 13% lower arterial oxygen content can be calculated for female subjects (184 mL O_2/L) when compared to males (210 mL O_2/L). Peripheral oxygen extraction potential is highly dependent upon training state but does not appear to be related to gender differences; thus, similar values for mixed-venous oxygen content have been reported for males and females (Mitchell et al., 1992).

The Cardiac Output Response To Dynamic Exercise

Under resting conditions cardiac output (Eq. 1) appears to be similar between genders, both in children and adults (Cumming, 1977, 1978; Sullivan et al., 1991; Younis et al., 1990). Comparisons of regression equations describing the relationship between $\dot{V}O_2$ and cardiac output between boys and girls (Bar-Or, 1983) or between adult men and women indicate similar patterns of increases in response to progressive maximal dynamic exercise; in general, however, higher maximal values for cardiac output are recorded in males (Åstrand et al., 1964; Åstrand & Rodahl, 1986; Bar-

Or, 1983; Cumming, 1978; Sullivan et al., 1991; Younis et al., 1990). There are no significant gender-related differences in cardiac index during exercise in either young or older subjects when exercise intensity is expressed as a percentage of $\dot{V}O_2$max (Bar-Or, 1983; Wirth et al., 1978; Younis et al., 1990). Thus, because girls or women have lower absolute values for $\dot{V}O_2$max, they exhibit greater cardiac indices than do men for any given $\dot{V}O_2$ (Åstrand et al., 1964; Bar-Or et al., 1971; Freedson et al., 1979). This is also apparent from more recent data obtained through right-sided cardiac catheterization and simultaneous radionuclide angiography (Sullivan et al., 1991). These studies showed identical cardiac outputs in men and women for any given submaximal work rate, but 8–20% lower $\dot{V}O_2$ values in women for matched work rates, thus implying higher cardiac outputs for any given $\dot{V}O_2$. Whether the higher cardiac outputs of women during exercise at a given $\dot{V}O_2$ reflect a compensatory mechanism for their lower arterial oxygen contents or merely reflect an effect of a smaller mitochondrial mass for oxygen utilization, and thus a need for greater transport, is not yet clear.

A wide variability in hemoglobin concentrations within genders causes much overlap in hemoglobin levels between genders. As a consequence it is difficult to isolate hemoglobin differences as the sole factor for the higher submaximal cardiac output of women (Freedson, 1981). In 11-y-old children, Bar-Or et al. (1971) found relatively higher cardiac outputs in girls than in boys of similar weight and body surface area at all work levels on a cycle ergometer, despite identical hemoglobin concentrations. Freedson et al. (1979) reported a similar observation in adult men and women subjects who were matched on $\dot{V}O_2$max. They noted an enhanced cardiac output in females versus males who cycled at given submaximal loads. However, this gender-related difference disappeared when cardiac output was expressed per unit of lean body weight, suggesting that the gender difference in cardiac output was a function of active muscle mass. Unfortunately, a comparison was only made for a low exercise intensity (50 W); at higher work rates a potential limitation in oxygen delivery would be more likely.

In a subsequent experiment to examine the relationship between circulating hemoglobin and submaximal cardiac output, Freedson (1981) found that blood withdrawal that reduced hemoglobin concentration by 18.6% in six men increased submaximal cardiac output by 12.6%. Thus, the drop in the oxygen-carrying capacity of blood appears to be at least partially offset by a compensatory increase in cardiac output. Because the second $\dot{V}O_2$max test was performed three days after blood withdrawal, when blood volume presumably had been restored, it is reasonable to assume that the increased cardiac output was a function of the decrease in hemoglobin concentration, not an altered blood volume (Warren & Cureton, 1989).

Peak or maximal heart rate does not appear to be affected by gender either in young or adult subjects (Åstrand et al., 1964; Bar-Or, 1983; Younis et al., 1990). Independent of gender, there is a maturity-onset decline in maximal heart rate of 0.7–0.8 beats·min^{-1}·y^{-1} from a range of 195–220 beats/min in children (Bar-Or, 1983). However, there is a gender-related difference in heart rate for submaximal work; preadolescent girls and adolescent girls and adult women exhibit higher heart rates than boys at the same absolute work loads (Bar-Or et al., 1983; Higginbotham et al., 1984; Sullivan et al., 1991; Younis et al., 1990). In adult women and post-pubertal girls this could reflect the higher relative intensity of work for females compared to males at given absolute exercise levels, but the cause of this relative tachycardia in young children matched for hemoglobin concentration and $\dot{V}O_2$max is not clear. Although they could be related to gender differences in habitual physical activity and fitness state, the higher heart rates of females can probably be best explained by relatively lower stroke volumes of females at standard workloads (Bar-Or, 1983; Higginbotham et al., 1984; Younis et al., 1990).

Stroke volume is determined to a significant extent by body size (Cunningham et al., 1984), in turn affecting end-diastolic ventricular dimensions (Blimkie et al., 1980; Feigenbaum, 1986). Examining the relationship between body weight and O_2 pulse (a reflection of stroke volume) at 140 beats/min, Cooper (1989) found a relatively steeper slope in the data from boys when compared to similar data from girls. However, when the O_2 pulse data were plotted as a function of the subjects' anaerobic threshold rather than body mass, gender-related differences disappeared, suggesting that the relationship between cardiorespiratory and musculo-skeletal growth is the same across genders.

The Regulation Of Exercise Stroke Volume. It is generally accepted from observations mainly in healthy male subjects that the exercise-induced rise in stroke volume results from a combination of an increase in ventricular contractility and heterometric regulation through the Frank-Starling mechanism (Casone et al., 1982; Crawford et al., 1979; Dickhuth et al., 1981; Higginbotham et al., 1986a; Mahler et al., 1985; Manyari et al., 1981; Péronnet & Perrault, 1985; Plotnik et al., 1986; Poliner et al., 1980; Rerych et al., 1980; Slutsky et al., 1979; Stein et al., 1978; Thadani & Parker, 1978; Upton et al., 1980). In response to upright progressive dynamic exercise up to roughly 40–50% $\dot{V}O_2$max, there is an increase in stroke volume, mainly attributed to an exercise-induced increase in end-diastolic ventricular filling; at greater exercise intensities a plateau in stroke volume is reached due to a decrease in ventricular diastolic filling coupled with a continuous decline in ventricular end-systolic volume (Higginbotham et al., 1986a; Plotnik et al., 1986; Poliner et al., 1980; Sullivan et al., 1991).

Challenging the widely accepted view of a plateau in stroke volume for exercise intensity above 50% $\dot{V}O_2$max, Gledhill et al. (1994) reported a continuous rise in stroke volume up to heart rates of 190 beats/min in young endurance-trained subjects when compared to untrained subjects, consequent to a higher rate of ventricular filling. Thus, in addition to an enhanced preload contributing to an increased exercise stroke volume, trained subjects may benefit from an enhanced ventricular diastolic function, enabling their stroke volumes to continue to increase beyond 50% $\dot{V}O_2$max. Also challenging the occurence of a plateau in exercise stroke volume, Spina et al. (1993a) reported a significant decrease between stroke volumes measured at 50% $\dot{V}O_2$max and 100% $\dot{V}O_2$max in healthy, older untrained men and women. A definite explanation for this observation was not provided; theoretically, an age-related decrease in both systolic and diastolic ventricular functions could explain difficulties in maintaining exercise stroke volume. It is noteworthy that the fall in exercise stroke volume was reversed by endurance training.

In addition to training state and aging, exercise hemodynamics are influenced by body position. A plateau in exercise stroke volume is also generally described in young, healthy untrained subjects exercising in the supine position. However, the exercise-induced contribution of the Frank-Starling mechanism to the increase in stroke volume is reduced on account of the higher basal end-diastolic volume consequent to the resting recumbent position (Crawford et al., 1979; Manyari et al., 1981; Poliner et al., 1980; Slutsky et al., 1979).

Gender-Related Differences In The Relative Contribution Of the Frank-Starling Mechanism. Using radionuclide angiography during upright progressive cycling exercise, Higginbotham et al. (1984) observed that the relative contribution of the Frank-Starling mechanism to the exercise-induced increase in stroke volume was significantly more important in women than in men of comparable age; under maximal exercise conditions women showed a 30% increase in end-diastolic radionuclide activity, whereas no significant difference from rest was found in men. Over the last 10 y, results of at least seven additional investigations of the gender-related differences in exercise stroke volume have been published (Figure 6-4). Most of the observations were obtained using radionuclide angiography in young or middle-aged subjects cycling to peak exercise intensity in an upright (Higginbotham et al., 1984; Sullivan et al., 1991; Younis et al., 1990) or supine position (Adams et al., 1987; Hanley et al., 1989; Pfisterer et al. 1985; Spina et al., 1993b; Weiss et al., 1979).

In terms of gender comparisons, the overall picture from these studies is at best controversial. In contrast to the original findings of Higginbotham et al. (1984), data obtained both by Sullivan et al. (1991) and Younis et al. (1990) reported that men and women showed similar exercise-induced increases in the end-diastolic volume index during upright

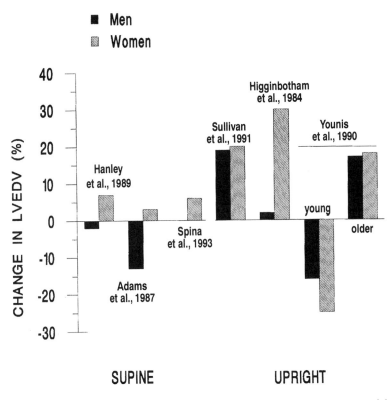

- ■ Men
- ▨ Women

FIGURE 6-4. *Summary of changes in left-ventricular end-diastolic volume from rest to maximal dynamic exercise reported in studies comparing healthy women and men.*

progressive maximal exercise, suggesting that gender is not an important determinant of left ventricular volume. In contrast, data obtained during supine exercise protocols suggest a gender-related difference in the end-diastolic volume response. In all three supine-exercise studies, a 5–10% increase in end-diastolic dimensions was observed in women from rest to peak exercise; the observation appeared independent of age because the age of subjects across the three studies varied between 30 and 63 y (Adams et al., 1987; Hanley et al., 1989; Spina et al., 1993a). In contrast end-diastolic volume decreased in male subjects in studies of both Hanley et al. (1989) and Adams et al. (1987) (Figure 6-4), a finding contrary to results of studies of exclusively male subjects (Crawford et al., 1979; Higginbotham et al., 1986b; Manyari et al., 1981; Poliner et al., 1980; Slutsky et al., 1979).

Therefore, considering all the factors affecting end-diastolic volume, namely, heart rate, central blood volume, and left-ventricular compliance, caution should be observed in any conclusions about gender effects on the Frank-Starling mechanism. Diastolic filling time, which is inversely related to heart rate, is an important determinant of end-diastolic volume, as can be seen during intensive dynamic exercise, when ventricular-filling time is reduced with increasing heart rate.

The influence of diastolic-filling time on end-diastolic volume may be illustrated by the findings of Younis et al. (1990) in young and older subjects. As can be seen from Figure 6-4, maximal exercise increased end-diastolic volume from rest in the older subjects, whereas a 15–25% reduction in end-diastolic volume occurred in young subjects. However, a comparison of maximal heart rates between groups reveals that younger subjects had a mean heart rate 20 beats/min higher than that of older subjects, which could account for a decrease in diastolic filling time at maximal exercise intensity and a fall in maximal end-diastolic volume below the resting value. In addition, because resting heart rate was not standardized in any of the studies, calculated changes in end-diastolic volume from rest could be accounted for by differences in resting diastolic filling time.

Also, a gender-related difference in ventricular compliance or ventricular distensibility, referred to as ventricular diastolic function, could conceivably account for a relatively greater involvement of the Frank-Starling mechanism in the regulation of stroke volume during supine exercise in women. The fact that in women, but not in men, end-diastolic volume increased during exercise in excess of the already enhanced ventricular filling associated with the supine position, may suggest that women benefit from a greater ventricular compliance than do men.

There is little information available on gender-related differences in ventricular diastolic function. In one investigation of gender differences in the left ventricular diastolic function response to isometric handgrip using M-mode echocardiography, postmenopausal women were found to have lower rapid atrial filling fractions than age-matched men, suggesting a lesser, not greater, left ventricular distensibility (Iwasaka et al., 1994). It is not known, however, whether a similar impairment in ventricular distensibility would be observed in younger premenopausal women or in postmenopausal women receiving estrogen replacement therapy.

Finally, gender-related differences in exercise-induced plasma fluid shifts could also contribute to the gender-related difference in end-diastolic volume response to supine exercise. In general, an acute bout of dynamic exercise induces a significant hemoconcentration in both men and women due to an 8–12% plasma fluid shift to the extravascular space (Convertino, 1991). However, plasma volume is also affected by the menstrual cycle. Plasma volume is lower during the luteal phase of the menstrual cycle (Stephenson & Kolka, 1993; Stephenson et al., 1989), more rapid and greater shifts of vascular fluid occur during exercise in the follicular phase,

and greater circulating concentrations of renin, angiotensin, and aldosterone are observed during the luteal phase (Gabelein & Senay 1982; Stephenson & Kolka, 1993). Thus, changes in cardiac output in response to
exercise in women should be interpreted in light of menstrual function,
but in the previously reported investigations of female end-diastolic volume responses to supine exercise, the phase of the menstrual cycle for
each subject was not reported, and neither hydration status nor mineral
balance was determined.

Differences in physical fitness status could also contribute to the
gender-related differences in end-diastolic volume responses to exercise.
Endurance-trained individuals generally exhibit higher resting blood volumes than do untrained subjects, and these greater blood volumes contribute to the higher stroke volumes and greater potential for heat dissipation in trained subjects (Convertino, 1991; Harrison, 1985; Hopper et
al., 1988; Kanstrup et al., 1992).

In summary, because of the incompleteness of the available evidence,
it is premature to conclude that there is a true gender-related difference
in the relative contribution of the Frank-Starling mechanism to the exercise-induced increase in stroke volume.

*Gender-Related Differences In The Relative Contribution Of Ventricular Contrac-
tility.* Similar to observations in men, an increase in ventricular contractility from rest to maximal exercise is generally observed in women. However, irrespective of body posture, changes in ventricular ejection fraction
induced by maximal dynamic exercise appear to be smaller in women than
in men (Figure 6-5) (Adams et al., 1987; Hanley et al., 1989; Higginbotham
et al., 1984; Pfisterer et al., 1985; Younis et al., 1990). There are two exceptions to this observation. Sullivan et al. (1991) reported only a tendency (P = 0.06) for the exercise-induced increase in ejection fraction to
be lower in women than in men, and a gender effect on ventricular ejection fraction was only reported for the group of older women (53 ± 2.5 y)
in the study by Younis et al. (1990). However, in both of these experimental groups, ejection fractions at rest were higher in women than in men,
whereas in all other investigations resting ejection fractions were similar
in male and female subjects. The discrepancies in findings of gender effects on ventricular ejection fraction cannot be ascribed simply to an influence of age because gender-related differences were reported in other
studies of young and middle-aged women compared to men (Adams et al.,
1987; Hanley et al., 1989; Higginbotham et al., 1984). Moreover, a regression analysis showed that gender, but not age, was a significant predictor
of changes in ejection fraction with exercise (Adams et al., 1987). Finally, a
gender effect on ventricular ejection was also reported in response to
isometric exercise. Young men exhibited significant increases in ejection
fraction and fractional shortenings in response to deadlift exercise at 30%

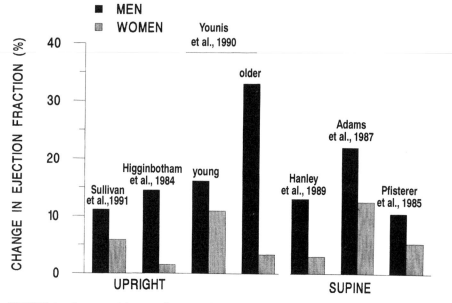

FIGURE 6-5. *Summary of changes in left-ventricular ejection fraction from rest to maximal dynamic exercise reported in studies comparing healthy women and men.*

of maximum voluntary contraction, whereas no such changes were found in young women (Sagiv et al., 1991).

Whether or not this apparent difference in ventricular function reflects an impairment in ventricular myocardial contractile reserve in women remains to be determined. A lesser increase in ventricular ejection fraction could be caused by a greater ventricular afterload in women than in men. Unfortunately, in previous reports there were no direct measurements of peripheral resistance and little information on diastolic blood pressure or other indices of arterial peripheral resistance. Mean arterial blood pressure during maximal exercise is usually similar in men and women, but the maximal exercise occurs at a lower absolute work load and cardiac output in females; whether this reflects a higher peripheral resistance cannot be clearly established.

Results of an investigation of peripheral vascular function in young and older men and women indicate a greater age-related reduction in peripheral vasodilatory capacity in women when compared to men, but not in women treated with estrogen replacement (Martin et al., 1991). Thus, gender-related differences in peripheral resistance during exercise could contribute to the lesser increase in ventricular contractility in postmenopausal women.

In light of the positive relationships between the changes in ejection fraction and peak work loads, differences in peak work loads between men and women could also explain some of the gender effects on ejection fraction (Adams et al., 1987). Another suggestion is that mitral valve prolapse, which might be more prominent in women, could alter the normal left ventricular ejection response to exercise (Hanley et al., 1989); this hypothesis remains controversial.

Gender-Related Differences In Reflex Control Of Circulation

Gender-related differences in reflex control of heart rate and blood pressure have been reported in age-matched normotensive males and females (Abdel-Rahman et al., 1994; Frey et al. 1986, 1988; Montgomery et al., 1977). For example, in children 6–8 y of age, boys exhibited greater increases in systemic vascular resistance and decreases in cardiac index in response to cold application to their foreheads, whereas girls showed a greater increase in heart rate during exercise and a quicker recovery in heart rate after exercise (Treiber et al., 1993). Similarly, in response to a bolus administration of phenylephrine that produced an abrupt rise in blood pressure, women exhibited lesser bradycardia than did men, suggesting lower baroreflex sensitivity in females and a lesser involvement of the cardiac vagal component in the baroreflex-mediated bradycardia (Abdel-Rahman et al., 1994). Results from investigations of cardiopulmonary baroreflex sensitivity using lower body negative pressure indicate an earlier and greater chronotropic response to orthostatic challenges in women than in men, concomitant with a lesser vasoconstrictor response (Frey et al., 1986, 1988; Montgomery et al., 1977). Considering that arterial and cardiopulmonary baroreflexes may be involved in the control of autonomic adjustments to exercise (Ray & Mark, 1993), gender-related differences in baroreflex sensitivity could potentially affect sympathetic nerve activity during exercise and contribute to the explanation of the reported gender-related differences in cardiovascular responses to exercise. Similarly, gender-related differences in the control of vasomotor tone affect blood flow redistribution during exercise. There is to date, however, no report of gender-related differences in the exercise-induced redistribution of cardiac output.

Oxygen Extraction During Exercise

The extent of peripheral oxygen extraction is dependent upon both the arterial oxygen content and the ability of the skeletal muscles to utilize the delivered oxygen. The arterial oxygen content may be somewhat lower in women than in men, providing the hemoglobin concentration is also lower. However, as shown by Cureton et al. (1986) following blood withdrawal from male subjects to equate their average hemoglobin concentration to that of a comparison group of women, the gender difference in hemoglobin accounts for only a small portion of the gender-related difference in absolute $\dot{V}O_2$max.

The lung continuously maintains a narrow range of arterial oxygenation. In most healthy individuals during dynamic exercise the arterial blood pH, PaO_2, and PCO_2 remain nearly constant during rest and exercise (Åstrand and Rodahl, 1986). In healthy individuals the exercise-induced alveolar hyperventilation is generally adequate to allow for maintenance of arterial oxygen content and oxyhemoglobin saturation, but there is increasing evidence that arterial hypoxemia and/or oxyhemoglobin desaturation may occur in response to high-intensity dynamic exercise (Babcock & Dempsey, 1994; Dempsey et al., 1990). Arterial hypoxemia observed through direct measurement of arterial oxygen partial pressure has predominantly been reported in 30–50% of highly trained endurance athletes exercising at very high levels of oxygen consumption (Dempsey et al., 1984). A clear explanation for this phenomenon still remains to be provided, especially on account of the selective nature of its occurrence. Ventilation-perfusion heterogeneity, relative hypoventilation, and diffusion limitations due to a markedly shortened mean pulmonary-capillary transit time or to an impairment in alveolar-capillary membrane diffusion are the most commonly proposed explanations (Dempsey et al., 1990). Because of their smaller body statures, women have lower pulmonary capacities and lower exercise ventilation volumes than do men (McGrath & Thompson, 1959).

There is little information concerning gender-related differences in pulmonary diffusion during exercise. However, in light of their smaller pulmonary capillary volumes, well-trained women who can generate maximal exercise cardiac outputs of considerable magnitude could be more susceptible to pulmonary diffusion limitations due to a marked reduction in pulmonary-capillary transit time. Using ear oximetry to monitor oxygen saturation, we have observed a significant fall in exercise-induced arterial saturation to below 91% in 20–38% of healthy untrained children, adolescents, and young adults during maximal cycling exercise (Gendron et al., 1994). The percentage of occurrence of oxyhemoglobin desaturation among 65 children aged 8–18 y was 17% in boys and 27% in girls. Because the total number of girls tested was slightly lower (29) than that of boys (36), it is perhaps premature to conclude that there is a female predominance of oxyhemoglobin desaturation. There is still insufficient evidence to clearly determine the conditions dictating the occurrence of exercise-induced arterial hypoxemia.

PHYSICAL TRAINABILITY IN FEMALES

In general, men and women shown similar qualitative physiological adaptations to aerobic physical training when training protocols are of similar intensity, duration, and frequency (Cunningham et al., 1979; Drinkwater, 1984; Mitchell et al., 1992). In addition, the influences of habitual physical activity and cardiovascular fitness on coronary artery disease risk factors such as high blood pressure, obesity, and smoking habits appear to be equally valid in female and male middle-aged individuals (Bovens et al., 1993). Both healthy men and women can adapt to endurance training with 15–20% increases in $\dot{V}O_2$max. Thus, improvements in $\dot{V}O_2$max have been reported at several points in the life spans of females, i.e., in young (Bar-Or, 1983; Cunningham et al., 1984), postmenopausal (Morrison et al., 1986; Spina et al., 1993b), and septuagenarian women (Warren et al., 1993). Earlier studies of cardiovascular adaptations to short-term training in women showed no change in arteriovenous oxygen content in women (Cunningham & Hill, 1975; Kilbom, 1971), but more recent studies indicate that the training-induced increases in $\dot{V}O_2$max seen in young women, similar to those in males, result from both central and peripheral adaptations (Cunningham et al., 1979; Spina et al., 1992b). The discrepancy between findings from earlier and more recent studies can probably be explained by differences in the initial fitness states of subjects, training intensity, or measurement techniques.

In young heathy subjects of both genders the increase in $\dot{V}O_2$max induced by endurance exercise training is partly explained by an increase in maximal cardiac output resulting from an increase in stroke volume (Saltin, 1990; Spina et al., 1992b). However, observations from Spina et al. (1993a) suggest an age-related difference in the stroke volume response to endurance training in women. They observed that in 60-y-old women, the entire posttraining 22% increase in $\dot{V}O_2$max was accounted for by a greater arteriovenous oxygen difference, whereas in age-matched men an increase in maximal stoke volume accounted for 66% of the increase in $\dot{V}O_2$max. There are insufficient data to provide a clear explanation for the apparent failure of stroke volume to increase in response to training in older women.

The training-induced increase in stroke volume, at least in young women, could be the result of an increase in ventricular filling consequent to plasma volume expansion (Convertino, 1991; Coyle et al., 1986), increased myocardial contractility (Saltin, 1990; Spina et al., 1992a), reduced ventricular afterload, or a combination of these factors. Similar to findings in male endurance athletes, greater total blood volumes primarily consequent to increased plasma volumes occur in endurance-trained female athletes (Drinkwater, 1984; Stevenson et al., 1994). In young women, endurance training seems to expand plasma volume to the same extent as in men but does not change the extent of exercise-induced hemoconcentration (Akgün et al., 1974; Convertino, 1991; Fortney & Senay, 1979; Maresh et al., 1985).

The absence of a training-induced plasma volume expansion in older women could account for the unchanged stroke volume observed after training in the study by Spina et al. (1993a) because their subjects exhibited no increase in resting end-diastolic left-ventricular diameter. In opposition to this argument is the finding by Morrison et al. (1986) of an increase in resting left-ventricular end-diastolic diameter in postmenopausal women, presumably because of an exercise training-induced plasma volume expansion. Similarly, observations in highly trained female endurance athletes who were 50–70 y old indicate significantly greater total blood volumes than in the age-matched non-athletes (Stevenson et al., 1994), suggesting that the potential for training-induced plasma volume expansion is retained across the life span.

It is also surprising that in the study by Spina et al. (1993a, b) the training-induced bradycardia reported in the older women was not associated with an increase in resting left-ventricular end-diastolic dimension. Using atrial pacing to increase heart rate over a range of 50–150 beats/min, De Maria et al. (1979), established that a 2.7% change in left-ventricular internal diameter could be predicted for every 10-beat change in heart rate. According to this prediction equation and the 9-beat decrease in resting heart rate reported by Spina et al. (1993a), a 1.3 mm increase in resting left-ventricular internal diameter would have been expected following training in these older women.

Failure of end-diastolic dimension to increase despite the increase in ventricular filling time could be related to an age-related decrease in ventricular compliance in women. As discussed previously, a restriction in left-ventricular diastolic function has been observed during isometric exercise in postmenopausal women (Iwasaka et al., 1994) similar in age to those studied by Spina et al. (1993a, b).

Gender-related differences in the ventricular inotropic response to endurance training could also contribute to the absence of a stroke volume adaptation seen in the older women studied by Spina et al. (1993a). Improvements in left ventricular systolic function or decreases in ventricular afterload could contribute to the training-induced increases in maximal stroke volume. An improvement in left-ventricular contractility following endurance training has been reported in response to beta-adrenergic stimulation with isoproterenol in young healthy male and female subjects (Spina et al., 1992a). Similarly, using M-mode echocardiography Morrison et al. (1986) reported a significant increase in resting left-ventricular ejection fraction following an 8-month, walk-jog training program in 50-y-old women, suggesting an improvement in ventricular systolic function with exercise training. It is noteworthy, however, that in the latter study, there were no significant differences in ejection fraction between trained and control subjects either before or after the training period. In the 60-y-old men and women studied by Spina et al. (1993a, b) exercise training increased exercise stroke work in men, but not in women. In men, this increase was not associated with changes in ventricular afterload, suggesting an improvement in myocardial contractility that could contribute to the training-induced increase in exercise stroke volume. The discrepancy in results between the studies of Morrison et al. (1986) and Spina et al. (1993 a, b) may reflect an age-dependent gender-related difference in the ventricular contractile adaptation to training. A similar age-related gender difference was reported for the arterial blood pressure response to submaximal exercise, i.e., systolic and mean arterial blood pressures were lower in physically conditioned subjects than in their sedentary age-and gender-matched counterparts, but not in older women (Martin III et al., 1991). Unfortunately, blood pressure and other cardiovascular effects of chronic endurance training have not been extensively studied in females. Thus, it is premature to speculate about other gender-related differences in these adaptations.

In summary, it seems that both women and men can benefit equally from endurance exercise training in terms of exercise performance.

MEDICAL AND SAFETY CONCERNS

Independent of age-related differences in body stature, the efficiency of the oxygen transport system in premenopausal women is limited by their reduced oxygen transport capacities consequent to lower concentrations of circulating hemoglobin when compared to men. The gender-related difference in hemoglobin concentrations may be compounded by a high incidence of iron deficiency in adolescent girls and women (Economos et al., 1993; Haymes, 1991; Sanborn & Jankowski, 1994). Found in greater prevalence in developing countries, iron deficiency is also common in affluent North American and European societies (Haymes, 1991; Weaver & Rajaram, 1992). In Western societies, the primary cause of iron deficiency in women is inadequate dietary intake of iron. In premenopausal women, recommended daily iron intakes are 13 mg in Canada and 18 mg in the United States (Newhouse & Clement, 1988). Considering that an average Western diet supplies 5–7 mg of iron per 1000 kcal, an adequate iron intake would require energy intakes of at least 2000 kcal. According to the Nutrition Canada Survey of 1973, 76% of women had iron intakes below the recommendation for the general population (Newhouse & Clement, 1988).

Iron Deficiency and Exercise

Bodily iron storage results from a positive balance between absorption of dietary iron and iron losses from sweat, urine, feces, and desquamation of cells. The average daily losses in men are 1.0 mg, whereas adult premenopausal women lose approximately 1.4 mg per day (Weaver & Rajaram, 1992). However, in athletic populations iron losses could be much more significant because of greater sweat losses, increased intravascular hemolysis, and potential gastrointestinal bleeding consequent to regular strenuous endurance training (Newhouse & Clement, 1988; Weight & Noakes, 1994). Accordingly, in the athletic population, subnormal serum concentrations have been reported in 9–82% of American female distance runners and in 8–9% of male middle- and long-distance runners (Weight & Noakes, 1994). However, findings of abnormalities in one of the three designated markers of body iron status, namely, serum ferritin concentration, red-cell protoporphyrin concentration, or percent transferrin saturation, are fairly common in the general American population (Cook et al., 1986). Using requirements of abnormalities in two or more of these indexes for the diagnosis of iron deficiency, it would appear that true iron-deficiency anemia is not as prominent as that predicted on the basis of a single measurement. Nevertheless, the incidence of iron-deficiency anemia in male endurance athletes may be slightly higher than that in the general population. In female endurance athletes, however, this condition does not appear to be more prominent than it is in the general Western population (Weight & Noakes, 1994).

The underlying causes for the iron deficiency in athletes appears to be gender specific. For many female athletes, iron deficiency is the result of low dietary intake of iron consequent to their relatively low total energy consumptions (Haymes, 1987; 1991; Nutter, 1991; Sanborn & Jankowski, 1994; Weight et al., 1992) and the low bioavailability of non-heme iron (Monsen, 1988). In female adolescents, hypoferritinemia was observed in 27% of non-athletic adolescents, in 40% of competitive runners, and in 47% of competitive swimmers; no statistical difference was found for differences in prevalence between athletic and non-athletic adolescents (Rowland et al., 1991). In contrast, whereas iron intake appears adequate in male endurance athletes, a state of relative iron deficiency may result from an increase in iron losses consequent to large sweat losses and intravascular hemolysis (Haymes, 1987; Newhouse & Clement, 1988; Weaver & Rajaram, 1992; Weight at al., 1992).

Iron supplementation may not improve $\dot{V}O_2max$ unless subjects suffer from a true anemia (Eichner, 1992; Fogelholm et al., 1992), but it effectively enhances iron stores in subjects with iron deficiency and/or anemia (Clarkson, 1991; Haymes, 1986, 1987, 1991). In light of the reported poor dietary habits of young active females, a first line of prevention for iron deficiency and iron store depletion might be the recommendation for regular monitoring of iron status and meeting the recommended dietary allowances for iron during exercise training.

DIRECTIONS FOR FUTURE RESEARCH

As we enter into the 21st century most of our ideas concerning the cardiorespiratory responses to exercise in women must be extrapolated from findings in men because these is a serious lack of experimental data on women. As more women choose to challenge the limits of endurance performance or adopt an active lifestyle for health benefits, there will be more opportunities to collect information on the cardiovascular and respiratory responses to exercise throughout the female life span. More specifically, much more information is needed on the cardiac response to exercise in women and how circulating sex hormones may affect the cardiovascular responses to exercise before and after menopause. Gender-related differences in cardiovascular regulatory mechanisms may exist, and we need to understand the causes, physiological significance, and health implications of these possible gender effects.

SUMMARY

The cardiorespiratory responses and adaptations of females to acute and chronic exercises, respectively, appear to be at least qualitatively, if not quantitatively, similar to those of men. Gender-related differences in endurance performance can predominantly be attributed to differences in body size. Somewhat lower oxygen-carrying capacities in some women may also contribute to such differences in performance. Gender-related differences in the regulation of end-diastolic volume have been observed, and a lesser increase of ventricular contractility has been reported in women than in men in response to both upright and supine dynamic exercise and to isometric exercise. There is too little information to firmly establish that women exhibit a gender-specific pattern of cardiovascular regulation during exercise. The available evidence, however, clearly establishes the need to further examine the issue. Gender-related differences in vasomotor and chronotropic responsiveness to orthostatic stress that reflect differences in neuro-hormonal regulation have been reported, but the functional significance of these differences or their implications in an exercise response remain to be determined. Exercise training causes similar cardiorespiratory fitness improvements in men and women, and trainability appears to be retained throughout the life span in both genders.

ACKNOWLEDGEMENTS

Special thanks are expressed to Eileen Leduc and Tammy Hughes for their skillful secretarial assistance.

Abdel-Rahman, A.R.A., R.H. Merrill, and W.R. Wooles (1994). Gender-related differences in the baroreceptor reflex control of heart rate in normotensive humans. *J. Appl. Physiol.* 77:606–613.

Adams, K.F., L.M. Vincen, S.M. McAllister, H. El-Ashmawy, and D.S. Sheps (1987). The influence of age and gender on left ventricular response to supine exercise in asymptomatic normal subjects. *Am. Heart J.* 113:732–742.

Akgün, N., N. Tartaroglu, F. Durusoy, and E. Kocatürk (1974). The relationship between the changes in physical fitness and in total blood volume in subjects having regular and measured training. *J. Sports Med.* 14:73–77.

Åstrand, I. (1960). Aerobic work capacity in men and women with special reference to age. *Acta Physiol. Scand.* 49 (suppl 169):1–92.

Åstrand, I., P-O Åstrand, I. Hallback, and A. Kilbom (1973). Reduction in maximal oxygen uptake with age. *J. Appl. Physiol.* 35:649–654.

Åstrand, P-O., and K. Rodahl (1986). *Textbook of Work Physiology: Physiological Bases of Exercise*, 3rd ed. New York: McGraw-Hill.

Åstrand, P-O., T.E. Cuddy, B. Saltin, and J. Stenberg (1964). Cardiac output during submaximal and maximal work. *J. Appl. Physiol.* 19:268–274.

Babcock, M.A., and J.A. Dempsey (1994). Pulmonary system adaptations: limitations to exercise. In: C. Bouchard, R.J. Shephard, and T. Stephens (eds.) *Physical Activity, Fitness and Health. International Proceedings And Consensus Statement.* Windsor, ON: Human Kinetics, pp. 320–330.

Bar-Or, O. (1983). *Pediatric Sports Medicine For The Practitioner: From Physiologic Principles To Clinical Application.* New York: Springer Verlag.

Bar-O., R.J. Shephard, and C.L. Allen (1971). Cardiac output of 10- to 13-year-old boys and girls during submaximal exercise. *J. Appl. Physiol.* 30:219–223.

Berg, U., B. Sjodin, A. Forsberg, and J. Svedenhag (1991). The relationship between body mass and oxygen uptake during running in humans. *Med. Sci. Sports Exerc.* 23:205–211.

Blimkie, C.J.R., D.A. Cunningham, and P.M. Nichol (1980). Gas transport capacity and echocardiographically determined cardiac size in children. *J. Appl. Physiol.* 49:994–999.

Bovens, A.M., M.A. Van Baak, J.G. Vrencken, J.A. Wijnen, W.H. Saris, and F.T. Verstappen (1993). Physical activity, fitness and selected risk factors for CHD in active men and women. *Med. Sci. Sports Exerc.* 25:572–576.

Bunc, V. and J. Heller (1989). Energy cost of running in similarly trained men and women. *Eur. J. Appl. Physiol.* 59:178–183.

Casone, R., S. Damiani, A. Lino, G. Germano, P. Corretti, S. Dalmaso, P. Chieco, C. Astorita, and V. Carsi (1982). Preliminary research regarding the application of echocardiography in the analysis of left ventricular function under dynamic conditions. *J. Sports Med.* 22:37–44.

Clarkson, P.M. (1991). Minerals: exercise performance and supplementation in athletes. *J. Sports Sci.* 9:91–116.

Conley, D.L., G.S. Krahenbuhl, L.N. Burkett, and A.L. Millar (1981). Physiological correlates of female road racing performance. *Res. Quart. Exerc. Sport* 52:441–448.

Convertino, V.A. (1991). Blood volume: its adaptation to endurance training. *Med. Sci. Sports Exerc.* 23:1338–1348.

Cook, J.D., B.S. Skikne, S.R.I. Lynch and M.E. Reusser (1986). Estimates of iron deficiency in the U.S. population. *Blood* 68:726–731.

Cooper, D.M. (1989). Development of the oxygen transport system in normal children. In: O. Bar-Or (ed). *Advances in Pediatric Sport Sciences, Vol. 3: Biological Issues.* Champaign, IL: Human Kinetics, pp. 67–100.

Costill, D.L., and E. Winrow (1970). Maximal oxygen consumption among marathon runners. *Arch. Phys. Med. Rehab.* 51:317–320.

Coyle, E.F., M.K. Hemmert, and A.R. Coggan (1986). Effects of detraining on cardiovascular responses to exercise: role of blood volume. *J. Appl. Physiol.* 60:95–99.

Crawford, M.H., D.H. White, and K.W. Amon (1979). Echocardiographic evaluation of left ventricular size and performance during handgrip and supine and upright bicycle exercise. *Circulation*, 59:1188–1194.

Cumming, G.R. (1977). Hemodynamics of supine bicycle exercise in "normal" children. *Am. Heart J.* 93:617–622.

Cumming, G.R. (1978). Supine bicycle exercise in pediatric cardiology. In: J. Borms and M. Hebbelinck (eds.) *Pediatric Work Physiology.* Basel: S. Karger, pp. 82–88.

Cunningham, D.A., and J.S. Hill (1975). Effect of training on cardiovascular response to exercise in women. *J. Appl. Physiol.* 39:891–895.

Cunningham, D.A., D. McCrimmon, and L.F. Vlach (1979). Cardiovascular response to interval and continuous training in women. *Eur. J. Appl. Physiol.* 41:187–197.

Cunningham, D.A., D.H. Paterson, and C.J.R. Blimkie (1984). The development of the cardiorespiratory system with growth and physical activity. In: R.A. Boileau (ed). *Advances In Pediatric Sport Sciences*, Vol 1. Champaign, IL: Human Kinetics, pp. 85–116.

Cureton, K.J., and P.B. Sparling (1980). Distance running performance and metabolic responses to running in men and women with excess weight experimentally equated. *Med. Sci. Sports Exerc.* 12:288–294.

Cureton, K., P. Bishop, P. Hutchinson, H. Newland, S. Viskery, and L. Zwiren (1986). Sex difference in maximal oxygen uptake. Effect of equating haemoglobin concentration. *Eur. J. Appl. Physiol.* 54:656–660.

Daniels, J., and N. Daniels (1992). Running economy of elite male and elite female runners. *Med. Sci. Sports Exerc.* 24:483–489.

Davies, C.T.M., and M.W. Thompson (1979). Aerobic performance of female marathon and male ultramarathon athletes. *Eur. J. Appl. Physiol.* 1:233–245.

De Maria, A.N., A. Neumann, P.J. Schubart, G. Lee, and D.T. Mason (1979). Systematic correlation of cardiac chamber size and ventricular performance determined with echocardiography and alterations in heart rate in normal persons. *Am. J. Cardiol.* 43:1–9.

Dempsey, J.A., S.K. Powers, and N. Gledhill (1990). Discussion: Cardiovascular and pulmonary adaptation to physical activity. In: C. Bouchard, R.J. Shephard, T. Stephens, R.J. Sutton, and B.D. McPherson (eds.) *Exercise Fitness and Health. A Consensus Of Current Knowledge*. Windsor, ON: Human Kinetics, pp. 205–214.

Dempsey, J.A., P.G. Hanson, and K.S. Henderson (1984). Exercise-induced hypoxemia in healthy human subjects at sea level. *J. Physiol.* 355:161–175.

Dickhuth, H.H., G. Simon, H.W. Weiss, M. Lehmann, K. Wybitui, and J. Keul (1981). Comparative echocardiographic examinations in sitting and supine position at rest and during exercise. *Int. J. Sports Med.* 1:178–181.

DiPrampero, P.E., C. Capelli, P. Pagliaro, G. Antonutto, M. Girardis, P. Zamparo and R.G. Soule (1993). Energetics of best performances in middle-distance running. *J. Appl. Physiol.* 74:2318–2324.

Drinkwater, B.L., S.M. Horvath, and C.L. Wells (1975). Aerobic power of females, ages 10 to 68. *J. Gerontol.* 30:385–394.

Drinkwater, B.L. (1984). Women and Exercise: Physiological Aspects. In: R.L Terjung (ed.) *Exercise and Sport Sciences Reviews*, Vol. 12. Lexington, MA: Collamore Press, pp. 21–51.

Economos, C.D., S.S. Bortz, and M.E. Nelson (1993). Nutritional practices of elite athletes. Practical recommendations. *Sports Med.* 16:381–399.

Eichner, E.R. (1992). Sports anemia, iron supplements, and blood doping. *Med. Sci. Sports Exerc.* 24:S315–318.

Feigenbaum, H. (1986). *Echocardiography*, 4th ed. Philadelphia: Lea and Febiger.

Fogelholm, M., L. Jaakkola, and T. Lampisjarvi (1992). Effects of iron supplementation in female athletes with low serum ferritin concentration. *Int. J. Sports Med.* 13:158–162.

Folkow, B., and A. Svanborg (1993). Physiology of cardiovascular aging. *Physiol. Rev.* 73:725–764.

Fortney, S.M., and L.C. Senay Jr. (1979). Effect of training and heat acclimation on exercise responses of sedentary females. *J. Appl. Physiol.* 47:978–984.

Freedson, P.S. (1981). The influence of hemoglobin concentration on exercise cardiac output. *Int. J. Sports Med.* 2:81–86.

Freedson, P., V.L. Katch, S. Sady, and A. Weltman (1979). Cardiac output differences in males and females during mild cycle ergometer exercise. *Med. Sci. Sports* 11:16–19.

Frey, M.A.B., K.L. Mathes, and G.W. Hoffler (1986). Cardiovascular responses of women to lower body negative pressure. *Aviat. Space Environ. Med.* 57:531–538.

Frey, M.A.B., K.L. Mathes, and G.W. Hoffler (1987). Aerobic fitness in women and responses to lower body negative pressure. *Aviat. Space Environ. Med.* 58:1149–1152.

Frey, M.A.B., and G.W. Hoffler (1988). Association of sex and age with responses to lower-body negative pressure. *J. Appl. Physiol.* 65:1752–1756.

Gaebelein, C.J. and L.C. Senay, Jr. (1982). Vascular volume dynamics during ergometer exercise at different menstrual phases. *Eur. J. Appl. Physiol* 50:1–11.

Gendron, R., R.A. Turcotte, J.E. Marcotte, and H. Perrault (1994). Prevalence of exercise-induced oxyhemoglobin desaturation and the effect of posture in healthy untrained young subjects. *Can. J. Appl. Physiol.* 19:S17P.

Gledhill, N., D. Cox, and R. Jamnik (1994). Endurance athletes' stroke volume does not plateau: major advantage is diastolic function. *Med. Sci. Sports Exerc.* 26:1116–1121.

Grande, F., and H.L. Taylor (1965). Adaptive changes in the heart, vessels and patterns of control under chronically high loads. In: W.F. Hamilton (ed.) *Circulation*, Volume III. Washington, D.C.: American Physiological Society, pp. 2615–2677.

Graves, J.E., M.L. Pollock, and P.B. Sparling (1987). Body composition of elite female distance runners. *Int. J. Sports Med.* 8:96–102.

Hanley, P.C., A.R. Zinsmeister, I.P. Clements, A.A. Bove, M.L. Brown, and R.J. Gibbons (1989). Gender-related differences in cardiac response to supine exercise assessed by radionuclide angiography. *J. Am. Coll. Cardiol.* 13:624–629.

Harrison, M.H. (1985). Effects of thermal stress and exercise on blood volume in humans. *Physiol. Rev.* 65:149-210.

Haymes, E.M. (1986). Nutrition for the female distance runner. In: B.L. Drinkwater (ed.) *Female Endurance Athletes.* Champaign, IL: Human Kinetics, pp. 81-92.

Haymes, E.M. (1987). Nutritional concerns: need for iron. *Med. Sci. Sports Exerc.* 19:S197-S200.

Haymes, E.M. (1991). Vitamin and mineral supplementation to athletes. *Int. J. Sport Nutr.* 1:146-169.

Heath, G.W., J.M. Hagberg, A.A. Ehsani, and J.O. Holloszy (1981). A physiological comparison of young and older endurance athletes. *J. Appl. Physiol.* 51:634-640.

Helgerud J. (1994). Maximal oxygen uptake, anaerobic threshold and running economy in women and men with similar performances level in marathons. *Eur. J. Appl. Physiol.* 68:155-161.

Helgerud J., F. Ingjer, and S.B. Stromme (1990). Sex differences in performance-matched marathon runners. *Eur. J. Appl. Physiol.* 61:433-439.

Higginbotham, M.B., K.G. Morris, E. Coleman, and F.R. Cobb (1984). Sex-related differences in the normal cardiac response to upright exercise. *Circulation* 70:357-366.

Higginbotham, M.B., K.G. Morris, R.S. Williams, P.A. McHale, R.E. Coleman, and F.R. Cobb (1986a). Regulation of stroke volume during submaximal and maximal upright exercise in normal man. *Circ. Res.* 58:281-291.

Higginbotham, M.B., K.G. Morris, R.S. Williams, R.E. Coleman, and F.R. Cobb (1986b). Physiologic basis for the age-related decline in aerobic work capacity. *Am. J. Cardiol.* 57:1374-1379.

Hopper, M.K., A.R. Coggan, and E.F. Coyle (1988). Exercise stroke volume relative to plasma-volume expansion. *J. Appl. Physiol.*64:414-408.

Hult, J.S. (1986). The female American runner: modern quest for visibility. In: B.L. Drinkwater (ed.) *Female Endurance Athletes.* Champaign, IL: Human Kinetics, pp. 2-30.

Iwasaka, T., K. Tamura, T. Tamura, K. Takahan, Y. Morita, T. Izuoka, T. Sugiura, N. Taruni, and M. Inada (1994). Effect of gender of the left ventricular diastolic performance during isometric handgrip exercise in normal individuals. *Cardiology* 84:255-260.

Joyner, M.J. (1994). Physiological limiting factors and distance running: influence of gender and age on record performances. In: J.O. Holloszy (ed.) *Exercise and Sport Sciences Reviews,* Vol. 21. Baltimore: Williams & Wilkins, pp. 103-135.

Kanstrup, I.L., J. Marving, and P.F. Holilund-Carlsen (1992). Acute plasma expansion: left ventricular hemodynamics and endocrine function during exercise. *J. Appl. Physiol* 73:1791-1796.

Kasch, F.W., and J.P. Wallace (1976). Physiological variables during 10 years of endurance exercise. *Med. Sci. Sports Exerc.* 8:5-8.

Kilbom, A. (1971). Physical training in women. *Scand. J. Clin. Lab. Invest.* 119 (Suppl.):1-34.

Kuscik, N. (1977). The history of women's participation in the marathon. *Ann. New York Acad. Sci.* 301:862-877.

Lacour J.R., S. Padilla-Magunacelaya, J.C. Barthélémy, and D. Dormois (1990). The energetics of middle distance running. *Eur. J. Appl. Physiol.* 60:38-43.

Mahler, D.A., R.A. Matthay, P.E. Snyder, L. Pytlik, B.L. Zret, and J. Loke (1985). Volumetric responses of right and left ventricles during upright exercise in normal subjects. *J. Appl. Physiol.* 58:1818-1822.

Malina, R.M., and C. Bouchard (1991). Aerobic power and capacity during growth. In: R.M. Malina and C. Bouchard, *Growth, Maturation and Physical Activity.* Champaign, IL: Human Kinetics, pp. 205-217.

Manyari, D.E., L.J. Melendez, A.A. Driedger, T.D. Cradduck, A.C. Macdonald, and W.J. Kostuk (1981). Left ventricular function and volume during supine exercise in subjects with coronary artery disease. *J. Appl. Physiol.* 50:636-642.

Maresh, C.M., B.C. Wang, and K.L. Goetz (1985). Plasma vasopressin, renin activity, and aldesterone responses to maximal exercise in active college females. *Eur. J. Appl. Physiol* 54:398-403.

Martin, W.H., III, T. Ogawa, W.M. Kohrt, M.T. Malley, E. Korte, P.S. Kieffer, and K.B. Schechtman (1991). Effects of aging, gender and physical training on peripheral vascular function. *Circulation* 84:654-664.

Matthews, P. (ed.) (1994). *The New Guinness Book of Records 1995.* Barcelona: Guinness Publishing, pp. 225-227; 292-294 .

McGrath, M.W., and M.L. Thomson (1959). The effect of age, body size and lung volume change on alveolar-capillary permeability and diffusing capacity in man. *J. Physiol.* 16:572-582.

Mitchell, J.H., C. Tate, P. Raven, F. Cobb, W. Kraus, R. Moreadith, M. O'Toole, B. Saltin, and N. Wenger (1992). Acute response and chronic acatation to exercise in women. *Med. Sci. Sports Exerc.* 24:S258-265.

Monsen, E.R. (1988). Iron nutrition and absorption: dietary factors which impact iron bioavailability. *J. Am. Diet. Assoc.* 88:786-790.

Montgomery, L.D., P.J. Kirk, P.A. Payne, R.L. Gerber, S.D. Newton, and B.A. Williams (1977). Cardiovascular responses of men and women to lower body negative pressure. *Aviat. Space Environ. Med.* 48:138-145.

Morrison, D.A., T.W. Boyden, R.W. Pamenter, B.J. Freund, W.A. Stini, R. Harrington, and J.H. Wilmore (1986). Effects of aerobic training on exercise tolerance and echocardiographic dimensions in untrained postmenopausal women. *Am. Heart J.* 112:561-567.

Newhouse, I.J., and D.B. Clement (1988). Iron status in athletes. An update. *Sports Med.* 5:337-352.

Noakes, T. (1986). *Lore of Running.* Cape Town: Oxford University Press.

Nutter J. (1991). Seasonal changes in female athletes' diets. *Int. J. Sport Nutr.* 1:395–407.

Padilla, S., M. Bourdin, J.C. Barthélémy and J.R. Lacour (1992). Physiological correlates of middle-distance running performance: A comparative study between men and women. *Eur. J. Appl. Physiol.* 65:561–566.

Pate, R.R., P.B. Sparling, G.E. Wilson, K.J Cureton, and B.J. Miller (1987). Cardiorespiratory and metabolic responses to submaximal and maximal exercise in elite women distance runners. *Int. J. Sports Med.* 8:S91–S95.

Paterson, D.H. (1992). Effects of aging on the cardiorespiratory system. *Can. J. Sport Sci.* 17:171–177.

Péronnet, F. (1993). Les records du monde de course à pied masculins et féminins: à propos d'un article de la revue Nature. *Rev. Sci. Tech. Activ. Phys. Sport.* 32:47–55.

Péronnet, F., and G. Thibault (1989). Mathematical analysis of running performance and world running records. *J. Appl. Physiol.* 67:453–465.

Péronnet, F., and H. Perrault (1985). Volumes ventriculaires à l'exercice dynamique en position debout et couchée: roles du mécanisme de Frank-Starling et de la contractilité du myocarde dans l'ajustement du volume d'éjection systolique: mise au point. *Med. Sport* 59:254–260.

Pfisterer, M.E., A. Battler, and B.L. Zaret (1985). Range of normal values for left and right ventricular ejection fraction at rest and during exercise assessed by radionuclide angiocardiography. *Eur. Heart J.* 6:647–655.

Plotnick, G.D., L.C. Becker, M.L. Fisher, G. Gerstenblith, D.G. Renlund, J.L. Fleg, M.L. Weisfeldt, and E.G. Lakatta (1986). Use of the Frank-Starling mechanism during submaximal versus maximal upright exercise. *Am. J. Physiol.* 251:H1101–H1105.

Plowman, S.A., B.L. Drinkwater, and S.M. Horvath (1979). Age and aerobic power in women: A longitudinal study. *J. Gerontol.* 34:512–520.

Poliner, L.R., G.J. Dehmer, S.E. Lewis, R.W. Parkey, C.G. Blomqvist, and J.T. Willerson (1980). Left ventricular performance in normal subjects: A comparison of the responses to exercise in the upright and supine positions. *Circulation* 61:528–534.

Pollack, S.J., S.T. McMillan, E. Mumpower, R. Wharff, W. Knopf, J.M. Felner, and A.P. Yoganathan (1987). Echocardiographic analysis of elite women distance runners. *Int. J. Sports Med.* 8:81–83.

Pollock, M.L. (1977). Submaximal and maximal working capacity of elite distance runners. Part 1: Cardiorespiratory aspects. *Ann. New York Acad. Sci.* 301:310–322.

Pollock, M.L., H.S. Miller, and J. Wilmore (1974). Physiological characteristics of champion American track athletes 40 to 75 years of age. *J. Gerontol.* 29:645–649.

Raine, C.A. (1978). An examination of men and women's Olympic performance since 1960. *Athl. Coach* 12:26–28.

Ramsbottom R., C. Williams, L. Boobis, and W. Freeman (1989). Aerobic fitness and running performance of male and female recreational runners. *J. Sports Sci.* 7:9–20.

Ray, C.A., and A.L. Mark (1993). Sympathetic adjustments to exercise: Insights from micromeurographic recordings. In: R. Hainsworth and A.L. Mark (eds.) *Cardiovascular Reflex Control In Health and Disease.* London: W.B. Saunders, pp. 137–164.

Rerych, S.K., P.M. Scholz, D.C. Sabiston, and R.H. Jones (1980). Effects of exercise training on left ventricular function in normal subjects: A longitudinal study by radionuclide angiography. *Am. J. Cardiol.* 45:244–252.

Riley-Hagan, M.R., R.M. Peshock, J. Stray-Gunderson, J. Katz, R.W. Ryschon, and J.H. Mitchell (1992). Left ventricular dimensions and mass using magnetic resonance imaging in female endurance athletes. *Am. J. Cardiol.* 69:1067–1074.

Rogers, M.A., J.M. Hagberg, W.H. Martin III, A.A. Ehsani, and J.O. Holloszy (1990). Decline in $\dot{V}O_2$max with aging in master athletes and sedentary men. *J. Appl. Physiol.* 68:2195–2199.

Rowland, T.W., I. Staff, and J.F. Kelleher (1991). Iron deficiency in adolescent girls. Are athletes at increased risk? *J. Adolescent Health* 12:22–25.

Sagiv, M., M.N. Fisher, E.Z. Fisman, and J.J. Kellermann (1991). Comparison of hemodynamic and left ventricular responses to increased after-load in healthy males and females. *Int. J. Sports Med.* 12:41–45.

Saltin, B. (1990). Cardiovascular and pulmonary adaptation to physical activity. In: C. Bouchard, R.J. Shephard, T. Stephens R.J. Sutton, B.D. McPherson (eds.) *Exercise Fitness and Health. A Consensus Of Current Knowledge.* Windsor: Human Kinetics, pp. 187–204.

Sanborn, C.F., and C.M. Jankowski (1994). Physiologic considerations for women in sport. *Clin. Sports Med.* 13:315–327.

Shvartz, E., and R.C. Reibold (1990). Aerobic fitness norms for males and females aged 6 to 75 years: A review. *Aviat. Space Environ. Med.* 61:3–11.

Slutsky, R., J. Karliner, D. Ricci, G. Schuler, M. Pfisterer, K. Peterson, and W. Ashburn (1979). Response of left ventricular volume to exercise in man assessed by radionuclide equilibrium angiography. *Circulation* 60:3:565–571.

Smith, H.L. (1928). The relation of the weight of the heart to the weight of the body and of the heart to age. *Am. Heart J.* 4:79–93.

Sparling, P.B. (1980). A meta-analysis of studies comparing maximal oxygen uptake in men and women. *Res. Quart. Exerc. Sport* 51:542–552.

Sparling, P.B., and K.J. Cureton (1983). Biological determinants of the sex difference in 12-min run performance. *Med. Sci. Sports Exerc.* 15:218-223.

Sparling, P.B., G.E. Wilson, and R.R. Pate (1987). Project overview and description of performance, training, and physical characteristics in elite women distance runners. *Int. J. Sports Med.* 8(Suppl. 2):73-76.

Spina, R.J., T. Ogawa, A.R. Coggan, J.O. Holloszy, and A.A. Ehsani (1992a). Exercise training improves left ventricular contractile response to B-adrenergic agonist. *J. Appl. Physiol* 72:307-311.

Spina, R.J., T. Ogawa, W.M. Kohrt, W.H. Martin, J.O. Holloszy, and A.A. Ehsani (1993a). Differences in cardiovascular adaptations to endurance exercise training between older men and women. *J. Appl. Physiol.* 75:849-855.

Spina, R.J., T. Ogawa, W.H. Martin, A.R. Coggan, J.O. Holloszy, and A.A. Ehsani (1992b). Exercise training prevents decline in stroke volume during exercise in young healthy subjects. *J. Appl. Physiol.* 72:2458-2462.

Spina, R.J., T. Ogawa, T.R. Miller, W.M. Kohrt, and A.A. Ehsani (1993b). Effect of exercise training on left ventricular performance in older women free of cardiopulmonary disease. *Am. J. Cardiol.* 71:99- 104.

Stamford, B.A. (1988). Exercise in the elderly. In: K.B. Pandolf (ed.) *Exercise and Sport Sciences Reviews*, Vol. 16. New York: Macmillan, pp. 341-379.

Stein, R.A., D. Michielli, E.L. Fox, and M. Krasnow (1978). Continuous ventricular dimensions in man during supine exercise and recovery: an echocardiographic study. *Am. J. Cardiol.* 41:655-661.

Stephenson, L.A., M.A. Kolka, R. Francesconi, R.R. Gonzalez (1989). Circadian variations in plasma renin activity, catecholamines and aldosterone during exercise in women. *Eur. J. Appl. Physiol.* 58:756-764.

Stephenson, L.A., and M.A. Kolka (1993). Thermoregulation in women. In: J.O. Hollosy (ed.) *Exercise and Sport Sciences Reviews*, Vol. 21. Baltimore, MD: Williams & Wilkins, pp. 231-262.

Stevenson E.T., K.P. Davy, and D.R. Seals (1994). Maximal aerobic capacity and total blood volume in higly trained middle-aged and older female endurance athletes. *J. Appl. Physiol.* 77:1691-1696.

Sullivan, M.J., F.R. Cobb, and M.B. Higginbotham (1991). Stroke volume increases by similar mechanisms during upright exercise in normal men and women. *Am. J. Cardiol.* 67:1405-1412.

Thadani, U., and J.O. Parker (1978). Hemodynamics at rest and during supine and sitting bicycle exercise in normal subjects. *Am. J. Cardiol.* 41:52-59.

Treiber, F.A., H. Davis, L. Musante, R.A. Raunikar, W.B. Strong, F. McCaffrey, M.C. Meeks, and R. Vandernoord (1993). Ethnicity, gender, family history of myocardial infarction and hemodynamic responses to laboratory stressors in children. *Health Psychol.* 12:6-15.

Upton, M.T., S.K. Rerych, J.R. Rochack, G.E. Newman, J.M. Douglas, A.G. Wallace, and R.M. Jones (1980). Effects of brief and prolonged exercise on left ventricular function. *Am. J. Cardiol.* 45:1154-1160.

Warren, G.L., and K.J. Cureton (1989). Modeling the effect of alterations in hemoglobin concentration on VO_2max. *Med. Sci. Sports Exerc.* 21:526-531.

Warren, B.J., D.C. Nieman, R.G. Dotson, C.H. Adkins, K.A. O'Donnell, B.L. Haddock, and D.E. Butterworth (1993). Cardiorespiratory responses to exercise training in septuagenarian women. *Int. J. Sports Med.* 14:60-65.

Weaver, C.M., and S. Rajaram (1992). Exercise and iron status. *J. Nutr.* 122(3 suppl.):782-787.

Weight, L.M., P. Jacobs, and T.D. Noakes (1992). Dietary iron deficiency and sports anemia. *Br. J. Nutr.* 68:253-260.

Weight, L.M. and T.R. Noakes (1994). Physical activity and iron metabolism. In: C. Bouchard, R. J. Shephard, and T. Stephens (eds.) *Physical Activity, Fitness and Health. International Proceeding And Consensus Statement.* Windsor, ON: Human Kinetics, pp. 456-470.

Weiss, J.L., M.L. Weisfeldt, S.J. Mason, J.B. Garrison, S.V. Livengood, and N.J. Fortuin (1979). Evidence of Frank-Starling effect in man during severe semisupine exercise. *Circulation* 59:655-663.

Wells, C.L., M.A. Boorman, and D.M. Riggs (1992). Effect of age and menopausal status on cardiorespiratory fitness in masters women runners. *Med. Sci. Sports Exerc.* 24:1147-1154.

Wells, C.L. (1991). Performance differences. In: C.L. Wells, *Women, Sport and Performance. A Physiological Perspective.* Champaign, IL: Human Kinetics.

Wells, C.L., L.H. Hecht, and G.S. Krahenbuhl (1981). Physical characteristics and oxygen utilization of male and female marathon runners. *Res Quart. Exerc. Sport* 52:281-285.

Whipp, B.J., and S.A. Ward (1992). Will women soon outrun men? *Nature* 355:25.

Wirth, A., E. Trager, K. Scheele, D. Mayer, K. Diehm, K. Reischle, and H. Weicker (1978). Cardiopulmonary adjustment and metabolic response to maximal and submaximal physical exercise of boys and girls at different stages of maturity. *Eur. J. Appl. Physiol.* 39:229-240.

Younis, L.T., J.A. Melin, A.R. Robert, and M.R. Detry (1990). Influence of age and sex on left ventricular volumes and ejection fraction during upright exercise in normal subjects. *Eur. Heart J.* 11:916-924.

DISCUSSION

BLIMKIE: Is there any information on how morphological changes in cardiac muscle that occur over the life span might influence the gender-related differences in cardiac function that you have highlighted?

PERRAULT: Myocardial hypertrophy may occur somewhat earlier in women than it does in men. This is also compatible with the observation that after menopause the rate of increase in diastolic blood pressure is higher in females than in men. I am not familiar with how ultrastructural changes might affect these phenomena.

BLIMKIE: Are there differences between genders in the specific tension of cardiac muscle tissue?

PERRAULT: I don't know.

DI PIETRO: I have some concern about the degree of adaptability with training in older women relative to younger or middle-aged women, especially when considering the possibility of selective survival in a healthy study population. Do you think it may take more of a training stimulus to cause adaptations in healthy older women than in younger women?

PERRAULT: I am not certain, but I suspect that the degree of training required to achieve an effect may not be the same across the life span.

WILMORE: In the work of Spina's group the magnitude of the change in $\dot{V}O_2$max cannot be totally explained on the basis of a change in a-v O_2 difference, so maximal cardiac output must be increasing. Also, recent data from Constance Mier might shed some light on the issue of potential gender differences in stroke volume during exercise. She conducted a unique study of groups of untrained and highly trained men and women and used beta-blockades to increase diastolic filling time and short-term training using high-intensity cycling exercise to expand plasma volume. In these individuals, who were between 20 and 35 y of age, the men and women essentially responded identically to these perturbations.

SPRIET: I have a concern about whether or not gender-related differences in endurance performance can predominantly be attributed to differences in body composition. First, you emphasized the study by Cureton that tried to match the hemoglobin concentrations in men and women. However, Bob Robertson's group blood-doped females and noted only small changes in $\dot{V}O_2$max and endurance performance. This is consistent with oxygen transport being the most important factor responsible for the gender performance changes.

Second, the body composition differences between the male and female athletes who are setting world records are much smaller than gender differences in body composition among the average population, and this again argues that body composition differences between genders probably are not crucial to the performance differences. I believe that oxygen transport is the most important factor.

PERRAULT: I think there is a series of factors determining $\dot{V}O_2$max that is probably the same for both genders. You are correct that there are only small differences in body composition between champion men and women distance runners. I would not go so far as to say that the oxygen-carrying capacity is the only determining factor; both it and body composition probably make contributions to performance differences between genders.

COYLE: There are two different ways to reduce hemoglobin concentration. One is to withdraw blood, and in the process blood volume will be reduced, although there will be some restoration of plasma volume. Another way to lower hemoglobin concentration is to increase plasma volume. Those are two very different approaches, but you seem to imply that both increase cardiac output largely by raising stroke volume. This seems strange. From the data of Cureton, you suggested that it was an increase in stroke volume that played a part in an increase in cardiac output. Furthermore, you cite work by Patty Freedson showing that blood withdrawal in men also increases their stroke volume, which is surprising. Perhaps Patty would comment on that.

FREEDSON: We withdrew blood from men and evaluated their cardiovascular responses to exercise with about a 10% decrease in hemoglobin concentration consequent to blood withdrawal. This condition was contrasted to the cardiovascular responses before the blood withdrawal, which represented our baseline. We observed an increase in cardiac output during submaximal exercise, as measured by CO_2 rebreathing. With this technique, stroke volume is not directly measured but rather is calculated from heart rate and cardiac output. We did observe an increase in stroke volume that explained the increased cardiac output under the blood withdrawal condition.

KANTER: Are there anatomical differences in the way that the hearts of men and women adapt to exercise? My assumption is that with aerobic training there would occur a volume-overload type of cardiac hypertrophy in the heart, whereas strength training would produce more of a pressure-overload type of hypertrophy. Do you see such changes in both males and females?

PERRAULT: The average changes in left-ventricular wall thickness before and after training are only about 0.4 mm, which is less than the resolution of the echocardiographic technique. Thus, I would not use the term "left-ventricular hypertrophy." As for the increased left-ventricular end-diastolic dimension that is found, it can probably be accounted for partly by dilation rather then eccentric hypertrophy. I think the adaptations in males and females to endurance training are the same.

BLIMKIE: Does the same correlation exist between end-diastolic volume and heart size in females and males? It seems to me that there is still a big difference in heart size between the two genders that may not be accounted for if there is a difference in the correlation between end-diastolic volume and heart size.

PERRAULT: I don't know about this correlation in a large population of females, but the clinical norms for heart size are the same for both men and women. The values are corrected for body surface area, but there does not appear to be the need for gender-specific norms.

7

Thermoregulation In Females From A Life Span Perspective

ODED BAR-OR, M.D.

INTRODUCTION

When climatic heat or cold stresses are added to exercise, the resulting physiological and perceptual strain is greater than that induced by exercise alone. Most of the literature on thermoregulation—during both rest and exercise—has focused on males. However, as early as the 1940s (Hardy & Dubois, 1940), studies have addressed gender-related differences in thermoregulation. A growing body of knowledge has been emerging since the 1970s regarding the responses of females to hot and, to a lesser degree, cold climates.

Evaluating the thermoregulatory response of females across the life span can be done by comparing the responses of females and males in discrete age groups or by assessing age-related differences among females. Most studies in the field have used a design that compares the thermoregulatory responses of females and males, so this chapter will focus on gender-related differences. However, in keeping with the "life span" theme of this volume, an attempt will be made to review the evidence that growth, maturation, age, and aging may modify the thermoregulatory characteristics of females. The discussion in most sections will therefore be divided into **gender-related differences** and **age-related patterns.**

Several factors, other than gender and age *per se*, affect the responses of females to the combined stresses of exercise and climate. These pose methodological constraints in comparing thermoregulation by gender or across age groups. The main challenge is equating the metabolic heat stress. Females on average have a lower maximal aerobic power than males. A scientist's dilemma is therefore whether to administer an exercise task that is equal in absolute intensity—thus having the females exercise at a higher relative intensity—or to equate the task as a percentage of maximal oxygen uptake ($\dot{V}O_2max$) or as $\dot{V}O_2/kg$ body mass. Using the latter two approaches, the females will be working at a lower absolute intensity. One approach to reconciling this dilemma is to select gender groups that are matched for body mass and maximal aerobic power. With such groups, both the relative and absolute intensities can then be equated. The drawback of this approach is that adult females whose $\dot{V}O_2max$ values are similar to those of males are often highly physically active; they do not represent the general female population. A similar dilemma emerges in comparing young and old adults because the latter have a lower $\dot{V}O_2$max on average.

Metabolic heat production is a function of body mass, whereas the rate of heat exchange with the environment through radiation, convection, conduction, and evaporation is a function of the surface area of the skin. A large surface area-to-mass ratio enhances heat dissipation when ambient temperature is cooler than the skin, and heat flows into the body when the ambient temperature exceeds skin temperature. The smaller the individual, the higher is the surface area-to-mass ratio. Thus, another challenge is to equate the metabolic load when subjects differ markedly in their body masses and surface area-to-mass ratios, as is the case with children, adolescents, and adults. Furthermore, females as a group have a higher percent body fat than do males; this adversely affects their thermoregulatory responses to heat but is an advantage during exposure to the cold. Finally, it is not always possible to select groups of subjects that are identically acclimatized to the heat or to the cold. For example, it is conceivable, but not proven, that elderly people, as a group, are less acclimatized than children or younger adults because the elderly are less exposed to outdoor climates.

This chapter will emphasize the combined stresses of climate and exercise. However, data related to resting conditions will also be mentioned because they constitute a major portion of the literature on thermoregulation in females.

Previous reviews on the thermoregulatory characteristics of females include those written by Burse (1979), Drinkwater & Horvath (1979), Haymes (1984), Kawahata (1960), Kenney (1985), Nunneley (1978), and Stephenson & Kolka (1988a). With the exception of studies by Drinkwater & Horvath (1979) and by Gonzalez et al. (1980) there has been little effort to address the life span from childhood to old age. This chapter represents an attempt to do this.

MORPHOLOGICAL AND PHYSIOLOGICAL FACTORS THAT AFFECT THERMOREGULATION IN FEMALES

Women have several morphological and physiological factors that affect their thermoregulatory effectiveness and heat tolerance. These factors include a large surface area-to-mass ratio, relatively great adiposity, low maximal aerobic power, the menstrual cycle, pregnancy, and menopause.

Larger Surface Area-to-Mass Ratio

Starting at puberty, and throughout old age, females as a group have a smaller body stature and body mass than males. One implication is that females have a larger ratio of skin-surface area to body mass. Thus, for any given temperature gradient between the skin and the environment, females have a faster heat exchange with the environment through convection, conduction, and radiation. The surface area-to-mass ratio also affects the rate of evaporative heat loss, but the latter is mostly determined by sweating rate, ambient water-vapor pressure, and wind velocity.

Greater Adiposity

Adolescent and adult females, as a group, have a higher percent body fat than do males. One implication of a higher adiposity is that adipose tissue has a low heat content relative to other body tissues (for details, see Bar-Or et al., 1969) and therefore requires less heat energy to raise its temperature by a given amount. Another implication, evident in marked obesity, is a greater mechanical and metabolic cost for any given physical activity, particularly if the activity is weight-dependent. Indeed, body fatness of females plays a considerable role in thermoregulatory effectiveness and heat tolerance. When walking at 4.8 km/h, lean young women (less than 18% body fat) on average worked at a lower % $\dot{V}O_2$max, had a lower heart rate and rectal temperature, and had a greater exercise tolerance time at high ambient temperatures than did their obese (31.5% fat) counterparts (Bar-Or et al., 1969).

Although the high insulative quality of body fat, particularly subcutaneous fat, can be detrimental to temperature regulation during exercise in the heat, fat plays a beneficial role during exposure to the cold. Subcutaneous skinfold thickness is probably the single most important factor that determines the rate of heat loss in a cold environment. In summary, the greater adiposity of females makes them less effective thermoregulators during exposure to heat stress and more effective thermoregulators during cold exposure.

Lower Maximal Aerobic Power

As a group, females have a lower maximal aerobic power ($\dot{V}O_2$max/kg body mass) than do males. Because T_{core} and cardiovascular strain during exercise in the heat are functions of the relative intensity of the exercise, i.e., % $\dot{V}O_2$max, a low $\dot{V}O_2$max implies a greater heat strain at any given absolute exercise task. Thus, females *a priori* are at a disadvantage during heat exposure. The role of maximal aerobic power during exposure to the cold is less obvious.

Menstrual Cycle

Core temperature at rest in a thermoneutral environment is higher by 0.3–0.6°C during the luteal phase of a woman's menstrual cycle, compared with the follicular phase (Hessemer & Bruck, 1985; Kleitman & Ramsaroop, 1948). This increase coincides with the surge in plasma progesterone during the luteal phase. A similar shift of core temperature according to the menstrual phase occurs during exercise in a hot environment (Figure 7-1) (Carpenter & Nunneley, 1988) or in a thermoneutral environment (Pivarnik et al., 1992). Heart rate and rating of perceived exertion are also higher during prolonged exercise during the luteal phase (Pivarnik et al., 1992); the decline of plasma volume during passive heating, but not during exercise, is also greater during the luteal phase (Stephenson & Kolka, 1988b).

The higher T_{core} during the luteal phase cannot be explained by a greater metabolic heat production (Frascarolo et al., 1990), but there seems to be a reduction in thermal conductance of the skin and in the calculated SkBF (Bittel & Henane, 1975; Frascarolo et al., 1990).

It has been suggested that during the luteal phase there is an elevation of the thermoregulatory set point, as evidenced by higher temperature thresholds for the onset of sweating (Bittel & Henane, 1975; Haslag & Hertzman, 1965; Hessemer & Bruck, 1985; Kolka & Stephenson, 1989; Stephenson & Kolka, 1985), for cutaneous vasodilatation (Hessemer & Bruck, 1985; Hirata et al., 1985; Stephenson & Kolka, 1985), and for the onset of shivering-induced heat production (Hessemer & Bruck, 1985). In addition, there may be an upward shift in the T_{core} that is perceived to be unpleasant (Cunningham & Cabanac, 1971) and an upward shift in the local skin temperature perceived as "cool" (Kenshalo, 1966).

The magnitude of increase in the thresholds for the above physiological variables is 0.3-0.5°C (Figure 7-2). In contrast, there is little or no in-

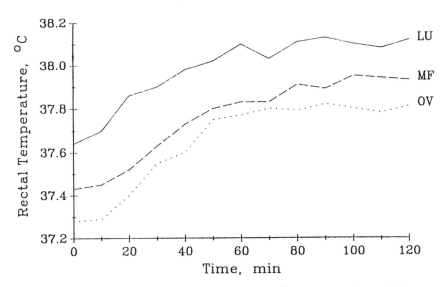

FIGURE 7-1. *Rectal temperature during exercise for 2 h at 30% $\dot{V}O_2max$ in a 48°C, 15% RH environment at three phases of the menstrual cycle: menstrual flow (MF), ovulation (OV), and mid-luteal phase (LU).* Values shown are means for seven, partially heat-acclimatized women aged 27.3 ± 7.1 y. Reproduced with permission from Carpenter & Nunneley (1988).

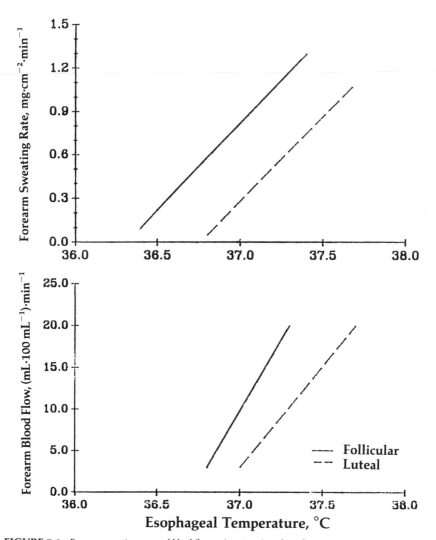

FIGURE 7-2. *Forearm sweating rate and blood flow as function of esophageal temperature in a woman exercising at 60% V̇O$_2$ peak in an environment characterized by a dry bulb temperature of 35°C and a water vapor pressure of 1.73 kPa, during the follicular and luteal phases of the menstrual cycle.* Measurement was made at 4:00 A.M. Adapted with permission from Stephenson & Kolka (1985).

crease during the luteal phase in the sensitivity of the sweating response (Bittel & Henane, 1975; Haslag & Hertzman, 1965; Stephenson & Kolka, 1985) or in the sensitivity of the peripheral vasodilatation response (Hirata et al., 1985; Stephenson & Kolka, 1985). Some data (Avellini et al., 1980) suggest that the higher core temperature during the luteal phase is limited to preacclimated women and does not appear following heat acclimation.

There is no clear understanding of the mechanism for the shift in set point associated with the menstrual cycle. Stephenson & Kolka (1988a) suggested that it might be triggered by a high progesterone activity or by a high interleukin-1 activity (Cannon & Dinarello, 1985). In contrast, Frascarolo e+ ꝫl. (1990) found no correlation between plasma progesterone concentration and either the higher T_{core} or the lower thermal conductance in the luteal phase. A possible effect of estrogen replacement therapy was explored by Tankersley et al. (1992), but the authors could not reach any conclusion regarding the role of estrogen in thermoregulation during the menstrual cycle.

In spite of the elevation of the thermal sudomotor and vasomotor thresholds during the luteal phase, there is no consistent evidence that the exercise-induced changes in T_{core}, sweating rate, or metabolic heat production are modified by the phase of the menstrual cycle, or that the heat tolerance of women who exercise in a hot environment is reduced in the luteal phase (Avellini et al., 1980; Bittel & Henane, 1975; Carpenter & Nunneley, 1988; Frye & Kamon, 1981; 1983; Senay, 1973; Wells & Horvath, 1974). Furthermore, the menstrual cycle does not appreciably affect substrate utilization (and hence metabolic heat production) during exercise (Bonen et al., 1983; Nicklas et al., 1989).

The only study that assessed the thermoregulatory responses of women to exercise in extreme cold (intermittent bouts of 45% $\dot{V}O_2$max at −5°C, for 3 h) found no effect of the menstrual cycle on core or skin temperatures (Graham, 1983).

The practical thermoregulatory effects of the menstrual cycle are therefore minimal, both during heat and cold stresses. Still, studies of women's thermoregulatory responses should attempt to control for the phase of the cycle. For further details on the effects of the menstrual cycle on thermoregulation see Stephenson & Kolka (1988a).

Pregnancy

The following is a brief summary of the factors that may affect thermoregulation during pregnancy and the major findings regarding thermoregulatory efficiency of the pregnant woman in hot and cold environments. For a detailed review of this topic see McMurray & Katz (1990). See also the final chapter in this volume (Clapp, 1996).

Pregnancy is accompanied by several morphological and physiological changes that may affect thermoregulation. For example, the decrease in surface-to-mass ratio reduces the rate of heat exchange with the environment, and the increase in body fat content decreases the average specific heat of the body. In addition, an increase in the women's basal metabolic rate and the growth of the fetus will both increase the overall metabolic heat that has to be dissipated by the pregnant woman.

The main concern is the safety of the fetus. Studies with several animals species have shown that hyperthermia, particularly during the first trimester of gestation, may induce teratogenic changes in the fetus. Retrospective studies in women suggest a greater prevalence of hyperthermia during pregnancy among those who gave birth to babies with congenital defects than among those giving birth to healthy children (McMurray & Katz, 1990). Hence the common medical recommendation that pregnant women reduce their exercise intensity and duration when exposed to ambient heat or when they are hypohydrated. It is generally believed that, particularly during the first trimester, rectal temperature should not exceed 38.5°C. Discussion of the possible mechanisms by which maternal hyperthermia may induce abnormal changes in the fetus is beyond the scope of this chapter.

For ethical reasons, most exercise-related thermoregulation studies of pregnant women have been limited to a thermoneutral environment. In spite of the above mentioned morphological and physiological constraints, there is no evidence that pregnant women are ineffective thermoregulators (Clapp, 1991; Jones et al., 1985; McMurray et al., 1990), particularly when allowed to exercise at their own pace. In fact, as pregnancy progresses, such women volitionally curtail their exercise intensities so that their T_{core} values during jogging are lower (Clapp, 1991).

Water-related activities have been recommended for pregnant women, mainly because the high thermal conductivity of the water will dissipate metabolic heat more effectively than air. This is true even when water temperature is as high as 30°C (McMurray et al., 1990). Indeed, when pregnant women in 30°C water rested for 20 min and then cycled for the same duration at 60% HRmax, their rectal temperatures remained practically unchanged at 37.2–37.4°C, and skin temperatures even decreased. When these women were tested periodically at the 15th, 25th, and 35th weeks of gestation the above pattern did not change. However, the decreases in skin and mean body temperatures were less pronounced at 8–10 wk after delivery—presumably representing a pre-pregnancy baseline—than during pregnancy. Average metabolic heat production and heat storage during exercise were greater during pregnancy, as was the sweating rate (McMurray et al., 1990).

Menopause

Although various studies have shown a lower thermoregulatory effectiveness and heat tolerance in menopausal women as compared with younger women, these studies were not designed to tease out the effects of menopause per se vs. the aging effect. As argued by Kenney & Hodgson (1987), it seems that menopause by itself has no effect, because amenorrhea does not affect thermoregulation (Frye et al., 1982). However, Tankersley et al. (1992) showed that estrogen (17 beta-estradiol) replacement therapy in 48-y-old menopausal women caused a reduction in heat strain during rest and exercise in a hot environment, downward shifts in temperature thresholds for both sweating and forearm blood flow, and a tendency for expansion of plasma volume.

THERMOREGULATORY EFFECTIVENESS IN THE HEAT

"Thermoregulatory effectiveness" denotes one's ability to prevent major shifts in core temperature (T_{core}) during exposure to any combination of climatic heat- or cold-stress and metabolic heat stress. Another often-used indicator of thermoregulatory effectiveness is one's ability to prevent major increases in heart rate (HR) during exposure to the heat.

Gender-Related Differences

Under equal climatic heat conditions women's T_{core} increases more on average than men's, both at rest (Bittel & Henane, 1975) and during exercise (e.g., Morimoto et al., 1967; Wyndham et al., 1965; Yousef et al., 1984). This is apparent even when the metabolic heat stress is equated as a percentage of $\dot{V}O_2$max (Frye & Kamon, 1981; Yousef et al., 1984) and can be observed over a wide age range among adults (Yousef et al., 1984).

Two major reasons for women's lower thermoregulatory effectiveness relative to that of men is their lower sweating rate and their higher sweating threshold (the core body temperature at which sweating is initiated). For details see the section on sweating rate. Another possible factor is the greater decrease in plasma volume of women during a combined exercise-climatic heat stress (Senay & Fortney, 1975). This difference, however, disappears if one compares women and men of a similarly high maximal aerobic power (Horstman & Christensen, 1982). It is noteworthy that women's thermoregulatory disadvantage is apparent mostly during exercise in dry heat, but less so in humid heat (Shapiro et al., 1980). This can be explained by the diminishing importance of sweating when its evaporation in a humid climate is limited. Under such conditions—particularly when ambient temperature is lower than skin temperature—women's higher surface area-to-mass ratio becomes an advantage. In a way, the higher sweating rate among men may become a liability during humid exposures because of the greater likelihood of dehydration (Shapiro et al., 1980).

Using multiple regression analysis Havenith & van Middendorp (1990) concluded that gender *per se* could not explain differences in thermoregulatory effectiveness in young adults once $\dot{V}O_2$max, body adiposity, and surface area-per-mass ratio were accounted for. However, such a conclusion may be premature unless confirmed by experiments in which subjects of both genders are selected such that they have equivalent body masses, surface areas, and $\dot{V}O_2$max values.

Lower thermoregulatory effectiveness in females may be one cause for a greater heat-related morbidity and mortality in elderly women compared with elderly men. In a recent study, Macey & Schneider (1993) reported that, of people 60 y of age or older who died in the U.S. of "excessive heat" exposure during 1979–1985, 54.6% were females. An even higher percentage (59%) of female heat-related mortality was reported during the 1988 heat wave at Allegheny County, Pennsylvania (Ramlow & Kuller, 1990). The extent to which this gender bias reflects the larger percentage of older women than men who are still alive, a lower thermoregulatory effectiveness of women, a diagnostic bias, gender differences in heat exposure time, or gender differences in behavior has yet to be discovered.

Age-Related Pattern

The most comprehensive study to date on the age- and aging-related differences in the thermoregulatory effectiveness of females was conducted by Drinkwater and Horvath (1979). Thirty-eight 12- to 68-year-old females were exposed to three levels of climatic heat stress (28°C, 45% relative humidity [RH]; 35°C 65% RH; and 48°C, 10% RH). Exercise consisted of a 50-min treadmill walk at approximately 30% $\dot{V}O_2$max, followed by 10-min rest and, depending on the subject's ability, a second exercise task identical to the first. Figure 7-3 summarizes the age-related pattern of rectal temperature, mean skin temperature, and sweating rate during exposure to 35°C, 65% RH. Final average rectal temperature for the older women, and to a lesser extent for the girls, was higher than for the younger women. The older women also had a higher average mean skin temperature and a lower average sweating rate than did their younger counterparts. In contrast to data from other authors (e.g., Kawahata, 1960), the sweating rate of the girls, when calculated per unit surface area, was not lower than that of the young adult women. It is evident from these data that older women are less effective thermoregulators than their younger counterparts. Girls under the conditions of the above study seem to effectively protect their T_{core}, but, as discussed in a later section, their tolerance times during exposure to a high heat stress are shorter than those of young adult women.

When performing an exercise task of equal intensity and duration, older women on average have a greater increase in T_{core} than do young women (Anderson & Kenney, 1987; Drinkwater & Horvath, 1979; Kenney & Anderson, 1988a; 1988b). One possible explanation for the above difference is the lower maximal aerobic power of the elderly. Indeed, when young and old women exercised at an equal %$\dot{V}O_2$max, with the latter performing at a lower absolute intensity, the two groups had similar increases in T_{core} (Drinkwater et al., 1977a; Yousef et al., 1984). However, by choosing younger and older women of a similar $\dot{V}O_2$max and thus equating both absolute and relative exercise intensities, Anderson & Kenney (1987) reported a higher increase in T_{core} among the older women

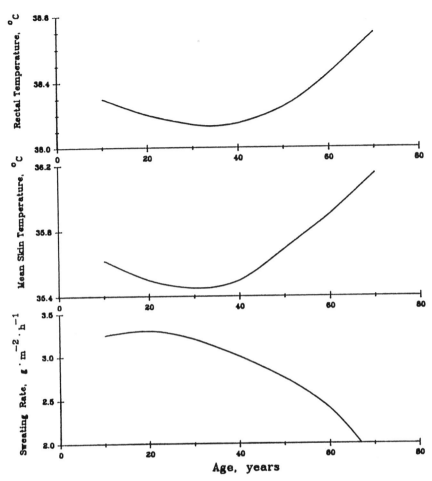

FIGURE 7-3. *Rectal temperature at the end of a 50-min exercise bout, mean skin temperature at 25-min of exercise, and sweating rate during exercise, as related to chronological age.* Thirty-eight 12- to 68-year-old females exercised at 30–35% $\dot{V}O_2$max in a 35°C, 65% RH environment. The curve was fitted by a second degree polynomial regression analysis. Reproduced with permission from Drinkwater & Horvath (1979).

(52–62 y). This suggests that the lower thermoregulatory effectiveness of older women is not merely due to their lower maximal aerobic power.

Such age-related differences in thermoregulatory effectiveness are more apparent during exposure to dry heat than to humid heat, which reflects the lower sweating rate of the elderly in dry, but not humid, heat (Kenney & Anderson, 1988b). It also reflects the greater contribution of evaporative heat loss to overall heat dissipation in a dry climate than in a humid climate.

HEAT TOLERANCE

"Heat tolerance" in the context of this chapter is the greatest heat stress or the greatest duration of a prescribed physical or mental task a person can sustain before predetermined physiological or perceptual endpoints are reached. Such limitations in tolerance time may have practical implications in prolonged sports events, industry, and the military.

Gender-Related Differences

Comparing 9–11-y-old girls and 9–12-y-old boys, Haymes et al. (1974, 1975) reported no differences in tolerance time when the two groups walked at 4.8 km/h up a 5% grade at 21.1, 26.7, and 29.4°C effective temperature (a heat-stress index that combines air temperature, humidity, and wind velocity). However, at 32.2°C boys sustained the exercise for the prescribed 60 min, compared with an average of only 43 min for girls. The lower tolerance time was accompanied by higher T_{core} readings and heart rates in the girls. On average the girls walked at a higher percentage of their $\dot{V}O_2$max (48% vs. 43%), so one cannot tell whether their shorter tolerance time reflects an actual gender difference or merely a difference in relative exercise intensity.

In the unacclimated state, women have shorter tolerance times than men (Frye et al., 1982; Wyndham et al., 1965). For example, Frye et al. (1982) compared the heat tolerance of young (21–27 y) women and men of equal maximal aerobic power who walked (25–30% $\dot{V}O_2$max) at 48°C, 15% RH, before and after heat acclimation. Before acclimation, the rise in rectal temperature was faster in the women than in the men (Figure 7-4). As a result, the men stayed in the chamber for 121 min until the endpoint of 39°C rectal temperature was reached, compared with only 79 min in the women. In contrast, following acclimation, rectal temperature of both groups reached a plateau within 60–90 min, and all subjects managed to complete the prescribed 3-h walk. For further details, see the later section on acclimation.

Another criterion for heat tolerance, used mostly in industry, is the threshold climatic heat stress (also termed "critical temperature") at which T_{core} starts rising, even if metabolic heat stress is constant. Using this criterion it was calculated (Bar-Or et al., 1969) that partially acclimated young adult women have an average critical temperature (26.5–27°C effective temperature) similar to that of partially acclimated young adult males.

Age-Related Pattern

In two separate studies, but using identical protocols, tolerance time of twelve 9–11-y-old girls (Haymes et al., 1974) was compared with that of twenty-nine 19–22-y-old women (Bar-Or et al., 1969). When both

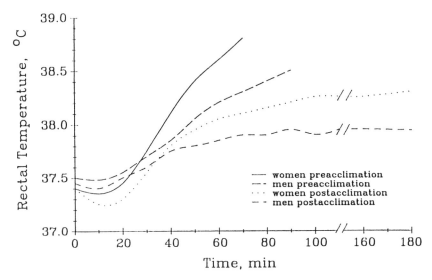

Figure 7-4. *Changes in rectal temperature of eumenorrheic women and of men during walking at 25-30% $\dot{V}O_2max$ in a 48°C, 15% RH environment before and after heat acclimation. Values for $\dot{V}O_2max$ for the four women and four men who served as subjects were similar, i.e., 54.1 mL·kg^{-1}·min^{-1} for the women and 56.3 mL·kg^{-1}·min^{-1} for the men. Reproduced with permission from Frye & Kamon (1981).*

groups walked at 4.8 km^{-1}) in the heat (50°C, 15% RH), the girls could sustain the task for only 45 min, compared to 70 min for the women (Figure 7-5). When the girls had to leave the chamber (due to dizziness, nausea, abdominal discomfort, or a heart rate exceeding 190 beats/min), their average T_{core} was 38.7°C, compared with 39°C in the women. This suggests that the lower tolerance time for the girls was not due to a greater body heat storage.

Drinkwater et al. (1977a) also found a lower heat tolerance in prepubertal girls than in young adult women. When the girls had to terminate the task of walking at 30% $\dot{V}O_2max$ in 48°C, 10% RH, only one of them had a rectal temperature in excess of 38.3°C. The authors suggested that the lower heat tolerance of the girls resulted from reduced central blood volumes (due to greater shifts to the periphery), as reflected by declines in stroke volumes and higher percentages of maximal heart rates, rather than from greater heat storage. For further discussion of this issue, see the subsequent section on age-related cardiovascular changes.

Figure 7-6A summarizes the tolerance time of thirty-eight 12–68-y-old females who exercised at approximately 30% $\dot{V}O_2max$ in 48°C 10% RH, as reported by Drinkwater & Horvath (1979). Both the girls and the older women had distinctly shorter tolerance times than did the young adults. A similar pattern was observed when the subjects exercised at

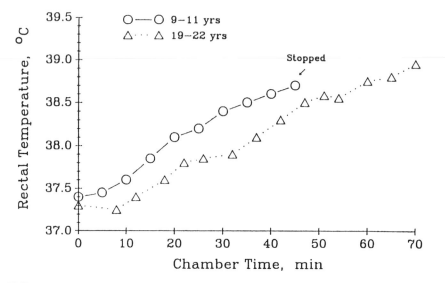

FIGURE 7-5. *Heat and exercise tolerance of girls (n = 12) and young women (n = 29).* Subjects walked intermittently et 4.8 km/h up a 5% grade in a 50°C, 15% RH environment. Rectal temperatures are group means. The girls could persist at the task for only about 45 min, whereas the women endured for 70 min. Based on data of Haymes et al. (1974) and Bar-Or et al. (1969). Reproduced by permission from Bar-Or (1980).

35°C, 65% RH, but there were no age-related differences in tolerance time at 28°C, 45% RH, when all subjects completed the prescribed 100-m n walk. Figure 7-6B shows that in each of the three climatic conditions, the girls and the older women exercised at a considerably higher % HRmax than did the young adult women. Indeed, using correlational analysis, the authors found that, regardless of age, the higher the % HRmax and the lower the resting stroke index (stroke volume divided by body surface area) the shorter the tolerance time. A higher % HRmax among older women, compared with young and middle-aged women, was also reported during walks in desert heat (40°C, 40% RH) (Yousef et al., 1986).

POPULATION DENSITY OF HEAT-ACTIVATED SWEAT GLANDS

Gender-Related Differences

Women have a greater population density (i.e., a greater number of activated glands per unit surface area) of heat-activated sweat glands (HASG) than do men (Bar-Or et al., 1968; Kawahata, 1960). The magnitude of this difference depends on a person's body size and adiposity, but the average density of HASG during rest in a hot climate (47°C 13% RH) is almost 50% greater in women than in men (Bar-Or et al., 1968). This

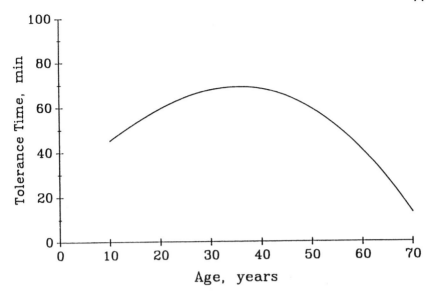

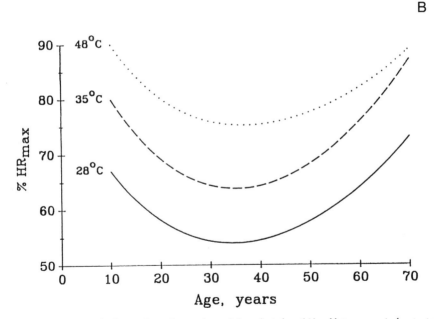

Figure 7-6. *Relationship between heat tolerance time and chronological age (A) and between exercise heart rate and chronological age (B).* Thirty-eight 12- to 68-year-old females exercised at 30-35% $\dot{V}O_2$max in three climatic conditions: 28°C, 45% RH; 35°C, 65% RH; and 48°C, 10% RH. Mean heart rates are presented as percentages of maximal heart rates (% HRmax). Data for tolerance time are presented only for the 48°C, 10% RH condition. The curves were fitted as described in Figure 7-1. Reproduced with permission from Drinkwater & Horvath (1979).

THERMOREGULATION IN FEMALES **263**

difference is not merely a reflection of the smaller body size of the women, because their calculated total number of HASG is also significantly larger than in men (Bar-Or et al., 1968), as shown in Figure 7-7. This gender-related pattern is not apparent before puberty (Bar-Or, 1976; Kawahata, 1960). The higher HASG in women is apparent during exposure to dry heat but not at high humidity (Morimoto et al., 1967). Calculating the HASG during exercise in dry heat as a percentage of maximal HASG (determined by methylcholine injected subcutaneously at increasing dosages), Frye & Kamon (1983) reported that young women activated some 90% of their available glands, compared with only 75% in young men. In a humid heat, on the other hand, the women activated only 80% of their glands and the men 75%. Such a reduction of HASG in the females was interpreted by these authors as a means to conserve body fluid during exposure to a humid environment, when evaporation of the sweat is reduced.

Age-Related Pattern

Girls have a higher density of HASG than do young women (Kawahata, 1960); however, there seems to be no further decline in HASG density between the third and the seventh decade when subjects exercise in the heat (Anderson & Kenney, 1987). Data during rest are less consistent: compared with young women (17–24 y), elderly women (72–84 y) had a lower sweat gland density in their fingers during "spontaneous" sweating and in response to a local adrenaline injection, but a considerably higher density in response to methylcholine injection (Silver et al., 1964).

HEAT–ACTIVATED SWEAT GLANDS

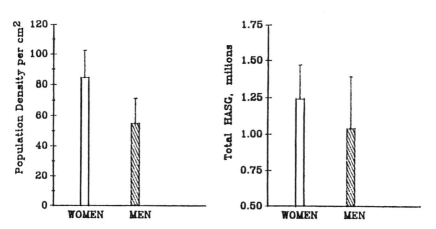

FIGURE 7-7. *Average population density and calculated total number of heat-activated sweat glands (HASG) in young women (18–27 y) and men (18–20 y).* Values are based on 46 skin sites and were obtained at rest. Both gender differences are significant (P<0.05). Vertical lines denote 1 SD. Based on data reported by Bar-Or et al. (1968).

SWEATING RATE

Gender-Related Differences

As a group, females have a lower sweating rate than do males, whether sweating is induced thermally (Avellini et al., 1980; Davies, 1979; Dill et al., 1983; Fox et al., 1969; Horstman & Christensen, 1982; Kawahata, 1960; Morimoto et al., 1967; Shapiro et al., 1980; Shoenfeld et al., 1978; Weinman et al., 1967; Wyndham et al., 1965), particularly in dry heat (Avellini et al., 1980), or by iontophoresis of sudorific substances (Gibson & Shelley, 1948; Main et al., 1991). This difference is most apparent in young adults, but it can also be seen during childhood (Kawahata, 1960; Main et al., 1991). Using pilocarpine iontophoresis, Main et al. (1991) found that, even before puberty, sweating rates of boys were approximately 50% higher than those in girls (Figure 7-8). In both gender groups sweating rates decrease at high humidity (Kenney & Anderson, 1988b; Morimoto et al., 1967; Shapiro et al., 1980). This lower sweat volume may reflect a subtle mechanism for the preservation of fluid when evaporation is limited. A greater rate of hidromeiosis (reabsorption of sweat when the skin is continuously wet) among females has been suggested as another possible mechanism (Brown & Sargent, 1965; Weinman et al., 1967). The authors, however, provided no proof that this indeed was the case.

Sweating threshold (Cunningham et al., 1978; Fox et al., 1969; Grucza et al., 1985) is higher in females. However, the sweating rate increase for a

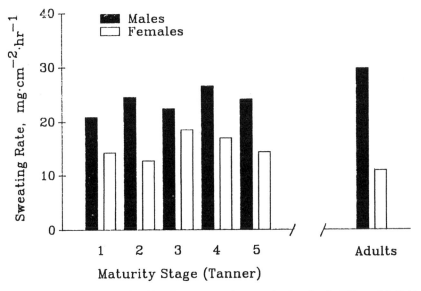

FIGURE 7-8. *Sweating rate induced by pilocarpine iontophoresis in female and male children subdivided by Tanner stage of puberty (Tanner 1 denotes prepuberty) and in adult females and males.* Based on data reported by Main et al. (1991).

given increment in mean body temperature (often called "sweating sensitivity") does not seem to differ between the sexes (Figure 7-9) (Gonzalez et al., 1980).

In a study of three women, initiation of sweating during exercise in a 30°C, 60% RH environment occurred faster after 60 d of training than before (Araki et al., 1981). However, no studies seem to have been reported that directly compare training-induced changes in sweating responses of males and females.

Because females' sweating rate is lower and they activate a greater number of sweat glands per cm² than do males, each gland produces less sweat than in males. For example, during rest at 34°C, 40% RH, sweat production per gland in men was more than three times that of women (Kawahata, 1960) (Figure 7-10). During exercise at 30% $\dot{V}O_2$max in dry and humid heat, acclimated men's sweating rate per gland was, respectively, 50% and 60% higher than that of acclimated women.

Age-Related Pattern

Although the sweating rate of boys is considerably lower than in young adult males (Bar-Or, 1989), there is a controversy in the literature as to whether girls sweat less than young adult women. Some authors (Drinkwater et al., 1977a) have found a similar sweating rate when calculated per

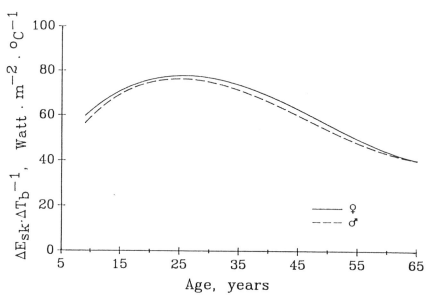

FIGURE 7-9. *Sweating sensitivity, expressed as the ratio between the increase in evaporative heat loss (ΔE) and the increase in mean body temperature (ΔT_b), in males and females ages 8 to 67 y who rested while exposed to a ramp increase in room temperature at 1.5°C/min.* Adapted with permission from Gonzalez et al. (1980).

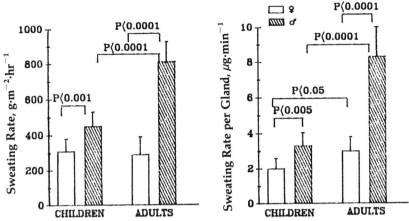

FIGURE 7-10. *Sweating rate and sweating rate per gland in 9-y-old girls (n = 7) and boys (n = 7) and in young adult women (n = 7) and men (n = 8) sitting at 34°C.* Vertical lines denote 1 SD. Based on data by Kawahata (1960). Reproduced by permission from Bar-Or (1989).

unit surface area, whereas others (Doupe et al., 1994) found a greater sweating rate among the young women. In a study comparing prepubescent, pubescent and young adult females who were matched for $\dot{V}O_2$max and exercised at 50% $\dot{V}O_2$max in a 42°C, 18% RH environment, the sweating rate per m² surface area of the adult women was some 50–70% higher than in the younger groups (Meyer et al., 1992). It thus appears that the largest developmental increase in sweating rate among females, as in males, occurs towards the latter stages of puberty.

Differences in sweating rate between young and elderly women seem to depend on whether the subjects rest or exercise and whether the climate is dry or humid. During rest at 40°C, 40% RH, there were no differences in sweating rate or sweating threshold between middle-aged and post-menopausal women (Drinkwater et al., 1982). Similarly, there were no differences in sweating rate of resting 20–27-y-old women and 78–94-y-old women, irrespective of whether sweating was elicited by local heating or by methylcholine injection (Foster et al., 1976). Sweating sensitivity during rest, in females and males alike, was higher in young adults than in children or in older adults (Figure 7-7). The authors (Gonzalez et al., 1980) found a strong relationship between sweating sensitivity and $\dot{V}O_2$max/kg body mass, irrespective of gender or age.

During exercise in dry heat (48°C dry bulb, 25°C wet bulb), on the other hand, 20–30-y-old women had consistently higher sweating rates than their older (52–62 y), post-menopausal counterparts (Anderson & Kenney, 1987). The groups in this study were matched for $\dot{V}O_2$max so that they exercised at the same absolute and relative (40% $\dot{V}O_2$max) intensities. In contrast with the dry heat experiment, there were no differences in sweating rates of these heat-acclimated younger and older women when they exercised in humid heat (37°C, 60% RH) (Kenney & Anderson, 1988b). The authors suggested that the lower sweating rates of the elderly in dry heat may not reflect a functional deficiency of the glands themselves, but may have resulted from insufficient drinking during exercise and a greater dehydration in the elderly group.

Possible Mechanisms

It is unclear why children and young women have lower sweating rates than do young men. One common characteristics of prepubescents and women is their lower plasma testosterone levels when compared with men. It is thus tempting to speculate that the above differences in sweating rate reflect differences in testosterone or testosterone-related hormonal activity. Indeed, some authors have suggested that testosterone is sudorific (Kawahata, 1960; Tanaka, 1956). Furthermore, using an isoelectric-focusing electrophoretic technique, Sens et al. (1985) found similar protein patterns in sweat for prepubescents of both genders and for women, but the pattern for men was different. The authors speculated that this difference may represent the activity of hormones that emerge after sexual maturation in the men. However, no experimental evidence confirms that a higher testosterone activity enhances sweating rate. For further review of this issue, see Bar-Or (1989).

Another possible reason for lower sweating rates in children and women may be lower rates of anaerobic energy turnover in their sweat glands. The total sweat lactate content per gland has been shown to be lower in prepubescent boys than in more mature boys (Falk et al., 1991); the authors suggested that this may reflect a lower rate of glycolysis in the glands of the prepubescents, in analogy to a lower rate of glycolysis in children's exercising muscles (Eriksson & Saltin, 1974). However, among 22–30-y-old females, sweat lactate concentrations and total sweat production were *greater* in those who were sedentary and had lower sweating rates when compared to those who were physically active and had higher sweating rates (Lamont, 1987). There is no published direct comparison of lactate production of females vs. males.

Finally, it is possible that lower sweating rates in females and children reflect their smaller sweat glands. Indeed, as found in cadaver data, both the duct lengths and the cross-sectional areas of the secretory coils are smaller in the glands of children than in adolescents (Landing et al., 1968). Sato & Sato (1983), using *in vitro* analysis of dissected glands, have shown a tight relationship between sweating rate per gland and the size of the gland in adult males (ages 22–43 y). However, it is not known whether the sweat glands of females are smaller than those of males or whether the sweating rate-to-size relationship, as described by Sato & Sato, also holds for females. Furthermore, in the above *in vitro* study, a tight relationship was also shown between sweating rate per gland and the sensitivity of the gland to injected methacholine. In conclusion, it is not clear whether the size of sweat glands *per se* is the cause of differences in their output.

SWEAT COMPOSITION

Knowledge of the composition of thermally-induced sweat may advance the understanding of the role of the sweat glands in the overall control of body electrolytes. It may also reveal practical information regarding the needs of the body for electrolyte replenishment during or following profuse sweating. Most data on this topic reflect measurements taken from a single skin site and thus may not represent total loss of electrolytes through sweat.

Gender-Related Differences

During exercise at 50% $\dot{V}O_2$max in dry heat (42°C, 18% RH) no gender-related differences emerged in the concentrations of Na^+, K^+, and Cl^- in sweat on the lower backs of prepubescents and pubescents (Meyer et al., 1992). In adults, there is inconsistent information about the sweat electrolyte content of men and women. Young women had significantly lower concentrations of Cl^- in sweat than did young men in some (Meyer et al., 1992; Robinson & Robinson, 1954) but not all (Dill et al., 1983; Morimoto et al., 1967) studies. One reason for the inconsistent results is the large intragroup variability. In the study by Dill et al. (1983), for example, the coefficients of variation for Cl^-, Na^+, and K^+ were as high as 50%. This variability may result from lack of control of dietary salt prior to the experiments or from genetic factors.

Concentrations of iron in sweat were higher in young adult females than in males but, because of the greater sweating rates among males, the total iron losses in sweat were similar for the two genders (Lamanca et al., 1988).

Age-Related Pattern

The concentrations of Na^+ and Cl^- in sweat seem to increase from childhood to adulthood. In contrast, sweat K^+ concentration is higher on average in children than in young adults. These age-related differences were statistically significant for all three electrolytes in the males, but only for K^+ in the females (Meyer et al., 1992). Postmenopausal women had higher concentrations of Na^+ in forearm sweat than did middle-aged women, all resting in a 40°C, 40% RH environment (Drinkwater et al., 1982). Even though the older women tended to have greater concentrations of Na^+ at other skin sites, the differences were non-significant; there were no differences in sweat K^+. It is unclear whether the above gender- and age-related differences in sweat composition have any practical importance, because the total electrolyte loss incurred in the above studies reflects a very small percentage of the total electrolyte pool in these subjects (Meyer & Bar-Or, 1994).

CARDIOVASCULAR RESPONSES TO THE HEAT

While sweat evaporation is the most important avenue for heat dissipation during exercise in the heat in humans, the cardiovascular system also plays a major role by transporting heat from body core to the skin. A higher skin blood flow (SkBF) can be achieved by redistributing the cardiac output ($\dot{Q}$) among body organs and regions, as well as by increasing $\dot{Q}$. For a detailed discussion of the cardiovascular adjustments during exercise in the heat, see the classic review by Rowell (1974).

In the cold, skin vasoconstriction is the first line of defense against heat loss. One constraint in studying the role of the cardiovascular system in thermoregulatory effectiveness and in heat and cold tolerance is that cardiovascular variables (heart rate and $\dot{Q}$ in particular) are strongly associated with maximal aerobic power. It is therefore important to equate aerobic fitness of the various groups if one is to discern differences that are due to gender or to age *per se*. If one cannot obtain subject groups with a similar aerobic fitness, a second best approach is to administer work rates at a similar % $\dot{V}O_2$max.

Gender-Related Differences

Relatively few studies of thermoregulation have monitored hemodynamic responses of both genders. Davies (1981) compared the thermoregulation of endurance-trained girls (13.8 ± 0.7 y) and boys (12.9 ± 0.8 y) who exercised for 1 h at 68% $\dot{V}O_2$max in a thermoneutral environment. Inferring from the girls' higher skin temperatures, he suggested that they had higher skin blood flows (SkBF) than did the boys. Unfortunately, there are no published studies that directly compared SkBF between girls and boys who exercised in a hot climate.

During rest and exercise in a thermoneutral environment cardiac outputs and stroke volumes of women are often lower than those of men (Spina et al., 1993). However, these differences are diminished when the two groups are matched for maximal aerobic power. In comparing young adult women and men of equally high $\dot{V}O_2$max values who exercised in a hot climate before and after acclimation, Horstman & Christensen (1982) found that the preacclimated women had on average a higher heart rate and a lower stroke volume than did the men, but cardiac output was almost identical in the two groups. Following a 10-d acclimation regimen, the women's mean heart rate was marginally higher than that of the men, as was the stroke volume. The end result was that $\dot{Q}$ tended to be higher in the women.

In a recent study (Havenith et al., 1995) 41 men and 15 women, 20–73 y of age, cycled at 60 W for 1 h in humid heat (35°C, 80% RH). There were no gender-related differences in $\dot{V}O_2$max. Even though the study was not designed to compare genders, the authors found no gender-related differences in heart rate, forearm blood flow, arterial blood pressure, or forearm vascular conductance.

Age-Related Pattern

Among boys, there is some indication that forearm SkBF during exercise in dry heat is higher in prepubescents, compared to early and late pubescents (Falk et al., 1992). There are no similar comparisons among females. However, Drinkwater et al. (1977a) compared SkBF at rest and following exercise in the heat in young women and in 12-y-old girls defined as prepubertal (although there was no indication that pubertal stage was actually determined). Neither at rest nor after exercise was there a significant difference in SkBF between the groups. However, the postexertional increase in SkBF in a 48°C, 10% RH environment tended to be greater among the girls. Although the cardiac index ($\dot{Q}$ divided by body surface area) was similar in both groups, the girls on the average had a consistently higher heart rate (Figure 7-6B) and a lower stroke volume. The authors argued that even though the relative increase in forearm SkBF was similar in both groups, a greater proportion of the girls' blood volume (and $\dot{Q}$) was diverted to the skin, because of their greater surface-area-to-mass ratio, and thus less blood was available for the central circulation. This pattern, coupled with the somewhat lower ratio of $\dot{Q}$:$\dot{V}O_2$ seen in children compared with adults (Bar-Or, 1983), may explain the lower heat tolerance of the girls.

As recently reviewed by Kenney (1995), SkBF during exercise in the heat declines with aging. Such a decline is apparent even when younger and older adults are equated for $\dot{V}O_2$max (Kenney, 1988; Tankersley et al., 1991) and seems to be similar in both gender groups (Havenith et al., 1995). The lower SkBF in the elderly does not depend on their state of hydration (Kenney et al., 1990). Both $\dot{Q}$ and arm blood flow were lower in 55–68-y-old women (n = 4) and men (n = 2), than in 19–30-y-old women (n = 4) and men (n = 2) matched for $\dot{V}O_2$max and exercising at the same % $\dot{V}O_2$max in a 37°C, 60% RH environment(Figure 7-11) (Kenney, 1988). In contrast to the above findings, Drinkwater & Horvath (1979) found no age-related differences in forearm blood flow when females exercised at 48°C, 10% RH. However, under these conditions no postmenopausal women completed the prescribed exercise task.

As recently reported (Martin & Kenney, in press) maximal arm SkBF, measured when the individual sits at 23°C with the arm exposed to 42°C, declines with age, particularly during the first two decades of life. This pattern does not differ between genders.

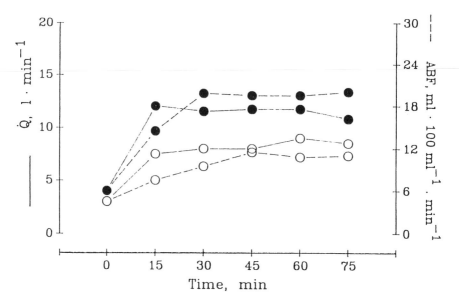

FIGURE 7-11. *Mean cardiac output (Q̇) and arm blood flow (ABF) in unacclimatized 55–68-y-old subjects (open circles) and 19–30-y-old subjects (filled circles); four women and two men comprised each group. Subjects were matched for V̇O₂max, and they exercised at 40% V̇O₂max in a 37°C, 60% RH environment. Adapted with permission from Kenney (1988).*

In conclusion, it seems that the cardiovascular adjustments during exercise in the heat are more effective in young adult women than in girls and elderly women. This may be an important reason for the lower heat tolerance in the latter two groups. Age *per se* seems to be the single most important factor that affects the differences between young adults and the elderly in their cardiovascular responses to exercise in humid heat (Havenith et al., 1995).

HEAT ACCLIMATIZATION AND ACCLIMATION

Heat *acclimatization* denotes physiological and perceptual changes that occur over several days or weeks in a person newly exposed to naturally occurring climatic heat. In general, these changes reflect an improved thermoregulatory effectiveness and heat tolerance. Heat *acclimation* is a term used when the above changes occur as a result of exposures to artificially produced climatic heat stress, as in a climatic chamber.

Gender-Related Differences

Like men, women benefit from acclimation to exercise in the heat (Avellini et al., 1980; Bar-Or et al., 1969, Buskirk et al., 1965; Frye & Kamon, 1981; Hertig et al., 1963; Horstman & Christensen, 1982; Morimoto et al., 1967; Sawka et al., 1983; Shapiro et al., 1980; Weinman et al., 1967; Wyndham et al., 1965). Judging from the reductions in T_{core} and heart rate, the degree of acclimation appears to be similar in the two genders (Wyndham et al., 1965). However, the increase in sweating rate, commonly considered a pivotal change during acclimation or acclimatization, may be greater in men than in women (Avellini et al., 1980; Weinman et al., 1967; Wyndham et al., 1965), but this finding is not universal (Frye & Kamon, 1981; Horstman & Christensen, 1982).

A major gender difference in acclimation is a markedly greater improvement in women's tolerance time, once they become acclimated (Figure 7-4) (Frye & Kamon, 1981; Horstman & Christensen, 1982; Wyndham et al., 1965). It thus appears that the practical effect of acclimation is greater for women than for men, especially when the combined metabolic and climatic heat stress is high and the exercise task is prolonged. Because women's greater improvement in tolerance time cannot be explained by a greater evaporative heat loss, it most probably reflects greater circulatory changes in the women. The possible effects of aerobic training *per se* are discussed in other sections of this chapter.

There are apparently no published data concerning gender-related differences in acclimation or acclimatization among children and among the elderly.

Age-Related Pattern

As reviewed by Kenney (1995), elderly men acclimate to heat as effectively as young men. There is very little information that similarly compares acclimation (or acclimatization) effectiveness of elderly women with young adult women. Henschel et al. (1968) tested 60–93-y-old women and men in the summer and in the winter, to assess their natural acclimatization to mild exercise in the heat. For both genders heart rate, $\dot{V}O_2$, and ventilation were lower in the summer than in the winter. These declines were similar to those found in middle-aged and young adult females and males. However, climatic and exercise conditions differed among the age groups. Neither body temperatures nor sweating rates were reported in the Henschel et al. study.

AEROBIC TRAINING

Some of the physiological changes ascribed to acclimation may in fact have been due to aerobic training *per se*. Among males, the respective effects of acclimation and training have been studied by several groups. Unfortunately, little information is available to help separate effects of these two factors in females.

Cross-sectional comparisons suggest that trained young women have a better thermoregulatory effectiveness on average than the general female population (Drinkwater et al., 1977b; Nunneley, 1978). As shown by Gisolfi & Cohen (1979) and Cohen & Gisolfi (1982), six 19-y-old women had marked reductions in heat strain and marked increases in tolerance time in dry heat (45°C 17% RH) following an 11-wk interval training regimen in a thermoneutral environment. These responses were similar to those achieved through acclimation. Likewise, Inbar et al. (1981) found that 8-10-y-old boys had similar reductions in heat strain following either acclimation to dry heat or training in a thermoneutral environment. There are no published reports that directly compare the thermoregulatory effects of training among gender or age groups.

THERMOREGULATORY RESPONSES TO THE COLD

Much less research has been conducted on the responses of females to cold stress than to heat stress. This may reflect the greater prevalence of questions posed to the applied environmental physiologist on thermoregulation during exercise in the heat than in cold environments.

Gender-Related Differences

Based on changes in T_{core} it seems that females thermoregulate as well as or even better than males when exposed to a cold environment. However, women's skin temperatures are often lower than men's. This pattern has been shown during exposures in air (DuBois et al., 1952; Graham, 1983; Wyndham et al., 1964a) and in water (Buskirk, 1966; Kollias et al., 1974; Sloan & Keatinge, 1973). Most cold-related gender differences have been observed in resting subjects. Only Graham (1983) and Sloan & Keatinge (1973) have studied the combined effects of cold stress and exercise.

Wyndham et al. (1964a) exposed resting women and men (18-24 y) to 5°C air for 1 h and found no differences in final T_{core} or in metabolic heat production. However, mean skin temperature was about 2°C lower in the women. Cunningham et al. (1978) reported that, when air temperature was cooled gradually from 48°C to 16°C, resting women started shivering earlier than men and at a higher T_{core}. While resting for 2 h in 10°C air , older (61 ± 3 y) women on the average maintained a near-constant rectal temperature, compared with a decline of about 0.4°C in an age-matched group of men (Wagner & Horvath, 1985b). The women also on the average had a faster increase in metabolic rate, which may have been facilitated by a greater availability of energy substrates (Wagner et al., 1987). Baum et al. (1976) have shown that, when exposed to a rapidly declining ambient air temperature, male distance runners started shivering at lower temperatures than did the untrained controls. It is thus possible that the higher shivering thresholds of women reflect lower fitness levels, rather than a true gender difference.

During a 3-h exposure to very cold conditions (intermittent exercise of 45% $\dot{V}O_2$max at $-5°C$), clothed young women and men had a similar "modest rise" in their rectal temperatures, but during the last hour, only the women had declines in rectal temperatures and significant increases in heat losses. The main gender difference was a greater decline in skin temperatures among the women (Figure 7-12). This greater decline could not be explained by body size or composition. It may have reflected a lower average absolute heat production in the women, who also had a smaller mean body mass (Graham, 1983).

Because thermal conductivity of water is some 25 times higher than that of air, thermoregulatory homeostasis is much more compromised in cool water than in cool air. Sloan & Keatinge (1973) compared the rates of body cooling (oral temperature) when 8–19-y-old boy and girl swimmers swam in 20.3°C water at metabolic rates of about 20 kJ/min. The authors did not provide a statistical analysis to compare intergender differences in the rates of cooling, but their individual data points suggest a somewhat faster cooling among the boys under 12 y of age than among the girls of that age group. These boys also had a greater surface area-to-mass ratio.

As reviewed by Kenney (1995), there has been less cold-related mortality among elderly women than among elderly men. For example, Macey & Schneider (1993) analyzed mortality data of people over 60 y of age in

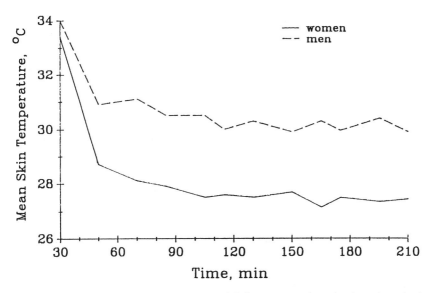

FIGURE 7-12. *Changes in mean skin temperature of clothed young women (n = 6) and men (n = 6), who exercised intermittently (six 20-min bouts at 45% $\dot{V}O_2$max) in a cold environment ($-5°C$, 40–50% RH). Values for the women are averages of those obtained during the luteal and follicular phases of the menstrual cycle. Adapted with permission from Graham (1983).*

the U.S. over a 7-y period (1979–1985). Of 3326 people whose cause of death was categorized as exposure to excessive cold, 65.2% were males. The authors suggested that one reason for the above gender bias might be the larger proportion of males among the homeless. Another suggested reason was "the greater care women take in responding to their illness symptoms with lay-care action and nutrition." Yet, many elderly women underestimate the need for heating their rooms, even on cold winter days (Fox et al., 1973; Watts, 1971).

Three morphological characteristics of females affect their ability to preserve body heat. As a group, adolescent and adult females (but not young girls) have greater body fat contents and subcutaneous fat thicknesses than do males. Because of the excellent insulative properties of fat, females can thus prevent heat loss more effectively than males. On the other hand, because of smaller average body size, adult women have a larger surface area-to-mass ratio on average than do their male counterparts. This causes a faster heat loss whenever ambient temperature is cooler than skin temperature. This detrimental effect of a large surface area-to-mass ratio is manifested mostly among lean individuals, and it disappears when men and women are obese (30% or more body fat) (Kollias et al., 1974). The above conclusion is based on the data of Figure 7-13 that were obtained from subjects immersed in 20°C water.

A third morphological difference between genders is the lower muscle mass in women. This characteristic is particularly important during

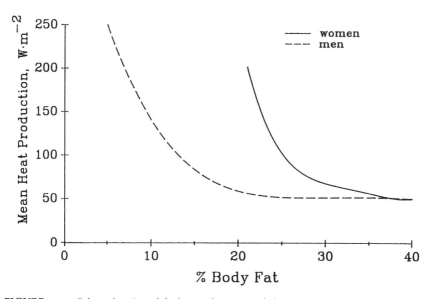

FIGURE 7-13. *Relationship of metabolic heat production to % body fat in young adult females and males immersed in cool (20°C) water for 45–60 min.* Adapted by permission from Kollias et al. (1974).

cold exposures because muscle—mostly in the limbs—provides thermal insulation. For a review of this topic see Kenney & Buskirk (1995).

In comparisons among women, the thermoregulatory effects of body adiposity and surface area-to-mass ratio are apparent mostly at rest. During exercise the main effect on core temperature is that of metabolic heat production (Gallow et al., 1984).

It is not clear whether factors other than morphological characteristics affect gender differences in response to the cold. It is possible that females have more effective peripheral vasoconstriction, as manifested by lower skin temperature in the chamber experiments by Wyndham et al. (1964a). An alternative explanation for the lower skin temperature in females is the thicker subcutaneous fat layer.

Age-Related Pattern

Based on scant information comparing children, adolescents, and young adults on the one hand, and between young adults and the elderly on the other, there seems to be an age-related pattern in the responses of females to the cold. This is summarized schematically in Figure 7-14. Prepubescent girls had a faster rate of cooling, compared with adolescents and young adult females, when swimming in 20.3°C water (Sloan & Keatinge, 1973). This difference reflected the larger surface area-to-mass ratio among the children and the rising body adiposity during and following puberty (the latter is typical for females but not for males). Whereas el-

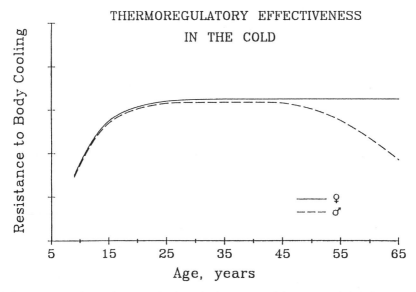

FIGURE 7-14. *Schematic depiction of the relationship between age and the resistance to body cooling of females and males exposed to a cold environment.*

derly men are less capable of maintaining core body temperature compared with younger men, there is little or no such age trend among females. This was first shown for resting subjects in mild cold conditions (17.5°C) (Bernstein et al., 1956) and subsequently for resting in conditions as cool as 10°C (Wagner & Horvath, 1985b). The effective preservation of body heat among elderly women may be explained by their body fat content, which is similar to or greater than that of younger women. In addition, older (61 ± 3 y) women responded to cool environments with a more rapid increase in metabolic rate than did younger (24 ± 1 y) women (Wagner & Horvath, 1985b). Another age-related difference is the markedly higher arterial systolic blood pressure and total peripheral resistance, but not the peripheral blood flow, in elderly people who are exposed to the cold (Wagner & Horvath, 1985a).

A finding of a practical relevance for clinical situations is that the oral temperatures of elderly people (60–102 y), men and women alike, drop to lower values after they drink iced water, compared with younger people. Furthermore, it takes longer for older people to regain their predrinking oral temperatures (Sugarek, 1986). The cause for this difference is not clear, but it may reflect a more sluggish peripheral blood flow response to thermal stimuli in the elderly (Kenney, personal communication; Rooke et al., 1994).

DIRECTIONS FOR FUTURE RESEARCH

Even though sex hormones have been suggested to affect sweating, only scant circumstantial evidence indicates that this may be the case. Research is needed to further study this issue and the role that female sex hormones play in the gender differences in sweating.

Likewise, an insight into the role of male sex hormones may help to explain why gender-related differences in sweating rate are greater in adults than in children.

Most studies on thermoregulation during pregnancy have been conducted in a thermoneutral environment or during water immersion. More information is needed on the acute responses to exercise in high ambient heat among pregnant women, as well as on the outcome of such pregnancies. The ethical constraints of such research are obvious, but it should be conducted because of the large numbers of pregnant women, particularly at the earlier stages of pregnancy, who exercise in hot environments at high intensities.

There is no information about thermoregulation during exercise in climacteric women. This issue is particularly interesting in light of speculation that hot flashes and the sensation of heat reflect a transitory decrease in the thermal setpoint. What is the mechanism for hot flashes, and do they occur exclusively in women?

Even though females depend more than males on adequate heat convection to the periphery, too few studies have compared the hemodynamic responses of the genders during exercise in the heat or during exposures to the cold.

SUMMARY

A major challenge for those wishing to ferret out the extent to which gender affects temperature regulation during exercise is to equate the metabolic heat stress for both genders. This goal can be approached if male and female subjects are matched according to body mass and absolute aerobic power and if they then exercise at identical percentages of that power. The downside of this approach is that women who satisfy these criteria are often much more fit than women selected from the general female population. Thus, most of the literature on how gender affects temperature regulation is confounded by important variables, e.g., body mass, body composition, aerobic power, training status, and menstrual status; these confounders can easily lead to erroneous conclusions about causes and effects.

Women—and especially older women—generally experience a greater rise in core body temperature than do men upon exposure to heat stress or prolonged exercise. Two major reasons for this reduced thermoregulatory effectiveness are that in women the onset of sweating occurs at a higher core temperature and the rate of sweat production is lower than in men. It is unclear whether the gender difference in sweat production is caused by differences in sex hormones, differences in anaerobic energy metabolism of the sweat glands, differences in sweat gland size, or some other factor. Exercise tolerance time in the heat is also lower in females than in males, at least in the unacclimated state; among females, exercise tolerance time is particularly brief in young girls and in older women. It remains uncertain whether low exercise tolerance times are caused more by excessive heat storage or by a relatively low cardiac output.

When subjects are matched on aerobic power, there seem to be few gender-related effects on cardiovascular function during exercise, but cardiac output and blood flow to the skin usually decline with aging in both genders. Young girls apparently divert more of their blood volumes to the skin during exercise in the heat than do young adult women so that heart rates are higher and cardiac outputs relative to oxygen uptakes are lower in the girls. Thus, cardiovascular adjustments during exercise in the heat are more effective in young adult women than in girls and elderly women. Also, age seems to be more important than gender in explaining differences in the cardiovascular responses to exercise in the heat between young adults and the elderly.

Women's exercise tolerance time in the heat increases to a greater extent than men's after acclimation to training in the heat. This exaggerated improvement in women cannot be explained by better evaporative cooling and seems more likely to be the result of enhanced cardiac output. The extent to which improvements in exercise tolerance time in women are caused by heat exposure vs. training has not been adequately studied.

In cold environments, women seem to regulate their core temperatures at least as well as, if not better than, men, but women's skin temperatures are often lower than those of men upon cold exposure. Women may start shivering earlier and increase their metabolic rates faster than men, thereby helping the women to better maintain their core temperatures. Whether this is a true gender effect or an effect of differences in training status is not known. Lower skin temperatures of women vs. men may be the result of more effective constriction of blood vessels serving the skin or of better insulation from a thicker subcutaneous fat layer. Young girls lose heat faster than adolescent girls or young women when swimming in cold water, and this is presumably explained by a greater ratio of surface area to body mass and a lesser accumulation of insulative subcutaneous fat in the young girls.

Core temperatures are higher in women during the luteal phase of the menstrual cycle both at rest and during exercise, at least in a preacclimated state. Associated with this elevation in core temperatures are higher thresholds required to elicit sweating and greater blood flow to the skin, but the mechanism responsible for these changes is uncertain. The effects of exercise on thermoregulation, including the magnitudes of increases in sweat rate and metabolic heat production, are unaffected by the menstrual cycle; exercise tolerance time is likewise unaffected. Thus, the practical effects of the menstrual cycle on thermoregulation during exercise are minimal.

ACKNOWLEDGEMENTS

I am indebted to W. Larry Kenney, Carl V. Gisolfi, and Ethan Nadel for their constructive critiques. Particular thanks to W. Larry Kenney for his substantial help in the literature search.

BIBLIOGRAPHY

Anderson, R.K., and W.L. Kenney (1987). Effect of age on heat-activated sweat gland density and flow during exercise in dry heat. *J. Appl. Physiol.* 63:1089–1094.
Araki, T., K. Matsushita, K. Umeno, A. Tsujino and Y. Toda (1981). Effect of physical training on exercise-induced sweating in women. *J. Appl. Physiol.* 51:1526–1532.
Avellini, B.A., E. Kamon, and J.T. Krajewski (1980). Physiological responses of physically fit men and women to acclimation to humid heat. *J. Appl. Physiol.* 49:254–261.
Bar-Or, O. (1980). Climate and the exercising child—a review. *Int. J. Sports Med.* 1:53–65.
Bar-Or, O. (1976). Distribution of heat activated sweat glands in 10- to 12-year-old Israeli girls and boys who differ in ethnic origin (in Hebrew). Research Report, Wingate Institute.
Bar-Or, O. (1983). *Pediatric Sports Medicine for the Practitioner.* New York: Springer.
Bar-Or, O. (1989). Temperature regulation during exercise in children and adolescents. In: C.V. Gisolfi, and D.R. Lamb (eds.). *Perspectives in Exercise Science and Sports Medicine, Vol. 2: Youth, Exercise, and Sport.* Indianapolis: Benchmark Press, pp. 335–367.

Bar-Or, O., H.M. Lundegren, and E.R. Buskirk (1969). Heat tolerance of exercising obese and lean women. *J. Appl. Physiol.* 26:403–409.

Bar-Or, O., M. Lundegren, L.I. Magnusson, and E.R. Buskirk (1968). Distribution of heat-activated sweat glands in obese and lean men and women. *Human Biol.* 40:235–248.

Baum, E., K. Bruck, and H.P. Schwenicke (1976). Adaptive modifications in the thermoregulatory system of long-distance runners. *J. Appl. Physiol.* 40:404–410.

Bernstein, L.M., L.C. Johnston, R. Ryan, T. Inouye, and F.K. Hick (1956). Body composition as related to heat regulation in women. *J. Appl. Physiol.* 9:241–256.

Bittel, J., and R. Henane (1975). Comparison of thermal exchanges in men and women under neutral and hot conditions. *J. Physiol.* 250:475–489.

Bonen, A., F.J. Haynes, W. Watson-Wright, M.M. Sopper, G.N. Pierce, M.P. Low, and T.E. Graham (1983). Effects of menstrual cycle on metabolic responses to exercise. *J. Appl. Physiol.* 55:1506–1513.

Brown, W.K., and F. Sargent, II (1965). Hidromeiosis. *Arch. Env. Health* 11:442–452.

Burse, R.L. (1979). Sex differences in human thermoregulatory response to heat and cold stress. *Human Factors* 21:687–699.

Buskirk, E.R. (1966). Variation in heat production during acute exposures of men and women to cold air or water. *Ann. N.Y. Acad. Sci.* 134:733–742.

Buskirk, E.R., H. Lundegren, and L. Magnusson (1965). Heat acclimatization patterns in obese and lean individuals. *Ann. N.Y. Acad. Sci.* 131: 637–653.

Cannon G.C., and C.A. Dinarello (1985). Increased plasma interleukin-1 activity in women after ovulation. *Science* 227:1247–1249.

Carpenter, A.J., and S.A. Nunneley (1988). Endogenous hormones subtly alter women's response to heat stress. *J. Appl. Physiol.* 65:2313–2317.

Clapp, J.F., III (1991). The changing thermal response to endurance exercise during pregnancy. *Am. J. Obstet. Gynecol.* 165:1684–1689.

Clapp, J.F., III (1996). Exercise during pregnancy. In O. Bar-Or, D.R. Lamb, and P. Clarkson (eds.) *Perspectives in Exercise Science and Sports Medicine, Vol. 9: Exercise and the Female: A Life Span Perspective.* Carmel, IN: Cooper Publishing Group, pp. 413–451.

Cohen, J.S., and C.V. Gisolfi (1982). Effects of interval training on work-heat tolerance of young women. *Med. Sci. Sports Exerc.* 14:46–52.

Cunningham, D.J., and M. Cabanac (1971). Evidence from behavioral thermoregulatory responses of a shift in setpoint temperature related to the menstrual cycle. *J. Physiol.* 63:236–238.

Cunningham, D.J., J.A.J. Stolwijk, and C.B. Wenger (1978). Comparative thermoregulatory responses of resting men and women. *J. Appl. Physiol.* 45:908–915.

Davies, C.T.M. (1981). Thermal responses to exercise in children. *Ergonomics* 24:55–61.

Davies, C.T.M. (1979). Thermoregulation during exercise in relation to sex and age. *Eur. J. Appl. Physiol.* 42:71–79.

Dill, D.B., M.K. Yousef, A. Goldman, S.D. Hillyard, and T.P. Davis (1983). Volume and composition of hand sweat of white and black men and women in desert walks. *Am. J. Phys. Anthropol.* 61:67–73.

Doupe, M.B., G.P. Kenny, M.D. White, and G.G. Giesbrecht (1994). Thermoregulation and rate of body warming during warm water (40°C) immersion in female children and adults. In: J. Frim, M.B. Ducharme, and P. Tikuisis (eds.) *Proceedings of the Sixth International Conference of Environmental Ergonomics.* York, Canada: DCIEM Publishers, pp. 12–13.

Drinkwater, B.L., and S.M. Horvath (1979). Heat tolerance and aging. *Med. Sci. Sports* 11:49–55.

Drinkwater, B.L., J.F. Bedi, A.B. Loucks, S. Roche, and S.M. Horvath (1982). Sweating sensitivity and capacity of women in relation to age. *J. Appl. Physiol.* 53:671–676.

Drinkwater, B.L., I.C. Kupprat, J.E. Denton, J.L. Crist, and S.M. Horvath (1977a). Response of prepubertal girls and college women to work in the heat. *J. Appl. Physiol.* 43:1046–1053.

Drinkwater, B.L., I.C. Kupprat, J.E. Denton, and S.M. Horvath (1977b). Heat tolerance of female distance runners. In: P. Milvy (ed.) *The Marathon: Physiological, Medical, Epidemiological and Psychological Studies.* New York: N.Y. Acad. Sci., pp. 777–792.

DuBois, E.F., F.G. Ebaugh, Jr., and J.D. Hardy (1952). Basal heat production and elimination of thirteen normal women at temperatures from 22°C to 35°C. *J.Nutr.* 48:257–293.

Eriksson, B.O., and B. Saltin (1974). Muscle metabolism during exercise in boys aged 11 to 16 years compared to adults. *Acta Paediatr. Belg.* 28 (Suppl.): 257–265.

Falk, B., O. Bar-Or, and J.D. MacDougall (1992). Thermoregulatory responses of pre-, mid-, and late-pubertal boys to exercise in dry heat. *Med. Sci. Sports Exerc.* 24:688–694.

Falk, B., O. Bar-Or, J.D. MacDougall, L. McGillis, R. Calvert, and F. Meyer (1991). Sweat lactate in exercising children and adolescents of varying physical maturity. *J. Appl. Physiol.* 71:1735–1740.

Foster, K.G., F.P. Ellis, C. Dore, A.N. Exton-Smith, and J.S. Weiner (1976). Sweat responses in the aged. *Age Aging* 5:91–101.

Fox, R.H., B.E. Lofstedt, P.M. Woodward, E. Eriksson, and B. Werkstrom (1969). Comparison of thermoregulatory function in men and women. *J. Appl. Physiol.* 26:444–453.

Fox, R.H., P.M. Woodward, A.N. Exton-Smith, M.F. Green, D.V. Donnison, and M.H. Wicks (1973). Body

THERMOREGULATION IN FEMALES **281**

temperatures in the elderly: a national study of physiological, social, and environmental conditions. *Br. Med. J.* 1:200-206.

Frascarolo, P., Y. Schutz, and E. Jequier (1990). Decreased thermal conductance during the luteal phase of the menstrual cycle in women. *J. Appl. Physiol.* 69:2029-2033.

Frye, A.J., and E. Kamon (1981). Responses to dry heat of men and women with similar aerobic capacities. *J. Appl. Physiol.* 50:65-70.

Frye, A.J., and E. Kamon (1983). Sweating efficiency in acclimated men and women exercising in humid and dry heat. *J. Appl. Physiol.* 54:972-977.

Frye, A.J., E. Kamon, and M. Webb (1982). Responses of menstrual women, amenorrheal women, and men to exercise in a hot, dry environment. *Eur. J. Appl. Physiol.* 48:279-288.

Gallow, D., T.E. Graham, and S. Pfeiffer (1984). Comparative thermoregulatory responses to acute cold in women of Asian and European descent. *Human Biol.* 56:19-34.

Gibson, T.E., and W.B. Shelley (1948). Sexual and racial differences in the response of sweat glands to acetylcholine and pilocarpine. *J. Invest. Dermatol.* 11:137-142.

Gisolfi, C.V., and J.S. Cohen (1979). Relationships between training, heat acclimation, and heat tolerance in men and women: the controversy revisited. *Med. Sci. Sports* 11:56-59.

Gonzalez, R.R., L.G. Berglund, and J.A.J. Stolwijk (1980). Thermoregulation in humans of different ages during thermal transients. In: Z. Szelenyi, and M. Szekely (eds.) *Proceedings of a Satellite Conference of the 28th Congress Physiological Sciences.* Pecs, Czechoslovakia: International Union of Physiological Sciences, pp. 357-361.

Graham, T.E. (1983). Alcohol ingestion and sex differences in the thermal responses to mild exercise in a cold environment. *Hum. Biol.* 55:463-476.

Grucza, R., J.L. Lecroart, J.J. Hauser, and Y. Houdas (1985). Dynamics of sweating in men and women during passive heating. *Eur. J. Appl. Physiol.* 54:309-314.

Hardy, J.D., and E.F. Dubois (1940). Differences between men and women in their responses to heat and cold. *Proc. Nat. Acad. Sci. (US).* 26:389-398.

Haslag, W.M., and A.B. Hertzman (1965). Temperature regulation in young women. *J. Appl. Physiol.* 20:1283-1288.

Havenith, G., Y. Inoue, V. Luttikholt, and W.L. Kenney (1995). Age predicts cardiovascular, but not thermoregulatory, responses to humid heat stress. *Eur. J. Appl. Physiol.* 70:88-96.

Havenith, G., and H. van Middendorp (1990). The relative influence of physical fitness, acclimation state, anthropometric measures and gender on individual reactions to heat stress. *Europ. J. Appl. Physiol.* 61:419-427.

Haymes, E.M. (1984). Physiological responses of female athletes to heat stress: A review. *Phys. Sportsmed.* 12(3):45-59.

Haymes, E.M., E.R. Buskirk, J.L. Hodgson, H.M. Lundegren, and W.C. Nicholas (1974). Heat tolerance of exercising lean and heavy prepubertal girls. *J. Appl. Physiol.* 36:566-571.

Haymes, E.M., R.J. McCormick, and E.R. Buskirk (1975). Heat tolerance of exercising lean and obese prepubertal boys. *J. Appl. Physiol.* 39:457-461.

Henschel, A., M.B. Cole, and O. Lyczkowskyj (1968). Heat tolerance of elderly persons living in a subtropical climate. *J. Gerontol.* 23:17-22.

Hertig, B.A., H.S. Belding, K.K. Kraning, D.L. Batterton, C.R. Smith, and F. Sargent (1963). Artificial acclimatization of women to heat. *J. Appl. Physiol.* 18:383-386.

Hessemer, V., and K. Bruck (1985). Influence of menstrual cycle on shivering, skin blood flow, and sweating responses measured at night. *J. Appl. Physiol.* 59:1902-1910.

Hirata, K., T. Nagasaka, A. Hirai, M. Hirashita, T. Takahata, and T. Nunomura (1985). Effects of human menstrual cycle on thermoregulatory vasodilation during exercise. *Eur. J. Appl. Physiol.* 54:559-565.

Horstman, D.H., and E. Christensen (1982). Acclimatization to dry heat: Active men vs. active women. *J. Appl. Physiol.* 52:825-831.

Inbar, O., O. Bar-Or, R. Dotan, and B. Gutin (1981). Conditioning vs. work-in-the-heat as methods for acclimatizing 8-10 year old boys to dry heat. *J. Appl. Physiol.* 50:406-411.

Jones, R.L., J.J. Botti, W.A. Anderson, and N.L. Bennett (1985). Thermoregulation during aerobic exercise in pregnancy. *Obstet. Gynecol.* 65:340-345.

Kawahata, A. (1960). Sex differences in sweating. In: H. Yoshimura, K. Ogata, and S. Itoh (eds.) *Essential Problems in Climatic Physiology.* Kyoto: Nankodo, pp. 169-184.

Kenney, W.L. (1995). Body fluid and temperature regulation as a function of age. In: D.R. Lamb, C.V. Gisolfi, and E.R. Nadel (eds.) *Perspectives in Exercise and Sports Medicine, Vol. 8: Exercise in Older Adults.* Carmel, IN: Cooper Publishing Group, pp. 305-345.

Kenney, W.L. (1988). Control of heat-induced vasodilation in relation to age. *Eur. J. Appl. Physiol.* 57:120-125.

Kenney, W.L. (1985). A review of comparative responses of men and women to heat stress. *Envir. Res.* 37:1-11.

Kenney, W.L., and R.K. Anderson (1988a). Heat balance during exercise in relation to age. In: C. Dotson (ed.) *Exercise Physiology: Current Selected Research, Vol. iii.* New York: AMS Press, pp. 113-120.

Kenney, W.L., and R.K. Anderson (1998b). Responses of older and younger women to exercise in dry and humid heat without fluid replacement. *Med. Sci. Sports Exerc.* 20:155–160.

Kenney, W.L., and E.R. Buskirk (1995). Functional consequences of sarcopenia: effects on thermoregulation. *J. Gerontol.* 50A:78–85.

Kenney, W.L., and J.L. Hodgson (1987). Heat tolerance, thermoregulation and aging. *Sports Med.* 4:446–456.

Kenney, W.L., C.G. Tankersley, D.L. Newswanger, D.E. Hyde, and S.M. Puhl (1990). Age and hypohydration independently influence the peripheral vascular response to heat stress. *J. Appl. Physiol.* 68:1902–1908.

Kenshalo, D.R. (1966). Changes in the cool threshold associated with phases of the menstrual cycle. *J. Appl. Physiol.* 21:1031–1039.

Kleitman, N., and A. Ramsaroop (1948). Periodicity in body temperature and heart rate. *Endocrinology* 43:1–20.

Kolka, M.A., and L.A. Stephenson (1989). Control of sweating during the human menstrual cycle. *Eur. J. Appl. Physiol.* 58:890–895.

Kollias, J., L. Bartlett, V. Bergsteinova, J.S. Skinner, E.R. Buskirk, and W.C. Nicholas (1974). Metabolic and thermal responses of women during cooling in water. *J. Appl. Physiol.* 36:577–580.

Lamanca, J.J., E.M. Haymes, J.A. Daly, R.J. Moffatt, and M.F. Waller. (1988). Sweat iron loss of male and female runners during exercise. *Int. J. Sports. Med.* 9:52–55.

Lamont, L.S. (1987). Sweat lactate secretion during exercise in relation to women's aerobic capacity. *J. Appl. Physiol.* 62:194–198.

Landing, B.H., T.R. Wells, and M.L. Williamson (1968). Studies on the growth of eccrine sweat glands. In B.D. Cheek (ed.) *Human Growth.* Philadelphia: Lea & Febiger, pp. 382–395.

Macey, S.M., and D.F. Schneider (1993). Deaths from excessive heat and excessive cold among the elderly. *Gerontologist* 33:497–500.

Main, K., K.O. Nilsson, and N.E. Skakkebaek (1991). Influence of sex and growth hormone deficiency on sweating. *Scand. J. Clin. Lab. Invest.* 51:475–480.

Martin, H.L., J.L. Loomis, and W.L. Kenney (1995). Maximal skin vascular conductance in subjects aged 5 to 85. *J. Appl. Physiol.* 79:297–301.

McMurray, R.G., and V.L. Katz (1990). Thermoregulation in pregnancy. Implications for exercise. *Sports Med.* 10:146–158.

McMurray, R.G., M.J. Berry, V.L. Katz, D.G. Graetzer, and R.C. Cefalo (1990). The thermoregulation of pregnant women during aerobic exercise in the water: a longitudinal approach. *Eur. J. Appl. Physiol.* 61:119–123.

Meyer, F., and O. Bar-Or (1994). Fluid and electrolyte loss during exercise: The pediatric angle. *Sports Med.* 18:4–9.

Meyer, F., O. Bar-Or, J. MacDougall, and J.F. Heigenhauser (1992). Sweat electrolyte loss during exercise in the heat: effect of gender and maturation. *Med. Sci Sports Exerc.* 24:776–781.

Morimoto, T., Z. Slabochova, R.K. Naman, and F. Sargent, II (1967). Sex differences in physiological reactions to thermal stress. *J. Appl. Physiol.* 22:526–532.

Nicklas, B.J., A.C. Hackney, and R.L. Sharp (1989). The menstrual cycle and exercise: performance, muscle glycogen, and substrate responses. *Int. J. Sports. Med.* 10:264–269.

Nunneley, S.A. (1978). Physiological responses of women to thermal stress: a review. *Med. Sci. Sports* 10:250–255.

Pivarnik, J.M., C.J. Marichal, T. Spillman, and J.R. Morrow, Jr. (1992). Menstrual cycle phase affects temperature regulation during endurance exercise. *J. Appl. Physiol.* 72:543–548.

Ramlow, J.M., and J.H. Kuller (1990). Effects of the summer heat wave of 1988 on daily mortality in Allegheny county, PA. *Publ. Health Rep.* 105:151–165.

Robinson, S., and A.H. Robinson (1954). Chemical composition of sweat. *Physiol. Rev.* 34:202–220.

Rooke, G.A., M.V. Savage, and G.L. Brengelmann (1994). Maximal skin blood flow is decreased in elderly men. *J.Appl. Physiol.* 77:11–14.

Rowell, L.B. (1974). Human cardiovascular adjustments to exercise and cardiovascular thermal stress. *Physiol. Rev.* 54:75–159.

Sato, K., and F. Sato (1983). Individual variations in structure and function of human eccrine sweat gland. *Am. J. Physiol.* 245:R203–R208.

Sawka, M.N., M.M. Toner, R.P. Francesconi, and K.B. Pandolf (1983). Hypohydration and exercise: effects of heat acclimation, gender, and environment. *J. Appl. Physiol.* 55:1147–1153.

Senay, L.C., Jr. (1973). Body fluids and temperature responses of heat-exposed women before and after ovulation with and without rehydration. *J. Physiol.* 232:209–219.

Senay, L.C., Jr., and S. Fortney (1975). Untrained females: effects of submaximal exercise and heat on body fluids. *J. Appl. Physiol.* 39:643–647.

Sens, D.A., M.A. Simmons, and S.S. Spicer (1985). The analysis of human sweat proteins by isoelectric focusing. I. Sweat collection utilizing the Macroduct system demonstrates the previously unrecognized sex-related proteins. *Pediatr. Res.* 19:873–878.

Shapiro, Y., K.B. Pandolf, B.A. Avellini, N.A. Pimental, and R.F. Goldman (1980). Physiological responses of men and women to humid and dry heat. *J. Appl. Physiol.* 49:1–8.

Shoenfeld, Y., R. Udassin, Y. Shapiro, A. Ohri, and E. Sohar (1978). Age and sex difference in response to short exposure to extreme dry heat. *J. Appl. Physiol.* 44:1–4.

Silver, A., W. Montagna, and I. Karacan (1964). Age and sex differences in spontaneous adrenergic and cholinergic human sweating. *J. Invest. Dermatol.* 43:255–265.

Sloan, R.E.G., and W.R. Keatinge (1973). Cooling rates of young people swimming in cold water. *J. Appl. Physiol.* 35:371–375.

Spina, R.J., T. Ogawa, W.M. Kohrt, W.M. Martin, J.O. Holloszy, and A.A. Ehsani (1993). Differences in cardiovascular adaptations to endurance exercise training between older men and women. *J. Appl. Physiol.* 75:849–855.

Stephenson, L.A., and M.A. Kolka (1988a). Effect of gender, circadian period and sleep loss on thermal responses during exercise. In: K. Pandolf, H. Sawka, and R. Gonzalez (eds.) *Human Performance Physiology Environmental Medicine at Terrestrial Extremes.* Indianapolis: Benchmark Press, pp. 267–304.

Stephenson, L.A., and M.A. Kolka (1985). Menstrual cycle phase and time of day alter reference signal controlling arm blood flow and sweating. *Am. J. Physiol.* 249:R186–R191.

Stephenson, L.A., and M.A. Kolka (1988b). Plasma volume during heat stress and exercise in women. *Eur. J. Appl. Physiol.* 57:373–381.

Sugarek, N.J. (1986). Temperature lowering after iced water. Enhanced effect in the elderly. *J. Am. Geriatr. Soc.* 34:526–529.

Tanaka, M. (1956). Studies on the important biological factors influencing the ability to perspire. Part I. Effect of age on the ability to perspire (in Japanese). *J. Physiol. Soc. Jap.* 18:390–394.

Tankersley, C.G., W.C. Nicholas, D.R. Deaver, D. Mikita, and W.L. Kenney (1992). Estrogen replacement in middle-aged women: thermoregulatory responses to exercise in the heat. *J. Appl. Physiol.* 73:1238–1245.

Tankersley, C.G., J. Smolander, W.L. Kenney, and S.M. Fortney (1991). Sweating and skin blood flow during exercise: effect of age and maximal oxygen uptake. *J. Appl. Physiol.* 71:235–242.

Wagner, J.A., and S.M. Horvath (1985a). Cardiovascular reactions to cold exposures differ with age and gender. *J. Appl. Physiol.* 58:187–192.

Wagner, J.A., and S.M. Horvath (1985b). Influences of age and gender on human thermoregulatory responses to cold exposures. *J. Appl. Physiol.* 58:180–186.

Wagner, J.A., S.M. Horvath, K. Kitagawa, and N.W. Bolduan (1987). Comparisons of blood and urinary responses to cold exposures in young and older men and women. *J. Gerontol.* 42:173–179.

Watts, A.J. (1971). Hypothermia in the aged: A study of the role of cold-sensitivity. *Environ. Res.* 5:119–126.

Weinman, K.P., Z. Slabochova, E.M. Bernauer, T. Morimoto, and F. Sargent III. (1967). Reactions of men and women to repeated exposure to humid heat. *J. Appl. Physiol.* 22:533–538.

Wells, C.L., and S.M. Horvath (1974). Responses to exercise in a hot environment as related to the menstrual cycle. *J. Appl. Physiol.* 36:299–302.

Wyndham, C.H., J.F. Morrison, and C.G. Williams (1965). Heat reactions of male and female Caucasians. *J. Appl. Physiol.* 20:357–364.

Wyndham, C.H., J.F. Morrison, C.G. Williams, G.A.G. Bredell, J. Peter, M.J. Von Rahden, L.D. Holdsworth, C.H. Van Graan, A.J. Van Rensburg, and A. Munro (1964a). Physiological reactions to cold of Caucasian females. *J. Appl. Physiol.* 19:877–880.

Wyndham, C.H., J.S. Ward, N.B. Strydom, J.F. Morrison, C.G. Williams, G.A.G. Bredell, J. Peter, M.J.E. Von Rahden, L.D. Holdsworth, C.H. Van Graan, A.J. Van Rensburg, and A. Munro (1964b). Physiological reactions of Caucasian and Bantu males in acute exposure to cold. *J. Appl. Physiol.* 19:583–592.

Yousef, M.K., D.B. Dill, T.S. Vitez, S.D. Hillyard, and A.S. Goldman (1984). Thermoregulatory responses to desert heat: age, race and sex. *J. Gerontol.* 39:406–414.

Yousef, M.K., S. Sagawa, and K. Shiraki (1986). Thermoregulatory responses of the elderly population. *J. Univ. Occup. Environ. Health* 8:219–227.

DISCUSSION

KENNEY: We did see much larger increases in skin blood flow consequent to a given increase in core temperature in postmenopausal women after estrogen replacement therapy. The next obvious question becomes, what is the mechanism? That is what we are looking into now. Not only does estrogen have the potential to exert its effect through direct cellular mechanisms, but there are catecholamine-like effects of estrogens, there are body fluid-retention effects of estrogen, etc.

NADEL: Gonzalez addressed sweat gland effectiveness, demonstrating that there are no differences between men and women in terms of the sweating rate per unit of internal temperature increase. This illustration impacts on some of your conclusions about differences between men and women in heat tolerance. The Frye and Kamon study in 1981, as well as a 1977 study by Roberts and colleagues, attributed differences between men and women to their state of heat acclimation or state of physical training, or in reality, their state of sweat gland training. Finally, there have been sophisticated studies over the years by Su Ki Hong showing that Ama divers of Korea and Japan, women who are acclimatized to cold water, reduce heat flow to the periphery to a greater extent than when they are unacclimatized.

BAR-OR: Real gender-related differences do exist. Indeed, men and women differ in $\dot{V}O_2$max, but studies that equated $\dot{V}O_2$max between the sexes still found differences in thermoregulatory effectiveness. Likewise, differences in sweating pattern are a real phenomenon. They are not merely related to different levels of aerobic fitness or body composition as you have suggested. Some of the differences are diminished if you normalize for such variables, but the differences do not disappear altogether.

KENNEY: Maybe, in an effort to bring those two points of view together, it is fair to say that the impact of both $\dot{V}O_2$max and heat acclimation on thermoregulatory responses by far outweigh any of the differences that people have attributed to either age or gender. For example, the effect of $\dot{V}O_2$max on sweating sensitivity is larger than the differential responses that people have attributed to gender and, in most cases, to age. Secondly, with respect to cold tolerance, it is important to note that adiposity in women across the life span is only part of the explanation of that tolerance. In fact, Michel Ducharme and Peter Tikuikis have demonstrated that when people are immersed in cold water or when the limbs are cooled, the lean tissue mass (i.e., muscle) contributes 70–80% to the total tissue insulation. Because the limbs are really what need to be protected first and foremost during cold exposure, we must address the issues of total body size and lean body mass—not just subcutaneous body fat.

NADEL: Larry, don't you agree that elevating $\dot{V}O_2$max in and of itself does not train sweat glands?

KENNEY: That is true for sweat gland function; however, with respect to other thermoregulatory effector responses, such as control of skin vasodilatation, there is an interactive influence of $\dot{V}O_2$max per se, heat acclimation, and training status, each of which plays a role.

NADEL: My point is that a swimmer who is trained in cold water may have a high $\dot{V}O_2$max but not necessarily a high heat tolerance.

KANTER: Have there been any studies done that attempted to diminish the sweat rate differences between men and women by hyperhydrating the women before exercise?

BAR-OR: I'm not familiar with any studies that have used that approach.

GISOLFI: Bass did a study on hyperhydration and showed that it can increase sweating rate.

BAR-OR: In females?

GISOLFI: No, not in females, but I suspect the response would be the same.

KANTER: When we develop fluid replacement guidelines for people, should we have different guidelines for women than for men? It seems to me that if hyperhydration enhances sweat rate, a woman might be better off if she drank relatively more than a man.

BAR-OR: The only related data that I can think of is a recent experiment in our laboratory (Wilk et al., in preparation) in which girls and boys were slightly hyperhydrated (+0.5% of initial body weight), but the boys still had a higher sweating rate.

HORSWILL: Ultimately, females or males are going to drink that which is palatable, and drink more of what they like. Do you think some component in the beverage, like sodium content, might be critical for stimulating additional fluid consumption in females?

BAR-OR: As far as the ability of the females to prevent dehydration, subjects in our early studies who drank grape-flavored beverages, irrespective of what the beverage content was, ended up with a positive water balance, which surprised us. Since then, we have compared responses to drinking water, flavored water, and flavored carbohydrate-electrolyte solutions. It seems that the addition of NaCl to flavored water does induce a greater intake, but the latter experiment was done with males only.

HORSWILL: So the recommendation for greater fluid intake in females may not be correct?

BAR-OR: I think it is still premature to say. We cannot state categorically at this stage that the addition of Na+ to water can prevent dehydration in females.

KENNEY: The link between drinking more fluid and sweating more relies on keeping that fluid in the vascular compartment. Unless that fluid is retained as part of the plasma volume, it cannot do much to enhance sweating. If the goal is to change the recommended volume or content of fluid replacement drinks to enhance thermoregulatory sweating, the key may be to come up with some way to retain the fluid within the vascular compartment longer.

MURRAY: Oded, are the gender-related differences you noted in sweating rate and sweating threshold also accompanied by a difference in actual evaporative cooling, and, if so, what other heat-loss mechanisms compensate for the difference?

BAR-OR: I can't cite specific studies that looked at that. However, my guess is that females and children may have a more efficient sweating pattern. They have a greater density of heat-activated sweat glands per square centimeter. Each of their drops is smaller than the sweat drops in the adult males.

TERJUNG: Are there differences in blood flow to the skin that bear upon differences in sweating rate?

BAR-OR: The methods that have been used so far have not given us a definitive answer to that question.

CLAPP: With regard to some of the information you discussed in the secion on pregnancy, I would like to make four points. First, all the malformation data from animals has been in response to thermal stresses that are unbelievably excessive in both their intensity and duration and are far removed from anything that a human being might experience except perhaps in an ultramarathon race. Secondly, in the retrospective studies in human beings, no one has ever measured the temperature of the women, let alone that of the fetus; the temperature of 38.5°C is arbitrary. Third, quite a few studies reported in the Scandinavian literature dealing with the thermal responses to sauna bathing in pregnancy found that pregnant women handled that heat stress very well. Fourth, in the article I wrote in 1991 the thermal stresses in terms of energy expenditure were identical in the women before and throughout pregnancy and clearly showed a change in both the magnitude and the rate of change of temperature during exercise in pregnancy.

BAR-OR: If I remember your 1991 study correctly, the women at the more advanced stages of pregnancy volitionally exercised at lower metabolic levels.

CLAPP: All the women exercised at 60–65% of their $\dot{V}O_2$max at each time point before and during pregnancy.

BAR-OR: But didn't they self-select the work rates during the experiments when you measured their rectal temperatures?

CLAPP: We kept them at 60–65% of their $\dot{V}O_2$max.

BAR-OR: Did the $\dot{V}O_2$max change during pregnancy?

CLAPP: The data indicate that for an untrained woman or a woman who maintains her exercise performance at a standard level, the $\dot{V}O_2$max is either unchanged or maybe slightly increased during pregnancy, but a significant increase has never been documented.

BLIMKIE: Is there any information on thermoregulatory changes in women who have eating disorders or menstrual cycle irregularities? Are they at additional risk for heat illness, particularly the runners who are generating extreme heat loads and often working in very extreme environments?

BAR-OR: Some 20 y ago Mervin Davies and Fohlin studied thermoregulation in girls with anorexia nervosa and found that both in hot climates and in cold climates these girls had a deficient thermoregulatory ability. I don't remember whether there was a control group or whether they compared responses once these girls had been nutritionally replenished. They concluded that it was not merely a reduction in subcutaneous fat that caused the temperature regulation deficiency. There may have been some hypothalamic dysfunction.

KENNEY: Thermoregulation is one area where we need to move away from the ubiquitous experimental design of taking all different types of people and exercising them at the same $\%\dot{V}O_2$max, assuming that solves a lot of ills of the experimental design. The calculable metabolic heat production is not a function of the $\%\dot{V}O_2$max; it is a function of the absolute $\dot{V}O_2$ for steady-state aerobic activities. However, the heat dissipation responses are more closely aligned to $\%\dot{V}O_2$max.

BAR-OR: Equating the conditions is an unresolved dilemma, especially when subjects differ markedly in body mass. You can do well on one end of it, but the blanket will be too short on the other end, and you cannot really satisfy both the absolute and the relative aspects of metabolic heat production and dissipation.

SUTTON: In epidemiological studies where males and females compete in races together, it is very interesting to note that there is no significant difference in the incidence of thermal illness between the males and females. In fact, where deaths have occurred, it has been only males who died. There are indices of motivation in the competitive environment showing that the males seem to be hell-bent on self destruction—more so than the females. Those motivational data have been published in the *Med. J. Aust.* by D. Lyle at the end of 1994.

8

Skeletal Muscle Function and Energy Metabolism

DIGBY G. SALE, Ph.D.

LAWRENCE L. SPRIET, Ph.D.

INTRODUCTION

The purpose of this chapter is to review gender differences in skeletal muscle structure and function and in energy metabolism throughout the life cycle. The emphasis is on strength performance and on adaptations to strength ("resistance") training. Its uniqueness will be the very fact that the whole life cycle is considered and that gender differences are highlighted. The chapter must review the growth and development literature, the extensive literature on young adults, and the growing body of literature on aging. Therefore, the present review must be less extensive than reviews devoted solely to one of the major life cycle periods. For more extensive reviews of muscle structure and function, the reader is referred to examples on growth and development (Blimkie, 1989; Malina & Bouchard, 1991) and aging (Booth et al., 1994; Cartee, 1994; Porter et al., 1995b; Rodgers & Evans, 1993; Vandervoort, 1992; White, 1995). There is a vast literature on skeletal muscle structure and function in young adults, but few reviews focus on gender differences, examples being those by Laubach (1976) and Holloway and Baechle (1990).

GENDER DIFFERENCES IN SKELETAL MUSCLE STRUCTURE THROUGHOUT THE LIFE CYCLE

Birth to Young Adulthood

Muscle Size/Mass. Muscles increase in length and cross-sectional area (CSA) throughout the growing years from birth to adulthood. Muscle CSA increases several-fold during this period (Imamura et al., 1983; Johnston & Malina, 1966; Kanehisa et al., 1995; Tanner et al., 1981). The gender difference in muscle CSA is small (~5–10%) until about age 14 y, after which the difference (males > females) increases markedly to ~30–50% by age ~20 y (Johnston & Malina, 1966; Parker et al., 1990; Tanner et al., 1981). The beginning of the growing gender difference in muscle CSA coincides with the marked increase in serum testosterone in the males (Winter, 1978). As the gender difference in muscle size develops, it becomes more marked in the upper than lower limbs so that when young adulthood is reached women have only about 50% of the upper body but about 70% of the lower limb muscle size of men.

Muscle Fiber Number and Area. It is generally thought that in humans maximal fiber number is fixed at or soon after birth (Gollnick et al., 1981; Malina & Bouchard, 1991). Thus, increases in muscle length and CSA during the growing years can be wholly accounted for by corresponding increases in muscle fiber length and CSA. Fiber area increases 15- 20- fold from birth through childhood, adolescence, and young adulthood (Aherne et al., 1971; Brooke & Engel, 1969; Colling-Saltin, 1980; Lexell et al., 1992), with up to half of the increase having occurred by 5 y (Colling-Saltin, 1980; Lexell et al., 1992).

There is little gender difference in fiber area in infancy and childhood (Aherne et al., 1971; Brooke & Engel, 1969). Males begin to show larger fibers during adolescence (Aherne et al., 1971; Costill et al., 1976; Glenmark et al., 1992; Malina & Bouchard, 1991; Saltin et al., 1977). There is a high correlation between fiber area and body height during the growing years, so it has been suggested that boys begin to overtake girls in height and fiber size at about the same time (age 15 y) (Aherne et al., 1971).

Some cross-sectional data suggest that in males mean fiber area increases to age 25 y (Lexell et al., 1992), whereas other cross-sectional (Malina & Bouchard, 1991) and longitudinal (Glenmark et al., 1992) data indicate that peak fiber size is already attained at age 16 y in both males and females.

In relation to fiber types, it is mainly the type II (fast-twitch) fibers that become larger in males. This is quite evident by age 16 y, at a time when there is little gender difference in type I (slow-twitch) area (Glenmark et al., 1992).

Muscle Fiber Types. Human skeletal muscle is composed of two main muscle fiber types: type I, also known as slow-twitch fibers, and type II, also known as fast-twitch fibers. Type II fibers are often classified into two subtypes—IIA and IIB. (There is also a small percentage of undifferentiated II "C" fibers.) The IIA fibers are also called fast, oxidative, glycolytic fibers (FOG); IIB fibers are called fast, glycolytic (FG). As their names imply, a major functional difference between the main fiber types is contraction speed. The IIB and IIA fibers may have 10 and 3 times, respectively, the maximum shortening velocity of type I fibers (Larsson & Moss, 1993). The large differences in shortening speed would be expected to influence velocity-dependent strength and power performance of muscles composed of different relative numbers of type I and II fibers (i.e., % type I or II fibers).

At birth, there is a relatively large (10–20%) proportion of undifferentiated IIC fibers. The percentage of IIC fibers decreases rapidly, and adult values of < 5% are attained by 1 y (Colling-Saltin, 1980; Elder & Kakulas, 1993). The percentage of type I fibers increases rapidly after birth at the expense of the undifferentiated fibers, which are decreasing in number. The increase in type I fibers may be most pronounced in postural, locomotory, and "anti-gravity" muscles (Elder & Kakulas, 1993; Vogler & Bove, 1985). By age 1 y, the adult percentage of type I fibers has been nearly attained; furthermore, there is some evidence that children may have higher percentages of type I fibers than do adults (Elder & Kakulas, 1993; Lexell et al., 1992; Oertel, 1988).

There appears to be little gender difference in muscle fiber distribution in infancy and childhood (Bell et al., 1980; Colling-Saltin, 1980; Malina & Bouchard, 1991; Vogler & Bove, 1985); however, in the teen years there is evidence of a greater percentage of type I fibers in males and a greater inter-individual variation in males (Glenmark et al., 1992; Komi & Karlsson 1978; Saltin et al., 1977). As will be discussed in the section on young adults, the evidence on gender difference in muscle fiber type distribution is equivocal.

Ultrastructure. Boys and girls aged 6 y have similar relative proportions of a muscle fiber occupied by myofibrils (83%), cytoplasm (11.5%), mitochondria (5%), and lipid droplets (0.5%). These proportions are similar to those found in young adults (Bell et al., 1980).

Muscle Composition. The chemical composition of muscle changes from birth through adolescence or young adulthood. The major changes are decreases in sodium and chloride ion content, and increases in potassium ion and phosphorus content as well as increases in sarcoplasmic and myofibrillar protein content. A large proportion of these changes are evident by 1 y of age (Dickerson & Widdowson, 1960). The changes reflect the large increase in muscle fiber size and large decrease in extracellular space that occurs from birth onward (Malina & Bouchard, 1991).

Young Adulthood

Muscle Size. Men have larger muscles than do women, especially in the upper limbs (Heyward et al., 1986). Compared to men, women have 50–60% of the upper arm and 65–70% of the thigh muscle CSA (Alway et al., 1990; Cureton et al., 1988; Kanehisa et al., 1994; Maughan et al., 1983a; Miller et al., 1993; Nygaard et al., 1983; O'Hagan et al., 1995; Sale et al., 1987; Schantz et al., 1983).

The gender difference in the sizes of upper vs. lower limb muscles corresponds to similar differences in skeletal size. Women have 65–75% of the humerus CSA and 85% of the femur CSA of men (Kanehisa et al., 1994; Miller et al., 1993; Sale et al., 1987). As with muscle size, the marked gender difference in bone size begins after age ~14 y (Johnston & Malina, 1966; Tanner et al., 1981).

Muscle Fiber Number. The greater muscle size of most men could be the result of both a greater fiber number and greater fiber area. The data on fiber number are contradictory. A gender difference in muscle fiber number might be most expected in upper limb muscles because gender effects on muscle size are greater in muscles of the upper body than in those of the lower body. In one study, women on average had only 69% of the number of fibers estimated in men's biceps brachii muscles, and these differences were statistically significant (Sale et al., 1987); others reported smaller, non-significant gender differences in fiber number for biceps (Alway et al., 1989; Miller et al., 1993) and triceps (Schantz et al. 1983).

In lower-limb muscles the results are also contradictory. Males seem to have more fibers in tibialis anterior muscles (Henriksson-Larsen, 1985) but not in the vastus lateralis (Miller et al., 1993; Schantz et al., 1981).

Interpretation of the fiber number data must consider the limitations of the method of *estimating* fiber number *in-vivo*, which consists of dividing mean whole muscle CSA by fiber area, which is usually measured in a single biopsy sample. The method assumes that all fibers run parallel to the long axis of the muscle and that all fibers run the whole length of the muscle and pass through the point where the scan is taken to obtain the measure of whole muscle CSA. A correction must also be made for non-contractile tissue (Alway et al. 1989; Henriksson-Larsen, 1985; Sale et al., 1987); this is especially relevant in a gender comparison because females have a greater relative amount of this tissue (Sale et al., 1987).

Regardless of whether or not a gender difference in fiber number exists, it is nevertheless clear that the larger sizes of the muscles of males are mainly due to their larger fiber areas. In five studies that reported both fiber number and mean fiber area, women had on average 84% of men's fiber number but only 65% of their fiber area (Alway et al., 1989; Henriksson-Larsen, 1985; Miller et al., 1993; Sale et al., 1987; Schantz et al., 1983). It is also evident that, regardless of gender or training status, fiber area correlates more strongly than fiber number with whole muscle CSA (Alway et al., 1989; MacDougall et al., 1984; Sale et al., 1987; Schantz et al., 1981).

Muscle Fiber Area. In the vastus lateralis, the muscle most studied, women have on average ~80, 70, and 60% of the type I, IIA, and IIB fiber areas of men, respectively (Figure 8-1, top). Gender differences also exist in the IIA/I, IIB/I, IIA/IIB area ratios (Figure 8-1, bottom). Men have greater IIA/I and IIB/I ratios, whereas women have a greater IIA/IIB ratio (Clarkson et al., 1981; Essen-Gustavsson, 1986; Glenmark et al., 1992; Klitgaard et al., 1990b; Nygaard, 1981; Saltin et al., 1977; Schantz et al., 1983; Simoneau & Bouchard, 1989; Simoneau et al, 1985; Staron et al., 1994).

There are limited data on other muscles. Relative to men, women have ~70% and 85% of the gastrocnemius type II and I fiber areas, respectively, and a greater II/I ratio (1.02 vs. 0.87) (Costill et al., 1976). This gender difference in II/I ratio is opposite that found in vastus lateralis, indicated previously, and in the biceps and triceps of the arms, in which the II/I ratio is greater in men (Miller et al., 1993; Schantz et al., 1983) (Figures 8-1 and 8-2, bottom).

The gender difference in whole muscle CSA is greater in the upper than lower limbs, as noted previously. Correspondingly, a greater gender difference in fiber area would be expected in upper than in lower limb muscles. To the contrary, the gender difference in fiber area between vastus lateralis and the biceps and triceps of the arms is much smaller than expected (Miller et al., 1993 [Figure 8-2, top]; Schantz et al., 1983). This suggests that the greater upper limb muscle size in men is due in part to a greater fiber number, an issue discussed previously. Consistent findings have been a greater II/I area ratio in upper than in lower limb muscles, and a greater gender difference (males > females) in this ratio in the upper limbs (Miller et al., 1993 [Figure 8-2, bottom]; Nygaard et al., 1983; Schantz et al., 1983; Sale et al., 1987).

Muscle Fiber Types. The vastus lateralis of the thigh is the muscle most studied in comparisons of muscle fiber type distributions between young women and men. The results of comparisons have not been consistent, no doubt due in part to sampling errors (i.e., both small vs. large subject samples and biopsy sample errors) and insufficient control for activity level, which may influence fiber type distribution. The study (Simoneau & Bouchard, 1989) with the largest sample sizes indicated a small

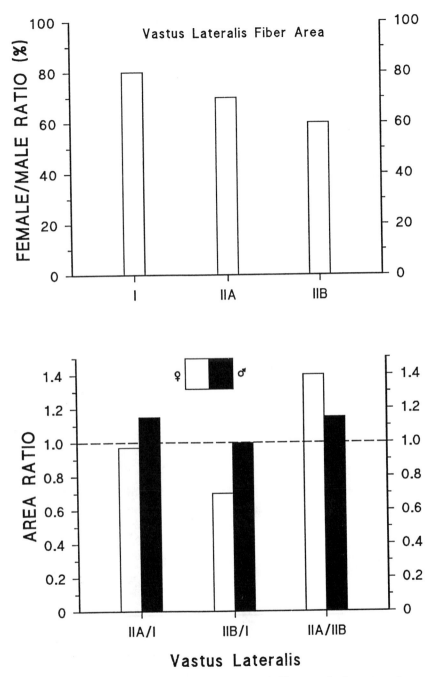

FIGURE 8-1. Gender difference in vastus lateralis muscle fiber area. In the top panel, women's values for the three fiber types are given as a percentage of men's values. In the bottom panel, women's and men's fiber area ratios are compared. See text for references.

SKELETAL MUSCLE FUNCTION AND ENERGY METABOLISM **295**

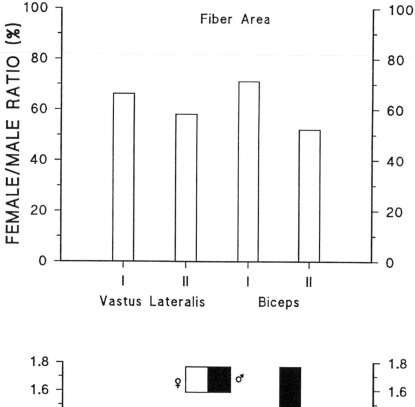

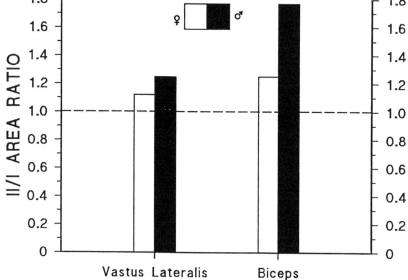

FIGURE 8-2. The top panel shows that the gender difference in fiber area is similar in vastus lateralis and biceps brachii. In both muscles, the gender difference is greater for type II than type I fibers. In regard to the type II/I area ratio (bottom panel), the ratio is greater in men in both muscles, especially biceps. See text for discussion. Based on Miller et al. (1993).

but significantly greater percentage of type I fibers in women (51 ± 13 vs. 46 ± 15) but a smaller percentage of IIB fibers (12 ± 9 vs 15 ± 9); there was no significant difference in type IIA fibers (37 ± 10 vs. 39 ± 12) (Figure 8-3, top). A greater percentage of type I fibers in women has also been found in studies with smaller samples (Miller et al., 1993; Simoneau et al., 1985), but others have failed to show a significant difference (Froese & Houston, 1985; Houston et al., 1988; Prince et al., 1976, 1977; Ryushi et al., 1988; Schantz et al., 1983; Staron et al., 1994).

Simoneau et al. (1985) suggested that part of the discrepancy in the literature regarding gender differences in muscle fiber composition is the result of lack of control for activity level. As activity level increases, the percentage of type I fibers tends to increase, but more so in women, thus decreasing the gender difference (Nygaard, 1981). When Simoneau et al. (1985) carefully controlled for activity level by ensuring that subjects in the sedentary group were very inactive, they found in general that the sedentary subjects on average had a smaller percentage of type I fibers and higher percentage of IIB fibers compared to a more active population (Figure 8-3 bottom vs. top). The gender difference in the percentage of type I fibers was similar in the sedentary and active subjects.

The fiber type distribution may differ between genders during the late teens and mid-20s. In a longitudinal study (Glenmark et al. (1992), 55 males and 28 females were examined at age 16 y and again at 27 y. At age 16, males on average had an insignificantly greater percentage of type I fibers (55 vs. 51%), confirming previous observations (Komi & Karlsson, 1978; Saltin et al., 1977). At age 27 the converse was true; women had a significantly greater percentage of type I fibers (55 vs. 48%), confirming previous observations (Miller et al., 1993; Simoneau & Bouchard, 1989; Simoneau et al., 1985). Thus, between the mid-teens and mid-20s, the percentage of type I fibers increased in females and decreased in males (Figure 8-4).

Compared to studies on the vastus lateralis, few studies of other muscles have reported the fiber type composition in men and women. No differences in percentage of type I fibers have been found in the brachial biceps (Miller et al., 1993; Nygaard et al., 1983; Sale et al., 1987), the triceps (Schantz et al., 1983), the tibialis anterior (Henriksson-Larsen, 1985), or the gastrocnemius (Costill et al., 1976). All of these studies had small sample sizes.

The functional significance of the small gender difference in fiber type distribution is open to question. More important than the percentage of type I and II fibers is the percent fiber area, i.e., the proportion of whole muscle CSA occupied by a given fiber type. An example of the latter is shown in Figure 8-5. Based on this example of vastus lateralis, women would be expected to have the advantage in muscle endurance (greater type-I-percent fiber area), whereas men would have the advantage in high

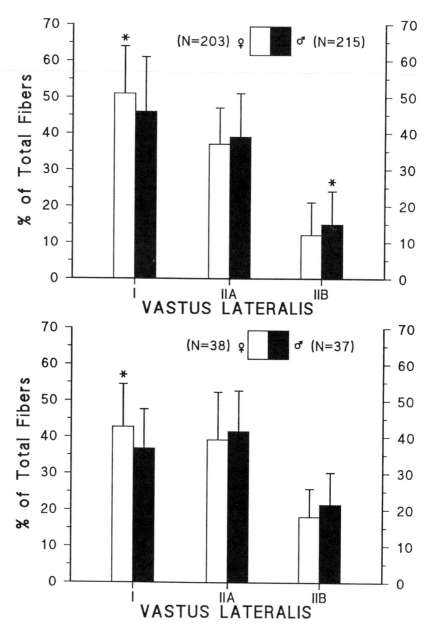

FIGURE 8-3. Top panel: Percentage of type I, IIA, and IIB fibers in vastus lateralis of large samples of women and men. Relatively small but significant differences (*) were found for type I and IIB fibers. Based on Simoneau and Bouchard (1989). Bottom panel: Percentage of type I, IIA, and IIB fibers in vastus lateralis of smaller samples of sedentary women and men. In these sedentary subjects, the %type I fibers was generally lower than in the more active sample in the top panel, but a gender difference (*) in %type I fibers was still observed. Based on Simoneau et al. (1985).

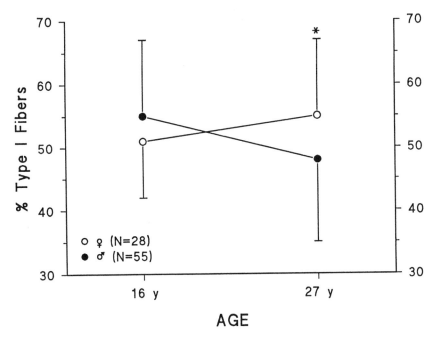

FIGURE 8-4. A longitudinal study of changes in %type I fibers in vastus lateralis between the ages of 16 and 27 years. At age 16 years there was no gender difference, but at 27 years females had a significantly (*) greater percentage of type I fibers. Based on Glenmark et al. (1992).

velocity concentric strength or isometric rate of force development (greater type-II-percent fiber area). Functional differences in strength will be considered later in the chapter.

Young Adulthood to Old Age

Muscle Size. Muscle size decreases from young adulthood onward. The decline in muscle size is relatively slow until age 60 y, then more rapid (Greig et al., 1993; Häkkinen & Häkkinen, 1991; Klitgaard et al., 1990a; Lexell et al., 1983; Overend et al., 1992; Phillips et al., 1992; Reed et al., 1991; Rice et al., 1989; Vandervoort & McComas, 1986; Young et al., 1984; 1985). For example, a cross-sectional study of women showed an 8% decrease in quadriceps CSA between ages 30–50 y and a more dramatic 20% reduction between ages 50–70 y (Häkkinen & Häkkinen, 1991; see Figure 8-25). The reported overall reduction in muscle size from young adulthood to old age varies somewhat depending on the actual ages of the subjects studied, the muscle groups studied, and the methods used to measure muscle CSA. In particular, the age range of the "old" subjects studied is a large influence, because the decline in muscle CSA accelerates beyond age 70 y. With consideration of these sources of variation, muscle size re-

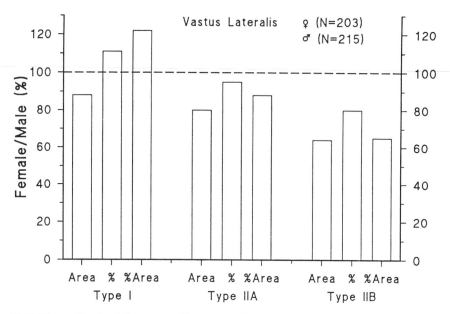

FIGURE 8-5. Gender differences in fiber area, %fiber type, and %fiber type area are shown for the vastus lateralis muscle. The %fiber area indicates the proportion of whole muscle CSA occupied by a given fiber type. The greatest differences are the women's greater %type I fiber area, and the men's greater type II area and %area. See text for further discussion. Based on Simoneau and Bouchard (1989).

ductions of ~10–35% have been reported between young adulthood and old age (Häkkinen & Häkkinen, 1991; Phillips et al., 1992; Vandervoort & McComas, 1986; Young et al., 1984).

Most studies relating advancing age to muscle atrophy have been cross-sectional, and caution has been recommended in interpreting these studies because there have been large changes in nutrition and health care over the life span of the oldest subjects used in these studies (Grimby & Saltin, 1983). Some of these influences may be offsetting. If more recent generations are attaining greater adult height and/or muscle mass (e.g., Häkkinen & Häkkinen, 1991), their absolute strength would be greater relative to previous generations, and the decline in strength with age would be exaggerated. On the other hand, subjects who survive into their 80s and 90s are a select population who perhaps had greater strength in their 50s, 60s, and 70s than did non-survivors; if so, data collected in their 80s and 90s data would tend to attenuate the decline in strength in these two decades. The few longitudinal studies reported show reasonably close agreement with the cross-sectional studies, suggesting that the previously discussed factors are offsetting. For example, Greig et al. (1993) observed a 6.4% decrease in quadriceps CSA in 4 men and 10 women examined at age ~74 y and again at age ~82 y. The yearly rate of loss (0.8%/y) in this group that consisted mostly of women was similar to that (~1%/y) reported in a cross-sectional study of women aged 50-70 y (Häkkinen & Häkkinen; 1991).

No consistent pattern of gender influence has emerged in relation to the decline in muscle size with aging. Reed et al. (1991) found greater losses of CSA in arm and thigh muscles of men than in women between the ages of 55-64 and 75+ y. In contrast, Vandervoort & McComas (1986) found a greater loss of calf muscle CSA in women than in men when comparing young adults to the very old (80-100 y). Finally, Phillips et al. (1992) reported a similar loss of adductor pollicis size in men and women in two groups whose mean ages were 28 y and 80 y, respectively.

Muscle Fiber Size and Number. The reduction in muscle size with advancing age appears to be more the result of a decline in fiber number than a decline in fiber area (Lexell & Downham, 1992; Lexell et al., 1988) (Figure 8-6). Based on cross-sectional studies in which direct muscle fiber counts have been made from whole vastus lateralis muscles, there may be a 30-50% loss of the number of muscle fibers in men by age 80 y. A loss of fibers is already evident by age 30 y, although the greatest loss seems to occur between ages 50 to 70 y (Lexell et al., 1988). The loss of muscle fib-

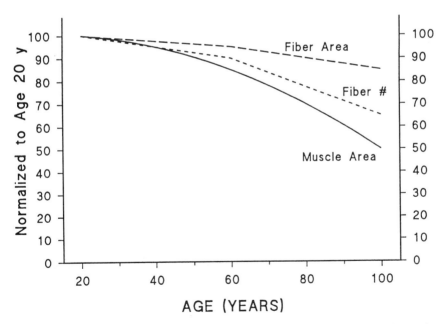

FIGURE 8-6. In vastus lateralis, loss of fibers contributes more than fiber atrophy to the whole muscle atrophy seen with aging (Lexell & Downham, 1992; Lexell et al., 1988). This pattern is depicted schematically in the figure.

ers is likely the result of the loss of motoneurons (motor units) that becomes especially evident after age 60 (Campbell et al., 1973). The loss of muscle fibers secondary to the loss of motoneurons is attenuated by the ability of surviving motoneurons to reinnervate fibers "orphaned" by deceased motoneurons. Thus, motor units of the elderly are enlarged, i.e., each motoneuron innervates a larger number of muscle fibers (Doherty et al., 1993b) (Figure 8-7).

It is not known whether the same pattern of fiber loss occurs in other muscles or in women and men; for example, in women the fiber loss in a chest muscle (pectoralis minor) was not as great as in vastus lateralis, and a decrease was not apparent in either muscle until after age 60 y (Sato et al., 1984).

To the extent that muscle fiber atrophy occurs with aging, it is more pronounced in type II fibers, resulting in a decrease in the II/I area ratio (Aniansson et al., 1986; Clarkson et al., 1981; Essen-Gustavsson & Borges, 1986; Klitgaard et al., 1990a, 1990b; Larsson, 1983; Larsson & Karlsson, 1978; Larsson et al., 1978, 1979; Lexell & Downham, 1992; Lexell et al.,

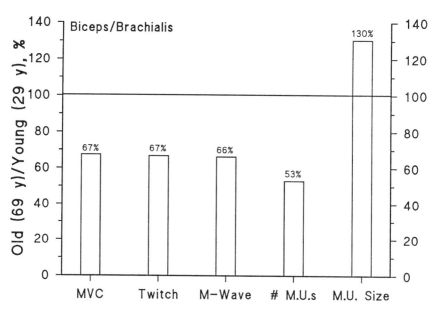

FIGURE 8-7. Effect of aging on voluntary isometric strength (MVC), evoked twitch force, compound muscle action potential amplitude (M-Wave), number of motor units (# M.U.s), and motor unit size (M.U. size) in biceps/brachialis. The values for the older adults ($\bar{X} = 69$ y) are expressed as a percentage of young ($\bar{X} = 29$ y) adult values. Subjects included both men and women. Note that the older adults had only about half the number of motor units of their younger counterparts, but surviving units were about 30% larger. These results indicate the loss of motoneurons with aging and the capacity of surviving neurons to adopt some of the "orphaned" muscle fibers. Based on Doherty et al. (1993b)

1988; Tomonga, 1977). In fact, some have reported no decrease in type I fiber area but substantial type II fiber atrophy in the elderly (Aniansson et al., 1986; Grimby et al. 1984; Jennekens et al. 1971; Lexell & Taylor, 1991). The rate of decrease in fiber size may accelerate after the age of 60 y (Essen-Gustavsson & Borges, 1986, Stalberg et al., 1989) (Figure 8-8).

In relation to a possible gender difference in aging-induced fiber atrophy, women show greater atrophy than men between the ages of 20 y and 70 y, particularly in type II fibers (Figure 8-9) (Essen-Gustavsson & Borges, 1986; Stalberg et al., 1989). Thus, the gender difference in fiber area is maintained or increased with advancing age (Aniansson et al., 1981; Grimby et al., 1982).

Muscle Fiber Types. There is lack of agreement in the literature on whether muscle fiber composition changes through adulthood to old age. As in young adults, vastus lateralis has been most studied in the elderly. Several cross-sectional studies have indicated an increase in the proportion of type I fibers with aging (Larsson, 1983; Larsson et al., 1979; Orlander et al., 1978), but others have shown no change (Clarkson et al., 1981; Essen-Gustavsson & Borges, 1986; Grimby et al., 1984; Klitgaard et al., 1990b; Lexell & Downham, 1992; Lexell et al., 1983, 1988) or even a decrease (Klitgaard et al., 1990a). The relatively small number of subjects,

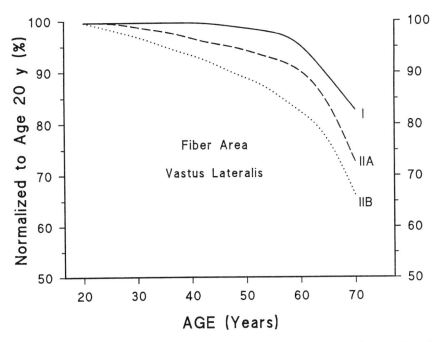

FIGURE 8-8. Decrease in vastus lateralis type I, IIA, and IIB fiber area with aging. Type II fibers are affected more than type I. Based on Essen-Gustavsson and Borges (1986).

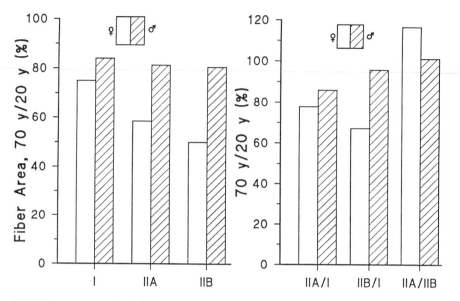

FIGURE 8-9. Age-related decline in vastus lateralis fiber area in men and women between 20 and 70 years. Left panel: Atrophy of all fiber types is more pronounced in women, particularly II fibers. Right panel: Fiber area ratios. The biggest changes in the elderly are the decreased IIB/I ratio in women, and the increased IIA/IIB ratio in women. Based on Essen-Gustavsson and Borges (1986).

the sampling error from single biopsy samples (Grimby & Saltin, 1983), and the varied activity levels of the subjects (Larsson, 1983) have likely contributed to the discrepancies.

Additional evidence suggests a transition from fast to slow muscle in the elderly. A rare longitudinal study reported an increase in percentage of type I fibers in gastrocnemius with age, and this increase was independent of activity level (Trappe et al., 1995) (Figure 8-10). The elderly show a greater interindividual variation in muscle fiber composition and a greater loss of type II fibers, based on whole muscle specimens (Lexell et al., 1983, 1988). Electrophysiological studies indicate a relatively greater loss of fast-conducting motoneurons in the elderly (Campbell et al., 1973). In some muscles there is slowing of the evoked-twitch contractile response in the elderly (Cupido et al., 1992; Davies et al., 1986; Petrella et al., 1989; Vandervoort & McComas, 1986). Finally, old muscles show striking changes in the co-expression of different types of myosin heavy chains (MHC) in single fibers; for example, old muscles have more fibers co-expressing types I and IIA MHC in vastus lateralis and biceps (Klitgaard et al., 1990b).

The few studies that have compared muscle fiber composition in el-

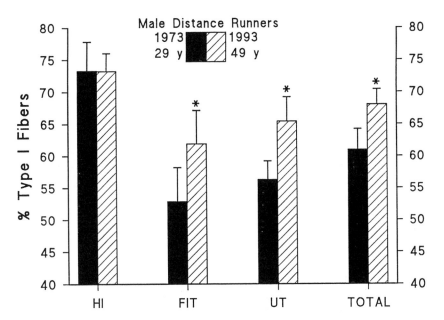

FIGURE 8-10. Influence of age on percentage of type I fibers in gastrocnemius. The subjects were male distance runners with an average age of ~29 years in 1973. Twenty years later, they had fallen into subgroups of those who had continued intensive training (HI, highly trained), continued running on a recreational basis (FIT, fitness trained), or retired from running (UT, untrained). After 20 years the HI group, with a high initial %type I fibers, showed no change in %type I fibers, but the other two groups increased their %type I fibers, irrespective of activity level. Based on Trappe et al. (1995).

derly women and men have produced contradictory findings (Aniansson et al., 1981; Essen-Gustavsson & Borges, 1986; Grimby et al., 1982, 1984).

Muscle Composition. Muscles are composed mainly of contractile tissue (muscle fibers) but also of connective tissue and fat. In young adults, women's muscles contain relatively more fat and connective tissue (Forsberg et al., 1991; Miller et al., 1993; Prince et al., 1977; Sale et al., 1987). Increased fat content of muscle is also observed in the elderly (Forsberg et al., 1991; Overend et al., 1992; Rice et al., 1989). In adulthood, muscle fat content does not change significantly between ages 20 y and 60 y, after which it increases; the greater fat content of female muscles is maintained into old age (Forsberg et al., 1991).

In a comparison of young (19–40 y), middle-aged (41–60 y), and older (61–85 y) adults, the muscles of the older adults had more water and less potassium, magnesium, and protein contents. In the two youngest groups combined, muscles of the women had more water but less sodium, creatine, and DNA content than did the muscles of the men (Forsberg et al., 1991). These differences may also reflect differences in fiber size.

GENDER DIFFERENCES IN SKELETAL MUSCLE STRENGTH THROUGHOUT THE LIFE CYCLE

Childhood to Young Adulthood

The development of strength from early childhood to late adolescence or early adulthood has been the subject of several reviews. Two excellent recent reviews are those by Blimkie (1989) and Froberg and Lammert (1995). Most data are cross-sectional and derived from isometric strength measurements; however, there are also data from dynamic strength measurements. These latter measurements have been made with velocity-controlled or "isokinetic" dynamometers that allow concentric or eccentric strength to be measured at various preset velocities.

Strength may be expressed as *absolute* values (e.g., newtons of force, newton meters of torque), or as *relative* values in relation to body mass or some other reference (e.g., muscle cross-sectional area). Absolute strength limits performance against external resistance or loads, whereas relative strength expressed as the strength/body mass ratio limits performance in lifting, supporting, or projecting one's own body mass.

Isometric and Low-Velocity Concentric Strength. Whether isometric or concentric strength is measured, the pattern is the same. Girls and boys increase strength linearly from early childhood (~5–7 y) until about 13–15 y (top panel of Figure 8-11). After this point, there is a marked acceleration in strength gain until the late teens in boys, whereas there is no clear evidence of a spurt in girls (Blimkie, 1989; Kanehisa et al., 1995; Parker et al., 1990).

As to the extent of the increase in absolute strength during this period, a good example is the study by Parker et al. (1990), in which elbow flexion strength and knee extension isometric strength were measured in 284 girls and 267 boys aged 5–17 y. In the girls, knee extension and elbow flexion strength increased 3.6- and 2.4-fold over this age span; the corresponding increases in the boys were 4.7- and 3.7-fold (top panel of Fig. 8-11).

The strength/body mass ratio does not increase as much over this age span because both body mass and absolute strength are increasing. The strength/body mass ratios are shown in the bottom panel of Figure 8-11. The boys managed about 20% and 60% increases for knee extension and elbow flexion, respectively; the girls increased about 35% in knee extension but suffered about a 15% decrease in elbow flexion. A decrease in the upper body strength/body mass ratio has also been shown by others (Montoye & Lamphiear, 1977), indicating that after age 10–12 y, girls have increasing difficulty performing strength activities that involve lifting and supporting their body weights with their arms.

The gender difference in strength is small until about age 14 y, after which boys become notably stronger than girls (e.g., Figure 8-11). In Fig-

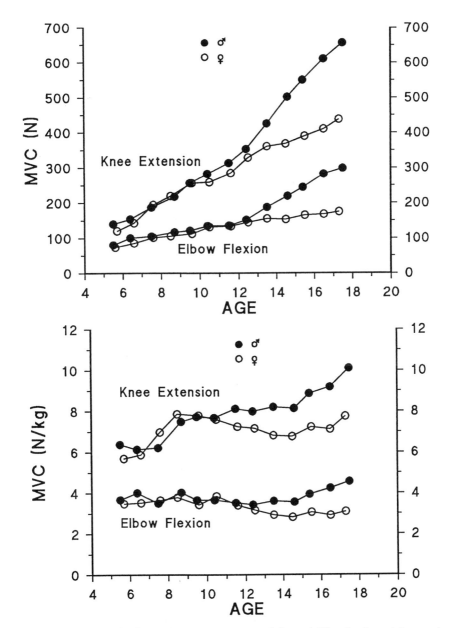

FIGURE 8-11. Example of increase in isometric strength from childhood to late adolescence/early adulthood. Absolute strength (top panel) increases linearly in boys and girls until about age 14, after which an acceleration, not shared by the girls, occurs in the boys. After age 14, a growing difference in strength develops between boys and girls. When strength is expressed as the strength/body mass ratio (bottom panel), the increase in strength/body mass ratio with age is not as great absolute strength because body mass is also increasing during this period. Indeed, girls tend to show a decrease in elbow flexion strength/mass ratio. Based on data of Parker et al. (1990).

ure 8-12, the data of Parker et al. (1990) described in Figure 8-11 are expressed as female-to-male (F/M) ratios. It can be seen that until 14 y the ratio is variable, ranging from 0.85-1.15. At age 14 the F/M ratio declines, reaching values at age 17-18 y that depend on muscle group and on how the strength is expressed, i.e., absolutely or relative to body mass. The data shown illustrate the general observation that the F/M ratio is lower for upper-body (~0.5-0.6) than lower-body (~0.65-0.75) muscle groups and lower for absolute strength than for the strength/body mass ratio.

High-Velocity Concentric Strength. Few studies have examined high-velocity concentric strength in children. Eleven-year-old boys were tested for knee extension concentric strength at velocities ranging from 1.05-4.2 rad/s; they had a strength-velocity relation similar to that of men (Burnie & Brodie, 1986). Boys and girls aged 7-13 y showed the expected decline in peak torque between velocities of 30°/s and 120°/s in knee and elbow flexion and extension. The female/male ratio was lower for upper-limb than for lower-limb strength, and it was slightly lower for higher-velocity strength than for lower-velocity strength (Gilliam, 1979). Miyashita and Kanehisa (1979) measured relatively high-velocity (210°/s)

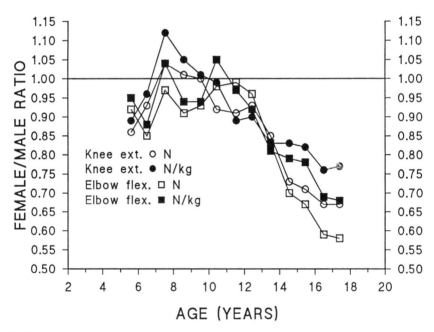

FIGURE 8-12. Data of Figure 8-11 are expressed as female to male ratios; that is, female values expressed as proportion of male values (F/M ratios). A ratio of 1.0 indicates equality of strength. Three trends are apparent: 1) until age 12 y the difference between girls and boys is not large; 2) after age 12 y the F/M ratio declines markedly; 3) the decline is greater for absolute strength than the strength/body mass ratio; and 4) the decline is greater for upper than lower limb strength. Based on data of Parker et al. (1990).

knee extension strength in boys and girls aged 13 to 17 y (Figure 8-13). The age and gender influence on strength was similar to that described previously for isometric strength, i.e., that absolute strength and the strength/mass ratio increased markedly in the boys throughout the age range but tended to reach a plateau in the girls after 14 y. Consequently, the female/male ratio for absolute strength decreased from 0.82 at 13 y to 0.62 at 17 y. In the study of isometric strength by Parker et al. (1990), the corresponding decline was from 0.85 to 0.67.

The literature indicates no striking change between childhood and late adolescence in the strength-velocity relationship for concentric muscle actions. It should be noted, however, that the "high" velocities studied represent less than 50% of maximum unresisted shortening velocity. Future studies incorporating the full range of velocities are needed to clarify any age or gender effect during this age span. Similarly, almost no data are available on eccentric strength; thus, it is not known whether the gender and age influences on eccentric strength apparent in adulthood are also present in childhood.

Role of Muscle Size. Because the patterns of age and gender influences on strength are similar to those for muscle size described in an earlier section, it would be reasonable to assume that the increase in muscle size from childhood to adulthood is largely responsible for the increase in strength through the same period. As reviewed by Blimkie (1989), this assumption is for the most part supported by the literature. For example, Davies (1985) measured plantarflexion strength and related it to muscle cross-sectional area in groups of girls and boys aged 10, 12, and 15 y and in young women and men aged 22 y. The previously described age and gender effects on absolute isometric strength were observed. When plantarflexor force was corrected for the angle of fiber pennation and for leverage, there was a very high correlation between isometric force and muscle cross-sectional area. Force per unit muscle cross-sectional area was similar in males and females and across age groups, indicating that age and gender differences in strength were related to quantity rather than quality of muscle. This was also shown in the earlier work of Ikai & Fukunaga (1968) with an upper limb muscle, as illustrated in Figure 8-14.

Role of Testosterone. The growing strength difference between girls and boys after age 14 y, as illustrated in Figure 8-11, is coincident with a surge in serum testosterone in boys (Gupta et al., 1975; Winter, 1978); the surge in this hormone is therefore probably responsible for the greater increases in muscle size and strength in males from age 14 y through early adulthood.

Young Adulthood

Taking into consideration muscle groups in the upper and lower limbs and trunk, young women have 60% of the absolute strength of men

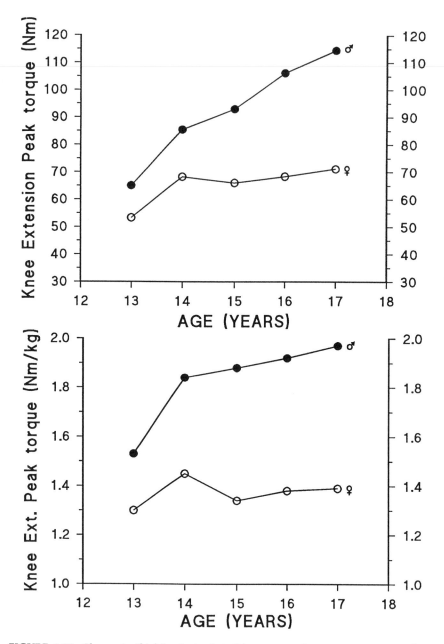

FIGURE 8-13. Change in "high" velocity (210°/s) concentric knee extension strength in boys and girls aged 13 to 17 y. The pattern is similar to that shown for isometric strength in Figure 8-11. In both absolute strength (top panel) and strength mass ratio (bottom panel), boys continue to increase after age 14, whereas girls tend to level off. As a result, the female/male ratio declines between ages 14 and 17 y. Based on data of Miyashita and Kanehisa (1979).

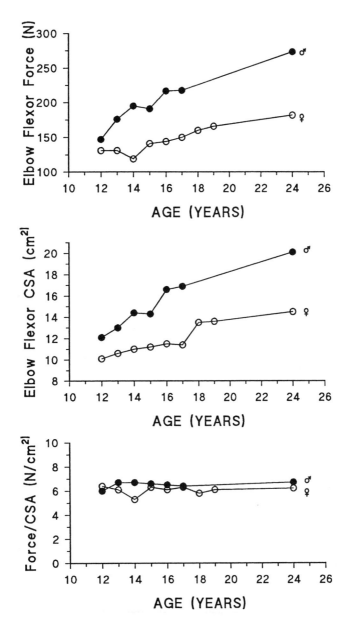

FIGURE 8-14. Influence of age (~12–~24 y) and gender on elbow flexion absolute isometric strength (top panel), elbow flexor muscle cross-sectional area (CSA, middle panel), and the ratio of force to muscle cross-sectional area ("specific tension," bottom panel). It is apparent that the age and gender influence on strength is a function of their influence on muscle size (CSA); that is, age and gender differences in strength are accounted for by corresponding differences in muscle CSA. On the other hand, there appear to be no age or gender differences in muscle "quality" ("specific tension," bottom panel). Based on data of Ikai and Fukunaga (1968).

(Nordgren, 1972). The gender difference is greatest in the upper limbs, where women have ~50–60% of men's strength (de Koning et al., 1985; Doherty et al., 1993b; Heyward et al., 1986; Laubach, 1976; Miller et al., 1993; Montoye & Lamphiear, 1977; Sale et al., 1987), and smallest in the lower limbs, with an F/M ratio of ~0.60–0.80 (Cioni et al., 1988; Davies, 1985; Froese & Houston, 1985; Heyward et al., 1986; Laubach, 1976; Laforest et al., 1990; Maughan et al., 1983a; Miller et al., 1993; Murray et al., 1980, 1985; Vandervoort & McComas, 1986).

Strength/Body Mass Ratio. In comparison to *absolute* strength, the gender difference is smaller when strength is expressed in relation to body mass because on average men have a greater body mass (Maughan et al., 1983a; Miller et al., 1993). This is evident in Figure 8-15, which shows a greater F/M ratio for the strength/body mass ratio than for absolute strength. The F/M ratio for strength expressed in relation to lean body mass (fat-free mass) is greater still. Figure 8-15 also illustrates the greater F/M ratios for lower-body than for upper-body strength, regardless of how strength is expressed.

Influence of Muscle Size. The F/M ratios for absolute strength are very similar to those for muscle size expressed as CSA. Thus, it is a natural conclusion that the greater absolute strength of men is due to a greater muscle mass, rather than to differences in muscle "quality" or the ability to fully activate muscles. This conclusion is consistent with the small or nonexistent differences between women and men in strength expressed per unit of muscle CSA (strength/CSA ratio), which is sometimes referred to as "specific tension" or "specific force" (Davies, 1985; Ikai & Fukunaga, 1968; Kanehisa et al., 1994; Maughan et al., 1983a; Miller et al., 1993; Sale et al., 1987; Schantz et al., 1983). It should be noted, however, that at least two studies have reported significantly greater knee extension strength/CSA ratios in men; the F/M ratio was ~0.80 (Kanehisa et al., 1994; Young et al., 1985). An F/M ratio of only 0.73 has been shown for knee flexion (Kanehisa et al., 1994). In Figure 8-15, which illustrates the data of Miller et al. (1993), there was no significant gender difference in either the knee extension or elbow flexion strength/CSA ratios. At the present time there is no explanation for the discrepant findings.

Concentric vs. Eccentric Strength. Most of the research comparing strength in women and men has focused on tests of isometric or relatively low-velocity concentric strength. However, one well-known study by Singh and Karpovich (1968) studied both concentric and eccentric muscle actions during elbow extension and flexion movements in young men and women. The concentric and eccentric actions were done at a single low velocity. As expected, eccentric force was greater than concentric force. The authors made no reference to a possible gender difference in the ratio of eccentric to concentric strength (now commonly referred to as the ECC/CON ratio); however, examination of their data indicates that the

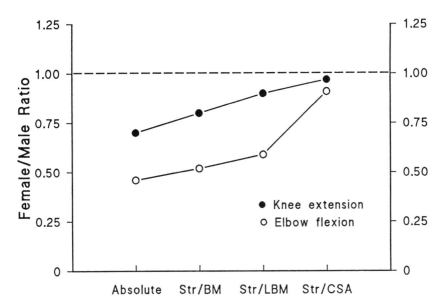

FIGURE 8-15. The female/male (F/M) ratios in young adults for isometric knee extension and elbow flexion strength expressed absolutely, per kilogram body mass (Str/BM), per kilogram lean body mass (Str/LBM), and per square centimeter of muscle cross-sectional area (Str/CSA). As also indicated in Figure 8-12, the F/M ratios are greater for lower than upper limb strength, and greater for Str/BM than absolute strength. The F/M ratio is greater still for Str/LBM. The F/M ratio for Str/CSA is close to equality; thus, unlike the other measures, women and men did not differ significantly in Str/CSA (see also Figure 8-14). It should be noted that strength *performance* is related to either absolute strength or Str/BM. Based on data of Miller et al. (1993).

elbow flexion ECC/CON ratio was higher in the women (1.69) than in the men (1.50).

In recent years the availability of eccentric loading dynamometers has allowed eccentric strength to be safely and reliably measured at low to moderately high velocities of lengthening, and more gender comparisons have been made. These comparisons have confirmed the data of Singh and Karpovich (1968). Women have greater ECC/CON ratios in elbow flexion and in knee extension and flexion (Colliander & Tesch, 1989; Griffin et al., 1993). The gender difference is more pronounced at higher velocities. These observations are illustrated in Figure 8-16.

The greater ECC/CON ratios in women, especially at higher velocities, could be the result of relatively enhanced eccentric strength in women or relatively diminished concentric strength. These alternatives will be discussed in the next section on the force-velocity relationship.

Force-Velocity Relation. The force-velocity relationship in isolated skeletal muscle has been well described: force decreases with increased velocity of concentric (shortening) actions, and increases (to a point) with

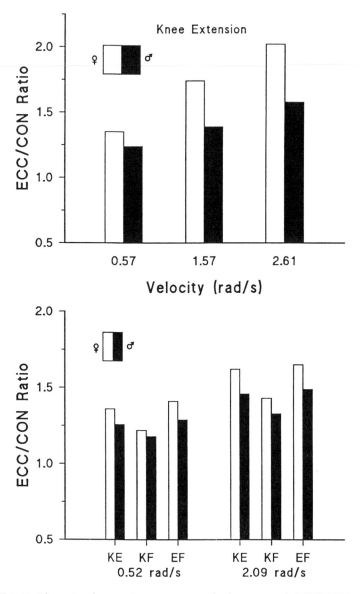

FIGURE 8-16. The ratio of eccentric to concentric absolute strength (ECC/CON ratio) in young women and men. In the top panel are data from knee extension concentric and eccentric strength measurements on an isokinetic (isovelocity) dynamometer at three knee joint angular velocities. As expected from the force-velocity relationship, the ECC/CON ratio increased as velocity increased. Young women had especially larger ECC/CON ratios at the two higher velocities. Based on data from Colliander and Tesch (1989). The bottom panel shows ECC/CON ratios determined at two velocities for knee extension (KE), knee flexion (KF), and elbow flexion (EF). In agreement with the top panel, the ECC/CON ratios were greater at the higher velocity and in women. These data (Griffin et al., 1993) are from subjects with a large range in age (21–67, $\bar{X} = 40$ y).

increased velocity of eccentric (lengthening) actions. This force-velocity relationship has to some extent been replicated in humans on the basis of maximal voluntary actions. However, there are discrepancies. Notably, in voluntary actions force may not increase as expected from high-velocity to low-velocity during concentric and isometric actions (Perrine & Edgerton, 1978; Wickiewicz et al., 1984). Furthermore, force may not increase as expected from isometric to eccentric nor from lower-velocity to higher-velocity eccentric actions (Colliander & Tesch, 1989; Dudley et al., 1990; Griffin et al., 1993; Westing & Seger, 1989; Westing et al., 1988). To put it in other terms, the previously discussed ECC/CON ratio increases more, as velocity increases, for artificially stimulated than for voluntary muscle actions (Dudley et al., 1990). These observations are illustrated in Figure 8-17.

It is of interest that the difference in the shape of the force-velocity relationship and the ECC/CON ratios between stimulated and voluntary muscle actions is remarkably similar to the differences observed between women and men, as illustrated in Figure 8-18 (and between young and old adults, to be discussed below). In this comparison, the women's voluntary force-velocity pattern is similar to that for artificial stimulation shown in Figure 8-17; in contrast, the men show the typical voluntary force-velocity relationship, also shown in Figure 8-17. The "flattening" of the voluntary force-velocity relation relative to the stimulated one has been attributed to some neural inhibition mechanism (Dudley et al., 1990; Perrine & Edgerton, 1978). The magnitude of inhibition is positively correlated with the magnitude of muscle force; hence, the inhibition is most evident in the low-velocity, high-force region of the force-velocity relationship for concentric muscle actions, and particularly throughout the force-velocity relationship for eccentric actions. Consequently, electrical stimulation superimposed on voluntary actions enhances force during eccentric actions the most (Westing et al., 1990), and motor-unit activity as estimated by electromyography (EMG) is less in eccentric vs. concentric actions (Westing et al., 1991).

These observations suggest that men may suffer more inhibition than do women in the high-force region of the force-velocity relationship, especially in eccentric actions. If this were so, men would show greater enhancement of eccentric force with stimulation superimposed on voluntary actions, and women would have greater ECC/CON ratios for EMG activity. Neither hypothesis has been tested on the knee extensors, the muscle most studied and the subject of Figures 8-17 and 8-18. However, a recent study of elbow flexion showed a greater ECC/CON ratio for EMG activity in women, but only a trend toward a greater ECC/CON force ratio (Davison et al., 1995). Why men might suffer greater inhibition than do women in the high-force region of the force-velocity relationship is not clear. If the inhibition is related to a tension-sensitive receptor in the ten-

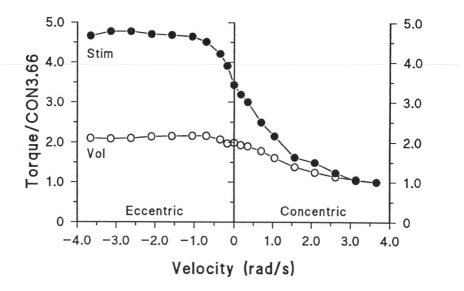

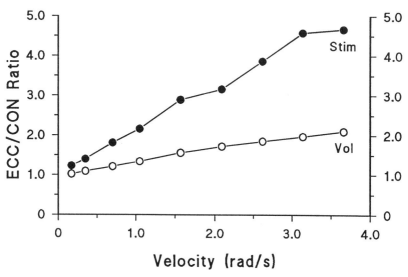

FIGURE 8-17. Comparison of the force-velocity relation produced by voluntary (Vol) and stimulated (Stim) muscle actions of the knee extensors in 6 men and 2 women. The top panel compares the torque produced relative to the concentric torque produced at 3.66 rad/s. A "flatter" voluntary force-velocity relation is evident. The bottom panel shows greater ECC/CON ratios in the stimulated vs. voluntary contractions. An ECC/CON ratio at each velocity is calculated as the eccentric torque divided by the concentric torque. Based on data of Dudley et al. (1990).

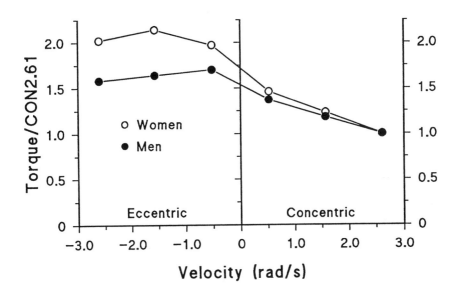

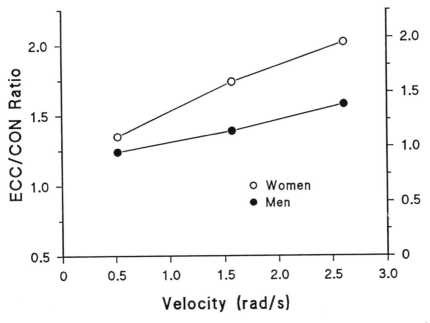

FIGURE 8-18. Comparison of force-velocity relation in women and men. The top panel compares the torque produced relative to the concentric torque produced at 2.61 rad/s. A "flatter" force-velocity relation is evident in the men. The bottom panel shows greater ECC/CON ratios in the women. An ECC/CON ratio at each velocity is calculated as the eccentric torque divided by the concentric torque. Note the similarity of the women's force-velocity relation to that induced by electrical stimulation in Figure 8-17. Based on data of Colliander and Tesch (1989).

dons, then perhaps the muscle force per unit cross-sectional area of *tendon* is greater in males, leading to greater inhibition. Earlier, it was pointed out that the literature is divided, at least for quadriceps, as to whether or not there is a gender difference in force per unit *muscle* cross-sectional area.

The ECC/CON ratio might also be influenced by muscle-fiber composition; a predominance of type I (slow) fibers may favor force production in lengthening (eccentric) actions and may partly account for the greater ECC/CON ratios observed in women and also the in the elderly (see next section).

A final consideration is whether or not women and men differ in the high-velocity region of the force-velocity relationship for concentric actions. In the commonly tested knee extension movement, some evidence indicates that men perform relatively better at higher velocities (Anderson et al., 1979; Froese & Houston, 1985; Griffin et al., 1993; Laforest et al., 1990). An example of this gender difference is shown in Figure 8-19. On the other hand, no such difference is observed in knee flexion or el-

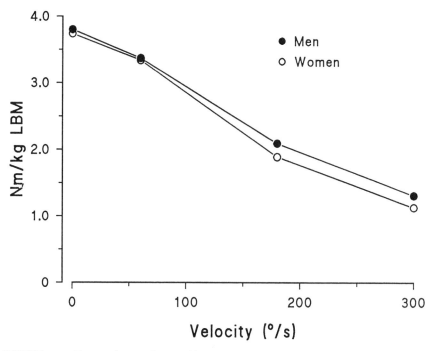

Velocity (°/s)

FIGURE 8-19. Force-velocity relation of knee extension in young women and men. Isometric and concentric strength (torque) values are shown, expressed per kilogram lean body mass (LBM). In isometric and 60°/s concentric there was no gender difference, but men produced significantly greater torque at the two higher velocities. Based on data of Anderson et al. (1979).

bow flexion (de Koning et al., 1985; Griffin et al., 1993; Laforest et al., 1990). Indeed, one study has shown relatively better elbow flexion performance in women than in men at high velocities (Sale et al., 1987). Measurements of maximal unresisted muscle-shortening velocity ($\dot{V}$max) have also been made, but again results vary according to muscle group. A study of elbow flexion in large samples of men and women showed that women had only 90% of the $\dot{V}$max of men (de Koning et al., 1985). In contrast, Houston et al. (1988) found no gender difference in knee extension $\dot{V}$max. When it has been observed, men's relatively greater high-velocity concentric performance or $\dot{V}$max may be related to their greater percent type II fiber area and/or to a greater percentage of type II fibers (see section on muscle fiber composition).

Young Adulthood to Old Age

Isometric and Low-Velocity Concentric Strength. The decline in strength from young adulthood to old age has been the subject of recent reviews (Doherty et al., 1993a; Porter & Vandervoort, 1995; Porter et al., 1995; Rodgers & Evans, 1993; Vandervoort, 1992; White, 1995). The extent of decline depends upon the muscle group tested, the type of muscle action, and the velocity of muscle action, as will be discussed below. The magnitude of the age-associated loss of strength reported in various studies is also affected simply by the age of the oldest subjects studied; studies with older subjects show greater losses. Taking these factors into consideration and focusing first on isometric and low-velocity concentric strength, the following general observations can be made: 1) there is a ~15–20% decline in strength between the mid-20s and age 60 y; 2) after age 60, the rate of decline increases, so by the mid- to late 80s only about 50–60% of the strength of young adulthood is retained; and 3) the pattern of strength loss is essentially similar in women and men. An example of the decline in absolute isometric and low-velocity concentric strength with age in a large population of women is shown in Figure 8-20. This study by Sandler et al. (1991) illustrates the different rates of strength loss in different muscle groups and the different patterns of strength loss. Figure 8-21 shows another example of age-related strength loss. This study by Vandervoort and McComas (1986) is notable in that subjects up to 100 y were included. The data shown are for ankle dorsiflexors and plantarflexors. The results of this study agree with the general observations made above, i.e., there was a strength loss of ~15% between the 3rd and 7th decades, increasing to a loss of ~40–50% by the 9th decade. The loss of strength was similar in women and men.

The data shown in Figure 8-21 notwithstanding, the issue has been raised as to whether or not there is a gender difference in the loss of strength with age. While there have been reports of a greater decline in men than in women (Davies et al., 1986; Murray et al., 1980; 1985 [top

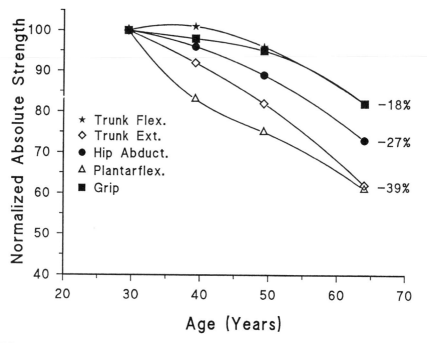

FIGURE 8-20. Decline in isometric and low-velocity concentric strength with age in women. Data were normalized (= 100) to values for the group with a mean age of 29 y. Based on data of Sandler et al. (1991).

panel of Figure 8-22]), most studies indicate a similar decline in both genders (Doherty et al., 1993b; Frontera et al., 1991; Montoye & Lamphiear, 1977; Phillips et al., 1992; Stalberg et al., 1989; Vandervoort & McComas, 1986; van Schaik et al., 1994; Young et al., 1984; 1985) or sometimes an even greater decline in women (Gerdle & Fugl-Meyer, 1985 [bottom panel of Figure 8-22]). At present no conclusive evidence exists of gender difference in the decline of isometric and low-velocity concentric strength. However, there may be gender differences in the loss of eccentric and high-velocity concentric strength, as well as in specific force or tension. These topics will be discussed in following sections.

As reviewed by Vandervoort et al. (1986), whether or not there is a significant loss of strength up to age 55–60 y has been questioned because some studies have failed to show a significant decline in isometric strength up to this age. On the other hand, other studies clearly show declines in both isometric strength and in low-velocity concentric strength between the mid-20s and mid-50s (Figure 8-22). Whether or not a significant strength loss is found during middle age may depend on the muscle group studied, as shown in Figure 8-20.

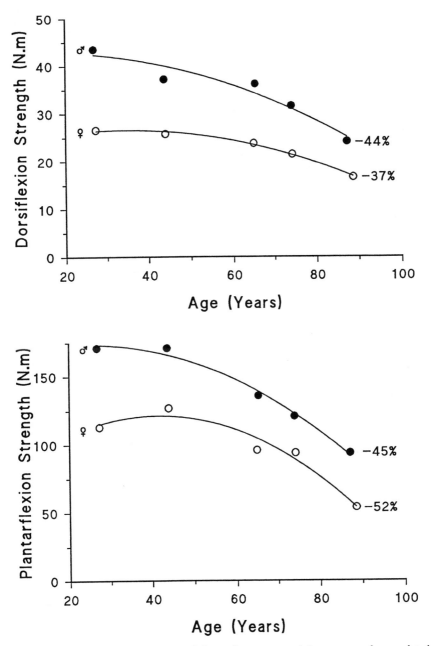

FIGURE 8-21. Isometric dorsiflexion and plantarflexion strength in women and men related to age. Subjects in this study ranged in age from 20 to 100 y, but were placed in subgroups with mean ages as shown. See text for discussion. Based on data of Vandervoort and McComas (1986).

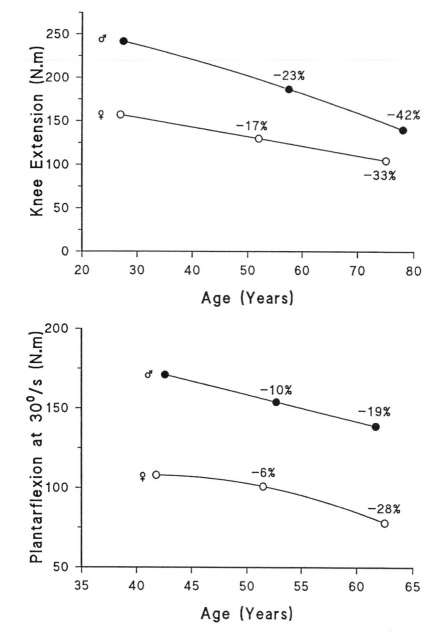

FIGURE 8-22. Decline in low-velocity concentric strength with age. The top panel, based on the data of Murray et al. (1980; 1985), shows a significant decline in knee extension strength from the mid-20s to the early and late 50s, and a further decline to the mid-70s. The bottom panel, based on the data of Gerdle and Fugl-Meyer (1985), shows a measurable decline in plantarflexion strength in the decade between the early 40s and 50s, and a further decline by the early 60s.

All of the foregoing discussion and most of what follows is based on data from cross-sectional studies because there have been only a few longitudinal studies. Two longitudinal studies have shown that the loss of strength in the 8th decade is close to what would be expected from the results of cross-sectional studies (Aniansson et al., 1983; 1986), whereas a third revealed a much smaller than expected loss (Greig et al., 1993). Finally, a recent report of a 12-y follow-up of some of the elderly subjects studied by Vandervoort and McComas (1986, Figure 8-21) indicated a loss of strength similar to that predicted from the cross-sectional data (Winegard et al., 1995).

Strength/Body Mass Ratio. As absolute strength is lost with advancing age, so is the strength/body mass ratio; that is, the ability to move and support body weight is progressively impaired. An example of the decline in the strength/body mass ratio in women is shown in Figure 8-23. Changes in height, mass (weight), and absolute strength over the same age span are also shown for comparison. If mass were to increase with age and if the increase were mainly in fat, then the decline in the strength/mass ratio would be expected to be greater than that for absolute strength. Figure 8-23 exemplifies this course of events. In the very old, however,

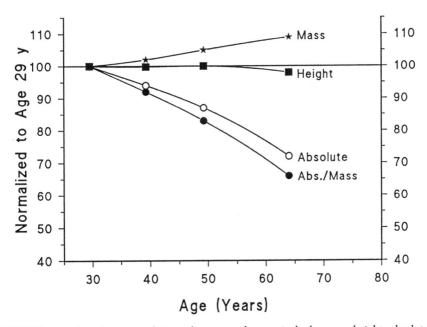

FIGURE 8-23. In a large population of women, changes in body mass, height, absolute strength, and the strength/mass ratio (Abs./Mass) over a 35-year period are shown. For the figure, isometric/low-velocity concentric strength data from 5 muscle groups were pooled. Based on Sandler et al. (1991).

the relative loss of absolute strength and strength/mass ratio is similar, suggesting that the fat gained in the "middle" years is lost in old age. Figure 8-24, which is based on a study of women and men up to the age of 100 y, shows the relatively greater loss of the strength/mass ratio compared to absolute strength up to the mid 70s, but in the 80s and 90s, the loss is similar for the two expressions of strength.

Role of Muscle Size. The changes in strength from young adulthood to old age are remarkably similar to those for muscle size, covered in an earlier section, i.e., a modest decline to age 60 y and then a more rapid decline. Most of the decline in strength might therefore be attributed to the decline in muscle mass that occurs with aging (Danneskiold-Samsoe et al., 1984; Frontera et al., 1991). An example of the close association between the loss of strength and muscle size in women is shown in Figure 8-25.

Specific Tension. If muscle atrophy is the only factor responsible for the age-related loss of strength, then *specific tension*, i.e., the force per unit muscle CSA, should remain constant throughout the life span. This appears to be the case in Figure 8-25. Another study of quadriceps had similar results for women (Young et al., 1984) but showed a decrease in specific tension in elderly men (Young et al. (1985). However, several studies have found a decreased specific tension in both elderly women and men in a variety of muscle groups (Bruce et al., 1989; Davies et al., 1986; Kallman et al., 1990; Pearson et al., 1985; Phillips et al., 1992; 1993; Reed et al., 1991; Vandervoort & McComas, 1986). Finally, in one longitudinal study, quadriceps-specific tension actually increased over an 8-y period during the 8th decade (Greig et al., 1993).

There are at least three possible explanations for the more commonly observed decrease in specific tension with aging. First, the ability to fully activate muscle with old age may decrease; however, research indicates that the elderly can fully activate their muscles, while still showing decreased specific tension (Phillips et al., 1992; Vandervoort & McComas, 1986). Moreover, tetanically stimulated muscles of the elderly show decreased specific tension, which could not be the result of reduced voluntary activation (Davies et al., 1986). Secondly, the reduction in specific tension may be related to the increased intramuscular fat and connective tissue that accumulates during aging (see section on muscle composition); this accumulation would "dilute" contractile tissue and thereby reduce specific tension. Thirdly, the decline in specific tension with aging in women is correlated with hormonal changes after menopause; the decline is attenuated by hormone therapy (Figure 8-26). The mechanism underlying the hormonal effect is unknown; however, because the ability to activate muscles is not impaired in these women (Phillips et al., 1992), the effect must be in the muscles.

Eccentric vs. Concentric Strength. Concentric strength declines to a greater extent than does eccentric strength with age in both women and

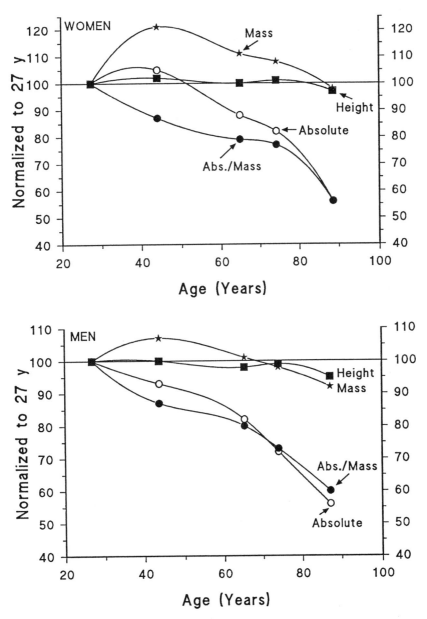

FIGURE 8-24. Changes in absolute strength, strength/body mass ratio (Abs./Mass), body mass, and height in women (top panel) and men (bottom panel). These cross-sectional data are from subjects aged 20–100 y; symbols denote mean ages of subgroups. Values for isometric dorsiflexor and plantarflexor strength have been combined. From young adulthood to middle age, mass increases with the effect that the strength/mass ratio declines more than absolute strength. By old age, however, mass has declined to a level similar to that of young adults, so that absolute strength and strength/mass ratio show similar impairment. Based on data of Vandervoort & McComas (1986).

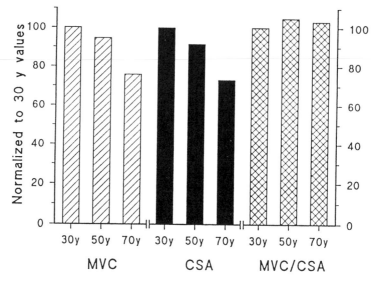

FIGURE 8-25. Knee extension isometric strength (MVC), quadriceps cross-sectional area (CSA), and specific force (MVC/CSA) in groups of women with mean ages of 30, 50, and 70 y. Strength and CSA decreased with age, particularly between 50 and 70 y. In contrast, specific force remained unchanged. Based on Häkkinen and Häkkinen (1991).

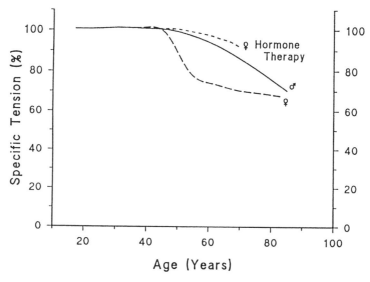

Age (Years)

FIGURE 8-26. Decline in specific tension of adductor pollicis with age in men, and women with and without hormone replacement therapy (HRT). Specific tension declined rapidly after age 45 in women not receiving HRT, and more rapidly than in men. Men did not "catch up" in their decline until age 80. Women on HRT were not investigated beyond about 70 y; until that age their pattern of loss was similar to that of the men. Based on the data of Phillips et al. (1993).

men (Poulin et al., 1992; Vandervoort et al., 1990), i.e., the ECC/CON force ratio increases (Figure 8-27). Eccentric strength is preserved more at moderately high than at low velocities; through this same velocity range concentric strength is affected equally by aging (Poulin et al., 1992). The greater ECC/CON ratio in young women than in men noted previously is preserved in the elderly (Porter et al., 1995a). However, the few studies to date suggest that women suffer greater losses of eccentric strength with aging than men (Porter et al., 1995a; Poulin et al., 1992; Vandervoort et al., 1990).

It is not known why eccentric strength is preserved more than concentric strength during aging. Studies of isometric actions indicate no loss of neural activation with age. On the other hand, neural activation in concentric and eccentric actions has not been studied in relation to aging. Therefore, one possible explanation is that activation becomes impaired in concentric relative to eccentric (and isometric) actions. This would not explain, however, why eccentric strength is better preserved than is isometric strength (Phillips et al., 1991). Moreover, changes within aging human muscle are probably involved, because electrically stimulated muscles of

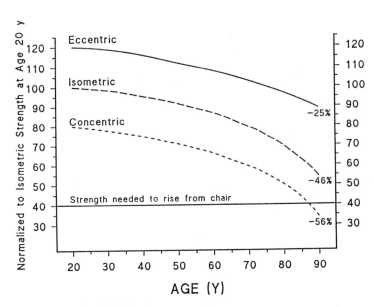

FIGURE 8-27. Schematic depiction of relative losses in eccentric, isometric, and concentric strength with aging. In old age, eccentric strength is better preserved than isometric or concentric strength. A task of daily living, such as rising from a chair without using the arms for assistance, requires a small proportion of a young adult's strength and therefore is easy to accomplish. By the 80s and 90s, however, this seemingly simple task may tax a high proportion of, or exceed maximal strength. Note that lowering into a chair (eccentric action) may be readily achieved at an advanced age; the problem is rising back out of the chair (concentric action). See text for further discussion.

aged mice show preservation of eccentric strength while isometric and concentric strength are reduced (Phillips et al., 1991). Increased concentrations of inorganic phosphate (P_i) and decreased intracellular pH reduce isometric and concentric force more than eccentric force, possibly by placing cross-bridges in a low-force state in concentric and isometric but not in eccentric actions. Thus, it has been suggested that aged muscle may have increased P_i and decreased pH, resulting in the observed pattern of strength loss (Phillips et al., 1991). Eccentric strength might also be spared if aged muscle contained increased amounts of less elastic connective tissue, which would help resist forced lengthening (Porter et al., 1995b). Finally, if in aged muscle a greater proportion of total mass consists of type I (slow) fibers, the lower rate of cross-bridge cycling may allow cross-bridges to be bound to actin longer during stretch, thereby causing a greater "braking" action.

Force-Velocity Relation. High-velocity concentric strength is lost to a greater extent than is low-velocity concentric strength as one ages (Aniansson et al., 1983; Harries & Bassey, 1990; Laforest et al., 1990), although this has not always been reported (Frontera et al., 1991; Gerdle & Fugl-Meyer, 1985; Larsson et al., 1979; Stanley & Taylor, 1993). The age range, velocity range, and the muscle group studied affect the results obtained. For example, one study found a greater loss of high-velocity strength in knee extensors but not in flexors (Laforest et al., 1990).

Recall that in young adults there is some evidence that women show a greater decline than do men in concentric strength from low to high velocities. This difference is also found in the elderly (Danneskiold-Samsoe et al., 1984; Grimby et al., 1982; Laforest et al., 1990), probably for the same reasons (see section on young adulthood). In the transition from young to old adulthood, this gender difference remains (Laforest et al., 1990).

The greater loss of high-velocity concentric strength during aging is consistent with results of those studies (discussed in an earlier section) showing a decline in the percentage of type II (fast) fibers with aging. Changes in connective tissue might also impair high-velocity performance in the elderly. Finally, the proportionally greater loss of large, fast-conducting motoneurons with age, as discussed in an earlier section, might impair neural activation in rapid ballistic movements.

GENDER DIFFERENCES IN SKELETAL MUSCLE METABOLISM THROUGHOUT THE LIFE CYCLE

Muscle Metabolic Capacity

The conversion of chemical energy to mechanical energy in skeletal muscles permits men and women to engage in all forms of exercise. The required chemical energy is provided through dietary intake of nutrients and their subsequent uptake and metabolism by the working muscles. The combustion of fat and carbohydrate (CHO), released from storage forms in the liver and adipose tissue and directly from within skeletal muscle, provide the vast majority of the substrate required to produce energy. Measurements of skeletal muscle substrates, including glycogen, triacylglycerol (TG), phosphocreatine (PCr), and adenosine triphosphate (ATP), reveal information about the capacities of muscle to produce both aerobic and anaerobic energy. Measurements of maximal enzyme activities provide information about the maximal rates that energy can be provided in the major energy-producing pathways. *In-vitro* determinations of respiratory capacity in skeletal muscle homogenates provide information about the potential rates that varying substrates may produce energy *in-vivo*.

It must be noted that the data discussed in the following section were derived from biopsies taken from the vastus lateralis and gastrocnemius muscles in human subjects. In addition, the data were derived from male and female subjects between the ages of 18–35 y, unless otherwise noted. In many cases there is little or no information about gender differences in skeletal muscle metabolism in other age cohorts.

Glycogen and Triacylglycerol. Although the substrate for exercise is most often a mixture of fat and CHO, the glycogen stored in the working muscles becomes the dominant substrate above power outputs of 50–70% $\dot{V}O_2$max (Hermansen et al., 1967; Saltin & Karlsson, 1971). The initial content of muscle glycogen is closely related to endurance time and race performance during prolonged aerobic exercise (Bergstrom et al., 1967; Hermansen et al., 1967; Karlsson & Saltin, 1971). This has led many authors to conclude that the depletion of muscle glycogen stores during prolonged aerobic exercise at 65–85% $\dot{V}O_2$max causes fatigue (for review, see Hultman & Spriet, 1988). Most studies examining the importance of muscle glycogen for energy production have employed only untrained and trained males. Many studies have had one or two women in their subject pool but have rarely examined an entire population of females. The assumption has always been that the important role of CHO in this type of exercise would be similar in females and males.

A gender difference in muscle glycogen might be expected because increases in plasma estrogen and progesterone concentrations during the luteal phase of the menstrual cycle enhance glycogen formation in rats (Ahmed-Sorour & Bailey, 1981; Carrington & Bailey, 1985). However, based on the limited amount of data, there appears to be no gender difference in resting or pre-exercise muscle glycogen content in humans. Nygaard (1985) reported resting glycogen of ~325 mmol/kg dry muscle (dm) in both untrained men and untrained women. Jansson (1986) also reported similar resting glycogen contents in 18 female and 15 male untrained subjects. Costill et al. (1979) examined 12 male and 12 female well-trained distance runners (80–115 km/wk) and reported resting glycogen values of ~510 and ~530 mmol/kg dm, respectively. These studies did not identify the menstrual status of the females, although none were taking oral contraceptives. Tarnopolsky et al. (1990) reported resting glycogen concentrations of ~450 mmol/kg dm in moderately trained males and females (35–40 km/wk) and ~400 mmol/kg dm in a similar group of endurance-trained male and female athletes in a subsequent study (Tarnopolsky et al., 1995). In these studies, females were tested in the follicular phase of the menstrual cycle.

Surprisingly, attempts at comparing muscle TG (TGm) stores between men and women do not exist. This may be partially explained by the difficulty in measuring this substrate in human skeletal muscles. Qualitative and quantitative estimates of TGm have been made using biopsies of human skeletal muscle from male subjects. Histochemical analyses revealed that lipid droplets are not stored in a homogenous manner (Hoppeler et al., 1985), raising the possibility that TGm measurements on biopsies of 50–100 mg may not accurately represent the entire muscle. An additional problem may be the inability to differentiate between interfiber and intrafiber TG. A recent study reported a coefficient of variation of 24% when comparing measurements performed on mixed muscle from three biopsies taken at the same time at rest and following exercise from the vastus lateralis (P.S. Wendling et al., unpublished manuscript). One study measured TGm on pools of single fibers from males but reported no variability data from repeated biopsies taken at the same time (Hurley et al., 1986). An alternate method to estimate TGm use during exercise is to predict the contribution of TGm to energy provision after estimating the energy contributions of total CHO and of exogenous-free-fatty acid (FFA) using indirect calorimetry and tracer techniques. In spite of these limitations, it is surprising that no gender comparisons of skeletal muscle TG contents have been attempted.

Circumstantial evidence in the literature suggests that TGm may be greater in females. Prince et al. (1977) reported that skeletal muscle of sedentary women had a large amount of fat between the muscle fascicles. Forsberg et al. (1991) found that the fat content in vastus lateralis muscle samples was 2.5-fold greater in women when comparing groups of 17 men and 23 women aged 19–40 y. Also, as discussed above, women appear to have a greater percentage of type I fibers than do men. Type I fibers of men and women appear equal in fiber diameter, whereas the type II fibers in muscles of females are smaller. This leaves women with a greater fractional volume of type I, slow-twitch, presumably more aerobic fibers. Because type I fibers have 2- to 3-fold more TG than do type II fibers in men (Essen, 1977), TGm stores may be greater in women.

Phosphocreatine and ATP. Few direct comparisons of PCr and ATP contents in resting human skeletal muscle of males and females exist. Esbjornsson et al. (1994) reported no gender differences in PCr and ATP contents measured in both type I and type II fibers. This is consistent with the fact that PCr and ATP measurements on whole biopsies from groups of females (Cheetham et al., 1986; Jacobs et al., 1982) appear similar to measurements on groups of males (Hultman et al., 1967; Spriet et al., 1987). There were also no gender differences in muscle PCr and ATP contents in older men (66–76 y) and older women (61–71 y)(Aniansson et al., 1981). Therefore, it seems reasonable to conclude that the potential for ATP resynthesis from PCr degradation during high-intensity exercise is similar in males and females.

Enzyme Activities. A number of investigations have compared the maximal activities of representative enzymes from the major energy-producing pathways in skeletal muscle samples of men and women. The activity of glycogen phosphorylase (PHOS), the rate-limiting enzyme in glycogenolysis, was similar in untrained males and females in two studies and 50% higher in males in another report (Table 8-1). In active and trained subjects, PHOS activity was 31–50% higher in the males. Activities of phosphofructokinase (PFK), triose-phosphate dehydrogenase (TPDH), and pyruvate kinase (PK), enzymes that predict the maximal flux through the glycolytic pathway in anaerobic situations, were generally higher in males, whether untrained, active, or trained (Table 8-1). The

TABLE 8-1. *A gender comparison of maximal enzyme activities of glycogenolytic, glycolytic, and high-energy phosphate degradation pathways. (I, type I fibers; II, type II fibers).*

		PHOS	PFK	TPDH	PK	LDH	HK	MK	CPK
UNTRAINED SUBJECTS									
Costill et al., 1976		ND				ND			
Cadefau et al., 1990		ND	75%		ND	68%			23%
Komi, Karlson, 1978		50%				ND	ND	ND	33%
Hedberg, Jansson, 1976			19%						
Bass, 1975				69%		100%	72%		
Simoneau et al, 1985		ND	26%			55%	20%		
ACTIVE SUBJECTS									
Essen-Gustavsson & Borges, 1986				ND		ND	ND		
Green et al., 1984		31%	20%		22%	47%	ND		
Esbjornsson et al., 1993			ND			33%			
Borges & Essen-	I					27%		ND	37%
Gustavsson, 1989	II					ND		ND	ND
TRAINED SUBJECTS									
Costill et al., 1976		50%				ND			
Cadefau et al., 1990		26%	33%		ND	26%			46%*

ND, no difference. Percent changes indicate higher enzyme activities in males. *, higher activity in females. PHOS, phosphorylase; PFK, phosphofructokinase; TPDH, triose phosphate dehydrogenase; PK, pyruvate kinase, LDH, lactate dehydrogenase; HK, hexokinase; MK, myokinase; CPK, creatine phosphokinase. Hedberg & Jansson, 1976 as cited by Komi and Karlsson, 1978. Data from Essen-Gustavsson & Borges, 1986 and Borges & Essen-Gustavsson, 1989 is a combination of untrained and active subjects.

findings for gender differences in lactate dehydrogenase (LDH) are not as clear. Evidence for higher LDH activity in males, again whether untrained, active, or trained, was as strong as the evidence reporting no gender difference. Hexokinase (HK) activity, indicative of the ability to phosphorylate glucose that has originated from outside the cell, has not been examined as frequently. Traditionally, alterations in this enzyme correlate better with activities of enzymes associated with the citric acid cycle (CAC) or with β-oxidation than with glycolytic enzyme activities. This seems logical because the maximal rate of glucose uptake and phosphorylation is consistent with the lower glycolytic flux experienced during aerobic exercise. Two of three studies reported greater HK activity in untrained males vs. females whereas two studies of active males and females reported no differences.

Comparisons of maximal activities of citrate synthase (CS), succinate dehydrogenase (SDH), and oxoglutarate dehydrogenase (OGDH), (all CAC enzymes) failed to demonstrate any gender differences in untrained subjects but did show higher levels of enzyme activities in active and trained males vs. females (Table 8.2). Costill et al. (1979) reported a 30% higher carnitine palmitoyl transferase (CPT) activity, the enzyme responsible for transporting FFA into the mitochondria, in trained males vs. females. Several groups examined the activity of a representative β-oxidation

TABLE 8-2. *A gender comparison of maximal enzyme activities of the citric acid cycle, B-oxidation, fatty acyl-CoA transferase, and ATP hydrolysis. (I, type I fibers; II, type II fibers).*

	CS	SDH	MDH	OGDH	HAD	CPT	Ca^{2+} Mg^{2+} ATPases
UNTRAINED SUBJECTS							
Costill et al., 1976	ND						
Cadefau et al., 1990		ND					
Komi, Karlson, 1978							67% ND
Bass, 1975	ND		ND		ND		
Simoneau et al., 1985		11%		ND	ND		
ACTIVE SUBJECTS							
Essen-Gustavsson &							
Borges, 1986	ND				ND		
Green et al., 1984		23%			ND		
Esbjornsson et al., 1993	ND				ND		
Borges & Essen-	I 60%				ND		
Gustavsson, 1989	II 53%				31%		
TRAINED SUBJECTS							
Costill et al., 1976		48%					
Costill et al., 1979		50%	ND			30%	
Cadefau et al., 1990		59%					

ND, no difference. Percent changes indicate higher enzyme activities in males. CS, citrate synthase; SDH, succinate dehydrogenase; MDH, malate dehydrogenase; OGDH, oxo-glutarate dehydrogenase; HAD, 3-hydroxyacyl CoA dehydrogenase; CPT, carnitine palmitoyl transferase. Data from Essen-Gustavsson & Borges, 1986 and Borges & Essen-Gustavsson, 1989 is a combination of untrained and active subjects.

enzyme, 3-hydroxyacyl CoA dehydrogenase (HAD), and all but one reported no gender difference in untrained and active subjects. Therefore, no gender differences exist in CAC and B-oxidation enzyme activities in untrained subjects. However, muscles of active and trained women vs. active and trained men exhibit lower activities of CPT and of enzymes of the CAC but similar potential for β-oxidation.

Maximal creatine kinase activity was generally higher in males, as was one examination of Ca^{2+} ATPase activity. No gender differences were reported for myokinase or Mg^{2+} ATPase activities (Tables 8-1, 8-2).

Correlations between fiber type analyses (histochemical) and maximal enzyme activities (biochemical) have been attempted to examine the relationship between the number of slow-twitch fibers (or ST fiber mass) in a muscle and the muscle's metabolic profile. Simoneau et al. (1985) reported that the covariance of fiber type distribution and enzyme activities in untrained males and females was low (~30%). Therefore, they suggested that the metabolic heterogeneity reported between males and females was independent of fiber type distribution. It seems reasonable, given the above findings, that this conclusion would also apply to active and trained males and females.

Several authors have examined the ratios of the activities of enzymes representative of the various metabolic pathways in an attempt to gain insight into the relative importance of pathways as they adapt to physiological stressors. For instance, Pette and Hofer (1980) reported that maximal activities of selected enzymes in some metabolic pathways maintain a constant proportion (or non-discriminative relation) to each other, in spite of changing absolute enzyme activities. Other representative enzymes of separate pathways exist in variable proportions. These discriminative enzyme ratios are thought to identify the relative importance of the different energy-producing pathways. Pette and Hofer (1980) confirmed these general relationships in several different tissues in a variety of altered metabolic states. Green et al. (1984) reported the most comprehensive analysis of these ratios as they relate to gender differences in active subjects. The non-discriminating ratios (PHOS/PFK, LDH/PFK, and PK/PFK) for the glycogenolytic/glycolytic enzymes and the (HK/SDH) ratio representing aerobic glycolytic/CAC relationships were similar between genders. However, the HAD/SDH ratio representing the β-oxidation/CAC relationship was significantly elevated in females, suggesting that they have a higher capacity for β-oxidation relative to CAC activity than do males. This phenomenon was also present in the data of Bass et al. (1975) and suggests a gender deviation from the concept that enzymes of various pathways change in constant proportion to one another. An examination of the discriminating ratios or the relative importance of the energy-producing pathways revealed no gender differences for relationships between glycogenolysis and glucose phosphorylation (PHOS/HK) and between glycolysis and the CAC (PFK/SDH, PK/SDH, and LDH/SDH). However, one exception was a lower glycolysis/ β-oxidation (PFK/HAD) relationship in females, implying a smaller difference between anaerobic and aerobic energy-generating pathways. Therefore, the enzyme ratio data generally strengthen the gender differences reported when examining the enzymes individually.

In summary, absolute activities of glycogenolytic/glycolytic enzymes are generally elevated in active and trained young adult males vs. active and trained young adult females. However, in untrained subjects the difference is less clear; about half the investigations have reported no gender differences. Higher activities of CAC enzymes are also generally present in active and trained males vs. females, with no gender differences in untrained subjects. The β-oxidation enzyme activities are unaffected by gender at all fitness levels. On a relative basis, females have a higher capacity for β-oxidation compared to CAC activity than do males, suggesting that they may be predisposed to using a greater proportion of fat (and less CHO) at a given percentage of $\dot{V}O_2$max as compared to men.

There have been attempts to examine maximal activities of key enzymes in older males and females. Many of the gender differences discussed above in young adults were not present in older adults examined in 10-y age cohorts. For example, there were no gender differences in the activities of HK and LDH in three or four separate comparisons of adults aged 70–80 y and in one study where comparisons were made in 10-y cohorts between the ages of 30 y and 80 y (Aniansson et al., 1981; Borges & Essen-Gustavsson, 1989; Essen-Gustavsson et al., 1986; Grimby et al., 1982). The activity of TPDH was not affected by gender in age groups 20–30 y and 60–70 y but was 9–33% higher in males in the age cohorts between 30 and 80 years of age (Essen-Gustavsson & Borges, 1986). Citrate synthase activities were not different in all 70–80-year-old gender comparisons, including one investigation examining both type I and II fibers, but was higher in males in the 10-y cohorts from 30 to 70 years of age (Borges & Essen-Gustavsson, 1989; Essen-Gustavsson & Borges, 1989; Grimby et al., 1982). The same studies also revealed that the activity of HAD was unaffected by gender in all age cohorts from 30–80 y. No gender differences were reported in MK and Mg^{2+} ATPase activities (Aniansson et al., 1981) and in MK and CK activities measured in both type I and type II fibers in 70–80-year-old individuals (Borges & Gustavsson-Essen, 1989). These findings suggest that reduced physical activity in the older males and females may be responsible for the loss of many of the gender differences reported in younger active and trained adults.

Borges and Essen-Gustavsson (1989) also reported that CS and HAD activities were higher in type I vs. type II fibers in all age groups in both men and women. Conversely, LDH and MK activities were higher in type II fibers in all age groups, but only in men.

Respiratory Capacity. In young trained male and female runners, Costill et al. (1979) examined the *in-vitro* capacities of gastrocnemius muscle homogenates to oxidize radiolabelled palmitoyl CoA. Trained males had a 50% greater rate of palmitoyl CoA oxidation than did similarly trained females. The authors concluded that males had a greater ability to increase absolute rates of fat oxidation following endurance training. However, this *in-vitro* finding did not predict the relative amounts of fat and CHO oxidized during a 60-min run at 70% $\dot{V}O_2$max, i.e., males and females had similar respiratory exchange ratios (RER). Presumably, this intensity of whole body aerobic exercise did not maximally challenge the capacity of the muscle to oxidize fat.

Aerobic Muscle Metabolism

A series of studies since 1980 suggests that females rely more heavily on fat oxidation than do men during prolonged aerobic exercise. Several investigations comparing untrained or recreationally active males and females reported lower RER values in females during submaximal exercise at the same relative intensity (Blatchford et al., 1985; Froberg & Pedersen, 1984; Jansson, 1986; Nygaard, 1985). However, three other studies reported no gender differences in RER during submaximal exercise in untrained subjects (Friedmann & Kindermann, 1989; Graham et al., 1986; Mendenhall et al., 1995). Nygaard (1985) also reported that women as compared to men used ~36% less glycogen during 60 min of cycling (20 min each at 50, 60, and 75% $\dot{V}O_2$max), and Jansson (1986) reported no gender difference in glycogen utilization during 25 min of cycling at 65% $\dot{V}O_2$max. The subjects in the above studies were aged 20–34 y and exercised at power outputs between 35% and 90% of $\dot{V}O_2$max for 21–90 min.

Similar comparisons using well-trained males and females matched for $\dot{V}O_2$max (58–61 mL·min^{-1}·kg^{-1} body mass) have been performed. Three studies reported no gender differences in exercise RER or venous plasma FFA concentration during 60–80 min of submaximal exercise at 70–80% $\dot{V}O_2$max (Costill et al. 1979; Friedmann & Kindermann, 1989; Powers et al., 1980). The athletes in these studies were aged 20–30 y and matched for gender, except for the Costill study, in which males averaged 35 y and females 23 y. There was also no indication of the menstrual status of the women, except that they were not taking oral contraceptives.

A series of recent studies from the laboratory of MacDougall and coworkers have challenged these findings. The initial study by Tarnopolsky et al. (1990) reported significantly lower RER values during 90 min of running at 63% $\dot{V}O_2$max in trained female runners vs. male runners. The calculated amounts of lipid and CHO utilization were 48 and 137 g in the females and 27 and 240 g in the males. No gender differences were reported in venous plasma FFA and glycerol concentrations, but females used 25% less glycogen during the 90 min of running. The authors recognized that many previous investigators had matched males and females on the basis of $\dot{V}O_2$max in $mL \cdot min^{-1} \cdot kg^{-1}$ and had not taken into account the dietary, menstrual, and hormonal status of the female subjects. Tarnopolsky et al. (1990) matched the subjects on the basis of $\dot{V}O_2$max in $mL \cdot min^{-1} \cdot kg^{-1}$ lean body mass (LBM), and training volume and intensity. The subjects also consumed identical, eucaloric diets for 3 d prior to testing, and the females were tested during the midfollicular phase of their menstrual cycles. Two potential concerns with this study were that the subjects fasted for 12 h before the running trial, and the RER values reported for the trained males appeared high (0.93–0.94) for exercise at 63% $\dot{V}O_2$max.

A subsequent study reported similar findings, although the absolute amount of fat oxidized (calculated from RER) was similar in males and females (60 g), whereas the CHO oxidized (127 vs. 72 g) was greater in the males (Phillips et al., 1993). Protein utilization and contribution to the total energy expenditure were low in both genders, but lower in the females. A third study compared the metabolic responses of males and females to 60 min of cycling at a higher intensity (75% $\dot{V}O_2$max) followed by cycling to exhaustion at 80–85% $\dot{V}O_2$max (Tarnopolsky et al., 1995). The subjects were given a meal in the hours preceding the exercise trial but were not matched for $\dot{V}O_2$max expressed as $mL \cdot min^{-1} \cdot kg^{-1}$ LBM, although both groups had high values (males, 75.5, and females, 65.2 $mL \cdot min^{-1} \cdot kg^{-1}$). Females had significantly lower RER values and venous plasma glycerol concentrations during cycling, but plasma FFA concentrations were not different. Again, fat contributed more to the total energy expenditure in the women (25%) than in the men (9%); therefore, because there were only small changes in the protein contribution, CHO contributed less (69% vs. 84%). However, the muscle glycogen data were not consistent with the RER calculations because glycogen utilization during the 60 min of cycling at 75% $\dot{V}O_2$max was not lower in the women as expected, but was similar in men and women.

In an attempt to explain the increased fat utilization by females during exercise at a given relative power output, Tarnopolsky et al. (1995) suggested that higher estrogen levels may be a contributing factor. This hormone increases the activity of lipoprotein lipase (LPL) in skeletal muscle and thus improves the ability to degrade plasma TG. Because estrogen simultaneously decreases LPL activity and lipolysis in adipose tissue, the increased ability of muscle to degrade plasma TG may direct FFA towards the working muscle. This may explain why increased fat utilization does not consistently coincide with increased venous plasma FFA and glycerol levels. However, muscle takes up only a fraction of the available FFA it receives, so it is questionable whether TG-FFA dynamics at the muscle would influence uptake.

According to the results of studies with trained subjects, it appears that females do rely less on CHO and more on fat during exercise intensities of 60–75% $\dot{V}O_2$max than do men. It may be that the data from those studies reporting no gender differences in metabolism were affected by the selection criteria for matching genders and by the lack of control of menstrual status. If the subjects were matched on the basis of LBM, would the results suggest more reliance on fat in the women? Alternately, it is possible that the *well*-trained males and females (e.g., Costill et al., 1979) had similar body compositions and that matching on the basis of LBM would make little difference in the interpretation of the results.

Anaerobic Muscle Metabolism

Early work by Jacobs et al. (1982, 1983) suggested that the maximal rate of muscle glycogenolysis during a 30-s cycle sprint test was lower in females than in males. The average power output during these sprints was ~3 times that required to elicit $\dot{V}O_2$max. Muscle lactate accumulation was 40–50% less in the females than in the males (Jacobs et al. 1982). Subsequently, Jacobs et al. (1983) reported muscle lactate levels of 25.2 and 47.4 mmol/kg dm after 10 and 30 s of sprinting in females and corresponding values of 46.1 and 73.9 mmol/kg dm in males. Average power outputs over the 30-s sprint were 440 W for the females and 604 W for the males. When power output was expressed per unit body mass, differences were reduced (7.5 and 8.5 W/kg body mass, respectively) and may have disappeared if power had been expressed per unit LBM.

In a more detailed experiment the contributions of muscle PCr, ATP, and glycogen breakdown to total energy provision in type I and type II fibers were assessed in males and females performing repeated bouts of 30 s of cycle sprinting (Bodin et al., 1994; Esbjornsson et al., 1994). Mean power output in this study was lower in the females even when normalized for body dimensions (7.0 vs. 8.7 W/kg$^{-2/3}$). The rates of energy provision from the degradation of PCr and of ATP (minor contribution) were not different between males and females in either fiber type during the cycle sprints (Bodin et al., 1994). The rates of ATP provision from glycogenolysis, measured during the first and third bouts of cycling, were also similar in males and females in type II fibers (Esbjornsson et al. 1994). However, the glycogenolytic rate in type I fibers was lower in the females during sprinting (1.2 vs. 3.4 mmol·kg dm^{-1}·s^{-1}). The lower energy provision by the glycogenolytic pathway of the type I fibers of the females appeared to contribute to their lower power outputs relative to the males, although cause and effect cannot be established with these data.

A recent study examining gender differences in anaerobic capacity using indirect methods reported results similar to those found with direct muscle measurements as discussed above. Hill and Smith (1993) measured the aerobic contribution to a 30-s cycle sprint and calculated the anaerobic contribution by assuming a muscular efficiency of 22%. The total work performed in 30 s was 30% lower in the females. The absolute aerobic energy contribution to the sprint was similar in males and females, but the anaerobic contribution was 35% lower in the females. Therefore, on a relative basis, the females provided a much lower proportion of the energy for a 30-s sprint from anaerobic metabolism than did the males.

NEUROMUSCULAR ADAPTATIONS TO STRENGTH TRAINING

Childhood

Adaptation to strength training in children has been the subject of recent reviews (Blimkie, 1989, 1993; Sale, 1989); therefore, only the main findings will be summarized. It was once questioned whether or not children would adapt to strength training, but many studies have now demonstrated that relative (percentage) increases in strength after comparable training regimens are similar in children and adults. In childhood, there is no evidence of a gender difference in trainability. A question that persists is whether or not training-induced muscle hypertrophy is possible in children. To date there is no clear evidence that hypertrophy occurs in preadolescence (Blimkie, 1993).

A final question is whether or not children in some way bear an increased risk of injury when participating in strength-training programs. There appears to be no increased risk, provided that children are adequately supervised (Blimkie, 1993). Special attention must be given to "fitting" children into weight training machines designed for adult body size.

Young Adults

In previous sections it was noted that after puberty and into young adulthood, males become substantially stronger and develop a larger muscle mass than do females. When young women and men participate in similar strength-training programs, does the gender difference in strength and muscle size increase, decrease, or remain the same? Indeed, there once was doubt about woman's ability to undergo hypertrophy in response to training; it is now well documented that women have this ability (Cureton et al., 1988; Krotkiewski et al., 1979; O'Hagan et al., 1995; Staron et al., 1989; Wang et al., 1993; Wilmore, 1974).

A consideration in comparing training responses in men and women is that pretraining absolute levels of muscle size and strength are greater in men. This raises the issue of whether the training responses in women and men should be compared on the basis of *absolute* increases in strength and muscle size or on *relative* increases (i.e., percentage increases). Similar relative increases in women and men would indicate greater absolute increases in the men, whereas similar absolute increases would indicate greater relative increases in the women. It has been argued that if muscle dimensions increase in a geometrically proportional manner, then a similar training adaptation in women and men would be indicated by the same relative increases in men and women but greater absolute increases in men (Cureton et al., 1988; Holloway & Baechle, 1990). Therefore, the "fair" comparison of trainability would be in terms of relative increases in strength and muscle size.

If the criterion for similar training responsiveness in women and men is similar *relative* increases in strength and muscle size, then the consensus of studies to date is that women and men have similar trainability (Colliander & Tesch, 1990; Cureton et al., 1988; O'Hagan et al., 1995; Weiss et al., 1988). There is no evidence of a markedly different training response. One additional way the trainability of women and men can be compared is to monitor any change in the ratio of women's to men's strength or muscle size during the course of training. An increase in this ratio would suggest greater trainability in women, whereas a decrease would suggest greater trainability in men. Most studies show no substantial training-induced change in this ratio (Cureton et al., 1988; O'Hagan et al., 1995). Similarly, cross-sectional studies have found the same ratios in highly trained women and men and in their untrained counterparts (Alway et al., 1989, 1990, 1992).

The similar training-induced muscle hypertrophy exhibited by men and women indicates that the net sum of all those factors that promote hypertrophy as an adaptation to resistance training is equal in both genders. However, individual factors may favor one gender. For example, men have greater resting blood testosterone concentrations than do women (Kraemer et al., 1991; Staron et al., 1994; Weiss et al., 1983), show greater increases in testosterone concentrations in response to a single session of resistance exercise (Kraemer et al., 1991; Staron et al., 1994; Weiss et al., 1983), and experience greater increases in testosterone concentrations at rest following a resistance training program (Staron et al., 1994). These differences with respect to this anabolic hormone *concentration* would seem to favor greater protein synthesis in men's versus women's muscles. In addition, although resting levels of cortisol (a catabolic hormone) are similar in untrained women and men, men's cortisol levels decrease after a training program, whereas women's levels do not change (Staron et al., 1994). This difference, combined with the increase in testosterone levels in men, results in an increased testosterone/cortisol ratio in the men, considered to be favorable for promoting muscle protein synthesis (Florini, 1985).

However, other hormones, including growth hormone, insulin, and insulin-like growth factor (IGF-1), also promote protein synthesis. Resting blood levels of growth hormone are greater in women than in men (Kraemer et al., 1991; Staron et al., 1994), but the acute response to a single session of resistance exercise is a greater increase in men (Kraemer et al., 1991). Resting levels of growth hormone are not altered by a short-term (9 wk) resistance training program (Staron et al., 1994). Resting IGF-1 levels are similar in men and women and increase transiently and similarly in women and men in response to a single session of resistance exercise (Kraemer et al., 1991). Resistance exercise has no acute effect on blood insulin levels in men (Chandler et al., 1994); gender comparisons related to resistance exercise have not been reported.

Taken together, the evidence related to anabolic hormones appears to favor men; however, the role of the various hormones, their interactions, and their influences on muscle hypertrophy remain unclear (Kraemer, 1992). Moreover, other as yet unidentified factors may favor women, allowing them to match men in *relative* increases in muscle cross-sectional area despite a seemingly less favorable hormonal environment.

It has been suggested that women's type II muscle fibers do not enlarge to the same extent as men's in response to training (Alway et al., 1990). Because preferential type II fiber hypertrophy is a typical response to resistance training (MacDougall, 1992), limited type II hypertrophy would reduce the overall hypertrophy in women. Previous research, however, has shown significant hypertrophy of type II fibers in women after resistance training and an increase in the II/I area ratio (Staron et al., 1989; Wang et al., 1993).

Another factor that may affect training-induced increases in muscle mass is initial muscle mass/size because a recent study has shown that in men, those with a greater initial level of fat-free body mass made greater absolute and relative increases in fat-free body mass after resistance training (van Etten et al., 1994). If people with larger muscles prior to training have greater muscle fiber numbers, this would bestow greater potential for hypertrophy in response to training. Women have, on average, a smaller fat-free body mass than do men, but the data on muscle fiber number are equivocal (see earlier section). Regardless, the training studies to date suggest that the correlation between fat-free mass and trainability, which might apply within men, does not apply across genders.

Yet another factor that has been raised in comparing training responses in women and men is the initial state of training. It has been suggested that women may have a lower initial state of training because of less experience with heavy resistance exercise, and this would predispose them to greater relative increases in strength and muscle size (Cureton et al., 1988). However, studies that have specifically controlled for initial state of training show similar relative gains in women and men (Cureton et al., 1988; O'Hagan et al., 1995).

A final consideration in comparing the training response of women and men is whether or not the optimal training program is the same for both. It has been suggested than men and women should train in the same way because they have similar responses to strength training from their pre-training baselines (Holloway & Baechle, 1990). However, it is not known, for example, whether women can tolerate a greater frequency of training than men can or vice versa. Nor is it known if there are gender differences in the optimal relative intensity or in the number of sets and repetitions done in each training session. One study has shown that women and men may differ in acute fatigue and recovery during resistance training sessions (Häkkinen, 1993). These issues need to be investigated to further clarify possible gender differences in the response to resistance training.

Older Adults

Retaining as much strength as possible with advancing age is important to maintaining an independent lifestyle. This fact, together with the growing number of older adults, has focused attention on the possible benefits of strength training in this population. Consequently, there has been an exponential growth of strength training studies in the elderly. The topic has been the subject of recent reviews (Porter & Vandervoort, 1995; Porter et al., 1995b; Rogers & Evans, 1993; White, 1995). It has been well established that the elderly are responsive to strength training even into the tenth decade. Increases in muscle strength, muscle cross-sectional area, and muscle fiber area have been observed. Strength increases proportionately much more than does muscle size; this pattern of results is also evident in young adults but seems to be more pronounced in the elderly. In both cases, the pattern indicates an important role for neural adaptation in improving strength.

Some studies have focused specifically on women, with the pattern of results as indicated (Charette et al., 1991; Connelly & Vandervoort, 1995; Nichols et al., 1993). Several studies have included both women and men, but few have specifically made a gender comparison (Fiatarone et al., 1990; Hicks et al., 1991; McCartney et al., 1995; Pyka et al., 1994). McCartney and colleagues (1995) found no gender effect on trainability, based on analysis of pre- and posttraining *absolute* values of strength and muscle size. No analysis was made of *relative* increases, but examination of their data indicates that the women made notably greater relative increases in most upper body strength measures but made similar increases in leg strength and in knee extensor muscle cross-sectional area. Another study by Häkkinen and Pakarinen (1994) found similar relative increases in leg strength in middle-aged and elderly women and men.

The various factors that could affect relative trainability in young women and men, discussed previously, for the most part apply equally to older adults. However, there are changes in endocrine function (hormone levels) with advanced age that could affect trainability (Häkkinen & Pakarinen, 1994). Moreover, it is assumed, as with young adults, that the optimal training stimulus is the same for older men and women; this assumption has never been tested. Similarly, it is assumed that the optimal training stimulus is the same for young and older adults.

METABOLIC ADAPTATIONS TO STRENGTH TRAINING

Energy Metabolism

No research examining potential gender differences in muscle metabolic responses to strength training was found. MacDougall et al. (1977) appear to be the only authors who examined aspects of muscle metabolism before and after heavy resistance training. They reported significant increases in resting contents of PCr (22%), total creatine (39%), ATP (18%), and glycogen (66%) in triceps brachii muscles of men following 5 mo of heavy resistance training. Because other forms of training do not induce increases in total Cr, PCr, and ATP contents, additional research is required to determine the significance of these findings.

HORMONAL AND NUTRITIONAL CONSIDERATIONS

Menstrual Status and Muscle Metabolism

It is well known that the plasma estrogen and progesterone concentrations are much higher in the luteal phase (LP) than in the follicular phase (FP) of the menstrual cycle (Bonen et al., 1981; 1991). Exercise also increases the concentrations of these hormones, especially during the LP, and it has been speculated that high levels of steroid hormones may alter the metabolic response to exercise (Bonen et al., 1983; Jurkowski et al., 1978). For example, a greater glycogen content in the LP might be expected based upon animal literature, in which glycogen formation was enhanced following increases in circulating estrogen and progesterone concentrations (Ahmed-Sorour & Bailey, 1981; Carrington & Bailey, 1985).

The literature that has carefully examined the metabolic responses of eumenorrheic (EUM) women to exercise during both phases of the menstrual cycle is sparse. The majority of studies examining the hormonal and metabolic responses of untrained women to light (40% $\dot{V}O_2max$) and intense (80% $\dot{V}O_2max$) walking and of moderately trained women to cycling at 70% $\dot{V}O_2max$ revealed few menstrual phase differences (Bonen et al., 1983, 1991; Kannely et al., 1992; Nicklas et al., 1989). There were no significant phase differences during exercise in RER and plasma or blood FFA, glycerol, lactate, and glucose concentrations. However, Hackney et al. (1991, 1994) reported significantly higher RER, and therefore lower fat utilization, in the FP during submaximal exercise. In the latter study, the lower RER in the FP was present during runs at 35 and 60% of $\dot{V}O_2max$ but not at 75% $\dot{V}O_2max$ (Hackney et al., 1994). Consistent with these findings, Hall-Jurkowski et al. (1981) reported higher blood lactate levels at 66% and 90% $\dot{V}O_2$max in the FP but did not report RER data.

Two studies examined concentrations of glycogen in muscles of resting subjects in both phases of the menstrual cycle; diet and physical activity in the 3 d preceding the biopsy sampling were controlled. The effect of the menstrual phase was minor; Nicklas et al. (1989) reported a nonsignificant trend for higher glycogen in the LP (~445 vs. 400 mmol/kg dm), and Hackney (1990) reported a significantly higher level of glycogen in the LP (~439 vs. 390 mmol/kg dm).

Menstrual Status and Exercise Performance

The effect of menstrual status on performance during exercise has not been extensively studied. Two reports examined performance recorded as time to exhaustion during an incremental $\dot{V}O_2$max test (10–12 min), with one reporting no effect of menstrual status in nonactive women (Dombovy et al., 1987) and the other a longer exercise time during the LP in untrained women (Schoene et al., 1981). Shorter exercise performance tests at or above 90% $\dot{V}O_2$max indicated a trend towards improved performance in the LP. Two studies examined time to exhaustion at ~90% $\dot{V}O_2$max following submaximal cycling at increasing exercise intensities in untrained women, with one reporting no change (Stephenson et al., 1982) and the other a longer time to exhaustion (2.97 vs. 1.57 min) in the LP (Hall-Jurkowski et al., 1981). Robertson and Higgs (1983) reported a longer run time to exhaustion at ~100% $\dot{V}O_2$max in the LP when preceded by a 12-min run at 90% $\dot{V}O_2$max in active/trained women. Lastly, in a well-controlled study by Lebrun et al. (1995), both run time to exhaustion at ~90% $\dot{V}O_2$max (~750 s) and sprint-run time to exhaustion (~28 s) were unaffected by menstrual phase in well-trained women.

Several studies have reported no change in $\dot{V}O_2$max or aerobic capacity between the menstrual phases in untrained, active, and trained women (Dombovy et al., 1987; Hall-Jurkowski et al., 1981; LeBrun et al., 1995; Schoene et al., 1981). Nicklas et al. (1989) examined the effect of the menstrual phase during cycling to exhaustion at 70% $\dot{V}O_2$max in moderately trained women. There were trends for a higher initial glycogen content, longer exhaustion time (139 vs. 127 min), and greater glycogenolysis during exercise in the LP, but these changes were not statistically significant.

Therefore, there is no consistent evidence that exercise performance is significantly affected by the phase of the menstrual cycle. Additional well-controlled studies are required to confirm this conclusion during prolonged aerobic exercise.

Maintaining or Increasing Aerobic and Anaerobic Power

Aerobic Muscle Metabolism. Experimental research has demonstrated that muscle glycogen stores in untrained individuals and trained athletes can be augmented prior to exercise through a series of exercise and diet regimens, leading to an improvement in performance during prolonged aerobic exercise (Bergstrom et al., 1967; Hermansen et al., 1967; Hultman & Bergstrom, 1967; Karlsson & Saltin, 1971; Sherman et al., 1981; Hultman & Spriet, 1988). There are also numerous reports demonstrating that ingestion of carbohydrate during intense aerobic exercise prevents decreases in blood glucose and improves performance, especially late in exercise (Coggan et al., 1988, 1989; Coyle et al., 1983, 1986)). The net result of this work has been to stress the importance of maximizing the muscle CHO store (and judging from blood glucose measurements, probably the liver CHO store) prior to engaging in prolonged, intense aerobic exercise. Almost without exception, these studies have examined only untrained and trained males. Many studies employed only one or two females in a much larger subject pool, precluding accurate conclusions about the similarity between male and female responses. Recently, attempts at addressing this problem have appeared.

O'Keefe et al. (1989) examined the effects of varying dietary CHO intake (13, 54, or 72% of total kJ) on cycling performance to exhaustion at $\sim$80% $\dot{V}O_2$max in well-trained female EUM cyclists. The diets were isocaloric and represented the normal intake for the subjects. Cycle time to exhaustion increased with increasing dietary CHO content. However, cycle times with the high- and moderate-CHO intake were not significantly different (113 vs. 98 min, respectively) but were significantly longer than those with the low-CHO diet (60 min). No muscle glycogen measurements were reported, and plasma glucose and blood lactates were not different between trials. The RER was significantly elevated in the high-CHO trial as compared to the other two diets. The authors concluded that female athletes benefit from a diet containing an ample quantity of CHO. However, increasing the dietary content above 54% did not result in improved performance, despite indications that more CHO was oxidized in the high CHO trial. One weakness of this study was that no control for menstrual status was attempted.

Tarnopolsky et al. (1995) improved on the previous study by comparing the abilities of the muscles of moderately trained male and female endurance athletes to enhance or "supercompensate" their glycogen stores. They measured muscle glycogen contents and controlled for menstrual status in the women by testing in the follicular phase. Surprisingly, the glycogen stores of the women did not increase following a glycogen-depleting ride and 4 d of tapering exercise plus dietary CHO consumption of $\sim$75% of total energy intake; the comparison control regimen included a diet with 55–60% of energy as CHO. Muscle glycogen concentrations in both trials in the women were $\sim$407 mmol/kg dm, whereas those for the men improved from $\sim$400 to 565 mmol/kg dm. The alterations in dietary CHO intake did not affect endurance performance at $\sim$85% $\dot{V}O_2$max

(~15 min to exhaustion) when preceded by 60 min of cycling at 75% $\dot{V}O_2$max in men or women.

Walker et al (1995) used a similar approach, as well-trained women ($\dot{V}O_2$max ~57 mL·min^{-1}·kg^{-1}) underwent a control and classic 7-d regimen of muscle glycogen supercompensation with a normal-CHO intake (50%) on one occasion and a high-CHO intake (> 75% of energy) in the final 3-4 d on another occasion. Subjects exercised to deplete muscle glycogen on day 1 and tapered the exercise duration while maintaining training intensity to no exercise on day 6, followed by a ride to exhaustion at ~85% $\dot{V}O_2$max on day 7. Menstrual status was carefully controlled by testing on both occasions in the luteal phase. Muscle glycogen levels following the 50% CHO regimen were already much higher (664 mmol/kg dm) than previously reported in untrained females and did not increase on the glycogen supercompensation regimen (685 mmol/kg dm). However, endurance performance at 85% $\dot{V}O_2$max increased significantly from 98 min and 15 s to 110 min and 25 s following the high-CHO diet. This suggests that the improved performance may be related to higher levels of liver glycogen prior to exhaustive exercise.

These studies indicate that the benefits of high-CHO diets and supercompensation regimens are less pronounced in trained female endurance athletes than in males. It should be noted, however, that with the lower energy intakes of female athletes (9,600–10,600 kJ), consuming diets containing 75% CHO succeeded in reaching CHO intakes of only 7.9–9.0 g/kg LBM or absolute amounts of 370–420 g (Tarnopolsky et al., 1995; Walker et al., 1995). These are less than the recommended amounts for maximizing glycogen levels to ~1000 mmol/kg dm in males, i.e., > 8.5 g CHO/kg LBM or, more importantly, 500–600 g/d (Roberts et al., 1988; Sherman et al., 1981). Achieving absolute daily CHO intakes in the 500–600 g range is probably unrealistic for female athletes because they would need to increase their total energy intakes substantially for a 3-4 d period.

Nicklas et al. (1989) exercised moderately trained women to exhaustion at 70% $\dot{V}O_2$max in both phases of the menstrual cycle with starting glycogen concentrations of 400–445 mmol/kg dm. Interestingly, fatigue in this study did not coincide with depletion of glycogen; ~210 and ~255 mmol/kg dm remained in the muscles at exhaustion in the LP and FP, respectively. These data suggested that the relationship between exhaustion and glycogen depletion during prolonged exercise in males did not exist in females. However, the studies discussed above demonstrated that muscle glycogen decreased to 65–80 and 115–120 mmol/kg dm in trained and motivated female athletes (Tarnopolsky et al., 1995; Walker et al., 1995). These muscle glycogen contents are as low following exhaustive exercise requiring 75–85% $\dot{V}O_2$max as has been reported in males (Bergstrom et al., 1967; Spriet et al., 1992).

Anaerobic Muscle Metabolism. Little has been done to examine the importance of nutrition for performance of intense resistance and sprint exercise as it relates to potential gender differences. However, it is known that repeated bouts of resistance exercise and sprint exercise degrade large amounts of glycogen in males (Gaitanos et al., 1993; McCartney et al., 1986; Robergs et al., 1991; Tesch et al., 1986). The literature also suggests that increasing or decreasing the initial muscle glycogen content prior to a single bout of short-term intense activity does not affect glycogenolysis or performance (Saltin et al., 1992: Spriet, 1992). However, it is important to maintain an adequate dietary intake of CHO to maintain optimal muscle glycogen levels and performance during repeated bouts of resistance and sprint exercise on a given day and during sequential days of activity (Pascoe et al., 1993).

DIRECTIONS FOR FUTURE RESEARCH

Neuromuscular Function

There is now a vast literature on neuromuscular function in both women and men throughout the life cycle. Although the majority of this literature still pertains to young adults, an increasing amount of research is being done with children, and even more with the elderly. Despite our increasing knowledge, many important problems remain unanswered. Some of these problems are enumerated below.

Women have only about half the upper body strength and muscle mass of men but about 75% of the lower body strength and muscle size, and the reason for this disparity is not known. The expectation that men would have a greater fiber number than women in upper limb muscles has not been convincingly fulfilled. This suggests a much greater fiber size in men's muscles, but it is not at all clear why muscle fibers, especially type II fibers, in males would be so much larger, specifically in the upper limbs.

Data are inconsistent in establishing age and gender influences on the concentric force-velocity relationship. In particular, further investigation of the "high" end of the velocity range is needed in children and the elderly.

Questions related to muscle fiber composition remain unresolved. Is there a difference in the percentage of type I and II fibers in males and females; if so, in which muscles does the difference occur? If there is a difference, when in the life cycle does it occur, does it have a functional impact, and does it account for any of the observed differences in strength? Is there really a decrease in the percentage of type II fibers with age in some or all muscles? Cross-sectional studies with large sample sizes and more longitudinal studies will be needed to answer these questions.

In addition to gender and age differences in muscle fiber number, size, and type, there may be ultrastructural differences underlying many of the functional differences observed. For example, gender and age effects on the sarcoplasmic reticulum could influence contractile speed.

Inasmuch as most of the age and gender differences in strength can be attributed to similar differences in muscle size, there remain reported age and gender differences in specific force, i.e., the force generated per unit of muscle cross-sectional area. Possible differences in specific force and the reasons for them require study.

There is no doubt that strength eventually declines with advancing age; however, there are intriguing contradictions in the literature. One is the age at which strength finally starts to decline, with studies showing starting points ranging from 25–50 y of age. When the loss begins, what roles do neural activation, muscle atrophy, and changes intrinsic to muscle play in the loss, and are there gender differences?

The recent availability of safe eccentric-loading dynamometers has spurred research that has raised more questions. For example, the ratio of eccentric to concentric strength (ECC/CON) is greater in women than in men, but the explanation for this difference is not clear, and it is unknown when in the life cycle the difference begins or why it is more evident in some muscle groups than in others. The ECC/CON ratio also increases with advanced age in both women and men. Research into the mechanisms of the increase is warranted, as well as investigation of a gender influence on the increase.

People of all ages respond favorably to strength training. Prepubescent children increase strength markedly but show little hypertrophy. The elderly show hypertrophy but perhaps not to the same extent as young adults. There is as yet no explanation for these different patterns of adaptation. Females appear to be as trainable as males throughout the life cycle, especially when relative improvements are compared. What remains to be investigated is whether or not the optimal training stimulus, in terms of training intensity, volume, and frequency, changes during the life cycle or differs between males and females.

Muscle Metabolism

The discussions in this chapter dealing with aerobic and anaerobic metabolism make it clear that investigation of possible gender differences in the ability of skeletal muscle to provide energy during various types of exercise has just begun. The assumption that female responses can be inferred from male results is now being severely tested. Information directly applicable to the female is lacking in many of the areas examined in this chapter. It is also clear that the gender information that does exist has been derived from the study of young adults between the ages of 18–30 y. Much of this information has come from measurements on muscle samples that require invasive techniques to obtain. Therefore, it may be more difficult to obtain similar information in younger and older individuals, unless the use of less invasive techniques such as metabolic tracers and magnetic resonance imaging and spectroscopy are improved and more widely accessible. A special area of interest is the lack of nutritional information directly applicable to the active female throughout the life span. Certainly, the interactions among nutrition, exercise training, and menstrual status as they relate to skeletal muscle energy metabolism and performance and whole body exercise performance require immediate attention.

SUMMARY

Neuromuscular Function

Absolute strength and muscle size increase several-fold in both genders, in a similar pattern, and almost linearly from early childhood to about age 13–14 y. Until this age there is little gender difference, but thereafter males show an acceleration of increased strength and muscle size not shared by the females, who show little further increase. By age 20 y, females have on average about 50% of the upper body strength and muscle size and 65% of the lower body strength and size of males. The increase in muscle size during growth and development is due to increasing muscle fiber size, rather than to increased fiber number. Similarly, males' greater muscle fiber size, particularly in upper limb muscles, and particularly the type II fibers, accounts for the gender difference in muscle size fully established at young adulthood.

The strength/body mass ratio, an indicator of the ability to support and move one's body weight, reaches its peak in females at about 10–12 y, after which it levels off or declines slightly. In contrast, this ratio increases in males until early adulthood.

The pattern described above for isometric and low-velocity concentric strength generally applies also to eccentric and high-velocity concentric strength. However, there is some indication that the ratio of eccentric to concentric strength (ECC/CON) is greater in women than in men, for reasons unknown.

Large-sample studies have indicated a higher percentage of type I fibers in females (vastus lateralis), but the gender difference is small. On the other hand, the percent type I fiber area is substantially higher in women, especially in upper limb muscles. This difference might be expected to enhance endurance but impair high-velocity concentric strength in females.

Isometric and low-velocity concentric strength values decline 15–20% between ages 20–60 y, after which the loss accelerates, yielding a 40–50% loss by 80 y. High-velocity concentric strength may suffer a greater loss over this period, whereas eccentric strength has been shown to be relatively spared. The loss of strength varies somewhat in different muscle groups. There is no striking gender difference in aging-induced strength loss.

Elderly women and men activate their muscles as well as young adults, so most of the loss in strength must be attributed to changes in muscle. The decline in muscle size parallels that of strength; thus, the former is likely the cause of the latter. Accordingly, *specific force*, the strength per unit of muscle cross-sectional area, differs little in old and young adults.

A decrease in both fiber number and size contributes to the decline in muscle size with aging. The decrease in fiber number may begin before age 50 y and makes the greater contribution to whole muscle atrophy, whereas fiber atrophy, which occurs most in type II fibers, occurs later. The research is equivocal whether one fiber type sustains a greater loss in number with aging; however, the preferential loss of fast-conducting motoneurons after age 60 y suggests that an increased proportion of type I fibers may be most likely. There is no gender difference in the pattern of fiber loss and atrophy nor in the change of fiber type distribution. The increased percent type I fiber area may account for both the preserved eccentric strength but deteriorated high-velocity concentric strength in the elderly.

The neuromuscular system is responsive to resistance (strength) training throughout the life cycle. Strength increases to a greater extent than does muscle size in response to training, and this lack of correspondence is generally attributed to "neural" adaptations that increase strength independently of hypertrophy. The capacity for muscle hypertrophy may be limited in children. Throughout adulthood, men make greater absolute but similar relative increases in muscle size and strength compared to women. A diminished, but still substantial, capacity for muscle hypertrophy is retained in old age. When it occurs, hypertrophy is characterized by a greater enlargement of type II than of type I fibers.

Muscle Metabolism

There is great interest in the possibility that gender differences in skeletal muscle metabolism may exist. Unfortunately, there has been no concerted effort to systematically examine this premise. There is limited gender information examining skeletal muscle energy-substrate stores, maximal enzyme activities representative of the major energy-producing pathways, and distribution of fiber types. There are also a few gender comparisons of muscle metabolism during prolonged aerobic exercise and short-term, high-intensity exercise. It is also apparent that gender comparisons have not been made throughout the life cycle; the existing information examines only young adult males and females (18–35 y).

Direct measurements of the skeletal muscle energy substrates, glycogen, phosphocreatine, and ATP, reveal no differences between males and females at rest. However, there is evidence to suggest that well-trained females are unable to increase their stores of muscle glycogen by "glycogen loading" regimens to the same extent as well-trained men. Circumstantial evidence also suggests that females have larger intramuscular stores of triacylglycerol (TG), but this has not been firmly established due to the difficulty in accurately measuring muscle TG. It has been well documented that females have, on average, greater stores of adipose tissue TG. Lastly, no gender information exists regarding the store of glycogen in the liver.

Absolute activities of glycogenolytic/glycolytic enzymes are generally elevated in active and trained young-adult males vs. their female counterparts. However, in untrained subjects the difference is much less pronounced. Higher citric acid cycle (CAC) enzyme activities are also common in active and trained males vs. females, with no gender differences in untrained subjects. Activities of β-oxidation enzymes are unaffected by gender at all fitness levels. However, on a relative basis, females have a greater capacity for β-oxidation compared to CAC activity than do males, suggesting they may be predisposed to oxidizing a greater proportion of fat (and less carbohydrate) at a given percentage of $\dot{V}O_2$max. Females also have a lower ratio of enzyme activities for glycolysis: β-oxidation than do males, implying a smaller difference between anaerobic and aerobic energy-generating pathways. Many of the above gender differences appear to be related to the tendency for greater proportions of type I fibers in women.

When examining exercise studies, indirect calorimetry data suggest that well-trained women, when compared with men matched on the basis of $\dot{V}O_2$max/kg LBM, oxidize less carbohydrate and more fat during aerobic exercise at intensities between 60% and 75% $\dot{V}O_2$max. These studies have carefully controlled for potential confounding factors such as diet, menstrual status, and the frequency, duration, and history of training, when comparing men and women. Therefore, the functional aerobic exercise studies confirm the greater use of fat by well-trained women vs. men that was predicted by the reports of greater proportion of type I fibers, larger stores of intramuscular and adipose tissue fat, and a greater ratio of enzyme activities in β-oxidation:CAC in the women. It is not known what role the hormones estrogen and progesterone may play in these findings, and many of the differences reported between well-trained males and females are not apparent or as pronounced in less active individuals.

Direct measurements of skeletal muscle anaerobic energy provision have been made in type I and II fibers of active males and females during repeated 30-s bouts of maximal cycling. The findings demonstrate no gender differences in the rates of energy provision from PCr degradation in either fiber type. Provision of ATP by glycogenolysis was also similar in males and females in type II fibers during sprinting, but lower in type I fibers of females. The lower glycogenolytic energy provision of the type I fibers in women was associated with lower power outputs as compared to males. Indirect estimates of anaerobic energy provision support the direct findings. These functional studies of sprinting exercise confirm the results predicted by the lower activities of glycogenolytic/glycolytic enzymes in females.

In conclusion, gender differences do appear to exist in skeletal muscle metabolism during exercise, but this area of metabolic research is clearly in its infancy. A major difficulty in conducting studies examining the effects of gender on skeletal muscle metabolism is the uncertainty of how best to match males and females. It is not clear what aspects of physiological function, including exercise and skeletal muscle performance, should be matched to represent a true comparison.

BIBLIOGRAPHY

Aherne, W., D.R. Ayyar, P.A. Clarke, and J.N. Walton (1971). Muscle fiber size in normal infants, children and adolescents: an autopsy study. *J. Neurol. Sci.* 14:171–182.

Ahmed-Sorour, H., and C.J. Bailey (1981). Role of ovarian hormones in the long-term control of glucose homeostasis, glycogen formation, and gluconeogenesis. *Ann. Nutr. Metab.* 25:208–212.

Alway, S.E., W.H. Grumbt, W.J. Gonyea, and J. Stray-Gunderson (1989). Contrasts in muscle and myofibers of elite male and female bodybuilders. *J. Appl. Physiol.* 67:24–31.

Alway, S.E., W.H. Grumbt, J. Stray-Gunderson, and W.J. Gonyea (1992). Effects of resistance training on elbow flexors of highly competitive bodybuilders. *J. Appl. Physiol.* 72:1512–1521.

Alway, S.E., J. Stray-Gunderson, W.H. Grumbt, and W.J. Gonyea (1990). Muscle cross-sectional area and torque in resistance-trained subjects. *Eur. J. Appl. Physiol.* 60:86–90.

Anderson, M.B., R.W. Coté III, E.F. Coyle, and F.B. Roby (1979). Leg power, muscle strength, and peak EMG activity in physically active college men and women. *Med. Sci. Sports* 11:81.

Aniansson, A., G. Grimby, M. Hedberg, and M. Krotkiewski (1981). Muscle morphology, enzyme activity and muscle strength in elderly men and women. *Clin. Physiol.* 1:73–86.

Aniansson, A., M. Hedberg, G.-B. Henning, and G. Grimby (1986). Muscle morphology, enzymatic activity, and muscle strength in elderly men: a follow-up study. *Muscle Nerve* 9:585–591.

Aniansson, A., L. Sperling, A. Rundgren, and E. Lehnberg (1983). Muscle function in 75-year-old men and women: a longitudinal study. *Scand. Rehab. Med.* (suppl. 9):92–102.

Bass, A., K. Vondra, R. Rath, and V. Vitek (1975). M. quadriceps femoris muscle of man, a muscle with an unusual enzyme activity pattern of energy supplying metabolism in mammals. *Pfluegers Arch.* 354:-249–255.

Bell, R.D., J.D. MacDougall, R. Billeter, and H. Howald (1980). Muscle fiber types and morphometric analysis of skeletal muscle in six-year-old children. *Med. Sci. Sports Exerc.* 12:28–31.

Bergstrom, J., L. Hermansen, E. Hultman, and B. Saltin (1967). Diet, muscle glycogen and physical performance. *Acta Physiol. Scand.* 71:140–150.

Blatchford, F.K., R.G. Knowlton, and D.A. Schneider (1985). Plasma FFA responses to prolonged walking in untrained men and women. *Eur. J. Appl. Physiol.* 53:343–347.

Blimkie, C.J.R. (1989). Age- and sex-associated variation in strength during childhood: anthropometric, morphologic, neurologic, biomechanical, endocrinologic, genetic, and physical activity correlates. In: C.V. Gisolfi and D.R. Lamb (eds.) *Perspectives in Exercise Science and Sports Medicine, Vol. 2: Youth, Exercise, and Sport.* Indianapolis: Benchmark Press, pp. 99–163.

Blimkie, C.J.R. (1993). Resistance training during preadolescence. Issues and controversies. *Sports Med.* 15:389–407.

Bodin, K., M. Esbjornsson, and E. Jansson (1994). Alactic ATP turnover rate during 30-s cycle sprints in females and males. *Clin. Sci.* 87 (Suppl.):125–126. (Abstract).

Bonen, A., A.N. Belcastro, W.Y. Ling, and A.A. Simpson (1981). Profiles of selected hormones during menstrual cycles of teenage athletes. *J. Appl. Physiol.* 50:545–551.

Bonen, A., F.W. Haynes, and T.E. Graham (1991). Substrate and hormonal responses to exercise in women using oral contraceptives. *J. Appl. Physiol.* 70:1917–1927.

Bonen, A., F.W. Haynes, W. Watson-Wright, M.M. Sopper, G.N. Pierce, M.P. Low, and T.E. Graham (1983). Effects of menstrual cycle on metabolic responses to exercise. *J. Appl. Physiol.* 55:1506–1513.

Booth, F.W., S.H. Weeden, and B.S. Tseng (1994). Effect of aging on human skeletal muscle and motor function. *Med. Sci. Sports Exerc.* 26:556–560.

Borges, O., and B. Essen-Gustavsson (1989). Enzyme activities in type I and II muscle fibres of human skeletal muscle in relation to age and torque development. *Acta Physiol. Scand.* 136:29–36.

Brooke, M.H., and W.K. Engel (1969). The histographic analysis of human muscle biopsies with regard to fiber types. Children's biopsies. *Neurology* 19:591–605.

Bruce, S.A., D. Newton, and R.C. Woledge (1989). Effect of age on voluntary force and cross-sectional area of human adductor pollicis muscle. *Quart. J. Exp. Physiol.* 74:359–362.

Burnie, J., and D.A. Brodie (1986). Isokinetic measurement in preadolescent males. *Int. J. Sports Med.* 7:205–209.

Cadefau, J., J. Casademont, J.M. Grau, J. Fernandez, A. Balaguer, M. Vernet, R. Cusso, and A. Urbano-Marquez (1990). Biochemical and histochemical adaptation to sprint training in young athletes. *Acta Physiol. Scand.* 140:341–351.

Campbell, M.J., A.J. McComas, and F. Petito (1973). Physiological changes in ageing muscles. *J. Neurol. Neurosurg. Psychiat.* 36:174–182.

Campbell, W.W., M.C. Crim, V.R. Young, and W.J. Evans (1994). Increased energy requirements and changes in body composition with resistance training in older adults. *Am. J. Clin. Nutr.* 60:167–175.

Carrington, L.J., and C.J. Bailey (1985). Effects of natural and synthetic estrogens and progestins on glycogen deposition in female mice. *Horm. Res.* 21:199–203.

Cartee, G.D. (1994). Aging skeletal muscle: response to exercise. *Exercise and Sport Sciences Reviews.* 22:91–120.

Chandler R.M., H.K. Byrne, J.G. Patterson, and J.L. Ivy (1994). Dietary supplements affect the anabolic hormones after weight-training exercise. *J. Appl. Physiol.* 76:839–845.

Charette, S.L., L. McEvoy, G. Pyka, C. Snowharter, D. Guido, R.A. Wiswell, and R. Marcus (1991). Muscle hypertrophy response to resistance training in older women. *J. Appl. Physiol.* 70:1912–1916.

Cheetham, M.E., L.H. Boobis, S. Brooks, and C. Williams (1986). Human muscle metabolism during sprint running. *J. Appl. Physiol.* 61:54–60.

Cioni, R., F. Giannini, C. Paradiso, N. Battistini, F. Denoth, C. Navona, and A. Starita (1988). Differences between surface EMG in male and female subjects evidenced by automatic analysis. *Electroenceph. Clin. Neurophysiol.* 70:306–312.

Clarkson, P.M., W. Kroll, and A.M. Melchionda (1981). Age, isometric strength, rate of tension development and fiber type composition. *J. Geront.* 36:648–653.

Coggan, A.R., and E.F. Coyle (1988). Effect of carbohydrate feedings during high-intensity exercise. *J. Appl. Physiol.* 65:1703–1710.

Coggan, A.R., and E.F. Coyle (1989). Metabolism and performance following carbohydrate ingestion late in exercise. *Med. Sci. Sports Exerc.* 21:59–65.

Colliander, E.B., and P.A. Tesch (1989). Bilateral eccentric and concentric torque of quadriceps and hamstring muscles in females and males. *Eur. J. Appl. Physiol.* 59:227–232.

Colliander, E.B., and P.A. Tesch (1990). Responses to eccentric and concentric resistance training in females and males. *Acta Physiol. Scand.* 141:149–156.

Colling-Saltin, A.-S. (1980). Skeletal muscle development in the human fetus and during childhood. In: K. Berg and B.O. Eriksson (eds.) *Children and Exercise IX.* Baltimore: University Park Press, pp. 193–207.

Connelly, D.M., and A.A. Vandervoort (1995). Improvement in knee extensor strength of institutionalized elderly women after exercise with ankle weights. *Physiother. Can.* 47:15–23.

Costill, D.L., J. Daniels, W. Evans, W. Fink, G. Krahenbuhl, and B. Saltin (1976). Skeletal muscle enzymes and fiber composition in male and female track athletes. *J. Appl. Physiol.* 40:149–154.

Costill, D., W. Fink, L. Getchell, J. Ivy, and F. Witzmann (1979). Lipid metabolism in skeletal muscle of endurance-trained males and females. *J. Appl. Physiol.* 47:787–791.

Coyle, E.F., A.R. Coggan, M.K. Hemmert, and J.L. Ivy (1986). Muscle glycogen utilization during prolonged strenuous exercise when fed carbohydrate. *J. Appl. Physiol.* 61:165–172.

Coyle, E.F., J.M. Hagberg, B.F. Hurley, W.H. Martin, A.A. Ehsani, and J.O. Holloszy (1983). Carbohydrate feeding during prolonged exercise can delay fatigue. *J. Appl. Physiol.* 55:230–235.

Cupido, C.M., A.L. Hicks, and J. Martin (1992). Neuromuscular fatigue during repetitive stimulation in elderly and young adults. *Eur. J. Appl. Physiol.* 65:567–572.

Cureton, K.J., M.A. Collins, D.W. Hill, F.M. McElhannon Jr. (1988). Muscle hypertrophy in men and women. *Med. Sci. Sports Exerc.* 20:338–344.

Danneskiold-Samsoe, B., V. Kofod, J. Munter, G. Grimby, P. Schnohr, and G. Jensen (1984). Muscle strength and functional capacity in 78–81-year-old men and women. *Eur. J. Appl. Physiol.* 52:310–314.

Davies, C.T.M. (1985). Strength and mechanical properties of muscle in children and young adults. *Scand. J. Sports Sci.* 7:11–15.

Davies, C.T.M., D.O. Thomas, and M.J. White (1986). Mechanical properties of young and elderly human muscle. *Acta Med. Scand.* 711:219–226.

Davison, K.S., G. Ioannidis, N. Tsunoda, D.G. Sale, J.D. MacDougall, and J. Moroz (1995). Influence of gender and training on muscle activation in eccentric and concentric actions. *Med. Sci. Sports Exerc.* 27(Suppl.):S89.

de Koning, F.L., R.A. Binkhorst, J.A. Vos, and M.A. van't Hof (1985). The force-velocity relationship of arm flexion in untrained males and females and arm-trained athletes. *Eur. J. Appl. Physiol.* 54:89–94.

Dickerson, J.W.T., and E.M. Widdowson (1960). Chemical changes in skeletal muscle during development. *Biochem. J.* 74:247–257.

Doherty, T.J., A.A. Vandervoort, and W.F. Brown (1993a). Effects of ageing on the motor unit: a brief review. *Can. J. Appl. Physiol.* 18:331–358.

Doherty, T.J., A.A. Vandervoort, A.W. Taylor, and W.F. Brown (1993b). Effects of motor unit losses on strength in older men and women. *J. Appl. Physiol.* 74:868–874.

Dombovy, M.L., H.W. Bonekat, T.J. Williams, and B.A. Staats (1987). Exercise performance and ventilatory response in the menstrual cycle. *Med. Sci. Sports Exerc.* 19:111–117.

Dudley, G.A., R.T. Harris, M.R. Duvoisin, B.M. Hather, and P. Buchanan (1990). Effect of voluntary vs. artificial activation on the relationship of muscle torque to speed. *J. Appl. Physiol.* 69:2215–2221.

Elder, G.C.B., and B.A. Kakulas (1993). Histochemical and contractile property changes during human development. *Muscle Nerve* 16:1246–1253.

Esbjornsson, M., K. Bodin, and E. Jansson (1994). Females have lower glycogenetic rate in type I muscle fibers than males during a 30-s wingate test. *Clin. Sci.* 87(Suppl):55–56. (Abstract).

Esbjornsson, M., C. Sylven, I. Holm, and E. Jansson (1993). Fast twitch fibers may predict anaerobic performance in both females and males. *Int. J. Sports Med.* 14:257–263.

Essen, B. (1977). Intramuscular substrate utilization during prolonged exercise. *Ann. N.Y. Acad. Sci.* 301:-30–44.

Essen-Gustavsson, B., and O. Borges (1986). Histochemical and metabolic characteristics of human skeletal muscle in relation to age. *Acta Physiol. Scand.* 126:107–114.

Fiatarone, M.A., E.C. Marks, N.D. Ryan, C.N. Meredith, L.A. Lipsitz, and W.J. Evans (1990). High intensity strength training in nonagenarians. *JAMA* 263:3029–3034.

Florini, J.R. (1985). Hormonal control of muscle cell growth. *J. Anim. Sci.* 61:21–37.

Forsberg, A.M., E. Nilsson, J. Werneman, J. Bergstrom, and E. Hultman (1991). Muscle composition in relation to age and sex. *Clin. Sci.* 81:249–256.

Friedmann, B., and W. Kindermann (1989). Energy metabolism and regulatory hormones in women and men during endurance exercise. *Eur. J. Appl. Physiol.* 59:1–9.

Froberg, K., and O. Lammert (1995). Development of muscle strength during childhood. In: O. Bar-Or (ed.) *The Encyclopedia of Sports Medicine. Vol. IV The Child and Adolescent Athlete.* London: Blackwell Scientific Publications, In Press.

Froberg, K., and P.K. Pedersen (1984). Sex differences in endurance capacity and metabolic response to prolonged, heavy exercise. *Eur. J. Appl. Physiol.* 52:446–450.

Froese, E.A., and M.E. Houston (1985). Torque-velocity characteristics and muscle fiber type in human vastus lateralis. *J. Appl. Physiol.* 59:309–314.

Frontera, W.R., V.A. Hughes, K.J. Lutz, and W. J. Evans (1991). A cross-sectional study of muscle strength and mass in 45- to 78-yr-old men and women. *J. Appl. Physiol.* 71:644–650.

Gaitanos, G.C., C. Williams, L.H. Boobis, and S. Brooks (1993). Human muscle metabolism during intermittent maximal exercise. *J. Appl. Physiol.* 75:712–719.

Gerdle, B., and A.R. Fugl-Meyer (1985). Mechanical output and IEMG of isokinetic plantar flexion in 40–64-year-old subjects. *Acta Physiol. Scand.* 124:201–211.

Gilliam, T.B., J.F. Villanacci, P.S. Freedson, and S.P. Sady (1979). Isokinetic torque in boys and girls ages 7 to 13: effect of age, height, and weight. *Res. Quart.* 50:599–609.

Glenmark, B., G. Hedberg, and E. Jannson (1992). Changes in muscle fibre type from adolescence to adulthood in women and men. *Acta Physiol. Scand.* 146:251–259.

Gollnick, P.D., B.F. Timson, R.L. Moore, and M. Riedy (1981). Muscular enlargement and numbers of fibers in skeletal muscles of rats. *J. Appl. Physiol.* 50:936–943.

Graham, T.E., J.P. VanDijk, M. Visanathan, K.A. Giles, A. Bonen, and J.C. George (1986). Exercise metabolic changes in men and eumenorrheic and amenorrheic women (Abstract). In: B. Saltin (ed.) *Biochemistry of Exercise VI.* Champaign: Human Kinetics, pp. 229–230.

Green, H.J., I.G. Fraser, and D.A. Ranney (1984). Male and female differences in enzyme activities of energy metabolism in vastus lateralis muscle. *J. Neurol. Sci.* 65:323–331.

Greig, C.A., J. Botella, and A. Young (1993). The quadriceps strength of healthy elderly people remeasured after eight years. *Muscle Nerve* 16:6–10.

Griffin, J.W., R.E. Tooms, R. Vander Zwaag, T.E. Bertorini, and M.L. O'Toole (1993). Eccentric muscle performance of elbow and knee muscle groups in untrained men and women. *Med. Sci. Sports Exerc.* 25:936–944.

Grimby G., and B. Saltin (1983). The ageing muscle. *Clin. Physiol.* 3:209–218.

Grimby, G., A. Aniansson, C. Zetterberg, and B. Saltin (1984). Is there a change in relative muscle fiber composition with age? *Clin. Physiol.* 4:189–194.

Grimby, G., B. Danneskiold-Samsoe, H. Kvid, and B. Saltin (1982). Morphology and enzymatic capacity in arm and leg muscles in 78–81-year-old men and women. *Acta Physiol. Scand.* 115:125–134.

Gupta, D., A. Attanasio, and S. Raaf (1975). Plasma estrogenand androgen concentrations in children during adolescence. *J. Clin. End. Metab.* 40:636–643.

Hackney, A.C. (1990). Effects of the menstrual cycle on resting muscle glycogen content. *Horm. Metab. Res.* 22:647.

Hackney, A.C., C.S. Curley, and B.J. Nicklas (1991). Physiological responses to submaximal exercise at the mid-follicular, ovulatory and mid-luteal phases of the menstrual cycle. *Scand. J. Med. Sci. Sports* 1:94–98.

Hackney, A.C., M.A. McCracken-Compton, and B. Ainsworth (1994). Substrate responses to submaximal exercise in the midfollicular and midluteal phases of the menstrual cycle. *Int. J. Sport Nutrition* 4:299–308.

Häkkinen, K. (1993). Neuromuscular fatigue and recovery in male and female athletes during heavy resistance exercise. *Int. J. Sports Med.* 14:53–59.

Häkkinen, K., and A. Häkkinen (1991). Muscle cross-sectional area, force production and relaxation characteristics in women at different ages. *Eur. J. Appl. Physiol.* 62:410–414.

Häkkinen, K., and A. Pakarinen (1994). Serum hormones and strength development during strength training in middle-aged and elderly males and females. *Acta Physiol. Scand.* 150:211–219.

Hall-Jurkowski, J.E., N.L. Jones, C.J. Toews, and J.R. Sutton (1981). Effects of menstrual cycle on blood lactate, O_2 delivery, and performance during exercise. *J. Appl. Physiol.* 51:1493–1499.

Harries, U.J., and E.J. Bassey (1990). Torque-velocity relationships for the knee extensors in women in their 3rd and 7th decades. *Eur. J. Appl. Physiol.* 60:187–190.

Henriksson-Larsen, K. (1985). Distribution, number and size of different types of fibers in whole cross-sections of female m tibialis anterior. An enzyme histochemical study. *Acta Physiol. Scand.* 123:229–235.

Hermansen, L., E. Hultman, and B. Saltin (1967). Muscle glycogen during prolonged severe exercise. *Acta Physiol. Scand.* 71:129–139.

Heyward, V.H., S.M. Johannes-Ellis, and J.F. Romer (1986). Gender differences in strength. *Res. Quart.* 57:154–159.

Hicks, A.L., C.M. Cupido, J. Martin, and J. Dent (1991). Twitch potentiation in the elderly: the effects of training. *Eur. J. Appl. Physiol.* 63:278–281.

Hill, D.W., and J.C. Smith (1993). Gender differences in anaerobic capacity: role of aerobic contribution. *Br. J. Sports Med.* 27:45–48.

Holloway, J.B., and T.R. Baechle (1990). Strength training for female athletes. A review of selected aspects. *Sports Med.* 9:216–228.

Hoppeler, H., H. Howald, K. Conley, S.L. Linstedt, H. Classen, P. Vock, and E.R. Weibel (1985). Endurance training in humans: aerobic capacity and structure of skeletal muscle. *J. Appl. Physiol.* 59:320–327.

Houston, M.E., R.W. Norman, and E.A. Froese (1988). Mechanical measures during maximal velocity knee extension exercise and their relation to fiber composition of the human vastus lateralis muscle. *Eur. J. Appl. Physiol.* 58:1–7.

Hultman, E., and Bergstrom, J. (1967). Muscle glycogen synthesis in relation to diet studied in normal subjects. *Acta Med. Scand.* 182:109–117.

Hultman, E., and L.L. Spriet (1988). Dietary intake prior to and during exercise. In: E.S. Horton, and R.L. Terjung (eds.) *Exercise, Nutrition, and Energy Metabolism.* Toronto: Collier Macmillan, pp. 132–149.

Hultman, E., J. Bergstrom, and N. McLennan-Anderson (1967). Breakdown and resynthesis of phosphorylcreatine and adenosine triphosphate in connection with muscular work in man. *Scand. J. Cli. Lab. Invest.* 19:56–66.

Hurley, B.F., P.M. Nemeth, W.H. Martin III, J.M. Hagberg, G.P. Dalsky, and J.O. Holloszy (1986). Muscle triglyceride utilization during exercise: effect of training. *J. Appl. Physiol.* 60:562–567.

Ikai, M., and T. Fukunaga (1968). Calculation of muscle strength per unit cross-sectional area of human muscle by means of ultrasonic measurement. *Int. Z. Angew. Physiol. Einschl. Arbeitsphysiol.* 26:26–32.

Imamura, K., H. Ashida, T. Ishikawa, and M. Fujii (1983). Human major psoas muscle and sacrospinalis muscle in relation to age: a study by computed tomography. *J. Geront.* 38:678–681.

Jacobs, I., O. Bar-Or, J. Karlsson, R. Dotan, P. Tesch, P. Kaiser, and O. Inbar (1982). Changes in muscle metabolites in females with 30-s exhaustive exercise. *Med. Sci. Sports Exerc.* 14:457–460.

Jacobs, I., P.A. Tesch, O. Bar-Or, J. Karlsson, and R. Dotan (1983). Lactate in human skeletal muscle after 10 and 30 s of supramaximal exercise. *J. Appl. Physiol.* 55:365–367.

Jansson, E. (1986). Sex differences in metabolic response to exercise. (Abstract). In: B. Saltin (ed.) *Biochemistry of Exercise VI.* Champaign: Human Kinetics, pp. 228–229.

Jennekens, F.G.I., B.E. Tomlinson, and J. Walton (1971). Histochemical aspects of five limb muscles in old age: an autopsy study. *J. Neurol. Sci.* 14:259–276.

Johnston, F.E., and R.M. Malina (1966). Age changes in the composition of the upper arm in Philadelphia children. *Human Biol.* 38:1–21.

Jurkowski, J.E., N.L. Jones, W.C. Walker, E.V. Younglai, and J.R. Sutton (1978). Ovarian hormonal responses to exercise. *J. Appl. Physiol.* 44:109–114.

Kallman, D.A., C.C. Plato, and J.D. Tobin (1990). The role of muscle loss in the age-related decline of grip strength: cross-sectional and longitudinal perspectives. *J. Geront.* 45:M82–M88.

Kanehisa, H., S. Ikegawa, T. Fukunaga (1994). Comparison of muscle cross-sectional area and strength between untrained women and men. *Eur. J. Appl. Physiol.* 68:148–154.

Kanehisa, H., S. Ikegawa, N. Tsunoda, and T. Fukunaga (1995). Strength and cross-sectional areas of reciprocal muscle groups in the upper arm and thigh during adolescence. *Int. J. Sports Med.* 16:54–60.

Kannely, J.A., R.A. Boileau, J.A. Bahr, J.E. Misner, and R.A. Nelson (1992). Substrate oxidation and GH responses to exercise are independent of menstrual phase and status. *Med. Sci. Sports Exerc.* 24:873–880.

Karlsson, J., and B. Saltin (1971). Diet, muscle glycogen and endurance performance. *J. Appl. Physiol.* 31:203–206.

Klitgaard, H., M. Mantoni, S. Schiaffino, S. Ausoni, L. Gorza, C. Laurent-Winter, P. Schnohr, and B. Saltin (1990a). Function, morphology and protein expression of ageing skeletal muscle: a cross-sectional study of elderly men with different training backgrounds. *Acta Physiol. Scand.* 140:41–54.

Klitgaard, H., M. Zhou, S. Schiaffino, R. Betto, G. Salviati, and B. Saltin (1990b). Ageing alters the myosin heavy chain composition of single fibers from human skeletal muscle. *Acta Physiol. Scand.* 140:55–62.

Komi, P.V., and J. Karlsson (1978). Skeletal muscle fiber types, enzyme activities and physical performance in young males and females. *Acta Physiol. Scand.* 103:210–218.

Kraemer, W.J.(1992). Endocrine responses and adaptations to strength training. In: P.V. Komi (ed.) *Strength and Power in Sport. The Encyclopaedia of Sports Medicine.* Oxford: Blackwell Scientific Publications, pp. 291–304.

Kraemer, W.J., S.E. Gordon, S.J. Fleck, L.J. Marichitelli, R. Mello, J.E. Dziados, K. Friedl, E. Harman, C. Maresh, and A.C. Fry (1991). Endogenous anabolic hormonal and growth factor responses to heavy resistance exercise in males and females. *Int. J. Sports Med.* 12:228–235.

Krotkiewski, M., A. Aniansson, G. Grimby, P. Bjorntorp, and L. Sjostrom (1979). The effect of unilateral isokinetic strength training on local adipose and muscle tissue morphology, thickness, and enzymes. *Eur. J. Appl. Physiol.* 42:271–281.

Laforest, S., D.M. St-Pierre, J. Cyr, and D. Gayton (1990). Effects of age and regular exercise on muscle strength and endurance. *Eur. J. Appl. Physiol.* 60:104–111.

Larsson, L. (1983). Histochemical characteristics of human skeletal muscle during aging. *Acta Physiol. Scand.* 117:469–471.

Larsson, L., and J. Karlsson (1978). Isometric and dynamic endurance as a function of age and skeletal muscle characteristics. *Acta Physiol. Scand.* 104:129–136.

Larsson, L., and R.L. Moss (1993). Maximum velocity of shortening in relation to myosin isoform composition in single fibers from human skeletal muscles. *J. Physiol.* 472:595–614.

Larsson, L., G. Grimby, and J. Karlsson (1979). Muscle strength and speed of movement in relation to age and muscle morphology. *J. Appl. Physiol.* 46:451–456.

Larsson, L., B. Sjodin, and J. Karlsson (1978). Histochemical and biochemical changes in human skeletal muscle with age in sedentary males, age 22–65 years. *Acta Physiol. Scand.* 103:31–39.

Laubach, L. (1976). Comparative strength of men and women: a review of the literature. *Aviat. Space Environ. Med.* 47:534–542.

Lebrun, C.M., D.C. McKenzie, J.C. Prior, and J.E. Taunton (1995). Effects of menstrual cycle phase on athletic performance. *Med. Sci. Sports Exerc.* 27:437–444.

Lennmarken, C., T. Bergman, J. Larsson, and L.-E. Larsson (1985). Skeletal muscle function in man: force, relaxation rate, endurance and contraction time-dependence on sex and age. *Clin. Physiol.* 5:243–255.

Lexell, J., and D.Y. Downham (1992). What is the effect of ageing on type 2 muscle fibers? *J. Neurol. Sci.* 107:250–251.

Lexell, J., and C.C. Taylor (1991). Variability in muscle fiber areas in whole human quadriceps muscle: effects of increasing age. *J. Anat.* 174:239–249.

Lexell, J., K. Henriksson-Larsen, B. Winblad, and M. Sjostrom (1983). Distribution of different fiber types in human skeletal muscles: effects of aging studied in whole muscle cross sections. *Muscle Nerve* 6:588–595.

Lexell, J., M. Sjostrom, A.-S. Nordlund, and C.C. Taylor (1992). Growth and development of human muscle: a quantitative morphological study of whole vastus lateralis from childhood to adult age. *Muscle Nerve.* 15:404–409.

Lexell, J., C.C. Taylor, and M. Sjostrom (1988). What is the cause of the ageing atrophy? Total number, size and proportion of different fiber types studied in whole vastus lateralis muscle from 15- to 83-year-old men. *J. Neurol. Sci.* 84:275–294.

MacDougall, J.D. (1992). Hypertrophy or hyperplasia. In: *Strength and Power in Sport.* P.V. Komi (ed.) London: Blackwell Scientific Publications, pp. 230–238.

MacDougall, J.D., D.G. Sale, S.E. Alway, and J.R. Sutton (1984). Muscle fiber number in biceps brachii in bodybuilders and control subjects. *J. Appl. Physiol.* 57:1399–1403.

MacDougall, J.D., G.R. Ward, D.G. Sale, and J.R. Sutton (1977). Biochemical adaptation of human skeletal muscle to heavy resistance training and immobilization. *J. Appl. Physiol.* 43:700–703.

Malina, R.M., and C. Bouchard (1991). *Growth, Maturation, and Physical Activity.* Champaign: Human Kinetics.

Maughan, R.J., M. Harmon, J.B. Leiper, D. Sale, A. Delman (1986). Endurance capacity of untrained males and females in isometric and dynamic muscular contractions. *Eur. J. Appl. Physiol.* 55:395–400.

Maughan, R.J., J.S. Watson, and J. Weir (1983a). Strength and cross-sectional area of human skeletal muscle. *J. Physiol.* 338:37–49.

SKELETAL MUSCLE FUNCTION AND ENERGY METABOLISM **355**

Maughan, R.J., J.S. Watson, and J. Weir (1983b). The relative proportions of fat, muscle and bone in the normal human forearm as determined by computed tomography. *Clin. Sci.* 66:683-689.

Mayhew, J.H., and P. Gross (1974). Body composition changes in young women with high resistance weight training. *Res. Quart.* 45:433-440.

McCartney, N., A.L. Hicks, J. Martin, and C.E. Webber (1995). Long-term resistance training in the elderly: effects on dynamic strength, exercise capacity, muscle, and bone. *J. Gerontol.: Biol. Sci.* 50A:B97-B104.

McCartney, N., L.L. Spriet, G.J.F. Heigenhauser, J.M. Kowalchuk, J.R. Sutton, and N.L. Jones (1986). Muscle power and metabolism in maximal intermittent exercise. *J. Appl. Physiol.* 60:1164-1169.

Mendenhall, L.A., S. Sial, A.R. Coggan, and S. Klein (1995). Gender differences in substrate metabolism during moderate intensity cycling. *Med. Sci. Sports Exerc.* 27:S213, Abstract.

Miller, A.E.J., J.D. MacDougall, M.A. Tarnopolsky, and D.G. Sale (1993). Gender differences in strength and muscle fiber characteristics. *Eur. J. Appl. Physiol.* 66:254-262.

Miyashita, M., and H. Kanehisa (1979). Dynamic peak torque related to age, sex, and performance. *Res. Quart.* 50:249-255.

Montoye, H.J., and D.E. Lamphiear (1977). Grip and arm strength in males and females, age 10 to 69. *Res. Quart.* 48:109-120.

Murray, M.P., E.H. Duthie, Jr., S.R. Gambert, S.B. Sepic, and L.A. Mollinger (1985). Age-related differences in knee muscle strength in normal women. *J. Geront.* 40:275-280.

Murray, M.P., G.M. Gardner, L.A. Mollinger, and S.B. Sepic (1980). Strength of isometric contractions. Knee muscles of men aged 20 to 86. *Phys. Ther.* 60:412-419.

Nichols, J.F., D.K. Omizo, K.K. Peterson, and K.P. Nelson (1993). Efficacy of heavy-resistance training for active women over sixty: muscular strength, body composition, and program adherence. *J. Am. Geriatr. Soc.* 41:205-210.

Nicklas, B.J., A.C. Hackney, and R.L. Sharp (1989). The menstrual cycle and exercise: performance, muscle glycogen, and substrate responses. *Int. J. Sports Med.* 10:264-269.

Nordgren, B. (1972). Anthropometric measures and muscle strength in young women. *Scand. J. Rehab.* 4:165-169.

Nygaard, E. (1985). Energy supply and utilization during exercise in women and men—a comparison. In: J. Vague, P. Bjorntorp, B. Guy-Grand, M. Rebuffe-Scrive, and P. Vague (eds.) *Metabolic Complications of Human Obesities.* Amsterdam: Elsevier, pp. 249-259.

Nygaard, E. (1981). Skeletal muscle fiber characteristics in young women. *Acta Physiol. Scand.* 112:299-304.

Nygaard, E., M. Houston, Y. Suzuki, K. Jorgensen, and B. Saltin (1983). Morphology of the brachial biceps muscle and elbow flexion in man. *Acta. Physiol. Scand.* 117:287-292.

Oertel, G. (1988). Morphometric analysis of normal skeletal muscles in infancy, childhood, and adolescence. *J. Neurol. Sci.* 88:303-313.

O'Hagan, F.T., D.G. Sale, J.D. MacDougall, and S.H. Garner (1995). Response to resistance training in young women and men. *Int. J. Sports Med.* 16:314-321.

O'Keefe, K.A., R.E. Keith, G.D. Wilson, and D.L. Blessing (1989). Dietary carbohydrate intake and endurance exercise performance of trained female cyclists. *Nutr. Res.* 9:819-830.

Orlander, J., K.-H. Kiessling, L. Larsson, J. Karlsson, and A. Aniansson (1978). Skeletal muscle metabolism and ultrastructure in relation to age in sedentary men. *Acta Physiol. Scand.* 104:249-261.

Overend, T.J., D.A. Cunningham, D.H. Paterson, and M.S. Lefcoe (1992). Thigh composition in young and elderly men determined by computed tomography. *Clin. Physiol.* 12:629-640.

Parker, D.F., J.M. Round, P. Sacco, and D.A. Jones (1990). A cross-sectional survey of upper and lower limb strength in boys and girls during childhood and adolescence. *Ann. Hum. Biol.* 17:199-211.

Pascoe, D.D., D.L. Costill, W.J. Kink, R.A. Robergs, and J.F. Zachwieja (1993). Glycogen resynthesis in skeletal muscle following resistance exercise. *Med. Sci. Sports Exerc.* 25:349-354.

Pearson, M.B., E.J. Bassey, and M.J. Bendall (1985). Muscle strength and anthropometric indices in elderly men and women. *Age Ageing* 14:49-54.

Perrine, J.J., and V.R. Edgerton (1978). Muscle force-velocity relationships under isokinetic loading. *Med. Sci. Sports* 10:159-166.

Petrella, R.J., D.A. Cunningham, A.A. Vandervoort, and D.H. Patterson (1989). Comparison of twitch potentiation in the gastrocnemius of young and elderly men. *Eur. J. Appl. Physiol.* 58:395-399.

Pette, D., and H. Hofer (1980). The constant enzyme proportion enzyme group concept in the selection of reference enzymes in metabolism. In: *Trends in Enzyme Histochemistry and Cytochemistry* (Ciba Foundation Symposium # 73). Amsterdam: Excerpta Medica, pp. 231-244.

Phillips, S.M., S.A. Atkinson, M.A. Tarnopolsky, and J.D. MacDougall (1993). Gender differences in leucine kinetics and nitrogen balance in endurance athletes. *J. Appl. Physiol.* 75:2134-2141.

Phillips, S.K., S.A. Bruce, D. Newton, and R.C. Woledge (1992). The weakness of old age is not due to failure of muscle activation. *J. Geront.* 47:M45-M49.

Phillips, S.K., S.A. Bruce, and R.C. Woledge (1991). In mice, the muscle weakness due to age is absent during stretching. *J. Physiol.* 437:63-70.

Phillips, S.K., K.M. Rook, N.C. Siddle, S.A. Bruce, and R.C. Woledge (1993). Muscle weakness in women occurs at an earlier age than in men, but strength is preserved by hormone replacement therapy. *Clin. Sci.* 84:95-98.

Porter, M.M., and A.A. Vandervoort (1995). High-intensity strength training for the older adult—a review. *Top. Geriatr. Rehabil.* 10:61-74.

Porter, M.M., A. Myint, J.F. Kramer, and A.A. Vandervoort (1995a). Concentric and eccentric knee extension strength in older and younger men and women. *Can. J. Appl. Physiol.* 20:429-439.

Porter, M.M., A.A. Vandervoort, and J. Lexell (1995b). Ageing of human muscle: structure, function and adaptability. *Scand. J. Med. Sci. Sports* 5:129-142.

Poulin, M.J., A.A. Vandervoort, D.H. Patterson, J.F. Kramer, and D.A. Cunningham (1992). Eccentric and concentric torques of knee and elbow extension in young and older men. *Can. J. Appl. Sport Sci.* 17:3-7.

Powers, S.K., W. Riley, and E.T. Howley (1980). Comparison of fat metabolism between trained men and women during prolonged aerobic work. *Res. Q. Exerc. Sport* 51:427-431.

Prince, F.P., R.S. Hikida, and F.C. Hagerman (1976). Human muscle fiber types in powerlifters, distance runners and untrained subjects. *Pflugers Arch.* 363:19-26.

Prince, F.P., R.S. Hikida, and F.C. Hagerman (1977). Muscle fiber types in women athletes and non-athletes. *Pflugers Arch.* 371:161-165.

Pyka, G., E. Lindenberger, S. Charette, and R. Marcus (1994). Muscle strength and fiber adaptations to year-long resistance training program in elderly men and women. *J. Gerontol.* 49:M22-M28.

Rantanen, T., S. Sipila, and H. Suominen (1993). Muscle strength and history of heavy manual work among elderly trained women and randomly chosen sample population. *Eur. J. Appl. Physiol.* 66:514-517.

Reed, R.L., L. Pearlmutter, K. Yochum, K.E. Meredith, and A.D. Mooradian (1991). The relationship between muscle mass and muscle strength in the elderly. *J. Am Geriatr. Soc.* 39:555-561.

Rice, C.L., D.A. Cunningham, D.H. Paterson, and M.S. Lefcoe (1989). Arm and leg composition determined by computed tomography in young and elderly men. *Clin. Physiol.* 9:207-220.

Rich, N.C. (1990). Electromyography of rapid forearm flexion and extension and aging. *Int. J. Aging Human Devel.* 31:11-29.

Robergs, R.A., D.R. Pearson, D.L. Costill, W.J. Fink, D.A. Pascoe, M.A. Benedict, C.P. Lambert, and J.F. Zachweja (1991). Muscle glycogenolysis during different intensities of weight-resistance exercise. *J. Appl. Physiol.* 70:1700-1706.

Roberts, K.M., E.G. Noble, D.B. Hayden, and A.W. Taylor. (1988). Simple and complex carbohydrate-rich diets and muscle glycogen content of marathon runners. *Eur. J. Appl. Physiol.* 57:70-74.

Robertson, L.A., and S.L. Higgs (1983). Menstrual cycle variations in physical work capacity, post-exercise blood lactate and perceived exertion. *Can. J. Appl. Sport Sci.* 8:220. (Abstract).

Rogers, M.A., and W.J. Evans (1993). Changes in skeletal muscle with aging: effects of exercise training. *Exercise and Sport Sciences Reviews.* 21:65-102.

Rutherford, O.M., D.A. Jones, and D.J. Newham (1986). Clinical and experimental application of the percutaneous twitch superimposition technique for the study of human muscle activation. *J. Neurol. Neurosurg. Psychiat.* 49:1288-1291.

Ryushi, T., K. Hakkinen, H. Kauhannen,, and P.V. Komi (1988). Muscle fiber characteristics, muscle cross-sectional area and force production in strength athletes, physically active males and females. *Scand. J. Sports Sci.* 10:7-15.

Sale, D.G. (1989). Strength training in children. In: C.V. Gisolfi and D.R. Lamb (eds). *Perspectives in Exercise Science and Sports Medicine*, Vol. II: Youth, Exercise, and Sport. Indianapolis: Benchmark Press, pp. 165-222.

Sale, D.G., J.D. MacDougall, S.E. Alway, and J.R. Sutton (1987). Voluntary strength and muscle characteristics in untrained men and women and male bodybuilders. *J. Appl. Physiol.* 62:1786-1793.

Saltin, B., and J. Karlsson (1971). Muscle glycogen utilization during work of different intensities. In: B. Pernow and B. Saltin (eds.) *Muscle Metabolism During Exercise.* New York: Plenum Press, pp. 289-299.

Saltin, B., J. Bangsbo, T.E. Graham, and L. Johansen (1992). Metabolism and performance in exhaustive intense exercise; different effects of muscle glycogen availability, previous exercise and muscle acidity. In: P. Marconnet, P.V. Komi, B. Saltin, and O.M. Sejersted (eds.) *Muscle Fatigue Mechanisms in Exercise and Training. Medicine and Sport Science,* Vol. 34. Basel: Karger, pp. 87-114.

Saltin, B., J. Henrikson, E. Nygaard, and P. Andersen (1977). Fiber types and metabolic potentials of skeletal muscles in sedentary men and endurance runners. *Ann. N.Y. Acad. Sci.* 301:2-29.

Sandler, R.B., R. Burdett, M. Zaleskiewicz, C. Sprowls-Repcheck, and M. Harwell (1991). Muscle strength as an indicator of the habitual level of physical activity. *Med. Sci. Sports. Exerc.* 23:1375-1381.

Sato, T., H. Akatsuka, K. Kito, Y. Tokoro, H. Tauchi, and K. Kato (1984). Age changes in in size and number of muscle fibers in human minor pectoral muscles. *Mech. Ageing Dev.* 28:99-109.

Schantz, P., E. Randall-Fox, W. Hutchisin, A. Tydén, and P.-O Åstrand (1983). Muscle fibre type distribution, muscle cross-sectional area and maximal voluntary strength in humans. *Acta Physiol. Scand.* 117:219-226.

Schantz, P., E. Randall-Fox, P. Norgen, and A. Tyden (1981). The relationship between the mean muscle fiber area and the muscle cross-sectional area of the thigh in subjects with large differences in thigh girth. *Acta Physiol. Scand.* 113:537-539.

Schoene, R.B., H.T. Robertson, D.J. Pierson, and A.P. Peterson (1981). Respiratory drives and exercise in menstrual cycles of athletic and nonathletic women. *J. Appl. Physiol.* 50:1300-1305.

SKELETAL MUSCLE FUNCTION AND ENERGY METABOLISM **357**

Sherman, W.M., D.L. Costill, W.J. Fink, and J.M. Miller (1981). Effect of exercise-diet manipulation on muscle glycogen utilization during performance. *Int J. Sports Med.* 2:114–118.

Simoneau, J.A., and C. Bouchard (1989). Human variation in skeletal muscle fiber-type proportion and enzyme activities. *Amer. J. Physiol.* 257:E567–572.

Simoneau, J.A., G. Lortie, M.R. Boulay, M.C. Thibault, G. Theriault, and C. Bouchard (1985). Skeletal muscle histochemical and biochemical characteristics in sedentary male and female subjects. *Can. J. Physiol. Pharmacol.* 63:30–35.

Singh, M., and P.V. Karpovich (1968). Strength of forearm flexors and extensors in men and women. *J. Appl. Physiol.* 25:177–180.

Spriet, L.L. (1992). Anaerobic metabolism in human skeletal muscle during short-term, intense activity. *Can. J. Physiol. Pharmacol.* 70:157–165.

Spriet, L.L., D.A. Maclean, D.J. Dyck, E. Hultman, G. Cederblad, and T.E. Graham (1992). Caffeine ingestion and muscle metabolism during prolonged exercise in humans. *Am. J. Physiol.* 262 (Endocrinol. Metab.):E891–E898.

Spriet, L.L., K. Soderlund, M. Bergstrom, and E. Hultman (1987). Anaerobic energy release in skeletal muscle during electrical stimulation in men. *J. Appl. Physiol.* 62:611–615.

Stalberg, E., O. Borges, M. Ericsson, B. Essen-Gustavsson, P.R.W. Fawcett, L.O. Nordesjo, B. Nordgren, and R. Uhlin (1989). The quadriceps femoris muscle in 20–70-year-old subjects: relationship between knee extension torque, electrophysiological parameters, and muscle fiber characteristics. *Muscle Nerve* 12:382–389.

Stanley, S.N., and N.A.S. Taylor (1993). Isokinematic muscle mechanics in four groups of women of increasing age. *Eur. J. Appl. Physiol.* 66:178–184.

Staron, R.S., D.L. Karapondo, W.J. Kraemer, A.C. Fry, S.E. Gordon, J.E. Falkel, F.C. Hagerman, and R.S. Hikida (1994). Skeletal muscle adaptations during early phase of heavy-resistance training in men and women. *J. Appl. Physiol.* 76:1247–1255.

Staron, R.S., M.J. Leonardi, D.L. Karapondo, E.S. Malicky, J.E. Falkel, F.C. Hagerman, and R.S. Hikida (1991). Strength and skeletal muscle adaptations in heavy-resistance-trained women after detraining and retraining. *J. Appl. Physiol.* 70:631–640.

Staron, R.S., E.S. Malicky, M.J. Leonardi, J.E. Falkel, F.C. Hagerman, and G.A. Dudley (1989). Muscle hypertrophy and fast fiber conversions in heavy resistance-trained women. *Eur. J. Appl. Physiol.* 60:71–79.

Stephenson, L.A., M.A. Kolka, and J.E. Wilkerson (1982). Metabolic and thermoregulatory responses to exercise during the human menstrual cycle. *Med. Sci. Sports Exerc.* 14:270–275.

Tanner, J.M., P.C.R. Hughes, and R.H. Whitehouse (1981). Radiographically determined widths of bone muscle and fat in the upper arm and calf from age 3–18 years. *Ann. Hum. Biol.* 8:495–517.

Tarnopolsky, M.A., S.A. Atkinson, S.M. Phillips, and J.D. MacDougall (1995). Carbohydrate loading and metabolism during exercise in men and women. *J. Appl. Physiol.* 78:1360–1368.

Tarnopolsky, L.J., J.D. MacDougall, S.A. Atkinson, M.A. Tarnopolsky, and J.R. Sutton (1990). Gender differences in substrate for endurance exercise. *J. Appl. Physiol.* 68:302–308.

Tesch, P.A., E.B. Collander, and P. Kaiser (1986). Muscle metabolism during intense, heavy-resistance exercise. *Eur. J. Appl. Physiol.* 55:362–366.

Tomonaga, M. (1977). Histochemical and ultrastructural changes in senile human skeletal muscle. *J. Am. Geriat. Soc.* 25:125–131.

Trappe, S.W., D.L. Costill, W.J. Fink, and D.R. Pearson (1995). Skeletal muscle characteristics among distance runners: a 20-yr follow-up study. *J. Appl. Physiol.* 78:823–829.

Vandervoort, A.A. (1992). Effects of ageing on human neuromuscular function: implications for exercise. *Can. J. Sport Sci.* 17:178–184.

Vandervoort, A.A., and A.J. McComas (1986). Contractile changes in opposing muscles of the human ankle joint with aging. *J. Appl. Physiol.* 61:361–367.

Vandervoort, A.A., K.C. Hayes, and A.Y. Belanger (1986). Strength and endurance of skeletal muscle in the elderly. *Physiother. Can.* 38:167–173.

Vandervoort, A.A., J.F. Kramer, and E.R. Wharram (1990). Eccentric knee strength of elderly females. *J. Geront.* 45:B125–B128.

van Etten, L.M.L.A., F.T.J. Verstappen, and K.R. Westerterp (1994). Effect of body build on weight-training-induced adaptations in body composition and muscular strength. *Med. Sci. Sports Exerc.* 26:515–520.

van Schaik, C.S., A.L. Hicks, and N. McCartney (1994). An evaluation of the length-tension relationship in elderly human ankle dorsiflexors. *J. Gerontol.* 49:B121–127.

Vogler, C., and K.E. Bove (1985). Morphology of skeletal muscle in children. *Arch. Path. Lab. Med.* 109:238–242.

Walker, J.L., G.J.F. Heigenhauser, E. Hultman, D. Friars, and L.L. Spriet (1995). Influence of dietary carbohydrate on muscle glycogen and exercise performance in well trained female endurance athletes. *Can. J. Appl. Physiol.* 20:56P. (Abstract).

Wang, N., R.S. Hikida, R.S. Staron, and J. Simoneau (1993). Muscle fiber types of women after resistance training—quantitative ultrastructure and enzyme activity. *Pflugers Arch-Eur. J. Physiol.* 424:494–502.

Weiss, L.W., F.C. Clark, and D.G. Howard (1988). Effects of heavy-resistance triceps surae muscle training on strength and muscularity of men and women. *Phys. Ther.* 68:208–213.

Weiss, L.W., K.J. Cureton, and F.N. Thompson (1983). Comparison of serum testosterone and androstenedione responses to weightlifting in men and women. *Eur. J. Appl. Physiol.* 50:413–419.

Westing, S.H., and J.Y. Seger (1989). Eccentric and concentric torque-velocity characteristics, torque output comparisons, and gravity effect torque corrections for the quadriceps and hamstring muscles in females. *Int. J. Sports Med.* 10:175–180.

Westing, S.H., A.G. Cresswell, and A. Thorstensson (1991). Muscle activation during maximal voluntary eccentric and concentric knee extension. *Eur. J. Appl. Physiol.* 62:104–108.

Westing, S.H., J.Y. Seger, E. Karlson, and B. Ekblom (1988). Eccentric and concentric torque-velocity characteristics of the quadriceps femoris in man. *Eur. J. Appl. Physiol.* 58:100–104.

Westing, S.H., J.Y. Seger, and A. Thorstensson (1990). Effects of electrical stimulation on eccentric and concentric torque-velocity relationships in man. *Acta Physiol. Scand.* 140:17–22.

White, T.P. (1995). Skeletal muscle structure and function in older mammals. In: D.R. Lamb, C.V. Gisolfi, and E. Nadel (eds.) *Perspectives in Exercise Science and Sports Medicine*, Vol. 8: Youth, Exercise, and Sport. Carmel, IN: Cooper Publishing Group, pp. 115–174.

Wickiewicz, T.L., R.R. Roy, P.L. Powell, J.J. Perrine, and V.R. Edgerton (1984). Muscle architecture and force-velocity relationships in humans. *J. Appl. Physiol.* 57:435–443.

Wilmore, J.H. (1974). Alterations in strength, body composition and anthropometric measurements consequent to a 10-week weight training program. *Med. Sci. Sports* 6:133–138.

Winegard, K.J., A.L. Hicks, A.A. Vandervoort, and D.G. Sale (1995). A 12-year follow-up study of ankle muscle function in older adults. *Med. Sci. Sports Exerc.* 27 (5, Suppl):S205.

Winter, J.S.D. (1978). Prepubertal and pubertal endocrinology. In: F. Falkner, and J.M. Tanner (eds.) *Human Growth 2. Postnatal Growth*. New York: Plenum Press, pp. 183–213.

Young, A. (1986). Exercise physiology in geriatric practice. *Acta Med. Scand.* 711:227–232.

Young, A., and D.A. Skelton (1994). Applied physiology of strength and power in old age. *Int. J. Sports Med.* 15:149–151.

Young, A., M. Stokes, and M. Crowe (1984). Size and strength of the quadriceps muscles of old and young women. *Eur. J. Clin. Invest.* 14:282–287.

Young, A., M. Stokes, and M. Crowe (1985). The size and strength of the quadriceps muscles of old and young men. *Clin. Physiol.* 5:145–154.

Young, A., M. Stokes, J.M. Round, and R.H.T. Edwards (1983). The effect of high-resistance training on the strength and cross-sectional area of the human quadriceps. *Eur. J. Appl. Physiol.* 13:411–417.

DISCUSSION

DESPRES: Do you think that the effect of age on muscle metabolism and morphology is overemphasized considering the trainability of skeletal muscle in the elderly population?

SALE: Not in terms of muscle mass. Although large increases in strength can be achieved in the elderly with training, these are largely due to neural adaptations. The experience in our lab is that while the elderly are capable of hypertrophy, it is less than that seen in young adults.

SPRIET: There isn't much information with respect to aging and metabolism. The major finding is that the gender differences decrease as people get older.

DESPRES: To what extent do you think that age-associated decrements in function are age specific vs. related to a sedentary lifestyle?

SPRIET: My intuition tells me that if one could control for physical activity differences, the aging effects would be relatively small.

SALE: To resolve the issue of relative trainability in young vs. old adults, a useful study would have healthy old and young people undergo identical strength-training programs. The hypothesis could be that if the loss of strength and muscle mass in the elderly is mainly due to physical inactivity, then old people should "close the gap" after a period of training. If inactivity in the elderly is not a factor, then the young and elderly should progress in parallel.

SMITH: Other than the apparent effect of androgens on strength development in young males, is there any information either in an individual age group or across the life span relating circulating androgen levels to either structure or metabolism of the muscle or to trainability?

SALE: I am not aware of data relating the loss of strength with aging to corresponding reductions in testosterone in males. In females, some evidence suggests that the loss of strength after menopause is related to reduced estrogen.

SPRIET: I do not believe that all metabolic responses in women are related to varying estrogen levels. In our study, whether they were eumenorrheic, amenorrheic, or using oral contraceptives, all the subjects showed the same results with little variability. Tarnopolsky's subjects were all in mid-follicular phase. Therefore, we decided to go for the mid-luteal phase because there is animal literature that suggests that more carbohydrate can be stored in muscle when the steroid hormones are higher. We didn't see anything in the luteal phase.

COYLE: Your women's average muscle glycogen values were about 700 mmol/kg dry weight, which is about 175 mmol/kg wet weight. It appears that the women were already supercompensated, even on the 50% CHO diet. I wouldn't expect their glycogen stores to increase much more, even with a greater carbohydrate intake.

SPRIET: We reported muscle glycogen contents that are about 200 mmol/kg dry muscle higher than in the Tarnopolsky report. I think there are several potential reasons for that. One is that they used an acid-extract method for measuring glycogen, and it gives values that are 15–17% lower than the amyloglucosidase technique that we used. Secondly, their study was performed in the follicular phase and we did ours in the luteal phase. While glycogen supercompensation wasn't evident in either study, it could be that the glycogen content is higher in the luteal phase than the follicular. The other point is that our women were better trained, and we were very careful to give them a full day off prior to participating in the study in the hope that we would mimic what they might do in a real athletic situation. Also, Mike Sherman and others reported values of muscle glycogen that are close to 1,000 mmol/kg dw in some cases. Their athletes also started at 500–600 mmol/kg dw in the so-called control trial or the low-carbohydrate situation.

SUTTON: Did you actually measure estradiol and progesterone?

SPRIET: Yes, we have made those measurements and they do appear to be consistent with people who are ovulating. There are a couple that are not as high as we thought they would have been for progesterone, but again I would stress that what has really impressed me is the consistency of the data. There were no women who showed a big increase in glycogen.

BLIMKIE: When we study children, we must be very careful to control for developmental stage. Often when data are expressed in terms of chronological age vs. developmental stage, quite different results can be obtained. Given that peak strength of young women occurs earlier than it does for males and that muscle morphology may stop changing earlier in females than in males, has anyone compared the trainability of strength in the elderly of both genders at the same number of years after peak strength was reached? At a given chronological age in later adulthood, males may have been aging for 5–10 fewer years than the females. Could such a phenomenon influence some of the results you have reported?

SALE: There is a lot of variability. Some studies show peak strength occurring by age 18 or 20 y, whereas others suggest that strength increases up to about 30 y of age.

KANTER: Because women in general tend to have substantially more body fat than men, it doesn't surprise me that women tend to oxidize more fat than men. It makes sense that women would have evolved as better fat burners based on their body composition.

SPRIET: Intuitively, you are correct, but we don't have any direct gender comparisons of the ability to mobilize the fat from the various adipose tissue sites and deliver the fatty acids to the skeletal muscle.

DESPRES: Women have more subcutaneous fat, and the metabolism of subcutaneous adipose tissue is different between men and women. The lipolytic response of adipose cells to epinephrine and norepinephrine is determined by the balance between $alpha_2$ and $beta_1$ adrenergic receptors. There is a greater proportion of $alpha_2$ adrenergic receptors in the femoral adipose tissue of women. Therefore, there is a biphasic response in lipolysis. First, at low catecholamine concentrations, there is an inhibition of lipolysis rather than a stimulation. Therefore, although there is more subcutaneous fat in women, it is much more difficult to mobilize this fat than in men. In one of my first Ph.D. studies, we trained men and women using the same regimen for 20 wk. They came to the lab, exercised 45 min, 5 sessions/wk, at 70% $\dot{V}O_2$max. The total energy expenditure generated by the training program may have been greater in the men than in the women, but it was quite a heavy exercise prescription for both groups. At the end of the program we found that the stimulation of lipolysis by catecholamines was greater in the trained men than in the women. There was a gender difference in the adaptation of subcutaneous lipolysis to the training program. To summarize this point, despite the fact that women have more subcutaneous fat, its metabolism is substantially different from that in men.

SPRIET: The studies just mentioned by Jean Pierre were *in-vitro* studies in which fat was biopsied and examined in a test tube. But there are numerous examples in which *in-vitro* work doesn't predict what will happen *in-vivo*. It is important to do some of these studies with a tracer technique and to measure the release of glycerol in exercising men and exercising women.

WILLIAMS: When you compared males and females and found similar concentrations of plasma fatty acids and glycerol concentrations but quite distinct R values, did you match the exercise intensity at the same relative exercise intensity?

SPRIET: Yes, the gender-comparison studies have matched on the basis of a similar relative power output.

WILLIAMS: It is difficult to equate exercise intensities in males and females whether on cycle ergometers or treadmills. I wonder if we are getting it wrong and should try equating exercise intensity according to something like fat-free mass. It is the lean body mass which is responsible for most of the aerobic metabolism.

SPRIET: That is what we did. The athletes were matched on their $\dot{V}O_2max/kg$ LBM. They were actually exercising at 63–75% of their gross $\dot{V}O_2max$. Possibly what has to be done are two or three comparisons in which subjects are matched on several different variables.

SPRIET: Perhaps all of this matching based on $\dot{V}O_2max$ is not what is important. Perhaps we should be matching on the basis of training intensity and training volume because this is what is going to stress the muscles involved. Obviously a problem with running males and females on a treadmill or riding them on a bicycle is that we are assuming the economy of the different subjects is similar and that they use the same proportions of quadriceps and buttocks muscles in performing the exercise.

WISWELL: With regard to apparently large strength gains in the elderly when they undertake a strength-training program, if you wait until 2 wk into the training session to record maximal strength, the magnitude of the strength gain later in the training is much more realistic. We have seen strength gains of 30–40% after only 2 wk of training in the elderly, and this must surely be related to motivation or some kind of release of inhibition. Also, some studies have found that after 26 wk of resistance training older people stopped increasing strength. This implies that perhaps the strength gain in the elderly is a very short-lived phenomenon, particularly in those over 70 y of age.

SALE: Neil McCartney at McMaster found that the elderly increased strength linearly over a 2-y period of resistance training. But extremely rapid strength gains would be more likely when the training exercises have a large motor-learning component. Bilateral, multijoint movements would fit into this category.

WISWELL: There have been 12 studies since 1990 that addressed the issue of strength gain in men and women over the age of 70. High-resistance training was used with at least 80% of one repetition-maximum training, and none of those studies showed a relation between muscle size increases and strength gain. This needs to be explained.

SALE: In fact, depending on the strength measures used, the correlation between strength and muscle mass gains are often poor in young adults, too. We have published a study in which there was no isometric strength gain in young adults, despite hypertrophy.

FREEDSON: What is the biological basis of gender differences in strength of the upper body musculature vs. the lower body musculature?

SALE: When males experience the surge in strength, it seems to be more pronounced in the upper limbs. By adulthood, females have 70% of the lower body strength of males, but only 50% of the upper body strength. The difference is also seen with bone dimensions, i.e., the female-to-male ratio for femur size is greater than for humeral size. Thus, I believe that the disparity between males and females in the upper body vs. the lower body is biological rather than a difference in behavioral patterns.

FREEDSON: How does the supposed effect of testosterone on strength development differentiate between the upper body and lower body muscles?

SALE: Although not convincing, there is some evidence that males have more muscle fibers in upper limb muscles. The gender disparity may occur when these fibers hypertrophy during adolescence.

MAUGHAN: Women body builders who use anabolic steroids can get great hypertrophy of their upper body musculature, which they don't get if they don't use steroids. The same is true in animal models, e.g., steers, which are castrated, do not get the large musculature that occurs in intact bulls. So it suggests very strongly that upper body development is entirely a function of hormonal milieu. The question is whether or not women body builders who get muscle hypertrophy with the use of steroids get corresponding gains in muscle strength?

FREEDSON: Not all women body builders take steroids. I think that a high-volume overload to women's upper body muscles will result in a narrowing of the gender differences in upper body strength. I don't believe that the larger gender difference in upper vs. lower body strength is biological.

MAUGHAN: I wasn't suggesting that all women body builders take steroids, but women who do use steroids have much greater hypertrophy than those who don't, as is the case for men.

SALE: In regard to the upper vs. lower body strength/muscle mass gender comparison, the work of Steve Alway indicates that the pattern seen in untrained subjects is also observed in highly trained body builders, i.e., female body builders have only about half the upper limb strength and size as highly trained males, whereas they have about 70–75% of the lower limb strength and size.

9

Exercise and Cardiovascular Health in Women

William L. Haskell, Ph.D.

Leslie Pruitt, Ph.D.

INTRODUCTION

Cardiovascular disease (CVD) is the leading cause of death in women in the United States and claims more lives of African-American and Caucasian women than all forms of cancer, accidents, and diabetes combined (Eaker et al., 1993). The age-adjusted death rates from diseases of the heart in women, primarily due to coronary heart disease (CHD), are four times higher in Caucasian women and six times higher in African-American women than the death rate for breast cancer. Furthermore, one in nine women aged 45–54 has some form of CVD, and after age 65 this ratio increases to one in three (American Heart Association, 1994). Despite the decline in age-adjusted CHD mortality rates in women of approximately 27% from 1980 to 1989, the total number of women dying of CHD in the United States continues to increase (American Heart Association, 1994). For other reviews of the issues regarding CVD in women see Wenger et al. (1993) and Eaker et al. (1993).

Coronary heart disease is still commonly perceived as a disease of men, probably because it strikes men much more often than women in the younger and middle years of life. For example, the Framingham study has shown that women develop the symptoms of CHD a decade later than men (Castelli, 1988). The mortality rate for CHD is 4.5 times greater in men than in women age 35–44 y. This difference then begins to narrow, so that by age 75–84 y the mortality rate is approximately 1.7 times greater in men, and after 85 y it decreases to a ratio of 1.2 (Figure 9-1A) (National Center for Health Statistics, 1990). However, due to the much larger population of older women, the total burden of CHD mortality is greater in women over age 80 y (Figure 9-1B). As life expectancy continues to increase in women and a much larger number of women reach these older ages as "the baby boom" cohort ages, the number of women at risk of CHD in the United States will greatly increase over the next 30 y. Effective programs to prevent CHD in women are needed as well as approaches to cardiac rehabilitation and secondary prevention that will effectively decrease the disability and financial burden of CHD in this most rapidly growing segment of the population.

THE PATHOBIOLOGY OF CORONARY HEART DISEASE IN WOMEN

The processes of atherosclerosis and thrombosis that lead to most clinical cardiac events appear to be similar in men and women. Differences

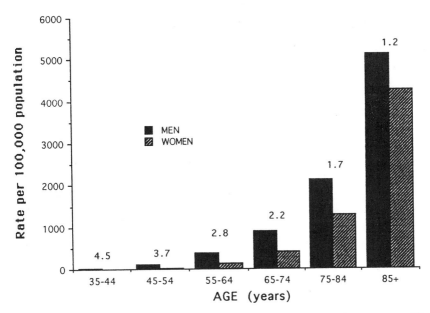

FIGURE 9-1A. *Death rates from ischemic heart disease in the U.S. by sex and age for 1990.* The numbers above each set of bars is the ratio of deaths in men versus those in women for that age.

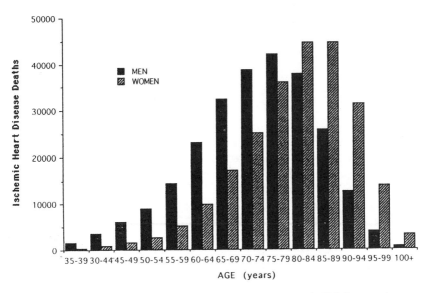

FIGURE 9-1B. *Number of deaths from ischemic heart disease in 1990 in the U.S. by sex and 5-y age intervals.*

that do exist are likely due to the effect of sex hormones on metabolic processes that contribute to atherosclerosis, thrombosis, and vascular wall function (Hong et al., 1992; Lieberman et al., 1994; Seed, 1994). Atherosclerotic plaques develop in coronary arteries when the amount of low-density lipoprotein cholesterol (LDL-C) entering the subintimal space exceeds that removed, resulting in the accumulation of LDL-C droplets in the form of cholesterol esters. The "response to injury" theory proposes that mechanical or chemical injury to the endothelium increases its permeability and exposes the subintimal and medial layers of the artery wall to the infiltration of LDL-C, monocytes, platelets, and other vasoactive factors (Raines & Ross, 1993). The accumulation of LDL-C in the subintima increases the tendency for monocytes to adhere to the endothelium and migrate into the subintimal space where they take up the extra cellular lipid as they become macrophages. Modification of LDL-C by oxidation and other processes facilitates its uptake by macrophages. Continued accumulation of lipid by macrophages leads to their conversion to foam cells, the major constituent of fatty streaks and the early lipid-filled plaque. The "lipid filtration" hypothesis assumes that at increased concentrations of LDL-C in the blood, LDL-C is filtered through the endothelium into the subintimal space, is followed by monocytes, and a series of events then occurs similar to that proposed by the "response to injury" theory. Steinberg and colleagues (1989) proposed a scheme that incorporates the major features of these two hypotheses (Figure 9-2).

Conversion of the plaque from a mainly lipid-filled unit to a complex structure involving smooth muscle cells, platelets, inert lipid crystals, and calcified material, all covered by a fibrous cap, is the result of a series of events currently under intense investigation (Levine et al., 1995). Platelets, macrophages, and modified LDL-C all release a variety of chemoattractants and growth factors resulting in the migration and proliferation of smooth muscle cells that contribute to the formation of raised lesions.

It now appears that many clinical cardiac events, including myocardial infarction, cardiac arrest, and unstable angina pectoris, occur when a plaque ruptures, releasing platelet aggregation factors into the artery lumen and stimulating the formation of a blood clot that rapidly occludes the artery (Fuster et al., 1992). These so-called "culprit lesions" that rupture tend to be the early lipid-filled plaques rather than the more advanced complex lesions. Thus, prevention of clinical cardiac events may be achieved by the reduction of new lesion formation, stabilization of existing lesions, reduction in the rate of existing lesion growth or progression, decrease in lesion size or regression, and the reduction of platelet aggregation or an increase in fibrinolysis.

Given the complex and multifactorial nature of the pathobiology of the events that contribute to the development, progression, regression, and stabilization of coronary artery lesions, there are several mechanisms

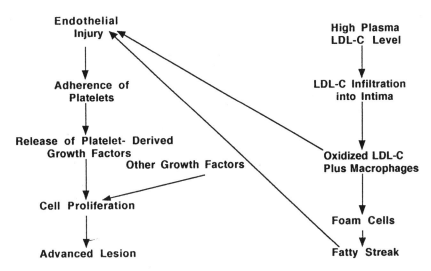

FIGURE 9-2. *Postulated linkage between lipid-infiltration and endothelial-injury hypothesis in the pathogenesis of coronary atherosclerosis.* The lipid-infiltration hypothesis (right column) may be sufficient to account for fatty streaks, and the endothelial-injury hypothesis (left column) may account for progression of the fatty streak to more advanced lesions. Reproduced from Steinberg et al. (1989).

by which a change in physical activity could cause a reduction in CHD morbidity and mortality. Also, it is possible the effect of exercise training on the myocardium instead of the coronary arteries might reduce the occurrence or severity of clinical cardiac events. This effect might include a reduction of myocardial work at rest and during exercise, an increase in myocardial electrical stability, or an enhancement of intrinsic myocardial contractility (Haskell, 1986). Most of these proposed mechanisms have been based primarily on data obtained from studies employing either the laboratory animal model or the male human model.

RISK FACTORS IN THE DEVELOPMENT OF CORONARY HEART DISEASE IN WOMEN

The identification of CHD risk factors specific to women has lagged behind such investigations in men. An inadequate representation of women in prospective studies has made it difficult to determine possible gender differences in heart disease risk. Nevertheless, there is now evidence that many of the CHD risk factors that have been identified in men are shared by women. These risk factors include hypertension, abnormal lipid and lipoprotein metabolism, cigarette smoking, obesity, sedentary lifestyle, glucose intolerance, and altered hemostatic factors. Additional factors that uniquely affect women include the use of oral contraceptives and the effects of postmenopausal hormones.

Our intent is not to discuss all CHD risk factors pertinent to women in this section; more inclusive reviews may be consulted on this topic (Corrao et al., 1990). Also, obesity and body composition are addressed in Chapter 5. The following review focuses primarily on those risk factors that appear to be influenced by physical activity or exercise training. A discussion of oral contraceptives and hormone replacement therapy is included because they may affect risk for heart disease and may modify the effects of exercise training on selected risk factors and the disease process. Although limited, information pertinent to young girls and adolescents is also addressed. Finally, the role that socioeconomic factors may play in CHD risk is briefly discussed because socioeconomic status is a major determinant of physical activity status.

Hypertension

Hypertension is strongly associated with CHD morbidity and mortality in men and women. Data from Framingham (Kannel, 1987; Wilson et al., 1991) and other prospective studies (Isles et al., 1992) provide evidence that elevated systolic or diastolic blood pressure is associated with CHD events in women in general, but data on hypertension and CHD risk in women of ethnic groups relevant to the United States are sparse. One 20-y follow-up study did evaluate 391 African-American women and 549 Caucasian women and found systolic blood pressure to be a risk factor among this cohort of African-American women (Johnson et al., 1986).

There is some evidence that elevated blood pressure may have greater relative importance among women with a predisposition for a CHD event. Several studies evaluated patients who had undergone myocardial infarctions (MI) and examined pre-infarction risk profiles (Greenland et al., 1991; Krueger et al., 1981; Rosenberg et al., 1983; Steingart et al., 1991). Greenland et al. (1991) evaluated 1525 women and 4315 men who had undergone acute MIs and found that the age-adjusted percentage of female patients who were hypertensive prior to the infarction (50.0%) was significantly greater than that observed for men (35.5%). Similarly, other studies have reported that women were more likely to be hypertensive than were men prior to a cardiac event (Rosenberg et al., 1983; Steingart et al., 1991) or by-pass surgery (Khan et al., 1990).

Evidence from Framingham suggests that the impact of hypertension as a risk factor for men and women varies according to the presence of other concurrent factors (Kannel, 1987; Lerner & Kannel, 1986). It is interesting to note, however, that at any level of combined risk, women fare better than their male counterparts in terms of CHD morbidity. Despite this apparent advantage, the attributable risk percentage for hypertensives compared with normotensives (the estimated percentage of CHD cases that could have been avoided by maintenance of normal blood pressure) is similar between men and women age 45–74 y. However, among the elderly (65–74 y), the attributable risk for women may exceed that for men (Anastos et al., 1991). The Framingham Study showed that more than 33% of the women aged 65 y and older had hypertension, compared to 20% of men (Kannel, 1987). It is clear from a public health perspective, prevention of hypertension is of particular importance for women, especially elderly women.

Lipids and Lipoproteins

Elevated total serum cholesterol has long been implicated as a major risk factor for CHD. Early work from the Framingham Study and others demonstrated a positive relationship between serum cholesterol levels and CHD risk for men and women (Brunner et al., 1987; Kannel, 1983; Stokes et al., 1987).

As laboratory methods for partitioning total cholesterol into its various lipoprotein moieties improved, the possible importance of these subfractions as independent risk factors emerged. Considerable work has focused on high-density cholesterol (HDL-C) and the particularly important role it may play for women. The inverse association between HDL-C and CHD incidence is well established, and this relationship appears especially strong in women (Gordon et al., 1977; Kannel, 1983). In the presence of high total cholesterol levels, high HDL-C concentrations may attenuate CHD risk (Castelli et al., 1986). One study found this to be true only in women (Brunner et al., 1987). For women, HDL-C and/or ratios that include this moiety may be of greater relative importance as risk factors for CHD morbidity than is total cholesterol. Hong et al. (1991) evaluated the risk factors of 108 women undergoing coronary angiography for suspected CHD. The ratio of total cholesterol:HDL-C was found to be the best predictor of the presence, severity, and extent of CHD. Total cholesterol or triglyceride levels did not significantly discriminate between those with CHD and those without disease. Similarly, Cooper and associates (1985) studied risk factors in African-American men and women undergoing catheterization and found that the TC:HDL-C ratio and HDL-C were the most powerful predictors of CHD among the women. However, HDL-C was a non-significant predictor among the male patients.

Certainly other lipids, lipoproteins, apoproteins, and ratios may relate to CHD risk. Triglycerides have been associated with CHD risk, particularly in women (Castelli, 1986), although the relation between triglycerides and CHD may not be as strong as that observed for HDL-C and CHD incidence. Four-year follow-up data from the Framingham cohort found that the strength of the association between triglycerides and CHD becomes nonsignificant when other lipids are analyzed concurrently (Gordon et al., 1977). Low-density lipoproteins (LDL-C) also play a role in CHD incidence. Higher levels of LDL are associated with greater risk. The ratio of LDL-C:HDL-C has been viewed as comparable to the total cholesterol:HDL-C ratio in identifying persons at increased risk for CHD (Kannel, 1983). Recent work by Kwiterovich and associates (1992) found that increased levels of apolipoprotein B, a major constituent of LDL particles, was the best predictor of CHD in women ≤ 60 y old. Neither LDL-C nor HDL-C were as powerful predictors.

Little doubt exists that lipids, lipoproteins, and their ratios to one another are associated with the incidence of CHD in women. The single best predictor in women, however, has yet to be established.

Glucose Intolerance and Non-Insulin Dependent Diabetes Mellitus

In women diabetes mellitus is a particularly harsh risk factor for CHD morbidity and mortality. Several prospective studies have found that the feminine advantage of reduced CHD incidence is eliminated in the presence of diabetes (Kannel & McGee, 1979; Pan et al., 1986). In general, diabetes has been found to be a consistent, independent risk factor for CVD events in women, with a greater relative impact apparent in women compared to men (Barrett-Connor & Wingard, 1983; Heyden et al., 1980; Kannel & McGee, 1979; Manson et al., 1991a, 1991b; Pan et al., 1986). According to 20-y follow-up data from Framingham, the attributable risk for CVD due to diabetes is 5.0% in women, compared to 3.9% in men. Similarly, Barrett-Connor and Wingard (1983) reported that the adjusted relative risk for CHD mortality in women was 3.5 in comparison to 2.4 for men. The adverse impact of diabetes is amplified in the presence of other risk factors as evidenced by a three-fold increase in attributable risk among female diabetic smokers and hypertensives (Manson et al., 1991a).

Although there is some evidence that diabetes may be an independent risk factor for CHD in men (Barrett-Connor & Wingard, 1983), there is consistent evidence that among women, the cardiovascular consequences of diabetes are more severe. Additional research is needed to provide insight as to why diabetes and associated sequelae intensify CHD risk in women.

Hemostatic Factors

Hemostatic factors have been evaluated as risk factors for CVD because both thrombogenesis and atherogenesis increase the risk of CHD. Published research on hemostatic factors and CHD risk among women is limited. Despite the paucity of data, there is some evidence of a positive association between plasma fibrinogen and CHD in women. There is also evidence linking exogenous and endogenous sex hormones with alteration of fibrinolytic and coagulation factors, which may help explain observed associations between CHD risk profiles and hormonal status (Meilahn, 1992). To date, Framingham has been the only large prospective study to report on hemostatic factors in women (Kannel et al., 1987). Based upon

12-y follow-up data, plasma fibrinogen levels were directly associated with CHD risk among women and men. The increased risk among women with the highest fibrinogen levels, relative to those with low levels, remained after adjustment for other risk factors. In a case-control study by Lee et al. (1991), women with high plasma fibrinogen levels were associated with a 35% greater risk of MI, or electrocardiographic evidence of MI, than were women with low plasma fibrinogen levels. In contrast to the above studies, Schmitz-Huebner and associates (1988) did not find a relation between fibrinogen and CHD documented by angiography, in men or women. In short, additional research is needed to characterize the role hemostatic factors play in risk for CHD among women.

Obesity

Obesity is strongly associated with the major metabolic and hemodynamic risk factors for CVD in both men and women. For example, the National Health and Nutrition Survey conducted from 1976 to 1980 found a strong association between a Body Mass Index (BMI) of 27.3 kg/m^2 or greater in women and hypertension, hypercholesterolemia, and non-insulin dependent diabetes mellitus (National Center for Health Statistics, 1981). High-density lipoprotein-cholesterol, a strong, independent predictor of CHD in women, is inversely associated with obesity (Glueck et al., 1980; Patterson et al., 1988; Van Horn et al., 1991). These relationships exist for both younger (Van Horn et al., 1991; Wing et al., 1989) and older women (Glueck et al., 1980; National Center for Health Statistics, 1973).

Obesity is also an independent predictor of CHD mortality in women. In the 26-y follow-up of the Framingham Heart Study, relative weight in women age 28–64 y was positively associated with CHD and CVD death, stroke, and congestive heart failure (Hubert et al., 1983). In Danish women, the CVD risk of obesity gradually increased as relative weight exceeded 103% (Schroll et al., 1981). The 10-y incidence of CVD doubled in women with a 120% relative weight as compared to women with a relative weight of 96% to 102%. At the 8-y follow-up of the U.S. Nurses' Health Study, elevated relative weight was inversely associated with each category of CHD (Manson et al., 1990). A significant increase in CHD clinical events was observed even with small increments of obesity. Women with a BMI >29 kg/m^2 had a rate of myocardial infarction (both fatal and nonfatal) three times that of women in the leanest tertile (BMI < 21 kg/m^2).

For the same degree of obesity, men have more abnormalities in their metabolic and hemodynamic risk factors and a higher risk for CVD than do women (Glueck et al., 1980; Hubert et al., 1983; Krotkiewski et al., 1983). This differential effect appears to be due the greater central (abdominal) obesity pattern in men (Lemieux et al., 1994; Vague, 1956). At the same overall level of obesity (i.e., percent body fat), women with greater abdominal obesity generally have higher levels of the major metabolic risk factors for CHD. For example, in a study of 32,856 women, Hartz and colleagues (1984) observed that waist-to-hip circumference ratio was significantly associated with the incidence of diabetes, hypertension, and gall bladder disease. Numerous other investigators, using a variety of measures to access total body and central obesity, have reported an independent association between degree of central obesity and abnormal lipid profiles (Anderson et al., 1988), glucose intolerance (Despres et al., 1989; Peiris et al., 1989), and hypertension (Blair et al., 1984).

Several initial studies have observed that central obesity is positively associated with clinical cardiovascular events in women. Waist-to-hip circumference ratio was independently associated with the 12-y incidence of myocardial infarction, angina pectoris, stroke, and CVD death in 1462 women aged 38–60 living in Gothenburg, Sweden (Lapidus et al., 1984). For women living in Framingham, Massachusetts, abdominal obesity contributed, independent of BMI, to the risk of CHD, CVD, and all-cause mortality (Kannel et al., 1991). For more comprehensive information on obesity, body fat distribution, and CHD risk see the review by Stefanick (1993). Additional data should be obtained with newer methods of measuring regional adiposity to assess the relation between body fat distribution patterns and CVD morbidity and mortality, especially in older women and in ethnic minorities because of their increased tendencies to become obese.

Estrogen Replacement Therapy

Estrogen has received considerable attention with regard to its role in potentially affecting CHD risk. It has been contended that the significantly lower risk of CHD enjoyed by premenopausal and early postmenopausal women is, in large part, due to an estrogenic effect. Early work in animal models suggested an anti-atherogenic effect of estrogen given to animals on a high-fat diet (Stamler et al., 1953). Despite the possibility of beneficial estrogen effects regarding CHD, no large-scale, long-term, randomized clinical trials have been reported for women.

At least 24 prospective and case-control studies have addressed the issue of noncontraceptive estrogen use and CHD risk. Most of the prospective studies reported a reduced risk of CHD morbidity and mortality among estrogen users compared to nonusers (Croft & Hannaford, 1989; Hammond et al., 1979; Henderson et al., 1988, 1991; Nachtigall et al., 1979; Petitti et al., 1987; Stampfer et al., 1985, 1991). Relative risks have ranged from 0.8–0.3, which is comparable to a 20%–70% reduction in risk among estrogen users compared to nonusers. Of nine prospective studies reviewed, four reported a statistically significant reduction for women on estrogen replacement therapy, amounting to a 40%–70% reduction in CHD risk (Henderson et al., 1988, 1991; Stampfer et al., 1985, 1991). The Framingham Study has been the only prospective study to report elevated CVD risk among estrogen users (Wilson et al., 1985). Data from the Framingham cohort was later reanalyzed, with angina excluded as an endpoint, and did not show increased CHD risk with estrogen use (Eaker & Castelli, 1987).

The Postmenopausal Estrogen/Progestin Interventions (PEPI) trial (The Writing Group for the PEPI Trial, 1995) is one of the first randomized, clinical trials conducted to evaluate the effect of estrogen alone, or in combination with progestin, on selected risk factors for heart disease. Seven clinical centers randomized 875 postmenopausal women (45–64 y) to one of five treatment arms: 1) placebo; 2) estrogen alone; 3) estrogen + cyclic medroxyprogesterone acetate (MPA); 4) estrogen + MPA 2.5 mg/d; or 5) estrogen + cyclic micronized progesterone (MP). Participants were followed for 3 y during which HDL-C, systolic blood pressure, fibrinogen, and serum insulin were measured. Results generally supported an improved CHD risk profile for women on hormonal therapy, compared to placebo. Estrogen alone, or in combination with a progestin regimen, was associated with an increase in HDL-C and a reduction in LDL-C and fibrinogen levels. Unopposed estrogen was most effective in elevating HDL-C; however, this regimen was associated with a high rate of endometrial hyperplasia, thus limiting its use in women with uteri. No significant treatment effects were noted for serum insulin levels or blood pressure.

Several case-control studies, using angiography to document CHD, provide additional evidence for a protective effect of estrogen (Gruchow et al., 1988; McFarland et al., 1989; Sullivan et al., 1988). For example, McFarland and associates (1989) found that the risk of significant coronary occlusion (>70% stenosis in 1 or more coronary artery) was reduced by 50% in users of estrogens. Statistical adjustments for other risk factors did not modify the result.

Evidence from a majority of prospective-cohort, case-control studies and from at least one clinical trial support a significant benefit of estrogen in the reduction of CHD risk, morbidity, and mortality. Although the evidence from observational studies strongly suggests causality between estrogens and risk reduction, there are limitations to such studies. Additional randomized clinical trials would refute or substantiate causality and shed light on the potential impact of combined-hormone therapy on coronary heart disease risk and incidence.

Oral Contraceptive Use

In contrast to the apparently beneficial effects of estrogen replacement therapy, oral contraceptive use has been associated with increased risk of CHD (Mann & Inman, 1975; Royal College of General Practitioners' Oral Contraception Study, 1981; Slone et al., 1981; Stampfer et al., 1988; Vessey et al., 1989). Eight-year follow-up data from the Nurses' Health Study (Stampfer et al., 1988) found a significant excess in fatal and nonfatal CHD among current oral contraceptive users (relative risk (RR)

= 2.5; 95% confidence interval (CI) = 1.3–4.9). Similarly, a study conducted in Great Britain found users of oral contraceptives to have a 3.3 times greater risk of fatal CHD compared to nonusers, although the excess risk was not statistically significant (Vessey et al., 1989).

Cigarette smoking appears to exacerbate CHD risk among oral contraceptive users. Salonen (1982) found that the risk of nonfatal MI among smokers who also used oral contraceptives was 7 times that of women who neither smoked nor used oral contraception. Furthermore, among all smokers, current oral contraceptive use was associated with 3.6 times the risk of smoking nonusers.

The adverse effects of oral contraceptives may be limited to current users. Most studies suggest that past oral contraceptive use is not significantly associated with increased risk of heart disease. Stampfer and others (1988) found the risk for fatal and nonfatal CHD among past users versus never users to be 0.91 (95% CI = 0.74–1.12). Relative risk was not significantly changed when adjusted for other potential risk factors. Furthermore, no significant trend was noted between increasing duration of past use and increased risk. In contrast, Slone et al. (1981) found duration of past use to be important. Increased duration of past use was associated with increased risk of nonfatal MI. However, this was true only among women in the age group 40–49 y.

The aforementioned studies evaluated oral contraceptives that contained higher doses of estrogen and progestin than do more recent oral contraceptive formulations. Because adverse effects of oral contraceptives may be dose dependent, newer preparations that contain less estrogen may not be associated with increased risk of heart disease. In fact, there is some evidence that more recent oral contraceptives may reduce CVD risk (Eaker et al., 1993). Additional work concerning low-dose oral contraceptive preparations and heart disease risk is warranted.

Socioeconomic Status

Coronary heart disease, once prevalent among the elite of the early 20th century, is now more of a problem among women and men of lower socioeconomic status. There is substantial epidemiologic evidence to suggest that socioeconomic status is an important factor in the etiology of CHD. Although the majority of literature in this area primarily has examined men, studies that have included a sufficient cohort of women generally conclude that socioeconomic status is a potentially important CHD risk factor for them.

Mathews and colleagues (1989) evaluated 541 women aged 42–50 y, residing in Allegheny County, PA. Measured risk factors included lipid/lipoprotein profiles, 2-h insulin and glucose levels, smoking history, and current physical activity levels (kcal/wk). Socioeconomic status was evaluated by educational attainment, current occupation, and partner's occupation.

After adjustment for possible confounders, less-educated women had a more atherogenic lipid/lipoprotein profile, had poorer exercise habits, and more often reported current or long-term use of cigarettes.

Other studies have focused on the relationship between socioeconomic status and a single risk factor. The Chicago Heart Association Detection Project in Industry evaluated blood pressure levels in more than 27,000 employed Chicagoans, of whom 9716 were white women and 1254 were black women (Dyer et al., 1976). Educational attainment was used as a measure of socioeconomic status. Among white women (25–44 y and 45–64 y), a significant inverse relation was reported for educational level and blood pressure. In contrast, data collected from black women were inconclusive, perhaps at least partly because the sample size was relatively small. In contrast, Kiel et al. (1981), who evaluated blood pressure in 226 black women for the Charleston Heart Study and classified education as low (0–7 y) or high (8 y or higher), did detect an association between high educational level and lower blood pressure.

Findings similar to those observed in the study of white female Chicagoans were reported for women living in a rural county in Sweden (Haglund, 1985). Nearly 3000 women were evaluated for blood pressure and socioeconomic status. Socioeconomic data were based on questions related to marital status, school education, place of residence, occupation, and place of work. Educational level was most strongly related to blood pressure; women with more education had lower blood pressures. This relationship was especially evident among the women compared to their male counterparts and was unchanged after adjustment for potential confounders.

Sorel et al. (1992) evaluated persons aged 25–74 y who participated in the Second National Health and Nutrition Survey and the Hispanic Health and Nutrition Examination Survey. This population included 4031 white, 597 black, and 1528 Mexican-American women. After adjustment for body mass index and age, the relationship between education and blood pressure was not consistent among the three groups of women. A negative association was found between education and systolic blood pressure for white and black women; a positive relationship was found between diastolic pressure and education among Mexican-American women. The lack of a consistent relationship between blood pressure and education is in contrast to many earlier studies. The authors provided possible reasons for their contrary findings: 1) the general educational level of the population may have increased since earlier investigations, and 2) treatment for hypertension has become more prevalent since early studies were conducted. As a result of these trends, the authors suggested that pharmacological treatment of hypertension may vary by social class, and educational level may not have exerted the same social leverage as it did in previous studies. Indeed, the validity of education as a measure of socioeconomic status across population subgroups has been questioned.

Level of physical activity has also been studied relative to socioeconomic status. Kaplan et al. (1991) evaluated the association between socioeconomic status and 9-y changes in leisure-time physical activity in a cohort of adult residents of Alameda County, CA. After adjustment for possible confounders, relative declines in physical activity were associated with lower educational attainment and lower income level.

Several other epidemiologic studies have investigated the relationship between socioeconomic status and other primary risk factors for CHD. Kaplan and Keil (1993) may be consulted to provide a more extensive review of literature in this area. It is clear from the research reviewed here that the relationship between socioeconomic status and CHD etiology is not consistent among women of different ethnic groups. Despite this shortcoming, there is substantial evidence to suggest that socioeconomic status is an important factor related to CHD among women. Future work should include adequate sample sizes to address this question among subpopulations.

CHD Risk Factors in Young Girls and Adolescents

Many of the risk factors that have been identified for adult women (abnormal lipid profile, hypertension, cigarette smoking, obesity, and physical inactivity) are already present in young girls (Berenson et al., 1988; Gilliam et al., 1977; Lauer et al., 1975). Furthermore, the adult phenomenon of risk factor clustering has also been reported in female youth (Raitakari et al., 1994; Webber et al., 1979). Considering the early presence of CHD risk factors, it should not be surprising that the atherosclerotic process is evident during infancy and early childhood (Pesonen et al., 1990). Although there are no definitive data that the presence of risk factors in childhood results in heart disease as a adult, some researchers have shown that certain CHD risk factors persist with time (Andersen & Haraldsdóttir, 1993; Clarke et al., 1978; Porkka et al., 1991). The "persistence" of a risk factor in children is referred to as "tracking" and has been defined as the correlation between repeated measures of a certain risk factor and/ or the relationship between percentile positions for a specific risk factor over an observed time period.

There is some evidence for a gender difference with regard to the tracking of both risk factor clusters and single risk factors (Andersen & Haraldsdóttir, 1993; Porkka et al., 1991). The Cardiovascular Risk in Young Finns Study (Raitakari et al., 1994) evaluated 1769 girls and 1688 boys (3–18 y) over a 6-y period. Sum of skinfolds, systolic blood pressure, and lipids were measured at baseline, after 3 y, and after 6 y. High-risk children were defined as those with a "cluster" of risk factors (serum lipid variable, obesity index, and blood pressure) at levels equal to or greater than the age- and gender-specific 75th percentile of the study cohort. The number of children with risk-factor clustering significantly increased with age among the boys, whereas this was not apparent with the girls. Among girls, clustering was most apparent only for those aged 9–12 y. Similar observations were reported by Anderson and Haraldsdóttir (1993) in 115 female and 88 male Danish adolescents (15-18 y) evaluated over an 8-y period. A risk factor score equal to the sum of systolic blood pressure, diastolic blood pressure, cholesterol, HDL-C, triglyceride, smoking, and skinfolds was calculated for each adolescent. Total risk score significantly increased in males (20.3 ± 4.2 to 25.5 ± 4.7, over the 8-y period, but not for the females (20.7 ± 2.2 to 21.6 ± 2.5). Furthermore, males in the upper quintile of risk score tended to remain there over time, whereas this was not the case for females.

Although it is not yet clear whether "high-risk" children become "high-risk" adults with clinical manifestations of heart disease, it is clear that the genesis of atherosclerosis occurs during childhood. Additional data collected in children of different ethnicities are needed to characterize risk factor profiles and the extent to which they track with time. Lifestyle patterns developed during childhood and adolescence may influence adult lifestyle patterns. Given the interaction of genetic and environmental influences on the manifestation of CHD, evaluation of CHD risk during childhood may serve as an important step toward early preventive measures.

THE EFFECTS OF EXERCISE ON CORONARY HEART DISEASE RISK FACTORS IN WOMEN

Over the past decade, an increasing number of studies has been published evaluating the relationship of physical activity or physical fitness to the major risk factors for CHD. In general, these relationships in women appear similar to those observed for men, but the data are still too limited to indicate if there are specific gender differences. The major confounder to this relationship is the hormonal status of the women.

Hypertension

Relatively few observational studies have examined the relationship between physical activity and hypertension among women. Often, separate analyses were not conducted in those studies that included men and women. Of the few studies that have focused on women, most support an inverse relation between blood pressure level and fitness or physical activity status (Ainsworth et al., 1991; Gibbons et al., 1983; Owens et al., 1990; Reaven et al., 1991). Although most studies have involved primarily Caucasian women, the apparently beneficial effects of an active lifestyle on blood pressure may hold true for African-American women as well. For example, Ainsworth and colleagues (1991) used a questionnaire to determine activity levels in 1096 African-American women and found that a sedentary lifestyle was associated with a 59% greater risk of diastolic hypertension than was an active lifestyle (performing work/exercise sufficient to produce sweating, 3 times/wk). This excess risk remained after adjustment for other factors related to hypertension. Considering the prevalence of hypertension among African-Americans, these results could have important implications for this high-risk group.

Studies in older women also suggest an influence of physical activity on blood pressure. Reaven et al. (1991) used a questionnaire to categorize the leisure-time activities of 641 women, aged 50–89 y, into light, moderate, or heavy exercise intensities. The prevalence of hypertension was lower at all levels of active women, compared to their sedentary peers. It is interesting to note that participation in either low-intensity activity (walking, gardening, bowling, etc.) or high-intensity activity (jogging, handball, racquetball, etc.) was associated with lower blood pressures. Some studies show no relationship between physical activity and blood pressure in younger (Ballor & Poehlman, 1992) or older women (Voorrips et al., 1993). In both cases, the lack of a relationship may have been due to small sample sizes that resulted in low statistical power.

Very few intervention studies have investigated the effect of exercise training in hypertensive women. To date, only three published reports have provided data specific to blood pressure adaptations in hypertensive women (Krotkiewski et al., 1979; Roman et al., 1981; Tanabe et al., 1988). All used modalities such as walking, jogging, or cycling as the primary exercise intervention, although one study (Krotkiewski et al., 1979) did include dancing and gymnastics in addition to the aforementioned activities. All three studies showed an average reduction in resting blood pressure of 11% (systolic) and 10% (diastolic) as a result of exercise training. Furthermore, Roman et al. (1981) noted an increase in resting blood pressure to near pretraining values, following 3 mo of detraining. The results of these studies should be interpreted cautiously because only one (Tanabe et al., 1988) included a non-exercising, hypertensive control group (which consisted of only two men and three women).

Limited data suggest that women may respond particularly well to endurance exercise training. Kinoshita and colleagues (1988) trained male and female hypertensives using cycling for 10 wk. They divided the group into responders (>10 mm Hg decrease in mean blood pressure after training) and nonresponders. Seventy-five percent of the responders were women; the composition of the nonresponders was not provided. Because responders differed from nonresponders in body weight prior to training, female gender may not have been the sole characteristic of a responder. Hagberg (1990) conducted a meta-analysis that included a small number of training studies in women and suggested that endurance exercise may evoke greater blood pressure reductions in women (−19/−14 mm Hg) than in men ($-7/-5$ mm Hg). However, the sample size for women was small so this conclusion should be viewed conservatively.

In general, the effectiveness of exercise training in reducing blood pressure in hypertensive women is not well established. Few studies have been conducted in female populations. Those that have focused on women have used a relatively small number of subjects and/or have lacked an appropriate control group. Those that have included men and women have had an inadequate number of female or male subjects to determine gender-specific adaptations. Despite these limitations, the evidence from cross-sectional and intervention studies to date does provide some groundwork for additional well-controlled studies on reducing the age-related rise in blood pressure by exercise.

Lipids and Lipoproteins

Cross-sectional research has generally shown a positive relationship between physical activity or physical fitness and HDL-C and an inverse relationship with LDL-C concentrations. Studies that have compared women runners and inactive peers have shown runners to have higher HDL-C levels (Moore et al., 1983; Morgan et al., 1986; Wood et al., 1977) and lower LDL-C (Hartung et al., 1986; Stamford et al., 1984; Wood et al., 1977). In a sample of women more representative of the general population, Gibbons et al. (1983) determined risk-factor status and fitness level by performance time on a maximal treadmill exercise test. At least 1700 healthy women, aged 18–65 y, were evaluated. After adjustment for potential confounders, treadmill time was inversely associated with levels of triglycerides as well as total cholesterol:HDL-C and was positively associated with HDL-C concentrations.

The extent to which menopausal status may affect the relationship between lipoproteins and exercise is unclear. In two studies (Hartung et al., 1984; Rainville & Vaccaro, 1984), menopausal status did not appear to modify the favorable effect on HDL-C observed among physically active women relative to their inactive counterparts. One report did show a differential effect of menopausal status on the HDL-C:LDL-C ratio (Hartung et al., 1984). Premenopausal women did not show a difference in HDL-C:LDL-C associated with activity, whereas postmenopausal women showed a higher ratio with increased exercise.

There is some evidence that the relationship between physical activity and lipoproteins is a function of body weight. Upton et al. (1984) found that significant differences in HDL-C between middle-aged marathoners and sedentary women were eliminated when adjusted for BMI. Similarly, Meilahn and associates (1988) used a physical activity questionnaire to categorize women according to energy expenditure and did not find energy expenditure to be a significant predictor of HDL, whereas BMI persisted as a significant predictor in this multiple-regression analysis. Body weight and related measures have not been consistently reported to be confounding factors, however. Haskell et al. (1980) found significantly higher HDL-C levels in active women, aged 20–39 y, compared to inactive women, despite adjustment for BMI. Similarly, Moore et al. (1983) reported that significantly greater HDL-C concentrations persisted among runners in comparison to inactive controls when body-fat percentage was statistically controlled.

Collectively, evidence from cross-sectional studies strongly suggests that regular physical activity can favorably affect lipoprotein profiles of premenopausal and postmenopausal women. These studies provide a foundation upon which prospective research may determine causality and identify appropriate exercise regimens for women across the age spectrum.

Unfortunately, the results of prospective studies have not been very consistent in documenting a lipid-lipoprotein adaptation to exercise training in women. Most intervention studies involving women have focused primarily on the effect of aerobic training on plasma HDL-C, LDL-C, and total cholesterol concentrations. Of the seven randomized, controlled investigations reviewed, two (Duncan et al., 1991; Hardman et al., 1989) reported an exercise effect of increased HDL-C concentrations, and one (Duncan et al., 1991) found lowered LDL-C levels with exercise. In a well-designed walking study conducted by Duncan et al. (1991), strollers (4.8 km/h) and aerobic walkers (8.0 km/h) covered the same distances during training and had similar significant increases in HDL-C (3 mg/dL). This suggests that volume of work may be more important than intensity in affecting HDL-C concentrations in premenopausal women. Training programs designed to maximize change in aerobic capacity may not be necessary to elicit meaningful changes in HDL-C levels.

The remaining randomized trials (with inactive controls) found aerobic training to be ineffective in changing HDL-C, LDL-C, or total cholesterol levels (Cauley et al., 1987; Franklin et al., 1979; Juneau et al., 1987; Suter & Marti, 1992; Williford et al., 1988). Other prospective studies have reported associations between aerobic training and increased HDL-C levels (Hill et al., 1989), decreased cholesterol levels (Moll et al., 1979; Shephard et al., 1980), and decreased LDL-C levels (Brownell et al., 1982), but the lack of concurrent inactive control groups and/or an absence of random assignment of subjects to groups limits the confidence one can place in the cause-and-effect nature of these results.

Factors unique to women, such as menstrual status, may modify possible exercise effects on plasma lipid levels. Blumenthal et al. (1991) conducted a 12-wk walk/jog program in 12 postmenopausal and 11 premenopausal women. A significant decline was reported for HDL-C (−11 mg/dL) and cholesterol (−4 mg/dL) in the postmenopausal women; premenopausal women had no change in either lipid variable.

Phase of the menstrual cycle may also affect plasma lipids and lipo-proteins. Plasma concentrations of cholesterol (Jones et al., 1988; Kim & Kalkhoff, 1979; Tangeny et al., 1991), HDL-C (Barclay et al., 1965; Jones et al., 1988), and triglyceride (Kim & Kalkhoff, 1979; Woods et al., 1987) fluctuate during the menstrual cycle. Although all reports do not support a menstrual phase effect on lipids and lipoproteins (Brideau et al., 1992; Lebech et al., 1990), it nonetheless seems prudent to control for phase of the menstrual cycle when investigating the relationship between exercise and lipids.

Few studies have examined whether or not oral contraceptives or hormone replacement therapy modify lipid-lipoprotein adaptations to ex-ercise training. One study (Suter & Marti, 1992) found that despite im-proved endurance capacity, oral contraceptive users did not show the favorable lipoprotein changes that were observed in exercising nonusers. For example, apolipoprotein A-I (a major constituent of HDL-C) signifi-cantly decreased (-0.19 mmol/L) in oral contraceptive users after train-ing, compared to an increase (0.15 mmol/L) observed in women not taking oral contraceptives.

In general, prospective aerobic training studies have reported equivo-cal findings with regard to changes in lipid and lipoprotein concentrations in women. This inconsistency is partly due to small sample sizes, un-known or poor compliance to the exercise regimen, inadequate exercise volume, changes in dietary intake, and lack of control for menstrual status or endogenous/exogenous hormone status. These factors must be con-trolled in order to delineate a causal relationship between physical activity and lipid-lipoproteins and to determine effective exercise regimens spe-cific to a woman's endocrine status and age.

Glucose Intolerance and Non-Insulin Dependent Diabetes Mellitus

Data reported over the past decade have increasingly demonstrated that higher levels of habitual physical activity or physical fitness in women are related to improved glucose tolerance, enhanced insulin-mediated glu-cose uptake, and a lower occurrence of non-insulin dependent diabetes mellitus (NIDDM) (Bogardus et al., 1984; Manson et al, 1991a). However, these relations have been somewhat more difficult to demonstrate in women than in men. For example, a population-based observational study demonstrated in men, but not in women, a significant inverse association between level of habitual physical activity and both fasting plasma insulin and c-peptide (Regensteiner et al., 1991). These data are in contrast to the data reported by Frisch et al. (1986) who compared the prevalence of NIDDM in former college athletes and non-athletes; the women athletes reported a lower prevalence of NIDDM (risk ratio of 2.24; 95% CI = 1.19–4.74). Similarly, Manson and colleagues (1991b) demonstrated that nurses who reported more habitual physical activity experienced less NIDDM. In the Nurses Health Study, 87,253 women aged 34–59 y were followed for an average of 9 y, during which time 1303 cases of NIDDM were reported. Women who engaged in vigorous activity at least once per week had a significantly lower occurrence of NIDDM than did the inactive women, both before and after adjustment for family history of diabetes and obesity. The apparent protective effect of activity existed for obese as well as for lean women.

Women who have elevated glucose and/or insulin responses to an oral glucose-tolerance test or glycemic-clamp procedure and women with NIDDM who undertake a program of endurance exercise training appear to improve their glucose tolerance and demonstrate less of a rise in plasma insulin concentrations in response to a glucose challenge (Björntorp et al., 1970; Krotkiewski et al., 1985; Ronnema et al., 1986; Seals et al., 1984; Tremblay et al., 1991). In all of these exercise training studies, both men and women were included, but no sex specific analyses were presented. However, in some of the studies the sample was predominately composed of women, and data presented on individuals indicated that the magnitude of the response was similar in men and women (Björntorp et al., 1970). The improvement in glucose tolerance with increased habitual exercise appears to be independent of weight loss in women (Björntop et al., 1970), but the effect is augmented when weight loss occurs either as a result of the exercise alone or the exercise plus restriction of dietary energy intake (Tremblay et al., 1991). Given the substantial role abnormal glucose metabolism appears to play in the risk of CHD in women, a much better understanding is needed of how different exercise regimens influence physiological and clinical measures of carbohydrate metabolism.

Hemostatic Factors

Cross-sectional and intervention studies of physical activity in relation to hemostatic variables in women are very limited. Four published cross-sectional investigations have provided information on women. The ARIC Study (Conlan et al., 1993) measured physical activity via questionnaire and two procoagulants (factor VIII and von Willebrand factor) in 6590 women and 5220 men aged 45–64 y. In women, only von Willebrand factor was inversely associated with sport activity score, whereas higher levels of von Willebrand factor and factor VIII were associated with lower levels of leisure activity. The CARDIA Study (Folsom et al., 1993) measured plasma fibrinogen levels and physical activity levels (by questionnaire) in 2260 African-American and Caucasian young adult women. Plasma fibrinogen levels were inversely associated with physical activity score.

The relationship between plasma fibrinogen concentration and leisure-time physical activity was assessed in 874 postmenopausal women participating in the Postmenopausal Estrogen/Progestin Interventions

Study (Stefanick et al., 1995). There was a significant negative association between level of reported activity and fibrinogen concentration as follows: inactive (2.84 g/L), light activity (2.89 g/L), moderate activity (2.8 g/L), and heavy activity (2.60 g/L). The fibrinogen concentration was significantly lower in the heavy-activity group, compared to all the other groups. However, the relationship between fibrinogen and activity was no longer significant in a multivariate analysis that included Body Mass Index.

Stevenson et al. (1995) measured plasma fibrinogen, plasminogen-activator-inhibitor type 1 (PAI-1), and tissue-type plasminogen activator (TPA) in a group of active (n = 14) and less active (n = 17) postmenopausal women. The active women were successful national-class road race participants, whereas the less active women were recruited from newspaper advertisements. Measurement of $\dot{V}O_2$max and estimated daily energy expenditure confirmed a higher energy expenditure and greater aerobic capacity among the active women compared to their less active peers. Levels of PAI-1 and TPA were significantly lower in the active women, whereas no significant group differences were noted for fibrinogen levels (Table 9-1). In addition to hemostatic factors, indices of glucose metabolism and lipid levels were also compared (Table 9-1). The more active women showed evidence of better glucose metabolism and more favorable HDL_2-C and triglyceride levels.

TABLE 9-1. *Hemostatic, metabolic, and androgenic risk factors for coronary heart disease in physically active and less active postmenopausal women.* See text for details; PAI-1 = Plasminogen-Activator-Inhibitor Type 1; TPA = Tissue-Type Plasminogen Activator. Based on data of Stevenson et al. (1995).

Variable	More Active Women (N = 14)	Less Active Women (N = 17)	P-Value
Hemostatic Factors			
Fibrinogen (g/L)	2.8 ± 0.2	2.9 ± 0.1	NS
PAI-1 Activity (Units/mL)	3.0 ± 0.9	9.1 ± 1.7	<0.005
TPA Antigen (ng/mL)	3.0 ± 0.5	5.4 ± 0.5	<0.005
Plasma Concentrations of Glucose and Insulin After Fasting			
Glucose (mmol/L)	4.5 ± 0.1	5.2 ± 0.1	<0.01
Insulin (pmol/L)	39 ± 1.0	49 ± 4.0	<0.01
Oral Glucose Tolerance Test Results (Area under the curve for 3-h test)			
Glucose Area	240 ± 40	500 ± 50	<0.01
Insulin Area	18,000 ± 2,000	44,000 ± 4,000	<0.01
Concentrations of Lipids in Blood Serum			
Total Cholesterol (mg/dL)	185 ± 7	200 ± 7	NS
LDL-Cholesterol (mg/dL)	98 ± 7	115 ± 8	NS
HDL-Cholesterol (mg/dL)	71 ± 5	61 ± 3	NS
HDL_2-Cholesterol (mg/dL)	19 ± 3	8 ± 1	<0.004
Triglycerides (mg/dL)	83 ± 5	118 ± 9	<0.004
Estimated Body Fat (%)	16.3 ± 1.0	31.7 ± 1.0	<0.001
Sex-Hormone-Binding Globulin (nmol/L)	53 ± 6	29 ± 5	<0.01

Because higher-dose oral contraceptive preparations have been associated with changes in hemostasis, De Paz and associates (1995) investigated whether low-dose oral contraceptives modified the response of the fibrinolytic system to acute exercise. Nine users and nine nonusers of low-dose oral contraceptives performed a maximal treadmill test. Pre- and post-test plasma samples were analyzed for TPA, fibrin degradation products (FbDP), and PAI. Acute exercise resulted in significant increases in TPA antigen, TPA activity, FbDP, and TPA/PAI complexes, but the magnitudes of the increases between users and nonusers did not differ.

No studies have reported the effects of increasing exercise participation on changes in hemostatic factors. Clearly, the relationship between altered hemostatic mechanisms and physical activity/exercise training in women has not been adequately investigated. Considering the multifactorial nature of CHD and the role thrombosis appears to play in this disease, further work in this area is needed.

Obesity

The effects of physical activity on adiposity have been addressed in Chapter 5 of this volume; thus, this topic will not be reviewed in detail here. In general, women who frequently participate in endurance exercise or who are generally more active are leaner than are sedentary women of a similar age (DiPietro et al., 1993; Martin et al., 1977), even though they consume more energy (Vodak et al, 1980). These more physically active women tend to have better cardiovascular risk profiles than sedentary women (Martin et al., 1977; Vodak et al., 1980). It has been more difficult to demonstrate that an increase in physical activity by sedentary women will result in loss of body fat (Hardman et al., 1992; Neiman et al., 1988). It is worthwhile, however, to recognize that participating in an exercise training program while adhering to an energy- and fat-restricted diet increases the effectiveness of a weight loss program in women and enhances improvements in their CHD risk profiles (Wood et al., 1991). A total of 112 overweight and sedentary women (25–49 y) were randomly assigned to the following groups for 1 y: control (no change in diet or exercise), weight loss diet only, or weight loss diet plus exercise training. The change in the overall lipid profile was greater in the diet-plus-exercise group compared to the diet group, as was the decrease in the estimated 12-y CHD risk (20% in the diet-only group and 35% in the diet-plus-exercise group).

Because abdominal obesity confers an increased risk of CVD in women that is independent of total obesity, physical activity could be of particular benefit if it contributed to a reduction in abdominal obesity in overweight women. This issue was addressed by Despres and colleagues (1991) in a long-term exercise training study of 13 overweight premenopausal women. Subjects trained for 90 min/d at approximately 55% of

$\dot{V}O_2$max for 4–5 d/wk for 14 mo. The training program significantly increased $\dot{V}O_2$max, decreased body fat mass by 4.6 kg, and did not affect lean body mass. As measured by computed tomography, there was a greater loss of abdominal fat than of midthigh adipose tissue. The training program also produced significant increases in HDL-cholesterol and apolipoprotein A-I and reductions in concentrations of LDL-cholesterol, total cholesterol, and apolipoprotein B, and lowered the insulinogenic index. Metabolic responses were correlated with the reduction in body fat mass and abdominal fat loss, but not with changes in $\dot{V}O_2$max.

Physical Fitness, Physical Activity, and CHD Risk Factors in Young Girls and Adolescents

Much of the literature in this area that has included girls has been cross-sectional in nature. Typically, physical fitness or physical activity has been assessed along with a host of other CHD risk factors. Findings have been mixed with regard to the relative importance of fitness versus physical activity on lipids, blood pressure, and adiposity indices. Stewart et al. (1995) evaluated blood pressure, body fatness, physical activity (7-d recall) and fitness (submaximal treadmill test) in 27 girls and 26 boys aged 9–10 y. Among the girls, body fatness measures (sum of skinfolds and BMI) were positively correlated only with systolic blood pressure. A rather unexpected finding was that heart rate during submaximal treadmill exercise was inversely correlated with TC and LDL-C, i.e., the more fit girls had greater levels of TC and LDL-C. Fitness was not correlated with HDL-C or triglyceride (TG) levels, and no correlation was found between habitual physical activity and blood pressure or lipid variables.

In contrast, Suter and Hawes (1993) evaluated 58 girls and 39 boys aged 10–15 y and found some small but significant associations between variables representing physical activity and body composition and risk factors for CHD. Fitness was measured by submaximal bicycle ergometry, and physical activity was estimated using a 7-d recall method. In girls, physical activity was correlated with HDL-C ($r = 0.28$, $P < 0.05$) but not with any other lipid variable. Estimated $\dot{V}O_2$max was not significantly associated with any lipid measure. Sums of skinfolds were inversely related to HDL-C ($r = -0.29$, $P < 0.05$) and apolipoprotein A-I ($r = -0.26$, $P < 0.05$) and directly correlated with apolipoprotein B ($r = 0.28$, $P < 0.05$). It is interesting that in this study, cardiovascular fitness was found to have little independent relationship to lipid levels, whereas physical activity and body composition measures were of greater importance.

However, in another study of slightly older (16–19 y) adolescents, *fitness* was found to be more related to lipid variables (Andersen & Haraldsdóttir, 1995). Andersen and Haraldsdóttir measured $\dot{V}O_2$max (bicycle ergometry), physical activity (1-y recall), and body fatness (bioelectric impedance analysis) in 115 female and 86 male adolescents. High- and low-fit groups were formed by dividing the cohort into tertiles based on $\dot{V}O_2$max values. In females, members of the high-fit group (highest tertile) had lower TC, higher HDL:TC ratios, and lower TG. In addition to the more favorable lipid profile, the high-fit females had lower body fat percentages and lower BMI scores. A comparison of low- versus high-physical-activity females found no difference in CHD risk factors.

Inconsistencies regarding the relative importance of physical activity versus aerobic fitness on CHD risk factors in children are likely due to a number of factors, e.g., different methodologies have been used to assess fitness and physical activity, the maturation level of the participants often has not been documented, and many studies have had small sample sizes. Andersen and Haraldsdóttir (1995) proposed that the relationship between physical activity and fitness can be portrayed by an s-shaped curve (Figure 9-3) and that in younger, more fit populations, high-intensity physical activity will have a greater impact on fitness level and, thus, possibly on CHD risk. This suggests that instruments used to investigate physical activity in a young, healthy population should be able to assess high-intensity physical activity levels. Clearly, more study is needed to: 1) characterize the fitness/physical activity relationship as it pertains to CHD risk in female youth and 2) determine whether or not a dose-response relationship

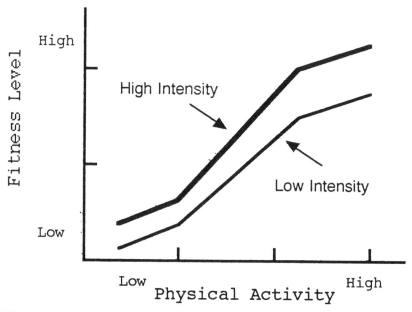

FIGURE 9-3. *Hypothesized relationship between fitness and physical activity in youth.* Choice of S-shaped curve will depend on individual's physical activity intensity. Adapted from Anderson and Haraldsdóttir (1995).

exists between fitness (and/or physical activity) and the presence of CHD risk factors in children.

Randomized, controlled, exercise-intervention trials that investigate the effect on CHD risk factors in youth are limited. There is some evidence for the efficacy of a school-based CVD risk-reduction program in high school students. Killen et al. (1988) randomly assigned one of two matched schools (total $N = 1447$) to receive a 20-session risk reduction intervention. The intervention group exhibited greater gains in knowledge in selected risk-factor domains, and a greater proportion of previously inactive students in the intervention group was participating in regular exerci at a 2-mo follow-up when compared to the control group. Additional large-scale randomized trials conducted in children are necessary to discern whether regular physical activity or aerobic exercise will produce changes in CHD risk factors similar to those observed in adults.

PHYSICAL ACTIVITY AND PHYSICAL FITNESS IN THE PREVENTION OF CORONARY HEART DISEASE MORTALITY IN WOMEN

Physical Activity and the Primary Prevention of CHD

Substantial data exist demonstrating that higher levels of physical activity (Berlin & Colditz, 1990; Powell et al., 1987) and endurance fitness (Blair et al., 1989; Ekelund et al., 1988; Sandvik et al., 1993) in men living in technologically advanced countries are significantly associated with reduced CVD mortality. For women, there are only limited data on sufficiently large samples collected over an extended period of time. However, the evidence that does exist shows lower all-cause and CHD mortality rates for more physically active (Brunner et al., 1974; Lapidus & Bengtsson, 1986; Magnus et al., 1979; Salonen et al., 1982) and fit (Blair et al., 1989; Ekelund et al., 1988) younger and older women and is consistent with data reported for men from these same as well as other studies.

Brunner and colleagues (1974) compared the ischemic heart disease rates in women and men engaged in sedentary and active occupations. All of these women (n = 5229) and men (n = 5288) lived in *kibbutzim* in Israel, thus having reasonably similar socioeconomic status and food availability. Of the women, 42% were considered sedentary and 58% non-sedentary. The incidences of first anginal symptoms, myocardial infarction, fatal ischemic heart disease, and total ischemic heart disease were followed for up to 15 y. The women with nonsedentary occupations had an incidence rate for total ischemic heart disease of 0.6 per 1000 person-years compared to 1.97 for the women with sedentary jobs. This lower rate for the nonsedentary women could be partially accounted for by their lower rates for angina pectoris, myocardial infarction, and fatal cardiac events. These differences in CHD rates between the two activity groups could not be accounted for by differences in body weight, plasma lipid concentrations, or leisure-time activity. Similar results were found for men.

In a study by Magnus and colleagues (1979) that evaluated walking, cycling, and gardening in relation to acute myocardial infarction, both women and men were included. This was a case-control study in which the specific activity habits of women aged 45–69 y who had acute myocardial infarctions were compared to those of a reference group of age-matched women who had not had infarctions. Information regarding the habitual physical activity of the cases over the preceding year was obtained by interviewing the women or their next of kin within 4 wk of their myocardial infarctions, and the controls were interviewed using the same questionnaire. The infarcted women reported significantly less walking, cycling, and gardening than did the controls; the rate ratio for occurrence of acute myocardial infarction was 0.19 (95% confidence limits = 0.10–0.38) when walking, cycling, or gardening was habitual, with a rate ratio of 0.25 for bouts of vigorous activity (95% confidence interval = 0.10–0.61). These rate ratios were somewhat smaller (more favorable for a protective effect of exercise) in women than in men. This relationship between activity and reduced risk of acute myocardial infarction did not appear to be due to cigarette smoking, hypertension, or diabetes.

Physical activity at work and during leisure time was studied in a random sample of women and men living in two counties in Eastern Finland (Salonen, et al., 1982). The study population consisted of 3688 women aged 35–59 y and 3978 men 30–59 y. Physical activity was assessed by an interviewer-administered questionnaire at baseline, and subjects were followed for approximately 7 y. In women free of CHD during the year prior to baseline, women reporting more activity on the job or during leisure time experienced fewer clinical manifestations of CHD than did less active women (Figure 9-4). Women reporting low physical activity both at work and in leisure time had an age-adjusted relative risk of acute myocardial infarction of 4.0 (95% CI = 2.1–7.9) and a relative risk for death of 3.5 (95% CI = 1.9–6.3). These results were similar to those observed in men.

In a prospective study of the relation between CVD and physical activity and socioeconomic status in women living in Oslo, Norway (Lapidus & Bengtsson, 1986), women who reported low physical activity at work or during leisure time over the preceding year had a higher rate of cardiovascular events during the next 12 y than did their more active peers. Low activity at work was a significant risk factor for stroke and overall mortality, whereas leisure-time activity was inversely related to the occurrence of myocardial infarction, stroke, and overall mortality.

To examine if women who performed more physical activity during leisure time have a lower risk of myocardial infarction, a population-based case control study was conducted among enrollees of a large pre-paid health insurance program (Lemaitre et al., 1995). The physical activity

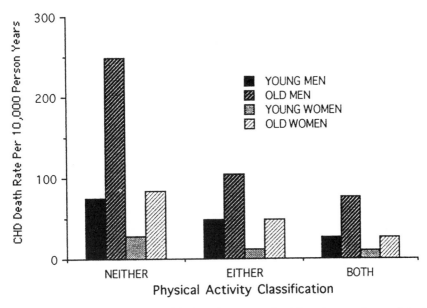

FIGURE 9-4. *Physical activity status and death rate from coronary heart disease in men and women living in eastern Finland.* NEITHER = no participation in physical activity at work or at leisure; EITHER = participation in physical activity either at work or at leisure; BOTH = participation in physical activity both at work and at leisure. See text for discussion of the data.

status over the previous month was assessed by a telephone interview of postmenopausal women who had sustained a nonfatal myocardial infarction (cases = 268) during 1986 through 1991 and of a random sample of women of a similar age with no evidence of CVD (controls = 925). After adjustment for potential confounding factors, the odds ratios for nonfatal myocardial infarction for women in the second, third, and fourth quartiles of total energy expenditure relative to women in the first quartile were 0.52 (95% CI = 0.34-0.80), 0.40 (95% CI = 0.26-0.63), and 0.40 (95% CI = 0.25-0.63), respectively. Similar odds ratios were associated with the energy expended in nonstrenuous leisure-time activity and with brisk walking. The amount of energy expenditure associated with a 50% lower risk of myocardial infarction was equivalent to 30-45 min of brisk walking 3 times/wk.

Several other longitudinal studies have included women and measures of physical activity but have provided little or no data specifically for women (Kannel & Sorlie, 1979; Kaplan et al., 1987). In an early report from the Framingham Study (Kannel & Sorlie, 1979), physical activity levels in women were not associated with overall mortality or cardiovascular morbidity or mortality over 14 y of follow-up with physical activity assessment performed in 1955-56. A major limitation of this study was that 71% of the women were classified in the middle tertile of activity, with very few deaths occurring among women in the other fitness categories. In a 17-y follow-up of 1454 women and men residents of Alameda County, California, who were age 60–94 y at baseline, habitual physical activity was inversely associated with all-cause mortality (relative hazard for slightly versus highly active = 1.38; 95% C.I. = 1.17–1.62 after adjustment for age, sex, baseline status, and six other risk factors). No gender-specific data were presented, but all indications are that the results were similar for women and men.

Physical Fitness and the Primary Prevention of CHD

So far, only Blair and colleagues (1989) have published a peer-reviewed report on the relationship between CHD mortality and cardiovascular fitness in women. The relationship between physical fitness, as determined by test duration during a symptom-limited treadmill exercise test, and all-cause and cause-specific mortality in 3120 women and 10,220 men was determined during an average follow-up period of 8 y. There were 240 deaths in men and 43 deaths in women. Levels of age-adjusted physical fitness were inversely associated with all-cause mortality and mortality for CVD and total cancer in women. When women were separated into fitness categories by quintile of treadmill-test duration, the women in the lowest quintile had a risk ratio for all-cause mortality of 4.65 (95% C.I. = 2.22–9.75) versus the women in the highest quintile (Figure 9-5). The major differences in all-cause mortality occurred between the first and second quintiles, with the relative magnitude of the differences in mortality rate across fitness categories similar for men and women. Given the small number of deaths due to CVD in women (7), one should place only limited confidence in the relationship detected between physical fitness and CVD, even though the tendency was for the more fit women to have lower age-adjusted death rates than did the moderately fit women or women with low levels of fitness (rate per 10,000 person years = 7.4, 2.9 and 0.8 for highly, moderately, and slightly fit categories, respectively). Given the low mortality rate in this group of women, a longer follow-up is required for more definitive data on the physical fitness versus CHD association.

Similar results have been published in an abstract on women participants in the Lipid Research Clinics Prevalence survey (Ekelund et al., 1988). During a 10.5 y follow-up of 2802 women age 30–69 y at baseline, the relative risk of CVD mortality was 2.4 for the least fit versus the most fit (as determined by heart rate during submaximal treadmill exercise).

Unfortunately, no randomized clinical trial of adequate size or duration in either men or women has been conducted to test the causality of the relationship between exercise and reduced CHD. However, selected features of the design and results of the various observational studies are consistent with the interpretation that a more physically active lifestyle

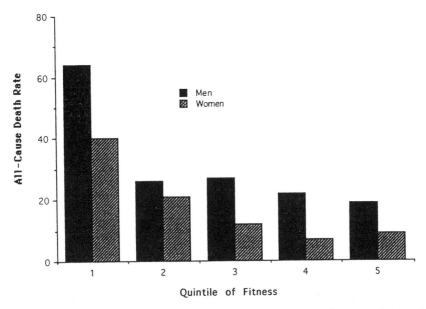

FIGURE 9-5. *All-cause mortality rates by physical fitness category for men and women evaluated at the Cooper Clinic.* The first fitness quintile represents the lowest fitness category, whereas the 5th quintile represents the highest fitness category. See text for discussion of the data.

independently contributes to reduced mortality from CVD. Such features include a proper sequence of events (physical activity or a higher level of fitness precedes the clinical event), a reasonable dose-response relationship between activity level or fitness and benefit, associations observed in relevant populations, independence of association from other established risk factors, and biological plausibility of a causal relationship.

In observational prospective studies where physical activity has been assessed for both younger (<65 y) and older men and women, follow-up for the next 8–20 y usually demonstrates that the risk ratio between sedentary and active persons for either coronary heart disease or all-cause mortality is at least as great or greater for the older as for the younger persons (Blair et al., 1989; Brunner et al., 1974; Salonen et al., 1982). It may be that this greater risk ratio is due to the higher overall mortality rate in the elderly, but it does indicate that the more favorable outcome observed in physically active younger persons is not lost with advancing age.

WOMEN IN CARDIAC REHABILITATION

Exercise-based cardiac rehabilitation, the restoration of medical, physical, and psychosocial function following a clinical cardiac event, is an important component of a comprehensive approach to the management of CHD. Most of the scientific data documenting the effects cardiac rehabilitation have been collected on middle and upper socioeconomic class white men. Very little information has been published on the participation rates, benefits, or special needs of women when they participate in the exercise component of cardiac rehabilitation. Preliminary data published over the past few years indicate that only a very small percentage of women with CHD participated in organized programs of cardiac rehabilitation, and the adherence rates for women were generally low compared to those for men.

The Benefits of Exercise-Based Cardiac Rehabilitation

The primary benefits credited to cardiac rehabilitation performed in-hospital (Phase I) following acute myocardial infarction or bypass surgery include decreased deconditioning, prevention of medical complications associated with prolonged bed rest, improved psychological status (less anxiety and depression), and earlier hospital discharge. During the out-patient phase of cardiac rehabilitation (Phases II & III) the major benefits appear to be an increase in physical working capacity, fewer symptoms at rest or during effort (angina and shortness of breath), improved psychological status, less cardiac morbidity and mortality, and enhanced return-to-work experience. These benefits have been primarily demonstrated in men and have been recently reviewed (Leon, 1990).

Morbidity and Mortality. In the reviews of the effects of cardiac rehabilitation on morbidity and mortality (O'Conner et al., 1989; Oldridge et al., 1988) that demonstrate reductions in all-cause mortality by 20–24% and CVD mortality by 23–25% in rehabilitation program participants, only 3 of the 22 studies included women, and they made up only 3% (143 of 4554 patients) of the entire sample (Kallio et al., 1979; Roman et al., 1983; Wilhelmsen et al., 1975). No separate analyses were performed evaluating the effects of participation in a cardiac rehabilitation program on clinical outcomes in these women. Thus, no data exist for determining if women experience reductions in CVD or all-cause mortality similar to those of men if they participate in cardiac rehabilitation.

Functional Capacity. In the few studies that have compared the changes in functional capacity in men and women during cardiac rehabilitation, most of them have reported similar responses when expressed as a percentage of baseline values. Oldridge and colleagues (1980) reported a 25% increase in power output over 12 mo in 12 women cardiac patients who participated in a medically supervised exercise training program, an increase similar to that achieved by men enrolled in the same program. In the relatively short (8 wk) program conducted by O'Callaghan et al. (1984), exercise test duration was significantly increased in both women (325 $\pm$ 140 to 490 $\pm$ 147 s, a 71.7% increase) and men (417 +158 to 568 $\pm$ 146 s; a 47.7% increase). This increase was not significantly different between the two groups. Also, heart rate during exercise was significantly decreased following training in both men (8.0%) and women (11.2%). These favorable changes were achieved by the women despite their somewhat lower rate of adherence to the program (women $= 77 \pm 16\%$; men $= 87 \pm 14\%$).

Women participating in a 12-wk cardiac rehabilitation program conducted by Cannistra et al. (1991) achieved an increase in exercise test duration of 31% (5.9 ± 1.6 to 7.7 ± 3.2 min), whereas men in the same program had a 21% increase (9.7 ± 3.0 to 11.7 ± 3.2 min). Peak METS increased from 3.7 to 4.8 in women and from 5.1 to 5.9 in men. As for other cardiac risk factors, there were no significant changes in blood lipids, body weight, or cigarette smoking status in either men or women.

The response of older women cardiac patients to a 12-wk cardiac rehabilitation program appears to similar that of older men (Ades, 1992b). In 17 women (mean age 70 ± 6 y) program participation resulted in a 31% improvement in $\dot{V}O_2$max from 16.5 ± 5 to 19 ± 5 mL·kg^{-1}·min^{-1} as compared to men aged 68 ± 5 y, who increased their $\dot{V}O_2$max values by 21% (20 ± 5 to 23 ± 5 mL·kg^{-1}·min^{-1}). During submaximal exercise (3 METS), heart rate, pulmonary ventilation, and rate-pressure product decreased significantly in both women and men following the program.

The results of the cardiac rehabilitation studies to date indicate that the physical working capacities of women patients respond to exercise training in a manner and magnitude that is similar to those for men patients of a similar age. In several studies, because the initial measures of exercise capacity are lower in women and the absolute magnitude of the increase is similar for men and women, the percent increase is greater for the women.

Participation by Women in Cardiac Rehabilitation

An analysis of the limited data available indicates that the percentage of CHD patients considered eligible for out-patient cardiac rehabilitation, the number of eligible patients that get referred to rehabilitation, and adherence to the program are all lower for women than for men (Ades et al., 1992a, 1992b; O'Callihan et al., 1984; Oldridge et al., 1980; Walling et al., 1988). In one of the earliest reports on the participation of women in cardiac rehabilitation, Oldridge et al. (1980) evaluated the participation and performance of 17 women in a medically supervised program for up to 21 mo. The dropout rate for women was "somewhat higher" than for male participants at the same institution. Boogaard (1984) reported on the experience of 20 cardiac patients, 10 women and 10 men aged 25–55 y, who had experienced myocardial infarctions in the previous 3–6 mo. A structured interview was used to determine the patient's participation in various activities, psychological status, and return-to-work experience. After discharge from the hospital, men tended to increase their activity primarily by walking, whereas women performed a variety of household chores.

Only 10% of the women enrolled in a cardiac rehabilitation program compared to approximately 50% of the men.

O'Callihan and colleagues (1984) evaluated the compliance and performance of 264 cardiac patients (men = 227; women = 37) enrolled in a medically supervised cardiac rehabilitation program. The dropout rate over the 8-wk program (3 sessions/wk) was approximately twice as great for the women (18.9%) as for the men (7.8%). Also, of those patients who did complete the program, the attendance rate was significantly higher for the men (men = 87 ± 14%; women = 77 ± 16%). The most common explanation cited for the lower compliance by the women was a greater commitment to domestic responsibilities. These Irish investigators also speculated that the women were less oriented to return-to-work because few women in that society were employed full-time outside of the home, the women tended to believe that they performed sufficient exercise around the home, and the women tended to receive less family support than did the men for participation in rehabilitation programs.

Walling and colleagues (1988) evaluated the rehabilitation potential of a large population of men and women following myocardial infarction. They evaluated the clinical profile of 1096 patients (men = 773; women = 323) and their eligibility to enter a low-risk phase-II cardiac rehabilitation program. The women were older (69 vs. 61 y), had a higher in-hospital mortality rate after adjustment for age (17% vs. 12%), and had an increased incidence of comorbid events that precluded their participation in exercise testing and cardiac rehabilitation. They considered only 5 of 323 (1.6%) women clinically and physiologically eligible for the rehabilitation training program versus 121 of the 773 (16%) men. These numbers are deceptive because one of the exclusion criteria was age > 65 y, and 180 (71%) of women were considered ineligible for this reason versus 281 (41%) of the men. More age-eligible women (55%) than men (38%) also were excluded for cardiac, medical, and psychiatric reasons. Because so few women were eligible for the rehabilitation program, adherence or dropout rates were not reported.

To determine whether women differ from men in their participation and responses to cardiac rehabilitation, 225 consecutive patients enrolled in an urban, multidisciplinary, exercise-based, cardiac rehabilitation program were prospectively evaluated (Walling et al., 1988). Participants included 51 women and 174 men with a mean age of 54 y, and most were white (84%). Compared with men, more women were nonwhite (35% vs. 10%), unemployed (61% vs. 30%), unmarried (71% vs. 26%), hypertensive 73% vs. 39%), or diabetic (33% vs. 11%); had higher cholesterol (257 vs. 230 mg/dL); and were more likely to report angina (45% vs. 29%). No data were presented on referral rates of patients to the rehabilitation program. The rehabilitation sessions were held 3 times/wk for 12 wk. Compliance rates were not significantly different for women (51%) and men (63%), and there were no differences with respect to the reasons given for lack of program completion, but more women tended to withdraw for medical reasons (32% vs. 20%). Rates of program dropout for logistical reasons were similar for women (20%) and men (22%) as were dropouts for work conflicts (women = 12%; men = 14%). Men tended to cite financial reasons as an additional reason for noncompliance (men = 9%; women = 0%). Univariate predictors for program noncompliance differed between women and men; smoking and older age among women were associated with lower compliance rates. Among men, those who smoked, had home stress, or had a positive family history of heart disease were less likely to complete the program.

Gender-related differences in cardiac rehabilitation referral patterns and responses to an aerobic conditioning program were examined in 226 (43% women and 57% men) hospitalized coronary patients (>61 y) living in or near Burlington, Vermont (Ades et al., 1992a, 1992b). All patients had acute myocardial infarction or coronary bypass surgery and had been hospitalized at the Medical Center Hospital of Vermont. Demographic, medical, and social data were collected during in-hospital guided interviews to determine predictors of participation of all patients who were candidates for the rehabilitation program. Patients were eligible to enter the program 4 wk after their cardiac events and after consultations with their physicians. Shortly after the patients' initial outpatient visits with their physicians, they were interviewed by project staff regarding cardiac rehabilitation participation and about the strength of their physicians' recommendation for participation. The 12-wk rehabilitation program consisted of 1-h sessions of telemetry-monitored treadmill, cycle, and rowing ergometer exercise (3/wk).

Older women were less likely than older men to enter the program (26% vs. 15%). Only 6% of women and 7% of men did not complete the program. Factors that influenced participation in both men and women (gender-specific responses not reported) included job type (blue collar—13%, white collar—13% and housewife—20%) and any chronic disease present (yes = 11%, no = 28%). Participants had shorter commute times to classes, higher educational levels, and less denial of the severity of their illnesses.

The strength of the physician recommendation was the most powerful predictor of participation for all patients (mean recommendation score = 4.7 ± 8 in participants and 1.9 ± 1.4 in nonparticipants). Physician recommendation scores were higher for men (3.0 ± 1.8) than for women (2.3 ± 1.7), despite similar clinical profiles. Other factors that may have influenced the lower rates of participation by women included their being older, less likely to drive cars, and more likely to have dependent spouses at home, as well as their having arthritis; however, these factors were not significant when entered into a multivariate analysis that included the strength of the physician's recommendation. Reasons for the lower rates at which physicians recommended participation by women in cardiac rehabilitation were not established, but physicians' perceptions that cardiac rehabilitation is less efficacious in women and that women are less inclined to exercise were considered.

Oldridge and colleagues (Oldridge et al., 1992) investigated the associations between the participation in cardiac rehabilitation and age, gender, major CVD risk factors, reasons for referral, and type on medical insurance coverage. They evaluated 492 patients (men = 337, women = 155) referred to a cardiac rehabilitation program in Milwaukee, Wisconsin, between January 1980 and December 1987. The "phase-II" rehabilitation program was hospital-based and lasted for 12 wk. Mean overall attendance to the program was 75%, with women having a significantly lower mean attendance (68%) than the men (78%). This lower attendance for women existed at all ages. The patients with the lowest program attendance were women less than 46 y who had Medicaid insurance. These data are consistent with the prior studies that generally found lower participation rates for women in cardiac rehabilitation, with the lowest rates occurring in women of low socioeconomic standing.

Nationwide Survey. In the early 1990s a survey of a random sample of cardiac rehabilitation programs throughout the U.S. evaluated the current involvement of women as patients in these programs and began to assess the specific needs of women for successful participation (Thomas et al., 1992). Data including such information as program phase, location, costs, size, gender specific enrollment, and gender-specific services and needs were collected from 173 programs. Each program also provided patient-specific data on a representative sample of men (n = 1603) and women (n = 1480) participants during 1990. This survey provided information on demographics, clinical/risk-factor status, and program participation. Preliminary analysis of the data from this survey demonstrated that only 25%–33% of program participants were women, who tended to be older than the men; 40% were not married. Women had slightly lower adherence and higher dropout rates than men. Very few programs provided any special services for women patients, although the majority of program directors sensed that such services were warranted. The results of this survey document the need for additional research on how to more effectively involve women in cardiac rehabilitation and secondary prevention programs and to evaluate the specific benefits derived by women.

DIRECTIONS FOR FUTURE RESEARCH

1. There is a need for more epidemiological studies on the relationship between habitual physical activity or physical fitness and the devel-

opment of CVD. Data related to older women and women of ethnicities relevant to the United States are particularly limited.

2. Inherent in the above recommendation is the need to develop a variety of reliable and valid physical/habitual activity questionnaires for use with women across the age spectrum and for women of different ethnicity.

3. Cross-sectional research and intervention trials on physical activity or fitness and CHD risk factors should be sufficiently inclusive to address how menopausal status and endogenous/exogenous hormone status may affect the exercise/fitness-risk factor relationship.

4. No studies have been published on the potential for exercise to reduce morbidity or mortality in women with established CHD. Large-scale, multicenter trials will be needed to determine if an increase in activity provides secondary prevention benefits to women. Also, no data have been presented on the safety of exercise in these high-risk women.

5. Intervention studies should be designed to address dose-response issues in both women and men. Recent work has indicated that moderate-intensity exercise training is associated with improved blood pressure and lipid-lipoprotein levels and with reduced CVD mortality. Well-designed intervention studies should build upon and expand this concept.

6. Most cross-sectional and intervention studies to date have focused on the effects of endurance training. Future studies should examine other exercise modalities such as resistance or strength training. There is some evidence that resistance or circuit-training may lower blood pressure (Tipton, 1991), although no studies have specifically addressed this hypothesis in women.

7. Future research must be more inclusive. Research on older women and women of various ethnicities relevant to the United States is practically nonexistent. The ability to generalize is obviously limited. In most cases, the aged and members of "minority" groups are particularly vulnerable to CHD and associated sequelae. Future studies that include diverse populations would make a significant contribution in providing a basis for health recommendations pertinent to women across all ages and ethnicities.

SUMMARY

Over the past half century, a majority of the research conducted to determine if and how physical activity might influence the development of CVD has been performed on men. Whereas more than 75 observational studies conducted in widely differing populations have reported on the relationship between CVD and physical activity or cardio-respiratory fitness in men, fewer than 10 have reported such information for women.

Also, none of the studies of the impact of exercise-based cardiac rehabilitation on morbidity or mortality has had adequate numbers of women patients to determine if the benefits that accrue to men are achieved by women. However, in the limited studies available, more active or fit women appear to receive some protection from CHD, and being more physically active seems to result in a more favorable CHD risk profile. Risk factors such as elevated blood pressure, increased platelet aggregation, glucose intolerance, abnormal lipid profiles, and adiposity are at more optimal values in active pre- and postmenopausal women. For all of these risk factors, there are still very few randomized, controlled trials that have included women or presented data for women separately. A major gap in our understanding is the interaction between the women's hormone status and the influence of physical activity on CVD risk. Of major concern is the paucity of data on older women and ethnic minorities.

BIBLIOGRAPHY

Ades, P.A., M.L. Waldmann, W.J. McCann, and S.O. Weaver (1992a). Predictor of cardiac rehabilitation participation in older coronary patients. *Arch. Intern. Med.* 152:1033–1035.
Ades, P.A., M.L. Waldmann, D. M. Polk, and J. Coflesky (1992b). Referral patterns and exercise response in the rehabilitation of female coronary patients aged greater than 62 years. *Am. J. Cardiol.* 69:1422–1425.
Ainsworth, B.E., N.L. Keenan, D.S. Strogatz, J.M. Garrett, and S.A. James (1991). Physical activity and hypertension in black adults: The Pitt County Study. *Am. J. Public Health* 81:1477–1479.
American Heart Association (1994). *1993 Heart and Stroke Facts Statistics.* Dallas, Texas: American Heart Association.
Anastos, K., P. Charney, R.A. Charon, E. Cohen, C.Y. Jones, C. Marte, D.M. Swiderski, M.E. Wheat, and S. Williams (1991). Hypertension in women: what is really known? *Ann. Intern. Med.* 115:287–293.
Andersen, L.B., and J. Haraldsdóttir (1993). Tracking of cardiovascular disease risk factors including maximal oxygen uptake and physical activity from late teenage to adulthood. An 8-year follow-up study. *J. Internal Med.* 234:309–315.
Andersen, L.B., and J. Haraldsdóttir (1995). Coronary heart disease risk factors, physical activity, and fitness in young Danes. *Med. Sci. Sports Exerc.* 27:158–163.
Anderson, A.J., K.A. Sobocinski, D.S. Freedman, J.J. Barboviak, A.A. Rimm, and H.W. Gruchow (1988). Body fat distribution, plasma lipids, and lipoproteins. *Arteriosclerosis* 8:88–94.
Ballor, D.L., and E.T. Poehlman (1992). Resting metabolic rate and coronary heart disease risk factors in aerobically and resistance-trained women. *Am J. Clin. Nutr.* 56:968–974.
Barclay, M., R. Barclay, V. Skipski, O. Trebus-Kehish, C. Mueller, E. Shah, and W. Elkins (1965). Fluctuations in human serum lipoproteins during the normal menstrual cycle. *Biochem. J.* 96:205–209.
Barrett-Connor, E., and D.L. Wingard (1983). Sex differential in ischemic heart disease mortality in diabetics: A prospective population-based study. *Am. J. Epidemol.* 118:489–496.
Berenson, G.S., S.R. Srinivasan, T.A. Nicklas, and L.S. Webber (1988). Cardiovascular risk factors in children and early prevention of heart disease. *Clin. Chem.* 34:B115–B122.
Berlin, J.A., and G.H. Colditz (1990). A meta-analysis of physical activity in the prevention of coronary heart disease. *Am. J. Epidemol.* 132:612–628.
Björntorp, P., K. De Jounge, L. Sjöstrom, and L. Sullivan (1970) The effects of physical training on insulin production in obesity. *Metabolism* 19:631–638.
Blair, D., J-P. Habicht, E.A.H. Sims, D. Sylwester, and S. Abraham (1984). Evidence for an increased risk for hypertension with centrally located fat and the effect of race and sex on this risk. *Am J. Epidemiol.* 119:526–540.
Blair, S.N., H.W. Kohl, R.S. Paffenbarger, D.G. Clark, K.H. Cooper, and L.W. Gibbons (1989). Physical fitness and all-cause mortality: A prospective study of healthy men and women. *J.A.M.A.* 262:2395–2401.
Blumenthal, J.A., K. Matthews, M. Fredrikson, N. Rifai, S. Schniebolk, D. German, J. Steege, and J. Rodin (1991). Effects of exercise training on cardiovascular function and plasma lipid, lipoprotein, and apolipoprotein concentrations in premenopausal and postmenopausal women. *Arterioscler. Thromb.* 11:912–917.

Bogardus, C., E. Ravussin, D.C. Robbins, R.R. Wolfe, E.S. Horton, and E.A.H. Sims (1984). Effects of physical training and diet therapy on carbohydrate metabolism in patients with glucose intolerance and non-insulin-dependent diaberes mellitus. *Diabetes* 33:311–318.

Boogaard, M.A.K. (1984). Rehabilitation of the female patient after myocardial infarction. *Nurs. Clin. North Am.* 19:433–440.

Brideau, M.A., J.-C. Forest, A. Lemay, and S. Dodin (1992). Correlation between ovarain steroids and lipid fractions in relation to age in premenopausal women. *Clin. Endocrinol.* 37:437–444.

Brownell, K.D., P.S. Bachorik, and R.S. Ayerle (1982). Changes in plasma lipid and lipoprotein levels in men and women after a program of moderate exercise. *Circulation* 65:477–484.

Brunner, D., G. Manelis, M. Modan, and S. Levin (1974). Physical activity at work and the incidence of myocardial infarction, angina pectoris and death due to ischemic heart disease. *J. Chronic Disease* 27:217–233.

Brunner, D., J. Weisbort, N. Meshulam, S. Schwartz, J. Gross, H. Saltz-Rennert, S. Altman, and K. Loebl (1987). Relation of serum total cholesterol and high-density lipoprotein cholesterol percentage to the incidence of definite coronary events: twenty-year follow-up of the Donolo-Tel Aviv Prospective Coronary Artery Disease Study. *Am. J. Cardiol.* 59:1271–1276.

Cannistra L., G.J. Balady, C.J. O'Malley, D.A. Weiner, and T.J. Ryan (1991) Clinical profile and outcome of women compared to men in phase II-III cardiac rehabilitation. *J. Am. Col. Cardiol.* 17:296a (abstract).

Castelli, W.P. (1988). Cardiovascular disease in women. *Am. J. Obst. Gyn.* 158:1553–1560 and 1566–1567.

Castelli, W.P. (1986). The triglyceride issue: A view from Framingham. *Am. Heart J.* 112:432–437.

Castelli, W.P., R.J. Garrison, and P.W.F. Wilson (1986). Incidence of coronary heart disease and lipoprotein cholesterol levels: The Framingham Study. *J.A.M.A.* 256:2835–2838.

Cauley, J.A., A.M. Kriska, R.E. LaPorte, R.B. Sandler, and G. Pambianco (1987). A two-year randomized exercise trial in older women: effects on HDL-cholesterol. *Atherosclerosis* 66:247–258.

Clarke, W.R., H.G. Schrott, P.E. Leaverton, W.E. Connor, and R.M. Lauer (1978). Tracking of blood lipids and blood pressures in school age children: The Muscatine Study. *Circulation* 58:626–634.

Conlan, M.G., A.R. Folsom, A. Finch, C.E. Davis, P. Sorlie, G. Marcucci, and K.K. Wu (1993). Associations of factor VIII and von Willebrand factor with age, race, sex, and risk factors for atherosclerosis. The Atherosclerosis Risk in Communities (ARIC) Study. *Thromb. Haemostas.* 70:380–385.

Cooper, R., C. Sempos, J. Ghali, and J. Ferlinz (1985). High-density lipoprotein cholesterol and angiographic coronary artery disease in black patients. *Am. Heart J.* 110:1006–1011.

Corrao, J.M., R.C. Becker, I.S. Ockene, and G.A. Hamilton (1990). Coronary heart disease risk factors in women. *Cardiology* 77(suppl 2):8–24.

Croft, P., and P.C. Hannaford (1989). Risk factors for acute myocardial infarction in women: evidence from the Royal College of General Practitioners' oral contraception study. *Br. Med. J.* 298:165–168.

De Paz, J.A., J.G. Villa, E. Vilades, M.A. Martin-Nuno, J. Lasierra, and J. Gonzalez-Gallego (1995). Effects of oral contraceptives on fibrinolytic response to exercise. *Med. Sci. Sports Exerc.* 27:961–966.

Despres, J.-P., A. Nadeau, A. Tremblay, M. Ferland, S. Moorjani, P.J. Lupien, G. Theriault, S. Pinualt, and C. Bouchard (1989). Role of deep abdominal fat in the association between regional adipose tissue distribution and glucose tolerance in obese women. *Diabetes* 38:304–309.

Despres, J.-P., M.-C. Pouliot, S. Moorjani, A. Nadeau, A. Tremblay, P.J. Lupien, G. Theriault, and C. Bouchard (1991). Loss of abdominal fat and metabolic response to exercise training in obese women. *Am. J. Physiol.: Endocrinology and Metabolism* 261:E159–E167.

Dipietro, L., D.F. Williamson, C.J. Caspersen, and E. Eaker (1993). The descriptive epidemiology of selected physical activities and body weight among adults trying to lose weight: The Behavorial Risk Factor Survelliance System Survey. *Int. J. Obesity* 17:69–76.

Duncan, J.J., N.F. Gordon, and C.B. Scott (1991). Women walking for health and fitness. How much is enough? *J.A.M.A.* 23:3295–3299.

Dyer, A.R., J. Stamler, R.B. Shekelle, and J. Schoenberger (1976). The relationship of education to blood pressure: findings on 40,000 employed Chicagoans. *Circulation* 54:987–992.

Eaker, E.D., and W.P. Castelli (1987). Coronary heart disease and its risk factors among women in the Framingham Study. In: E. Eaker, B. Packard, N.K. Wenger, T.B. Clarkson, and H.A. Tyroler (eds.) *Coronary Heart Disease in Women.* New York: Haymarket Doyma, pp. 122–132.

Eaker, E.D., J.H. Chesbro, F.M. Sacks, N.K. Wenger, J.P. Whisnant, and M. Winston (1993). Cardiovascular disease in women. *Circulation* 88:1999–2009.

Ekelund, L., W.L. Haskell, Y.L. Troung, E.H. Gordon, and D.S. Shepps (1988). Physical fitness as predictor of cardiovascular (CVD) mortality in asymptomatic females. *Circulation* 78:(supplement)II–110 (abstract).

Folsom, A.R., H.T. Qamhieh, J.M. Flack, J.E. Hilner, K. Liu, B.V. Howard, and R.P. Tracy (1993). Plasma fibrinogen: levels and correlates in young adults. *Am. J. Epidemiol.* 138:1023–1036.

Franklin, B., E. Buskirk, J. Hodgson, H. Gahagan, J. Kollias, and J. Mendez (1979). Effects of physical conditioning on cardiorespiratory and serum lipids in relatively normal-weight and obese middle-aged women. *Int. J. Obes.* 3:97–109.

Frisch, E., G. Wyshak, T.E. Albright, N.L. Albright, and I. Schiff (1986). Lower prevalence of diabetes in female former college athletes compared with nonathletes. *Diabetes* 35:1101–1105.

Fuster, V., J.J. Badmion, L. Badmion, and J.H. Chesebro (1992). The pathogenesis of coronary artery disease and acute coronary syndrome. *N. Engl. J. Med.* 326:310–318.

Gibbons, L.W., S.N. Blair, K.H. Cooper, and M. Smith (1983). Association between coronary heart disease risk factors and physical fitness in healthy adult women. *Circulation* 67:977–983.

Gilliam, T.B., V.L. Katch, and A. Weltman (1977). Prevalence of coronary heart disease risk factors in active children, 7 to 12 years of age. *Med. Sci. Sports* 9:21–25.

Glueck, C.J., H.L. Taylor, D.R. Jacobs, J.A. Morrison, R. Beaglehole, and O.D. Williams (1980). Plasma high-density lipoprotein cholesterol: association with measurements of body mass: The Lipid Research Clinics Program Prevalence Study. *Circulation* (suppl. IV) 62:62–69.

Gordon, T., W.P. Castelli, M.C. Hjortland, W.B. Kannel, and T.R. Dawber (1977). High-densisty lipoprotein as a protective factor against coronary heart disease. The Framingham Study. *Am. J. Med.* 62:707–714.

Greenland, P., Reicher-Reiss, U. Goldbourt, and S. Behar (1991). In-hospital and 1-year mortality in 1524 women after myocardial infarction. *Circulation* 83:484–491.

Gruchow, H.W., A.J. Anderson, J.J. Barboriak, and K.A. Sobocinski (1988). Postmenopausal use of estrogen and occlusion of coronary arteries. *Am. Heart J.* 115:954–963.

Hagberg, J.M. (1990). Exercise, fitness and hypertension. In: C. Bouchard, R.J. Shephard, T. Stephens, J.R. Sutton, and B.D. McPherson (eds.) *Exercise, Fitness and Health.* Champaign, IL: Human Kinetics, pp. 455–456.

Haglund, B.J.A. (1985). Geographical and socioeconomic distribution of high blood pressure and borderline high blood pressure in a Swedish rural county. *Scand. J. Soc. Med.* 13:53–66.

Hammond, C.B., F.R. Jelovsek, K.L. Lee, W.T. Creasman, and R.T. Parker (1979). Effects of long-term estrogen replacement therapy. *Am. J. Ob. Gyn.* 133:525.

Hardman, A.E., A. Hudson, P.R.M. Jones, and N.G. Norgan (1989). Brisk walking and plasma high-density lipoprotein cholesterol concentration in previously sedentary women. *Br. Med. J.* 299:1204–1205.

Hardman, A.E., P.R.M. Jones, N.G. Norgan, and A. Hudson (1992). Brisk walking improves endurance fitness without changing body fatness in previously sedentary women. *Eur. J. Appl. Physiol.* 65:354–359.

Hartung, G.H., C.E. Moore, R. Mitchell, and C.M. Kappus (1984). Relationship of menopausal status and exercise level to HDL cholesterol in women. *Exp. Aging Res.* 10:13–18.

Hartung, G.H., R.S. Reeves, J.P. Foreyt, W. Patsch, and A.M. Gotto (1986). Effect of alcohol intake and exercise on plasma high-density lipoprotein cholesterol subfractions and apolipoprotein A-I in women. *Am. J. Cardiol.* 58:148–151.

Hartz, A.J., D.C. Rupley, A.A. Rimm (1984). The association of girth measurements with disease in 32,856 women. *Am. J. Epidemiol.* 119:71–80.

Haskell, W.L. (1986). Mechanisms by which physical activity may enhance the clinical status of cardiac patients. In: M.L. Pollock and D. H. Schmidt (eds.) *Heart Disease and Rehabilitation* (2nd ed.) New York: John Wiley and Sons, pp. 303–324.

Haskell, W.L., H.L. Taylor, P.D. Wood, H. Schrott, and G. Heiss (1980). Strenuous physical activity, treadmill exercise test performance and plasma high-density lipoprotein cholesterol. The Lipid Research Clinics Program Prevalence Study. *Circulation* 62:IV-53–IV-61.

Henderson, B.E., A. Paganini-Hill, and R.K. Ross (1988). Estrogen replacement therapy and protection from acute myocardial infarction. *Am. J. Ob. Gyn.* 159:312–317.

Henderson, B.E., A. Pananini-Hill, and R.K. Ross (1991). Decreased mortality in users of estrogen replacement therapy. *Arch. Intern. Med.* 151:75–78.

Heyden, S., G. Heiss, A.G. Bartel, and C.G. Hames (1980). Sex differences in coronary mortality among diabetics in Evans County, Georgia. *J. Chron. Dis.* 33:265–273.

Hill, J.O., J. Thiel, P.A. Heller, C. Markon, G. Fletcher, and M. DiGirolamo (1989). Differences in effects of aerobic exercise training on blood lipids in men and women. *Am. J. Cardiol.* 63:254–256.

Hong, M.K., P.A. Romm, K. Reagan, C.E. Green, and C.E. Rackley (1992). Effects of estrogen replacement therapy of serum lipid values and angiographically defined coronary artery disease in postmenopausal women. *Am J. Cardiol.* 69:176–178.

Hong, M.K., P.A. Romm, K. Reagan, C.E. Green, and C.E. Rackley (1991). Usefulness of the total cholesterol to high-density lipoprotein cholesterol ratio in predicting angiographic coronary artery disease in women. *Am. J. Cardiol.* 68:1646–1650.

Hubert, H.B., M. Feinleib, P.M. McNamara, and W.P. Castelli (1983). Obesity as an independent risk factor for cardiovascular disease: A 26-year follow-up of participants in the Framingham Heart Study. *Circulation* 67:968–977.

Isles, C.G., D.J. Hole, V.M. Hawthorne, and A.F. Lever (1992). Relation between coronary risk and coronary mortality in women of the Renfrew and Paisley survey: Comparison with men. *Lancet* 339:702–706.

Johnson, J., E. Heineman, G. Heiss, C.G. Hames, and H.A. Tyroler (1986). Cardiovascular disease risk factors and mortality among black women and white women aged 40–64 years in Evans County, Georgia. *Am. J. Epidemiol.* 123:209–220.

Jones, D.Y., J.T. Judd, P.R. Taylor, W.S. Campbell, and P.P. Nair (1988). Menstrual cycle effect on plasma lipids. *Metabolism* 37:1-2.

Juneau, M., F. Rogers, V. De Santos, M. Yee, A. Evans, A. Bohn, W.L. Haskell, C.B. Taylor, and R.F. De-Busk (1987). Effectiveness of self-monitored, home-based, moderate-intensity exercise training in middle-aged men and women. *Am. J. Cardiol.* 60:66-70.

Kallio, V., H. Hâmalainen, J. Hâkkila, and O.J. Luuria (1979). Reduction of sudden deaths by a multifactorial intervention programme after acute myocardial infarction. *Lancet* 2:1091-1094.

Kannel, W.B. (1983). High density lipoproteins: Epidemiologic profile and risks of coronary artery disease. *Am. J. Cardiol.* 52:9b-72b.

Kannel, W.B. (1987). Status of risk factors and their consideration in antihypertensive therapy. *Am. J. Cardiol.* 59:80A-90A.

Kannel, W.B., and D.L. McGee (1979). Diabetes and glucose tolerance as risk factors for cardiovascular disease: The Framingham study. *Diabetes Care* 2:120-126.

Kannel, W.B., and P. Sorlie (1979). Some health benefits of physical activity: The Framingham Study. *Arch. Intern Med.* 139:857-861.

Kannel, W.B., L.A. Cupples, R. Ramaswami, J. Stokes, B.E. Kreger, and M. Higgins (1991). Regional obesity and risk of cardiovascular disease: The Framingham Study. *J. Clin. Epidem.* 44:183-190.

Kannel, W.B., P.A. Wolf, W.P. Castelli, and R.B. D'Agostino (1987). Fibrinogen and risk of cardiovascular disease: The Framingham Study. *J.A.M.A.* 258:1183-1186.

Kaplan, G.A., T.E. Seeman, R.D. Cohen, L.P. Knudsen, and J. Guralink (1987). Mortality among the elderly in the Alameda County Study: Behavorial and demographic risk factors. *J. Pub. Health* 77:307-312.

Kaplan, G.A., and J.E. Keil (1993). Socioeconomic factors and cardiovascular disease: A review of the literature. *Circulation* 88:1973-1998.

Kaplan, G.A., N.B. Lazarus, R.D. Cohen, and D. Leu (1991). Psychosocial factors in the natural history of physical activity. *Am. J. Pre. Med.* 7:12-17.

Keil, J.E., S.H. Sandifer, C.B. Loadholt, and E. Boyle (1981). Skin color and education effects on blood pressure. *Am. J. Pub. Health* 71:532-534.

Khan, S.S., S. Nessim, R. Gray, L.S. Czer, A. Chaux, and J. Matloff (1990). Increased mortality of women in coronary artery bypass surgery: evidence for referral bias. *Ann. Intern. Med.* 112:561-567.

Killen, J.D., M.J. Telch, T.N. Robinson, N. Maccoby, B. Taylor, and J.W. Farquhar (1988). Cardiovascular disease risk reduction for tenth graders. A multiple-factor school-based approach. *J.A.M.A.* 260:1728-1733.

Kim, H.-K., and R.K. Kalkhoff (1979). Changes in lipoprotein composition during the menstrual cycle. *Metabolism* 23:663-668.

Kinoshita, A., H. Urata, Y. Tanabe, M. Ikeda, H. Tanaka, M. Shindo, and K. Arakawa (1988). What types of hypertensives respond better to mild exercise therapy? *J. Hypertens.* 6:S631-S633.

Krotkiewski, M., P. Björntorp, L. Sjostrom, and U. Smith (1983). Impact of obesity on metabolism in men and women: importance of regional adipose tissue distribution. *J. Clin. Invest.* 72:1150-1162.

Krotkiewski, M., P. Lönnroth, K. Mandrokas, Z. Wroblewski, and M. Rebuffé-Scrive (1985). The effects of physical training on insulin secretion and effectiveness and on glucose metabolism in obesity and and Type 2 (non-insulin-dependent) diabetes mellitus. *Diabetologia* 28:881-890.

Krotkiewski, M., K. Mandroukas, L. Sjostrom, L. Sullivan, H. Wetterqvist, and P. Bjorntorp (1979). Effects of long-term physical training on body fat, metabolism, and blood pressure in obesity. *Metabolism* 28:650-658.

Krueger, D.E., S.S. Ellenberg, S. Bloom, B.M. Calkins, R. Jacyna, D.C. Nolan, R. Phillips, J.C. Rios, R. Sobieski, R.B. Shekelle, K.M. Spector, B.V. Stadel, P.D. Stolley, and M. Terris (1981). Risk factors for fatal heart attack in young women. *Am. J. Epidemol.* 113:357-370.

Kwiterovich, P.O.J., J. Coresh, H.H. Smith, P.S. Bachorik, C.A. Derby, and T.A. Pearson (1992). Comparison of the plasma levels of apolipoproteins B and A-1, and other risk factors in men and women with premature coronary disease. *Am. J. Cardiol.* 69:1015-1021.

Lapidus, L. and C. Bengtsson (1986). Socioeconomic factors and physical activity in relation to cardiovascular disease and death: A 12-year follow-up of participants in a population study of women in Gothenburg, Sweden. *Br. Heart. J.* 55:295-301.

Lapidus, L., C. Bengtsson, B. Larsson, L. Penwert, E. Rybo, and L. Sjostrom (1984). Distribution of adipose tissue and risk of cardiovascular disease and death: A 12-year follow-up of participants in the population study of women in Gothenburg, Sweden. *Br. Med. J.* 289:1257-1261.

Lauer, R.M., W.E. Connor, P.E. Leaverton, M.A. Reiter, and W.R. Clarke (1975). Coronary heart disease risk factors in school children: The Muscatine study. *J. Pediatrics* 86:697-706.

Lebech, A.M., A. Kjaer, and P.E. Lebech (1990). Metabolic changes during the menstrual cycle: A longitudinal study. *Am. J. Obstet. Gynecol.* 163:414-416.

Lee, A.J., G.D.O. Lowe, M. Woodward, and H. Tunstall-Pedoe (1991). Plasma fibrinogen and indicators of coronary heart disease. *Perfusion* 4:432. Abstract.

Lemaitre, R.N., S.R. Heckbert, B.R. Psaty, and D.S. Siscovick. (1995). Leisure-time physical activity and the risk of nonfatal myocardial infarction in postmenopausal women. *Arch. Intern. Med.* 155:2302-2308.

Lemieux, S., J.P Depres, S. Moorjami, A Nadeau, G. Thériault, D. Prud'homme, A. Tremblay, C. Bouchard, and P.J. Lupien (1994). Are gender differences in cardiovascular disease risk factors explained by the level of visceral adipose tissue? *Diabetologia* 37:757-764.

Leon, A.S. (Chairman) (1990). Position Paper of the American Association of Cardiovascular and Pulmonary Rehabilitation. Scientific evidence of the value of cardiac rehabilitation services with emphasis on patients following myocardial infarction—Section 1. Exercise conditioning component. *J. Cardiopul. Rehab.* 10:79-87.

Lerner, D.J., and W.B. Kannel (1986). Patterns of coronary heart disease morbidity and mortality in the sexes: A 26-year follow-up of the Framingham population. *Am. Heart J.* 111:383-390.

Levine, G.N., J.F. Keaney, and J.A. Vita (1995). Cholesterol reduction in Cardiovascular Disease. *New Engl. J. Med.* 332:512-520.

Lieberman, E.H., M.D. Gerhard, A. Uehata, B.W. Walsh, A.P. Selwyn, P. Ganz, A.C. Yeung, and M.A. Creager.(1994). Estrogen improves endothelium-dependent, flow-mediated vasodilation in postmenopausal women. *Ann. Intern. Med.* 121:936-941.

Magnus, K., A. Matroos, and J. Strackee (1979). Walking, cycling, or gardening, with or without seasonal interruptions, in relation to acute coronary events. *Am. J. Epidemiol.* 110:724-733.

Mann, J.I., and W.H.W. Inman (1975). Oral contraceptives and death from myocardial infarction. *Br. Med. J.* 2:245-248.

Manson, J.E., G.A. Colditz, M.J. Stampfer, W.C. Willett, B. Rosner, R.R. Monson, F.E. Speizer, and C.H. Hennekens (1990). A prospective study of obesity and risk of coronary heart disease in women. *N. Eng. J. Med.* 322:882-889.

Manson, J.E., G.A. Colditz, M.J. Stampfer, W.C. Willett, A.S. Krolewski, B. Rosner, R.A. Arky, F.E. Speizer, and C.H. Hennekens (1991a). A prospective study of maturity-onset diabetes mellitus and risk of coronary heart disease and stroke in women. *Arch. Intern. Med.* 151:1141-1147.

Manson, J.E., E.B. Rimm, M.J. Stampfer, G.A. Colditz, W.C. Willett, E.F. Krolewski, B. Rosner, C.H. Hennekens, and F.S. Speeizer (1991b). Physical activity and incidence of non-insulin-dependent diabetes mellitus in women. *Lancet* 338:774-778.

Martin, R.P., W.L. Haskell and P.D. Wood. (1977). Blood chemistry and lipid profiles of elite distance runners. *Ann. NY Acad. Sci.* 301:346-360.

Matthews, K.A., S.F. Kelsey, E.N. Meilahn, L.H. Kuller, and R.R. Wing (1989). Educational attainment and behavioral and biologic risk factors for coronary heart disease in middle-aged women. *Am. J. Epidemiol.* 129:1132-1144.

McFarland, K.F., M.E. Boniface, C.A. Hornung, W. Earnhardt, and J.O. Humphries (1989). Risk factors and noncontraceptive estrogen use in women with and without coronary disease. *Am. Heart J.* 117:1209-1214.

Meilahn, E.N. (1992). Hemostatic factors and risk of cardiovascular disease in women. *Arch. Pathol. Lab. Med.* 116:1313-1317.

Meilahn, E.N., L.H. Kuller, E.A. Stein, A.W. Caggiula, and K.A. Matthews (1988). Characteristics associated with apoprotein and lipoprotein lipid levels in middle-aged women. *Arteriosclerosis* 8:515-520.

Moll, M.E., R.S. Williams, R.M. Lester, S.H. Quarfordt, and A.G. Wallace (1979). Cholesterol metabolism in non-obese women. Failure of physical conditioning to alter levels of high density lipoprotein cholesterol. *Atherosclerosis* 34:159-166.

Moore, C.E., G.H. Hartung, R.E. Mitchell, C.M. Kappus, and J. Hinderlitter (1983). The relationship of exercise and diet on high-density lipoprotein cholesterol levels in women. *Metabolism* 32:189-196.

Morgan, D.W., R.J. Cruise, B.W. Girardin, V. Lutz-Schneider, D.H. Morgan, and W.M. Qi (1986). HDL-C concentrations in weight-trained, endurance-trained, and sedentary females. *Phys. Sportsmed.* 14:166-181.

Nachtigall, L.E., R.H. Nachtigall, R.D. Nachtigall, and E.M. Beckman (1979). Estrogen replacement therapy II: a prospective study in the relationship to carcinoma and cardiovascular and metabolic problems. *Obstet. Gynecol.* 54:74-79.

National Center for Health Statistics (1973). Plan and Operation of the Health and Nutrition Examination Survey, United States—1971-1973. Vital and Health Statistics. Series 1, No. 10. DHEW publication no. (HSM) 73-1310. Washington, D.C.: U.S. Government Printing Office.

National Center for Health Statistics (1981). Plan and Operation of the Second National Health and Nutrition Examination Survey, 1976-1980. Vital and Health Statistics. Series 1, No. 15. DHEW publication no. (PHS) 81-1317. Washington, D.C.: U.S. Government Printing Office.

National Center for Health Statistics, Bureau of Vital Statistics (1990). Death From Diseses of the Circulatory System. DHHS Publication No. (PHS) 90-11-1. Washington, D.C.: U.S. Public Health Service. pp. 44-47.

Nieman, D.C., J.L. Haig, E.D. DeGula, G.P. Aizon, and V.D. Register (1988). Reducing diet and exercise training effects on resting metabolic rate in mildly obese women. *J. Sports Med.* 28:79-88.

O'Callihan, W.G., K.K. Teo, J. O'Riordan, H. Webb, T. Dolphin, and H. Horgan. (1984). Comparative response of male and female patients with coronary artery disease to exercise rehabilitation. *Eur. Heart J.* 5:649-651.

O'Conner, G.T.J., J.E. Buring, S. Yusuf, S. Goldhaber, E.M. Olmstead, R.S. Paffenbarger, and C.H. Hennekens (1989). An overview of randomized trials of rehabilitation with exercise after myocardial infarction. *Circulation* 80:234-244.

Oldridge, N.B., H.G. Gordon, M.E. Fischer, and A.A. Rimm (1988). Cardiac rehabilitation after myocardial infarction: combined experience of randomized clinical trials. *J. Am. Med. Assoc.* 260:945-950.

Oldridge, N.B., D. LaSalle, and N.B.Jones (1980). Exercise rehabilitation of female patients with coronary heart disease. *Amer. Heart. J.* 100:755-765.

Oldridge, N.B., B. Ragowski, and M. Gottlieb (1992). Use of outpatient cardiac rehabilitation services: Factors associated with attendance. *J. Cardiopul. Rehab.* 12:25-31.

Owens, J.F., K.A. Matthews, R.R. Wing, and L.H. Kuller (1990). Physical activity and cardiovascular risk: a cross-sectional study of middle-aged premenopausal women. *Prev. Med.* 19:147-157.

Pan, W.H., L.B. Cedres, K. Liu, A. Dyer, J.A. Schoenberger, R.B. Shekelle, R. Stamler, D. Smith, P. Collette, and J. Stamler (1986). Relationship of clinical diabetes and asymptomatic hyperglycemia to risk of coronary heart disease mortality in men and women. *Am. J. Epidemol.* 123:504-516.

Patterson, C.C., E. McCrum, D. McMaster, M. Kerr, D. Sykes, and A.E. Evans (1988). Factors influencing total cholesterol and high-density lipoprotein cholesterol concentrations in a population at high coronary risk. *Acta Med. Scand.* (suppl) 728:150-158.

Peiris, A.N., M.S. Sothmann, M.I. Hennes, M.B. Lee, C.R. Wilson, A.B. Gustafson, and A.H. Kissebah (1989). Relative contribution of obesity and body fat distribution to alterations in glucose insulin homeostasis: predictive values of selected indices in premenopausal women. *Am. J. Clin. Nutr.* 49:758-764.

Pesonen, E., R. Norio, J. Hirvonen, K. Karkola, V. Kuusela, H. Laaksonen, M. Mottonen, T. Nikkari, J. Raekallio, J. Viikari, S. Yla-Herttuala, and H.K. Akerblom (1990). Intimal thickening in the coronary arteries of infants and children as an indicator of risk factors for coronary heart disease. *Eur. Heart J.* 11(Supl. E):53-60.

Petitti, D.B., J.A. Perlman, and S. Sidney (1987). Noncontraceptive estrogens and mortality: long-term follow-up of women in the Walnut Creek Study. *Obstet. Gynecol.* 70:289-293.

Porkka, K.V., J.S. Viikari, and H.K. Akerblom (1991). Tracking of serum HDL-cholesterol and other lipids in children and adolescents: the Cardiovascular Risk in Young Finns Study. *Prev. Med.* 20:713-724.

Powell K.E., P.D. Thompson, C.J. Casperson, and J.S. Kendrick (1987). Physical activity and the incidence of coronary heart disease. *Ann. Rev. Public Health* 8:253-287.

Raines, E.W., and R. Ross (1993). Smooth muscle cells and the pathogenesis of the lesions of atherosclerosis. *British Heart J.* 69, Suppl 1:S30-S37.

Rainville, S., and P. Vaccaro (1984). The effects of menopause and training on serum lipids. *Int. J. Sports Med.* 5:137-141.

Raitakari, O.T., K.V.K. Porkka, J.S.A. Viikari, T. Ronnemaa, and H.K. Akerblom (1994). Clustering of risk factors for coronary heart disease in children and adolescents. The Cardiovascular Risk in Young Finns Study. *Acta Paediatr.* 83:935-940.

Reaven, P.D., E. Barrett-Connor, and S. Edelstein (1991). Relation between leisure-time physical activity and blood pressure in older women. *Circulation* 83:559-565.

Regensteiner, J.G., E.J. Mayer, S.M. Shetterly, R.H. Eckel, W. L. Haskell, J.A. Marshall, J. Baxter, and R.F. Hamman (1991). Relationship between habitual physical activity and insulin levels among nondiabetic men and women. *Diabetes Care* 14:1066-1074.

Roman, O., A.L. Camuzzi, E. Villalon, and C. Klenner (1981). Physical training program in arterial hypertension. A long-term prospective follow-up. *Cardiology* 67:230-243.

Roman, O., M. Guitierrez, and I. Luksic (1983). Cardiac rehabilitation after myocardial infarction: Nine-year controlled follow-up study. *Cardiology* 70:223-231.

Rônnemaa, T., K. Mattila, A. Lehtonen, and V. Kallio (1986). A controlled randomized study on the effect of long-term physical exercise on the metabolic control in Type 2 diabetic patients. *Acta Med. Scand.* 220:219-224.

Rosenberg, L., D.R. Miller, D.W. Kaufman, S.P. Helmrich, S. Van De Carr, P.D. Stolley, and S. Shapiro (1983). Myocardial infarction in women under 50 years of age. *J.A.M.A.* 250:2801-2806.

Royal College of General Practitioners' Oral Contraception Study (1981). Further analyses of mortality in oral contraceptive users. *Lancet* 1:541-546.

Salonen, J.T. (1982). Oral contraceptives, smoking and risk of myocadial infarction in young women. *Acta Med. Scand.* 212:141-144.

Salonen, J., P. Puska, and J.Tuomilehto (1982). Physical activity and risk of myocardial infarction, cerebral stroke and death. *Am. J. Epidemiol.* 115:526-537.

Sandvik, L., J. Erikssen, J. Thaulow, G. Erikssen, R. Mundal, K. Rodahl (1993). Physical fitness as a predictor of mortality among healthy, middle-aged Norweigian men. *New Engl. J. Med.* 328:533-537.

Schmitz-Huebner, U., S.G. Thompson, L. Balleisen, C. Fechtrup, W. Grosse-Heitmeyer, B. Kirchhof, E. Most, U.S. Muller, C. Seiffert, D. Seiffert et al. (1988). Lack of association between haemostatic variables and the presence or the extent of coronary atherosclerosis. *Br. Heart J.* 59:287-291.

Schroll, M. (1981). A longitudinal epidemiologic survey of relative weight at age 25, 50, and 60 in Glostrup population of men and women born in 1914. *Dan. Men. Bull.* 28:106-116.

Seals, D.R., J.M. Hagberg, B.F. Hurley, an J.O. Holloszy (1984). Effects of endurance training on glucose tolerance and plasma lipid levels in older men and women. *J.A.M.A.* 252:645–649.

Seed, M. (1994). Postmenopausal hormone replacement therapy, coronary heart disease and plasma lipoproteins. *Drugs* 47:25–34.

Shephard, R.J., P.E. Youldon, M. Cox, and C. West (1980). Effects of a 6-month industrial fitness programme on serum lipid concentrations. *Atherosclerosis* 35:277–286.

Slone, D., S. Shapiro, D.W. Kaufman, L. Rosenberg, O.S. Miettinen, and P.D. Stolley (1981). Risk of myocardial infarction in relation to current and discontinued oral contraceptive use. *New Engl. J. Med.* 305:420–424.

Sorel, J.E., D.R. Ragland, S.L. Syme, and W.B. Davis (1992). Educational status and blood pressure: the Second National Health and Nutrition Examination Survey, 1976–1980, and the Hispanic Health and Nutrition Examination Survey, 1982–1984. *Am. J. Epidemiol.* 135:1339–1348.

Stamford, B.A., S. Matter, R.D. Fell, S. Sady, M. Cresanta, and P. Papanek (1984). Cigarette smoking, physical activity, and alcohol consumption: Relationship to blood lipids and lipoproteins in premenopausal females. *Metabolism* 33:585–590.

Stamler, J., R. Pick, and L.N. Katz (1953). Prevention of coronary atherosclerosis by estrogen-androgen administration in the cholesterol-fed chick. *Circ. Res.* 1:94–98.

Stampfer, M.J., G.A. Colditz, W.C. Willett, J.E. Manson, B. Rosner, F.E. Speizer, and C.H. Hennekens (1991). Postmenopausal estrogen therapy and cardiovascular disease: ten-year follow-up from the Nurses' Health Study. *New Eng. J. Med.* 325:756–762.

Stampfer, M.J., W.C. Willett, G.A. Colditz, B. Rosner, F.E. Speizer, and C.H. Hennekens (1985). A prospective study of post menopausal estrogen therapy and coronary heart disease. *New Engl. J. Med.* 313:1044–1049.

Stampfer, M.J., W.C. Willett, G.A. Colditz, F.E. Speizer, and C.H. Hennekens (1988). A prospective study of past use of oral contraceptive agents and risk of cardiovascular diseases. *New Engl. J. Med.* 319:1313–1317.

Stefanick, M.L. (1993). The roles of obesity, regional adiposity, and physical activity in coronary heart disease in women. In: N.K. Wenger, L. Speroff, and B. Packard (eds.) *Cardiovascular Health and Disease in Women* Greenwich, CT: Jacq Communications, Inc., pp. 149–156.

Stefanick, M.L., C. Legault, R.P. Tracy, G. Howard, C.M. Kessler, D.L. Lucas, T.L. Bush (1995). Distribution and correlates of plasma fibrinogen in middle-aged women: Inital findings of the postmenopausal estrogen/progestin interventions (PEPI) Study. *Arterioscler. Thromb. Vasc. Biol.* 15:2085–2093.

Steinberg, D., S. Parthasarathy, T.E. Carew, J. C. Khoo, and J.L. Witztum (1989). Beyond cholesterol: Modifications of low-density lipoproteins that increase its atherogenicity. *New Engl. J. Med.* 320:915–923.

Steingart, R.M., M. Packer, P. Hamm, M.E. Coglianese, B. Gersh, E.M. Geltman, J. Sollano, S. Katz, L. Moye, L.L. Basta, et. al (1991). Sex differences in the management of coronary artery disease. *New Engl. J. Med.* 325:226–230.

Stevenson, E.T., K.P. Davy, and D.R. Seals (1995). Hemostatic, metabolic, and adrogenic risk factors for coronary heart disease in physically active and less active postmenopausal women. *Arterioscler. Thromb. Vasc. Biol.* 15:669–677.

Stewart, K.J., C.S. Brown, C.M. Hickey, L.D. McFarland, J.J. Weinhofer, and S.H. Gottlieb (1995). Physical fitness, physical activity, and fatness in relation to blood pressure and lipids in preadolescent children. Results from the FRESH Study. *J. Cardiopul. Rehab.* 15:122–129.

Stokes, J., W.B. Kannel, P.A. Wolf, L.A. Cupples, and R.B. D'Agostino (1987). The relative importance of selected risk factors for various manifestations of cardiovascular disease among men and women from 35–64 years: 30 years of follow-up in the Framingham Study. *Circulation* 75(suppl V):V65–V73.

Sullivan, J.M., R.V. Zwaag, G.F. Lemp, J.P. Hughes, V. Maddock, F.W. Kroetz, K.B. Ramanathan, and D.M. Mirvis (1988). Postmenopausal estrogen use and coronary athersclerosis. *Ann. Intern. Med.* 108:358–363.

Suter, E., and M.R. Hawes (1993). Relationship of physical activity, body fat, diet, and blood lipid profile in youths 10–15 yr. *Med. Sci. Sports Exerc.* 25:748–754.

Suter, E., and B. Marti (1992). Little effect of long-term, self-monitored exercise on serum lipid levels in middle-aged women. *J. Sports Med. Phys. Fit.* 32:400–411.

Tanabe, Y., J. Sasaki, H. Urata, A. Kiyonaga, H. Tanaka, M. Shindo, and K. Arakawa (1988). Effect of mild aerobic exercise on lipid and apolipoprotein levels in patients with essential hypertension. *Jpn. Heart J.* 29:199–206.

Tangeny, C., C. Brownie, and S.-M. Wu (1991). Impact of menstrual periodicity on serum lipid levels and estimates of dietary intakes. *J. Am. Coll. Nutr.* 10:107–113.

Thomas, R. J., C. Lamendola-Rudd, N. Houston Miller, B. Hedback, W. Haskell, J.L. Durstine, K. Berra (1992). National survey of cardiac rehabilitation: A comparison of women and men (abstract). Proceedings of the Seventh Annual Meeting of the American Association of Cardiovascular and Pulmonary Rehabilitation. Chicago, Il. October 22, 1992.

Tipton, C.M. (1991). Exercise, training and hypertension: An update. In: J.O. Holloszy (ed.) *Exercise and Sport Sciences Reviews*, Vol. 19. Baltimore: Williams & Wilkins, pp. 447–505.

Tremblay, A., J.-P. Dueprés, J. Maheux, M.C. Pouliot, A. Nadeau, S. Moorjani, P.J. Lupien, and C. Bouchard (1991). Normalization of the metabolic profile in obese women by exercise and a low fat diet. *Med. Sci Sports Exerc.* 23:1326–1331.

Upton, S.J., D. Hagan, B. Lease, J. Rosentswieg, L.R. Gettman, and J.J. Duncan (1984). Comparative physiological profiles among young and middle-aged female distance runners. *Med. Sci. Sports Exerc.* 16:67–71.

Vague, J. (1956). The degree of masculine differentiation of obesities: A factor determining predisposition to diabetes, atherosclerosis, gout, and uric calculous disease. *Am. J. Clin Nutr.* 4:20–34.

Van Horn, L.V., D. Ballew, K. Liu, K. Ruth, A. Mcdonald, J.E. Hilner, G.L. Burke, P.J. Savage, C. Bragg, B. Caan, D. Jacobs, M. Slattery, and S. Sidney (1991). Diet, body size, and plasma lipids-lipoproteins in young adults: Differences by race and sex: The Coronary Artery Risk Development in Young Adults (CARDIA) Study. *Am. J. Epidemiol.* 133:9–23.

Vessey, M.P., L. Villard-Mackintosh, K. McPherson, and D. Yeates (1989). Mortality among oral contraceptive users: 20-year follow-up of women in a cohort study. *Br. Med. J.* 299:1487–1491.

Vodak, P.A., P.D. Wood, W.L. Haskell, and P.T. Williams (1980). HDL-cholesterol and other plasma lipid and lipoprotein concentrations in middle-aged male and female tennis players. *Metabolism* 29:745–752.

Voorrips, L.E., K.A.P.M. Lemmink, M.J.G. Van Heuvelen, P. Bult, and W.A. Van Staveren (1993). The physical condition of elderly women differing in habitual physical activity. *Med. Sci. Sports Exerc.* 25:1152–1157.

Walling, A., J.L. Tremblay, J. Jobin, J. Charest, F. Delage, M.-H. LeBlanc, Y. Tessler, and I. Villa (1988). Evaluating the Rehabilitation Potential of a large population of post-myocardial infarction patients: Adverse prognosis in women. *J. Cardiopulmonary Rehab.* 8:99–106.

Webber, L.S., A.W. Voors, S.R. Srinivasan, R.R. Frerichs, and G.S. Berenson (1979). occurrence in children of multiple risk factors for coronary artery disease: the Bogalusa Heart study. *Prev. Med.* 8:407–418.

Wenger, N.K., L. Speroff, and B. Packard (1993). Cardiovascular health and disease in women. *New Engl. J. Med.* 329:247–256.

Wilhelmsen, L., H. Sanne, and D. Elmfeld (1975). A controlled trial of physical training after myocardial infarction: effects on risk factors, nonfatal infarction, and death. *Prev. Med.* 4:491–508.

Williford, H.N., D.L. Blessing, J.M. Barksdale, and F.H. Smith (1988). The effects of aerobic dance training on serum lipids, lipoproteins and cardiopulmonary function. *J. Sports Med. Phys. Fit.* 28:151–157.

Wilson, P.W., K.M. Anderson, and W.P. Castelli (1991). Twelve-year incidence of coronary heart disease in middle-aged adults during the era of hypertensive therapy: the Framingham Offspring Study. *Am. J. Med.* 90:11–16.

Wilson, P.W.F., R.J. Garrison, and W.P. Castelli (1985). Postmenopausal estrogen use, cigarette smoking, and cardiovascular morbidity in women over 50: The Framingham Study. *New Engl. J. Med.* 315:1038–1043.

Wing, R.R., D.H. Bunker, L.H. Kuller, and K.A. Matthews (1989). Insulin, body mass index, and cardiovascular risk factors in premenopausal women. *Arteriosclerosis* 9:479–484.

Wood, P.D., W.L. Haskell, M.P. Stern, S. Lewis, and C. Perry (1977). Plasma lipoprotein distributions in male and female runners. *Ann. New York Acad. Sci.* 301:748–763.

Wood, P.D., M. Stefanick, P.T. Williams, and W.L. Haskell (1991). The effects on plasma lioproteins of a prudent weight-reducing diet with or without exercise, in overweight men and women. *New Engl. J. Med.* 325:461–466.

Woods, M., E.J. Schaefer, A. Morrell, B. Golden, C. Longcope, J. Dwyer, and S. Gorbach (1987). Effect of menstrual cycle phase on plasma lipids. *J. Clin. Endocrin. Metab.* 65:321–323.

Writing Group for the PEPI Trial (1995). Effects of estrogen or estrogen/progestin regimens on heart disease risk factors in postmenopausal women: the Postmenopausal Estrogen/Progestin Interventions (PEPI) Trial. *J. Am. Med. Assoc.* 273:199–208.

DISCUSSION

GISOLFI: Is it known how areas of low shear stress develop?

HASKELL: Depending upon the curvature at the bifurcation of the arterial tree there are areas of low shear stress throughout all vessels. If there is turbulent flow at a bifurcation, that produces low shear stress versus nice laminar flow that causes significant shear stress. Early lesion formation is almost exclusively initiated in areas of low shear stress in the coronary bed. With shear stress, substantial changes occur in nitric oxide release from the endothelium, ability to dilate, and in the release of factors that contribute to endothelial integrity. Increasing evidence suggests that growth of arteries is dependent on flow, not pressure, so arterial growth during fetal development and throughout life is determined by changes in flow. Flow has a major impact on artery size and possibly on endothelial integrity.

FREEDSON: How might estrogen protect the endothelial lining?

HASKELL: Estrogen alters the release of nitric oxide and a variety of growth factors from the endothelium. In fact, if one administers adenosine, typically an endothelial-dependent vasodilator, to postmenopausal women with very limited coronary atherosclerosis who have not had hormone replacement therapy, the adenosine causes constriction of coronary arteries. But after hormone replacement therapy, adenosine once again acts as a vasodilator. This phenomenon does not occur with vasodilators such as nitroglyceride that act directly on the arterial smooth muscle and not through the endothelium. Estrogen plays a significant role in women in enhancing the endothelium-mediated dilating capabilities of the arteries.

MAUGHAN: Are you saying that there is a purely hemodynamic component to the protective effect of exercise and that anything that elevates cardiac output will cause coronary arterial growth?

HASKELL: We don't know. It is hypothesized that increased blood flow through arteries will increase artery size very rapidly. In rabbit models in which pressure is maintained constant for 4 wk while flow through one carotid artery is increased and that through the other is decreased, a larger artery develops where there was increased flow and a smaller artery where flow was decreased flow; this is not just dilatation, but actually angiogenesis. There could be a direct hemodynamic effect of increasing coronary blood flow via increased cardiac output that might help protect the arteries, but this has not yet been proven.

GREGG: Is it known what causes the damage to the endothelium?

HASKELL: At least within physiologic ranges, flow *per se* doesn't seem to create major damage to the endothelium. If flow were increased without a concomitant decrease in resistance, increased pressure could produce damage. If there were a situation where a more rigid vascular bed developed due to diffuse atherosclerosis, e.g., in diabetic patients, increased flow would increase pressure and might produce damage. Chemicals, e.g., nicotine, may also cause injury to the endothelium. But, I think the filtration theory will demonstrate at the cellular level that particularly high concentrations of relatively small LDL particles will migrate through a healthy endothelium. So, you don't need what has traditionally been thought of as a damaged endothelium in order to have filtration of LDL into the subintimal space. I think that we may move more and more away from the injury hypothesis that has been so prevalent in textbooks.

GISOLFI: What is the difference between the use of oral contraceptives and estrogen therapy?

HASKELL: In hormone replacement therapy the hormone(s) used, i.e., estrogen only or estrogen plus progesterone, depends on the uterine status of the woman. Also, the amounts of estrogen and progesterone in oral contraceptives are substantially different than those used in hormone replacement therapy for postmenopausal women.

GISOLFI: What is the relative protective effect of oral contraceptives as opposed to estrogen therapy?

HASKELL: This is not clear. In fact, the biggest concern with oral contraceptives is increased blood clotting that occurs.

EICHNER: The newer oral contraceptive pills with lower doses of estrogen are associated with much less of a risk of blood clotting than earlier formulations. I think that blood rheology and viscosity, not only the level of fibrinogen, but also platelet function and even hematocrit, which tends to be lower in women and is lowered in both genders by regular exercise, are key hemostasis concerns in cardiovascular disease. It is better to have a lower hematocrit, because when blood goes through arterioles, red cells tend to stream in the middle and create a "Waring blender" effect; the higher the hematocrit, the more forcefully platelets are flung against the endothelium.

LOUCKS: Would you comment on the mechanism by which progesterone may be acting on cells?

HASKELL: So far, there seems to be little evidence that adding progesterone to estrogen has a significant effect, at least, from the cardiovascular status. About the only systematic data are the early published PEPI study, in which there was a randomized investigation of about 600 women either on placebo, estrogen only, or one of three different estrogen-progestin compounds. No differences among these compounds were detected with regard to effects on the major cardiovascular risk factors. These data are probably the best we'll have for some time. Surely, progestin has major effects on other tissues, particularly the uterus, in preventing hyperplasia.

FREEDSON: Has anyone ever administered estrogen to men?

HASKELL: Oh, yes.

EICHNER: They used large doses of estrogen in the initial Veterans Administration coronary drug study, and estrogens increased the heart attack risk in men with the doses used.

HASKELL: The side effects were considered to be greater than the disease in men. Given some of the new hormone regimens and synthetic preparations that are very specific, that question probably needs to be looked at again.

CLAPP: If a woman undergoes hormone replacement therapy and exercises until she is 70 y of age and then reduces her hormones and her exercise, will she undergo risk reversal?

HASKELL: I don't know much about hormone replacement therapy, but it surely seems that the early postmenopausal years are most critical, at least in terms of maintaining bone mass. The recent data on breast cancer risks suggest that after only 5 y on hormone replacement therapy there may be an increase in breast cancer incidence.

CLAPP: If a woman undergoes hormone replacement therapy for 5 y, starting at the critical time when there is usually a large loss in bone mass, does she eventually lose that bone mass anyway, just beginning 5 y later?

HASKELL: I don't know. One of the arguments is that if she delays the bone loss by 5 y, she is still be better off because the critical level of decreased bone density is going to be reached at a later age.

KANTER: What is the current status of the research being undertaken to try to minimize the oxidation of LDL-cholesterol?

HASKELL: There is an enormous amount of this research underway. Oxidation of LDL seems to occur quite rapidly once it stays around the subintimal space. I'm actually more impressed that some of the molecular-level research is turning out to be very positive as compared to the epidemiological evidence that so far has been quite weak, in terms of whether increases in dietary beta-carotene, vitamin C, and/or vitamin E are associated with lower coronary heart disease mortality rates.

KANTER: What compounds seem to be the most promising?

HASKELL: The epidemiologic data goes back and forth between beta-carotene and vitamin E, but in the more basic work, it looks like there is a cascade effect with vitamins C and E acting in conjunction with one another. I think it is way too early to conclude that one is better than another.

DESPRES: The mechanistic aspect of LDL oxidation is a very exciting field that will generate a lot of very relevant data. Having said that, however, I believe that when it comes to the therapeutic implications, i.e., using antioxidants versus lipid lowering therapy, there is a step here that we should not take too quickly. The susceptibility of LDL particles to oxidation is one thing, but the actual concentration of those LDL particles is another important point. For example, people in Guatemala eat 20–25% of their energy as fat, and they have higher triglyceride concentrations than do North Americans. They also often have low concentrations of HDL and are characterized by the dense LDL phenotype. But if you look at the prevalence of heart disease there, it's much lower than here. However, they have a very small number of LDL particles in their blood plasma, i.e., a low concentration of apoliprotein b.

HASKELL: I fully agree. All of the clinical data we have suggest that lowering LDL, in particular, small, dense LDL, would be the initial strategy. I agree with you that it is probably the total number of LDL particles that we should deal with first.

DESPRES: I know you're very much aware of that, but I wanted to raise this point because the dense-LDL phenotype has been over-emphasized if we do not consider the number of those particles.

DIPIETRO: With advancing age some of the established risk factors for coronary heart disease, e.g., total cholesterol and cigarette smoking, lose some relative impact. Would you predict that aging will eventually be shown to also reduce the importance of physical activity as a CVD risk factor for both men and women?

HASKELL: There is no current evidence for a decline in the risk ratio for active versus inactive men as age increases. In fact, in the two or three studies that have men across three to four decades, that ratio actually increases so that there appears to be greater benefit, in a sense, for older men versus younger. The absolute mortality rate changes, and that may influence those ratios in some way. The only data we have on younger and older women is from Finland, and it doesn't look like there is a lot of difference between younger and older individuals. The other intriguing factor about physical activity as a risk factor for coronary disease is that it tends to lose its potency when you look at all-cause mortality. So, in men total cholesterol is reasonably well associated with coronary heart disease mortality, but when you look at all-cause mortality, that relationship is very weak or almost disappears. That's been one of the major criticisms of considering cholesterol as an important risk factor for general health and not just cardiovascular health. But this does not hold true for physical activity, regardless of whether activity status or fitness level are considered. The risk ratios for physical activity and all-cause mortality are nearly as strong as for CHD disease mortality.

DIPIETRO: I think it is very important that we give the message that physical activity maintains its relative importance with regard to other risk factors throughout the life span.

10

Exercise During Pregnancy

JAMES F. CLAPP, III, M.D.

INTRODUCTION

Physical Activity in Women of Reproductive Age

Approximately 38% of women of reproductive age regularly engage in some form of sustained, recreational exercise, and the public health goal is to increase participation to 90% by the year 2000 (McGinnis, 1992). Roughly half of these women perform one or more forms of sustained, moderate- to high-intensity exercise (e.g., aerobics, running, stair climbing, cross-country skiing, and rowing) three or more times a week, and most plan to continue at that level during pregnancy and lactation (Clapp & Dickstein, 1984; Sady & Carpenter, 1989).

The Physiological Basis for Clinical Concern

In the nonpregnant state, sustained, moderate- to high-intensity exercise reduces splanchnic blood flow by 50% or more (Rowell et al., 1965), often raises core temperature more than 1.5°C (Clapp, 1991a; Clapp et al., 1987; Saltin & Hermansen, 1966), and depletes glycogen stores (Bonnen et al., 1992; Clapp & Capeless, 1991a; Clapp et al., 1987). The obstetrical concern is that a reduction in visceral blood flow of this magnitude coupled with decreased substrate levels could produce fetal hypoxia (Clapp et al., 1995b) and/or growth retardation (Clapp, 1991b), while increased maternal temperature could initiate fetal malformation (Milunsky et al., 1992). There is also concern that vigorous exercise may increase the risk of fetal or placental injury from accidental blunt abdominal trauma or motion-induced shear stress (Clapp, 1991b). Finally, there is concern that the information obtained to date may not be representative because it has been gathered in a fairly select populace that does not include substantial numbers of women younger than 25 years of age, truly sedentary women, African-American women, or women of lower educational attainment. Therefore, although the American College of Obstetricians and Gynecologists Guidelines (1994) support regular physical activity during pregnancy, they caution that the duration, intensity, and type of exercise should be limited. Nonetheless, as will be discussed in some detail, none of the evidence currently available demonstrates any increased risk when women regularly exercise throughout pregnancy without adhering to these cautionary measures.

To clarify the basis of this inconsistency, the chapter will focus on the interaction between the physiological adaptations to pregnancy and to regular, sustained exercise. The information will then be used to: assess the validity of the concerns, develop a rational approach to exercise prescription during pregnancy and lactation, and identify several directions for future research.

MEDICAL AND SAFETY CONCERNS

Mother

Musculoskeletal Injury. Several reviews focusing on accidental injury and biomechanics during pregnancy comment that there is no evidence that exercise during pregnancy increases the incidence of accidental injury and that case reports are rare (Karzel & Friedman, 1991; McNitt-Gray, 1991; Sherer & Schenker, 1989). While this conclusion is contrary to what might be expected, it concurs with our finding that the rate of exercise-induced injury is actually decreased during pregnancy (Clapp, 1994). The reason for this is not entirely clear, but simple observation suggests that fit pregnant women pay greater attention, exert more control, and avoid factors that increase injury risk.

Premature Labor And Premature Membrane Rupture. Most women who regularly perform sustained exercise note symptoms suggestive of increased uterine activity during and immediately after exercise throughout middle and late pregnancy. However, most studies of sustained aerobic activity have not been able to objectively confirm an exercise-induced alteration in uterine activity (Durack et al., 1990; van Doorn et al., 1992; Veille et al., 1985). Likewise, other investigators have not found evidence that regular exercise during pregnancy increases the risk of premature labor or pre-term rupture of the membranes (Clapp, 1994; Lokey et al., 1991).

Fetus

Substrate Availability and Hypoxia. There is concern that the decrease in circulating maternal glucose levels coupled with reduced placental blood flow (Bonnen et al., 1992; Clapp & Capeless, 1991a) may reduce fetal glucose and oxygen delivery to critical levels during exercise. This concern is accentuated when considering intense, prolonged exercise in which both the extravascular fluid shift and sweating reduce blood volume, resulting in a further reduction in blood flow. Ultimately, this could result in growth retardation, low birth weight, and/or developmental abnormalities after birth. However, the data (Clapp, 1991b, 1994; Lokey et al., 1991) do not support the concern.

Cord Entanglement. The ballistic motion and sudden postural changes associated with a variety of exercises could produce equally sudden postural changes in the fetus, who is tethered by the umbilical cord. The end result might well be either an overhand true knot in the umbilical cord or loops of the cord lying around the fetal neck, extremities, or trunk, leading to reductions in blood flow and fetal compromise. Most studies have not examined this possibility.

Direct Fetal Trauma. Either direct abdominal trauma or shear stress, the result of the acceleration and deceleration forces associated with sudden motion, can produce fetal tissue injury (Sherer & Schenker, 1989). However, at present, there are no case reports documenting this type of event in association with accidental injury during exercise.

Placenta and Membranes

Early Pregnancy. It is possible that the mechanical and hormonal changes associated with regular exercise might result in an increased incidence of abnormal implantation (e.g., ectopic pregnancy or abortion) and that the metabolic and cardiovascular effects of exercise might limit placental as well as fetal growth. Again, there are no reports in humans that document the existence of such an association.

Late Pregnancy. During exercise the placenta and membranes are subject to the same physical forces as the uterus and fetus. Significant shear stress or direct compressive forces generated by exercise could manifest themselves as placental separation with hemorrhage or membrane rupture. However, a causal association between exercise and these disorders remains to be documented.

MATERNAL RESPONSES TO EXERCISE DURING PREGNANCY

An expanding body of information suggests that the cardiovascular, metabolic, thermal, and endocrine adaptations to pregnancy and regular exercise generally enhance one another and interact to protect the fetus from multiple potential sources of injury. This is reflected in the changes observed in a woman's physiological response to exercise during pregnancy, the fetal responses to maternal exercise, the placental response, and the outcomes observed.

Cardiovascular Adaptations To Pregnancy

During pregnancy there are large (40%) increases in blood volume and cardiac output, with 2- to 20-fold increases in regional blood flow within the cutaneous, renal, and uterine circulations. These are initiated within two weeks of conception by a generalized and persistent decrease in vascular tone and reactivity that reduces both preload and afterload, increases heart rate, and triggers salt and water retention. Concomitantly, end-diastolic volume and stroke volume increase by 15–20%, vascular compliance increases, and total peripheral resistance falls 40% or more (Capeless & Clapp, 1989; Duvekot et al., 1993; Lees et al., 1967; Pivarnik et al., 1990; Robson et al., 1987, 1989). These dramatic changes appear to be induced by the changing hormonal milieu (Duvekot et al., 1993; Giraud et al., 1993; Hart et al., 1985; Veille et al., 1986) and persist for an undetermined time interval after delivery (Capeless & Clapp, 1991; Clapp et al., 1995a; Hart et al., 1986). In addition, both catecholamine release to physical stress and adrenergic vascular sensitivity are down-regulated during pregnancy. Circulating catecholamine levels are lower during and after postural stress, hemorrhage, thermal stress, and both hand-grip and whole-body exercise (Barron et al., 1986; Clapp & Capeless, 1991a; Clapp et al., 1994; Nisell et al., 1985b), and vascular responsiveness to a standard dose of agonist is depressed (Crandall et al., 1990; Davidge & McLaughlin, 1992; Nisell et al., 1985a).

Cardiovascular Adaptations to Exercise

The classic studies of Saltin et al. (1968) demonstrate that regular endurance exercise has similar effects on blood volume and ventricular volumes. It also increases the cross-sectional area of the muscle capillary bed; lowers resting heart rate, cardiac output, and arterial blood pressure; and attenuates the decrease in visceral blood flow during exercise (Andersen & Henriksson, 1977; Saar et al., 1986; Saltin et al., 1968; Tipton, 1991). Total peripheral resistance at rest appears either unchanged or increased, and regional perfusion patterns are unchanged (Blomqvist & Saltin, 1983;

Saltin et al., 1968; Tipton, 1991). All changes rapidly revert to baseline values if the exercise regimen is interrupted for an extended period. Training also lowers the catecholamine secretion at any given absolute work load, but the change is minimal when the work load is normalized to a given percent of $\dot{V}O_2$max.

Interactive Effects and the Resultant Maternal Cardiovascular Response

When regular exercise is continued during pregnancy, it appears that many of the cardiovascular adaptations are complementary, producing a physiological environment that reduces the risk of fetal hypoxia (Table 10-1). For example, at rest, the exercise-induced increases in end-diastolic volume and stroke volume are further enhanced (> 10%) by pregnancy (Capeless & Clapp, 1989), and the same is true for blood volume (Pivarnik et al., 1994). These and other complementary cardiovascular effects (Pivarnik et al., 1990) act to maintain fetal oxygenation, apparently by minimizing the need for flow redistribution away from the uterine bed during sustained exercise or other hemodynamic stress (Clapp et al., 1993, 1994, 1995b).

The maternal cardiovascular responses to exercise during pregnancy have not been extensively studied but appear to differ with fitness status, exercise type, and the stage of pregnancy in which the measurements are obtained. For example, once one corrects basal and maximum heart rate for genetic variability, the pregnancy-related changes in exercise heart rate over a wide range of exercise type and intensity appear to be inversely related to fitness, time point in pregnancy, and current exercise volume measured as the product of weekly exercise time and intensity (Clapp et al., 1993). Indeed, during pregnancy the documented subject range in exercise intensity at a heart rate of 140 beats/min is between 31 and 76% of $\dot{V}O_2$max (Clapp, 1990), and pulse rates up to 170 beats/mind occur at exercise intensities < 50% of $\dot{V}O_2$max (Clapp et al., 1993). Thus, sub-maximal exercise heart rates are either increased, decreased, or unchanged; stroke volumes and cardiac outputs are increased; and maximum heart rates are either unchanged or decreased slightly (Clapp et al., 1993; Knutt-

TABLE 10-1. *The cardiopulmonary interactions between the physiological adaptations to regular exercise and to pregnancy.*

Variable	Exercise	Pregnancy	Combination
Blood Volume	↑	↑	↑↑
Stroke Volume	↑	↑	↑↑
Heart Rate	↓	↑ or ↓	↑ or ↓
Vascular Tone	UC	↓	↓?
O_2 Availability	↑	↑	↑↑

(↑ = increased, ↓ = decreased, UC = unchanged)

gen & Emerson, 1974; Lotgering et al., 1991; Sady et al., 1989; Veille et al., 1994; Watson et al., 1991). The most detailed study of cardiovascular responses to date (Sady et al., 1989) indicates that the coupling between cardiac output and oxygen consumption during exercise is unchanged, suggesting that the balance between oxygen consumption and blood flow is also unchanged in the exercising muscles of pregnant women.

Respiratory Adaptations To Pregnancy

Minute ventilation and, more importantly, alveolar ventilation, rise by 40–50% or more due to an increase in tidal volume in response to a downward shift in the sensitivity of the respiratory center to pCO_2 caused by sex-steroids (DeSwiet, 1991). This is often associated with subjective symptoms of dyspnea (breathlessness) at rest or during mild exertion as well as an increase in the ventilatory equivalent for oxygen. While maximum breathing capacity is unchanged, the changes in rib-cage configuration cause a slight increase in vital capacity and inspiratory capacity with a concomitant reduction in residual volumes and functional residual capacity. The change in alveolar ventilation coupled with the decrease in residual volumes more than offset the small decrease in diffusing capacity and increase in a-A gradient. As a result, arterial pO_2 is increased by 5–10 torr, and pCO_2 is decreased by a similar amount. Both enhance gas exchange at a tissue level (DeSwiet, 1991).

Respiratory Adaptations To Exercise

Regular exercise has minimal impact on pulmonary function, but its cardiovascular and cellular effects clearly improve the capacity for oxygen transport to, and utilization by, tissue (Saltin & Rowell, 1980; Saltin et al., 1968). The metabolic and muscular adaptations to training also reduce the ventilatory equivalent for oxygen during moderate exercise, and maximal breathing capacity is increased.

Interactive Effects and the Resultant Maternal Respiratory Response

Respiratory adaptations appear adequate when regular exercise is continued during pregnancy. The heterogeneity of reported values for specific ventilatory parameters during exercise appear to be related to characteristics of the study populace and exercise regimen (Artal et al., 1986b; Lotgering et al., 1991; Pernoll et al., 1975a, 1975b; Pivarnik et al., 1990, 1992). The same is true for the subjective symptom of dyspnea on exertion. However, it is clear that peak minute ventilation and absolute $\dot{V}O_2$max (mL/min) are not reduced (Lotgering et al., 1991) and may actually be increased when regular exercise is continued during pregnancy (Clapp & Capeless, 1991b). The effect of regular exercise on the metabolic cost of exercise during pregnancy remains controversial, and, as there are good data supporting both increases and decreases in that cost, the effect is probably populace-specific (Artal et al., 1986b; Carpenter et al., 1990; Clapp, 1989a; Pernoll et al., 1975b; Pivarnik et al., 1990; Prentice et al., 1989; van Raaij et al., 1990).

Thermoregulatory Adaptations to Pregnancy

During pregnancy there is a progressive decrease in rectal temperature at rest and a marked increase in body mass and skin blood flow (Clapp, 1991a; Katz & Sokal, 1980). In all probability, the first is due to the hormonally induced 5- to 6-fold increase in skin blood flow and the associated 5°C increase in skin temperature in the extremities, which results in an imbalance between heat production and heat loss at rest. In any case, the first two adaptations reduce the probability of thermal stress by increasing the capacity for heat storage, and the latter adaptation, along with the increase in minute ventilation, improves heat dissipation.

Thermoregulatory Adaptations to Exercise

Regular, sustained exercise increases blood volume and decreases the core temperature threshold for both cutaneous vasodilatation and sweating (Roberts et al., 1977; Saltin et al., 1968). All improve the capacity for heat dissipation in response to thermal stress. Estrogen also enhances both heat storage capacity and heat dissipation by reducing resting core temperature and the thresholds for vasodilation and sweating (Stephenson & Kolka, 1985; Tankersley et al., 1992).

Interactive Effects and the Resultant Maternal Thermal Response

When regular sustained exercise is continued during pregnancy, the thermoregulatory adaptations appear to complement one another, reducing the possibility of significant, exercise-associated, thermal stress for both mother and fetus (Clapp, 1991a). These changes are summarized in Table 10-2.

This reduction in thermal stress during exercise is ironic as early morning basal body temperature is increased by 0.2–0.6°C throughout early and mid pregnancy (Benjamin, 1960), and peak rectal temperature during exercise often exceeds potentially teratogenic levels (> 39–$39.5°C$) in nonpregnant women runners (Clapp, 1991a; Palone et al., 1978; Rozycki, 1984). Therefore, it was surprising when reports appeared that the thermal stress associated with strenuous exercise was either unchanged or decreased during pregnancy, depending on the environmental conditions (Clapp, 1991a; Jones et al., 1985). There are at least three physiological bases for this conclusion.

First, the early marked increases in skin blood flow, skin temperature, and minute ventilation improve heat dissipation to the point where oxy-

TABLE 10-2. *The thermoregulatory interactions between the physiological adaptations to regular exercise and to pregnancy.*

Variable	Exercise	Pregnancy	Combination
Blood Volume	↑	↑	↑↑
Vasodil Threshold	↓	↓↓	↓↓↓
Sweat Threshold	↓	↓	↓↓
Resting Temp	UC	↓	↓
Storage Capacity	↓	↑↑	↑
Respiratory Cooling	UC	↑	↑

(↑ = increased, ↓ = decreased, UC = unchanged)

gen consumption increases by 10–15% during quiet standing by the eighth week of pregnancy (Burt, 1949; Clapp et al., 1988; Katz & Sokal, 1980), apparently to maintain rectal temperature near nonpregnant levels. This trend is accentuated with advancing pregnancy such that resting rectal temperature falls progressively under these conditions at a rate of 0.05°C each lunar month to an average level of 37.3°C near term (Clapp, 1991a).

Second, the progressive increase in body mass acts as a thermal buffer by increasing the amount of heat necessary to raise the temperature of the entire tissue mass.

Third, the central thermoregulatory set point for sweating progressively decreases throughout pregnancy at a rate of 0.08°C each lunar month. This also improves heat dissipation (Clapp, 1991a). The end result is that, relative to the preconceptional measurements, the maternal thermal response is reduced by at least 20–30% in early pregnancy and by as much as 70% near term. As a result, the peak rectal temperature achieved during 20 min of exercise at 60–65% of $\dot{V}O_2$max at term is often less than that observed at rest in the nonpregnant state (Clapp, 1991a).

Metabolic and Endocrine Adaptations to Pregnancy

The major characteristic of pregnancy is the formation of new tissue that increases resting metabolic rate by 15–20% (Pernoll et al., 1975b). In Western society, there is a dramatic increase in maternal fat mass early in pregnancy that averages 3.5–5 kg, whereas feto-placental growth dominates late pregnancy (Clapp & Little, 1995; Goldberg et al., 1993; Hytten et al., 1966, King et al., 1994). Total maternal weight gain is populace-dependent but averages in excess of 12 kg in Western society (Clapp & Little, 1995). Another characteristic of pregnancy is a progressive rise in insulin resistance that increases utilization of fat for maternal energy needs, assuring the availability of glucose for feto-placental growth (Freinkel et al., 1974; Ryan et al., 1985). However, the resultant increase in postprandial glucose levels may be primarily an artifact created by the usual Western diet (Fraser et al., 1988). Finally, the endocrine changes of pregnancy reduce both the resting tone and reactivity of smooth muscle, thereby suppressing uterine contractility to ensure maintenance of the pregnancy (Hodgen & Iskovitz, 1988).

Metabolic and Endocrine Adaptations to Exercise

Regular exercise has no consistent effect on resting metabolic rate but increases both absolute $\dot{V}O_2$max and lean body mass without a consistent effect on total weight (Saltin et al., 1968; Schultz et al., 1992; Stephanick, 1993). Exercise training reduces insulin resistance and improves glucose availability by simply increasing the use of fat as energy substrate both at rest and during exercise (Coggan et al., 1990; Gollnick, 1985). Training reduces the catecholamine response to a standard work load, and, although unstudied, exercise training should also decrease or eliminate any uterine smooth muscle irritability associated with flow redistribution at all except extremely intense levels of activity.

Interactive Effects and the Resultant Maternal Metabolic and Endocrine Response to Exercise

Again the metabolic and endocrine adaptations to both pregnancy and exercise appear to complement one another, and, as detailed in Table 10-3, their effects on the stress response and fetal glucose availability should be feto-protective.

Body Composition. Most studies have not evaluated the impact of regular exercise on weight gain and fat deposition during pregnancy. However, several studies have reported that beginning a sanctioned exercise program during pregnancy reduced maternal weight gain more than a kilogram in the third trimester (Beckmann & Beckmann, 1990; Kulpa et al., 1987). As illustrated in Figure 10-1, one additional study noted a 3–kg reduction of body weight in women who continued to perform aerobics and/or run throughout pregnancy at levels well above those typically recommended (Clapp & Little, 1995). Note that the reduced rate of weight gain was limited to the latter portion of pregnancy. The same study is the only report that addresses the impact of exercise on fat deposition. As shown in Figure 10-2, it demonstrated that subcutaneous fat deposition,

TABLE 10-3. *The metabolic and endocrine interactions between the physiological adaptations to regular exercise and to pregnancy.*

Variable	Exercise	Pregnancy	Combination
Insulin Resistance	↓	↑	↑ or ↓
Maternal Glucose Oxidation	↓	↓	↓↓
Hepatic Glucose Release	↓	↓	↓
Maternal Lipid Oxidation	↑	↑	↑
Catecholamine Response	↓	↓	↓

(↑ = increased, ↓ = decreased)

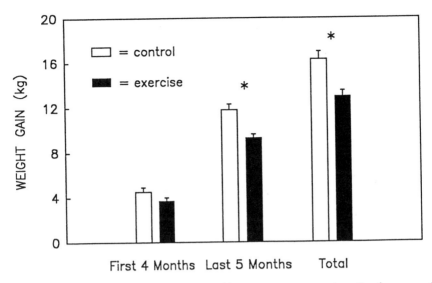

FIGURE 10-1. *The weight gain observed in early and late pregnancy in women who continued a program of regular, sustained, antigravitational exercise throughout pregnancy and a group of matched physically active controls (adapted from Clapp & Little, 1995).* Data are presented as means ± S.D. Significant between-group differences are noted by an asterisk.

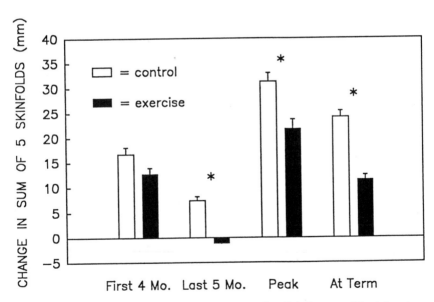

FIGURE 10-2. *The changes observed in the sums of five site skinfold thicknesses at different times in pregnancy in women who continued a program of regular, sustained, antigravitational exercise throughout pregnancy and a group of matched physically active controls (adapted from Clapp & Little, 1995).* Data are presented as means ± S.D. Significant between-group differences are noted by an asterisk.

as assessed by five site skinfold thicknesses, was significantly curtailed in mid pregnancy and decreased more rapidly in late pregnancy in exercising women. This difference was primarily due to the changes in the three skinfolds surrounding the pelvic girdle and explained about two thirds of the difference in weight gain between the two groups.

However, regular sustained exercise does not appear to enhance postpartum weight loss. Although a single small study suggests that lactation may increase the rate of weight loss and lower body fat loss after delivery (Kramer et al., 1993), participation in regular, sustained, fairly intense exercise during the period of lactation does not alter the rate of change in skinfolds, fat mass, or total body mass (Dewey et al., 1994; Little et al., 1994; Lovelady et al., 1990) because energy intake spontaneously rises to match the increased energy expenditure of the exercise.

Substrate Utilization. The data on the impact of regular exercise on substrate utilization are conflicting (Wolfe & Mottola, 1993). It appears that this conflict is due to variation in the exercise regimens and the fitness of the populations studied. It is unlikely that clear answers will be obtained until methodology is developed that can separate the substrate utilization of the uterus, placenta, and fetus from that of the maternal organism.

During pregnancy, the respiratory exchange ratio at the same absolute $\dot{V}O_2$max during both treadmill and cycle exercise is lower than it is after childbirth (Lotgering et al., 1991). Others report similar findings during lower intensity exercise (Wolfe et al., 1994). Both suggest a greater reliance on lipid oxidation during exercise in pregnancy. However, additional studies indicate that glucose utilization is either unchanged (Pernoll et al., 1975a; Sady et al., 1989) or increased (Clapp et al., 1987; Clapp & Capeless, 1991a; Knuttgen & Emerson, 1974), suggesting that dependence on glucose as energy substrate during exercise is either unchanged or increased when substrate utilized by the utero-placental and fetal tissues is included. These differences are hard to explain definitively, but they may be due in part to the fact that many of the studies used either a cross-sectional design or inappropriately used postpartum values rather than values obtained prior to pregnancy to represent the nonpregnant state.

All studies concur that multiple types of sustained exercise conducted at intensities of 40–85% of $\dot{V}O_2$max during pregnancy produce a decrease in the circulating levels of glucose, indicating an imbalance between glucose appearance and utilization (Bonnen et al., 1992; Clapp & Capeless, 1991a; Hauth et al., 1982). In individual cases, the fall in blood glucose concentration ranges between 0.3 and 2.3 mmol/L, appears to vary with exercise intensity in early pregnancy, but is most marked after the 20th week at exercise intensities less than 60% of $\dot{V}O_2$max. This occurs despite a similar fall in circulating insulin levels. In late pregnancy the fall in blood glucose with exercise is associated with a concomitant blunting of the catecholamine response to exercise. As such, the fall in glucose concentration probably represents both an increase in peripheral utilization due to fetal and placental demands coupled with a reduction in hepatic glucose release, the latter being more important in early gestation.

Musculoskeletal Adaptations to Pregnancy

With the exception of ligamentous laxity of the pelvic girdle (Abramson et al., 1934), the musculoskeletal adaptations to pregnancy are poorly studied. Clearly, body mass increases by 15–25%, and in late pregnancy the protuberant abdomen coupled with lumbar lordosis changes the center of gravity, increases the loading of most joints, and is thought to be responsible for an increased incidence of low back pain (Berg et al., 1988; Clapp & Little, 1995; Ellis et al., 1985). The limited information on changes in bone mineral content and bone density indicates that both calcium absorption and bone turnover are increased and that bone density is maintained (Heaney & Skillman, 1971; Little et al., 1993; Sowers et al., 1991). Although often mentioned as a major change, objective evidence of an increase in ligamentous laxity around peripheral joints is minimal and probably not functionally significant (Calganeri et al., 1982). Changes in muscle mass, as well as the force and velocity of contraction of specific muscle groups, have not been documented, but the increase in body mass and the variable results obtained for oxygen demand during physical activity suggest that these may well be altered.

Musculoskeletal Adaptations to Exercise

Regular exercise improves bone density, muscle mass and strength, and ligamentous tensile strength in a site-specific fashion that is highly dependent on the training regimen (Drinkwater et al., 1984; Gollnick et al., 1981; Henriksson, 1977; Saltin & Rowell, 1980; Tipton et al., 1986). In women there is an additional interaction with the ovarian steroids, estrogen and progesterone. Both act to retain bone mineral but have opposite actions on bone remodeling, i.e., progesterone activates and estradiol inhibits remodeling (Drinkwater et al., 1984; Prior, 1990).

Interactive Effects and the Resultant Maternal Musculoskeletal Adaptations

These are poorly studied at present, but it appears that the endocrine changes of pregnancy probably enhance the effects of exercise on bone and that the effects of exercise act to balance the pregnancy-induced changes in mass, posture, and ligamentous laxity. The latter conclusion is based on the findings that regular exercise during pregnancy reduces the incidence of musculoskeletal complaints and may actually reduce the incidence of musculoskeletal injury as well (Clapp, 1994; Karzel & Freidman, 1991; Wallace et al., 1985).

The available data indicate that the interactive effects on bone are specific to time, site, and exercise regimen (Drinkwater & Chestnut, 1991; Little et al., 1993), with remodeling being dominant in early pregnancy and the femoral neck a potentially vulnerable site for injury. The impact of exercise during pregnancy on maternal muscle strength and function has not been assessed.

Potential Enhancement and Limitation of Performance During Pregnancy

This is an area where there is an abundance of anecdotal data and opinion but very little definitive information. Individual experiences with competition in early pregnancy suggest that the endocrine and blood volume changes of early pregnancy may enhance performance in field and track events (Clapp & Capeless, 1991b; Cohen et al., 1989; Higdon, 1981; Sady & Carpenter, 1989). The same is true for pregnancy *per se* as there is evidence that both $\dot{V}O_2$max and running performance are improved after childbirth in women who continue exercise throughout pregnancy (Clapp & Capeless, 1991b; Villarosa, 1985). However, no study has serially assessed the impact of pregnancy on competitive performance, and the findings in the four longitudinal studies of physically active women that have addressed physiological issues related to performance have not been independently confirmed.

The first of these indicates that continuing regular exercise throughout pregnancy significantly improves both absolute (mL/min) and relative $(mL\cdot kg^{-1}\cdot min^{-1})$ $\dot{V}O_2$max after childbirth, despite a decrease in training volume (Clapp & Capeless, 1991b). The second indicates that continuing regular exercise during pregnancy decreases absolute oxygen consumption during standardized low- and moderate-intensity treadmill exercise (Clapp, 1989a). The third indicates that pregnancy-induced changes in thermoregulation reduce the thermal stress of exercise when women continue to exercise during pregnancy (Clapp, 1991a), and the fourth study demonstrates that the enhanced cardiovascular adaptations to pregnancy persist for at least 1 y after childbirth (Capeless & Clapp, 1991; Clapp et al., 1995a). All of these studies support the idea that both short- and long-term performance should be improved after pregnancy if regular exercise is continued during pregnancy.

Despite the fact that $\dot{V}O_2$max is unchanged (Lotgering et al., 1991), the spontaneous decrease in exercise performance experienced by most physically active women during pregnancy suggests that the pregnancy-associated changes in mass, abdominal contour, center of gravity, and pelvic girdle do limit aspects of performance such as speed, balance, acceleration, coordination, and sudden lateral motion to some degree (Clapp et al., 1987; Clapp & Capeless, 1991a, 1991b; Cohen et al., 1989; Dale et al., 1982). However, as illustrated in Table 10-4, these and other issues have

TABLE 10-4. *The exercise performance interactions between the physiological adaptations to regular exercise and to pregnancy.*

Parameter	Exercise	Pregnancy	Combination
Maximal Power Output	↑	UC	↑
Maximal Workload	↑	↓	↑, ↓, or UC
Fitness	↑	UC or ↑	↑
Submaximal Efficiency	↑	↓ or ↑	↑?
Limitations	↓	↑?	↑, ↓, or UC

(↑ = increased, ↓ = decreased, UC = unchanged)

not been specifically addressed, and it is probable that beginning a regular training program during pregnancy actually decreases a previously sedentary individual's limitations in terms of physical performance.

There are two studies of the limitation imposed by pregnancy weight gain in previously untrained women who undertake weight-bearing versus nonweight-bearing exercise during submaximal and maximal performance (Carpenter et al., 1990; Lotgering et al., 1991). Both studies indicate that maximal power output is maintained during treadmill exercise with only a minimal (4%) reduction occurring in late pregnancy during cycle ergometry. However, absolute submaximal and maximal work loads were reduced in proportion to weight gain. The maximal work load data in four moderately trained women were similar (Lotgering et al., 1991). However, longitudinal data gathered in both untrained women and regularly exercising women with $\dot{V}O_2$max values > 50 mL·kg^{-1}·min^{-1} indicate that regular exercise during pregnancy may actually improve the efficiency of oxygen utilization during low- and moderate-intensity treadmill exercise (Clapp, 1989a; Prentice et al., 1989; van Raaij et al., 1990).

Finally, numerous reports indicate that previously sedentary women may begin a variety of progressive training regimens during pregnancy without limitations other than those detailed above, and the data indicate that their fitness is improved (Beckmann & Beckmann, 1990; Collings et al., 1983; Kulpa et al., 1987; Sibley et al., 1981; South-Paul et al., 1988; Wong & McKenzie, 1987). This includes light-to-moderate circuit training and resistance training with machines, but as yet there are no reports dealing with free-weight training. However, the American College of Obstetricians and Gynecologists Guidelines (1994) recommend avoidance of most activities other than swimming and stationary cycling to minimize theoretical risk. Likewise, although unstudied, exercise in the supine position is not recommended to avoid potential hemodynamic compromise from aorto-caval compression.

FETAL RESPONSES TO MATERNAL EXERCISE

To date, the fetal responses that have been observed during and after maternal exercise suggest that either beginning or continuing a regular exercise regimen during pregnancy does not produce biologically significant fetal stress.

Heart Rate

The reports of the impact of exercise on fetal heart rate have been inconsistent, probably because of differences in the intensity, duration, and type of exercise regimen, as well as the subject's fitness and the gestational age at which the study was carried out (Artal et al., 1986a; Carpenter et al., 1988; Clapp et al., 1993; Collings & Curet, 1985; Erkkola et al., 1992; Hauth et al., 1982; Jones et al., 1985; Katz et al., 1988; Morrow et al., 1989; Pipers et al., 1984; Pomerance et al., 1979; Sibley et al., 1981; Sorensen & Borlum, 1986; Sovia et al., 1964; Steegers et al., 1988; Veille et al., 1985, 1992; Watson et al., 1991).

One of these studies (Clapp et al., 1993) examined data from a large number of subjects to determine if this interpretation was correct. We studied 120 fit women with uncomplicated pregnancies who performed their chosen forms of exercise for 20 min at intensities ranging between 40 and 83% of $\dot{V}O_2$max on two or mored occasions between the 16th and 39th gestational week, and we observed that the fetal heart rates increased during and after exercise about 95% of the time. However, in order to obtain a consistent response, the measurements had to be made with the fetus quiescent, and the exercise had to be continued for 10 or more min at an intensity above 40% of the woman's $\dot{V}O_2$max. The magnitude of the response varied widely (increases of 1–55 beats/min) and was influenced by the muscle mass utilized (cycle ergometry $<$ than treadmill exercise), exercise intensity and duration, and gestational age. For example, the fetal heart rate response increased 4 beats/min for each 10% increase in exercise intensity above 40% of $\dot{V}O_2$max, and cycle ergometry had to be performed at 60% of $\dot{V}O_2$max to produce the response observed during treadmill exercise at 40% of $\dot{V}O_2$max. These relationships suggest that the fetal heart rate response to exercise represents a sympathetic response to a minor decrease in pO_2 secondary to a fall in uterine blood flow and that the magnitude of the response reflects maturation of the fetal autonomic nervous system and the magnitude of the reduction in uterine blood flow and pO_2. The fact that exercise does not elevate erythropoietin levels in amniotic fluid and cord blood is consistent with this interpretation as it indicates that this fetal heart rate response is not associated with evidence of tissue hypoxia within the fetal compartment (Clapp et al. 1995b).

However, other studies noted that approximately 15% of the time, the fetuses of healthy but relatively unfit women experience decreases in heart rate during and immediately after exercise, including sustained cycle ergometry at a moderate intensity, rapidly progressive submaximal cycle ergometry, and tethered swimming (Artal et al., 1986a, Carpenter et al., 1988; Veille et al., 1992; Watson et al., 1991). These may represent the classic, baroreceptor-mediated, autonomic response to an abrupt decrease in pO_2, suggesting that protracted or intense exercise in this populace may reduce flow and fetal pO_2 significantly.

Breathing Movements, Body Movements, and Velocity-Flow Profiles

Several studies have examined the impact of exercise on fetal breathing and/or motion (Clapp, 1985; Clapp et al., 1993; Hauth et al., 1982; Katz et al., 1988; Marsal et al., 1979) with inconsistent, minor, and transitory findings. Likewise, Doppler studies have not demonstrated changes in the velocity-flow profile in either the fetal aorta or the umbilical circulation following short bouts of cycle ergometry at unmeasured but apparently moderate to very high intensities (Erkkola et al., 1992; Morrow et al., 1989; Pipers et al., 1984). These findings, coupled with the erythropoietin data and the absence of reports of exercise being associated with unexpected fetal demise or distress, suggest that the normal fetus is not significantly perturbed by exercise at usual training levels during pregnancy. However, the same cannot be said for the pregnancy with uteroplacental insufficiency. In the limited number of cases studied, short duration, apparently moderate- to high-intensity stepping exercise produced abnormal fetal heart rate patterns in most cases (Pomerance et al., 1979).

Growth Rate

Multiple studies have assessed the impact of beginning various exercise regimens during mid-pregnancy on birth weight (Beckmann & Beckmann, 1990; Collings et al., 1983; Hall & Kaufmann, 1987; Kulpa et al., 1987; Lokey et al., 1991; Sibley et al., 1981). The results indicate that starting a program of cycle ergometry, swimming, stretching, or multimodality exercise has not had a significant impact on birth weight. Multiple retrospective and epidemiological studies, in which the consistency, intensity, and duration of the exercise was not measured, indicate that the same is true when regular walking or running is continued during pregnancy (Clapp, 1994). However, birth weight is reduced by about 300 g when fit women maintain a regimen of vigorous, sustained exercise (three or more sessions/week at >50% $\dot{V}O_2$max for a minimum of 20 min) throughout pregnancy which, as illustrated in Figure 10-3, shifts the frequency distribution of birth weight for gestational age to the left in the exercise group. Conversely, in those who exercise throughout the first and second trimester and then stop, birth weight is increased above control levels by a similar amount (Clapp, 1994; Clapp & Capeless, 1990). The changes in birth weight are due primarily to changes in fat mass and are not associated with changes in either head circumference or axial length; the reduction in birth weight is directly related to the rigor or the moth-

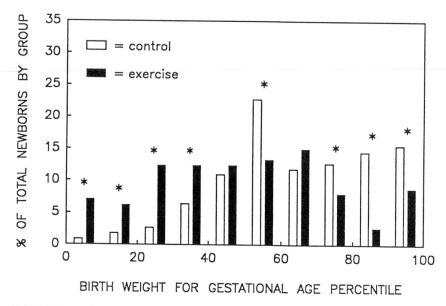

FIGURE 10-3. *The frequency distribution of birth weight for gestational age by birth weight percentiles in women who continued a program of regular, sustained, antigravitational exercise throughout pregnancy and a group of matched physically active controls (adapted from Clapp, 1994).* Significant between-group differences are noted by an asterisk.

er's exercise in the third trimester (Clapp & Capeless, 1990). To date, childhood follow-up indicates that the same morphometric pattern (normal height and circumferences, with a decrease in weight and subcutaneous skinfold thicknesses) is present at the age of 5 y (Clapp et al., 1995c).

PLACENTAL RESPONSES TO MATERNAL EXERCISE

Regular exercise during pregnancy does not increase placental tissue weight at term (Clapp & Capeless, 1990), but it does increase the growth rate of placental volume, as measured by B-mode ultrasound, in mid-pregnancy by about a third (Clapp & Rizk, 1992). This suggests that the main effect of exercise is to increase the volume of blood, blood flow, and surface area in both the maternal and fetal placental circulations, which should improve the transfer of gases and substrates between mother and fetus. A recent detailed histomorphometric study demonstrates that this is indeed the case (Jackson et al., 1995). As illustrated in Figure 10-4, regular exercise increased the total volume of functional placental parenchymal tissue, with increases in villous and vascular volumes as well. The same is true for surface areas. These adaptations are clearly feto-protective and probably explain why it has been difficult to obtain descriptive data doc-

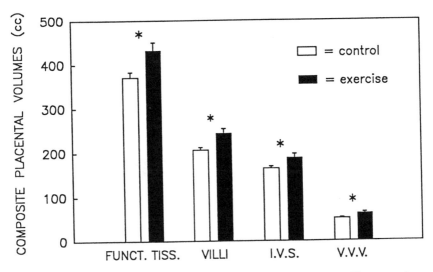

FIGURE 10-4. *The differences in placental composition between the placentae delivered by women who continued a program of regular, sustained, antigravitational exercise throughout pregnancy and a group of matched physically active controls (adapted from Jackson et al., 1994).* Funct. Tiss. = functional tissue, I.V.S. = intervillous space vascular volume, and V.V.V. = villous vascular volume. Data are presented as means ± S.D. Significant between-group differences are noted by an asterisk.

umenting adverse fetal effects of continuing fairly intense and sustained exercise throughout pregnancy.

NUTRITIONAL CONCERNS

Energy Intake

There is concern that women who regularly exercise during pregnancy and lactation need to increase their energy intakes significantly to provide adequate calories for both the growth process and the exercise. All sanctioned nutritional recommendations reflect this concern (Food & Agriculture Organization, 1985; Institute of Medicine, 1990). However, recent data clearly indicate that both individual and societal variations are so great that general recommendations are simply not justified at this time (Dewey & McCrory, 1994; Goldberg et al., 1993; Heini et al., 1989; King et al., 1994; Prentice et al., 1989). For example, studies with both whole body calorimetry and doubly-labeled water indicate that the total increase in energy cost due to normal pregnancy in well-nourished, healthy women ranged from 34–1192 MJ (Goldberg et al., 1993; Prentice et al., 1989) and that the individual components of daily energy expenditure changed within an individual woman at different times during the pregnancy. For example, a decreased basal metabolic rate in early pregnancy may have been followed by an increased efficiency in physical activity in late pregnancy. This is particularly true for lean, hard-working populaces with marginal energy intakes who develop a marked increase in energy efficiency during pregnancy. The best example of this phenomenon comes from studies done with Gambian women who become so efficient during pregnancy that the energy demands of pregnancy range between -460 kJ/d to $+150$ kJ/d (Heini et al., 1989; Lawrence et al., 1987). Similar observations have recently been made during physical activity in the nonpregnant state (Leibel et al., 1995). Furthermore, the differences observed appear to be related to individual energy balance with a chronic negative balance decreasing the energy cost of a given physical task and visa versa. Thus, it appears that the most practical approach for assessing energy intake during pregnancy is the use of incremental weight gain coupled with estimates of maternal fat deposition and uterine growth. This approach would appear to be even more important in women who choose to maintain a vigorous exercise regimen during pregnancy.

Energy Mix, Iron, Calcium, Vitamins, and Micronutrient Content

While it is clear that nutrient composition and mix should be important during pregnancy and lactation, there is little objective data confirming exactly how much of what is actually required. Thus, while helpful, the current nutritional guidelines represent populace estimates only (King et al., 1994). These uncertainties are highlighted in areas such as the need for iron (Barton et al., 1994), calcium (Heaney & Skillman, 1971; Prentice, 1994) and folic acid (Rush, 1994) supplementation. Unfortunately, the same issues exist in the exercise arena.

Based on current knowledge (Heaney & Skillman, 1971; Institute of Medicine, 1990; King et al., 1994; Prentice, 1994), it would appear that a high-carbohydrate, low-fat diet containing 100 g of protein and 1–1.5 g of calcium daily should be adequate. Standard supplementation with iron and folic acid appears to offer some value, and additional basic, low-dose supplements of vitamins and micronutrients should provide protection, especially in complete vegetarians and in those with marginal dietary intakes.

Feeding Frequency and Timing of Exercise Relative to Nutrient Intake

During pregnancy, gastrointestinal symptomatology, i.e., the changes in anatomic configuration, gastric secretion, sphincteric tone, and transit times, coupled with a propensity for fasting hypoglycemia, suggests the need for a change in dietary habits (Freinkel et al., 1974; Hytten, 1991). As one might expect, small, frequent, low-fat feedings are usually well tolerated and ideal for most pregnant women. Likewise, scheduling exercise sessions at times when insulin levels are low (immediately before or three or more hours after food intake) promotes glycogenolysis and gluconeogenesis which, coupled with energy intake after exercise, should minimize the hypoglycemic response.

Breast Milk Composition and Infant Weight Gain

During lactation, there is concern that a regular exercise regimen may alter the quality and quantity of the milk and impair growth of the newborn. This has been accentuated by the dairy literature indicating that moderate exercise decreases milk production (Lamb et al., 1979) as well as by a study that noted a decrease in human infant suckling after a bout of maximal exercise due to lactic acid accumulation in breast milk (Wallace et al., 1992). However, high-intensity training studies in both rodents and humans clearly demonstrate that the quantity and quality (i.e. protein, fat, and mineral content) of milk and infant growth are not adversely affected by maternal exercise (Dewey et al., 1994; Dewey & McCrory, 1994; Karasawa et al., 1981; Lovelady et al., 1990; Treadway & Lederman, 1986).

EXERCISE, FITNESS, AND THE COURSE AND OUTCOME OF PREGNANCY

Conception and Early Pregnancy

Although there is very little information regarding the impact of regular exercise on either a woman's ability to conceive or early pregnancy events, it has been clearly documented that sudden increases in exercise load and/or the high levels of training found in elite athletes produce both ovulatory dysfunction and infertility (Bullen et al., 1985; Loucks et al., 1989). Nonetheless, in an ongoing prospective study, we have been unable to detect an increased incidence of infertility, abortion, ectopic implantation, or congenital malformation in more than 200 women who continued vigorous, endurance exercise regimens at a recreational level while attempting conception and throughout early pregnancy (Clapp, 1994). All exercised a minimum of three times weekly at intensities in excess of 50% $\dot{V}O_2$max for 20 min or more. The range in exercise rigor among subjects was wide, with mean values for frequency exceeding four times a week (range: 3–11); for intensity, 64% $\dot{V}O_2$max (range: 51–90%); and for duration, 47 min per session (range: 20–135 min).

There is no published information on the impact of beginning an exercise regimen during the periconceptional period. However, the work of Bullen et al. (1985) suggests that it is probably not the optimal time to start an intense training program because training clearly disrupts the normal rhythms of the hypothalamic-pituitary-ovarian axis as evidenced by ovulatory and menstrual dysfunction.

Physical and Emotional Well-Being

There is only one report of the effect of exercise on maternal well-being during pregnancy (Wallace et al., 1985). This study found that regular exercise clearly reduced the usual musculoskeletal complaints of pregnancy and improved self-esteem, and our findings indicate a virtual absence of discomfort of the low back or extremities as well as improved productivity and self-image as determined by direct interview (Clapp, 1994). However, about one in five women who continue with weight-bearing exercise develop a noticeable and bothersome degree of lower abdominal and/or pelvic discomfort during exercise, which is usually relieved almost completely by lower abdominal support with one of a variety of homemade or commercially available belts crafted for that purpose. The latter suggests that the etiology of the discomfort is related to uterine mobility, creating tension on the round ligaments and/or some degree of pelvic instability.

Gestational Length

Beginning or continuing regular exercise during pregnancy does not increase the incidence of either premature labor or premature rupture of the membranes (Clapp, 1994; Hatch et al., 1993; Lokey et al., 1991). However, as shown in Figure 10-5, when fit women continue regular, sustained exercise throughout late pregnancy, there is a shift to the left in

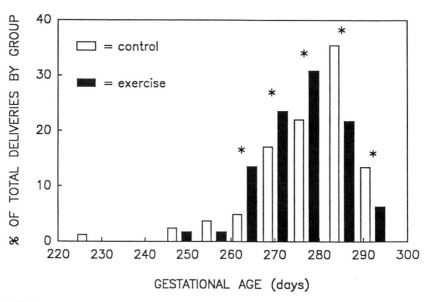

FIGURE 10-5. *The mean duration of pregnancy in women who continued a program of regular, sustained, antigravitational exercise throughout pregnancy and a group of matched physically active controls (adapted from Clapp, 1994).* Data are presented as the percent of total deliveries. Significant between-group differences are noted by an asterisk.

the timing of the onset of labor at term. As a result, their deliveries occur an average of five days earlier at term; e.g., 70% deliver on or before their estimated dates of confinement. This is viewed as a beneficial effect of exercise by most women and by those who care for them.

Length of Labor and Mode of Delivery

Most investigators find that exercise during pregnancy does not influence the course and outcome of labor, but two reports suggest that the expulsive phase of labor may be prolonged to some extent in Olympic athletes (Erdelyi, 1962; Hatch et al., 1993; Lokey et al., 1991; Zaharieva, 1972). Others note that the duration of labor is shorter in women who have continued a regular exercise program in late pregnancy (Beckmann & Beckmann, 1990; Clapp, 1990, 1994; Wong & McKenzie, 1987). However, the differences in the duration of labor noted in these studies are likely due to inaccuracies in methods used for data collection, sampling error, and differences in the various exercise variables.

Our study (Clapp, 1994) has eliminated most of these confounders and clearly demonstrates that fit women who continue vigorous exercise throughout late pregnancy, at the performance levels mentioned earlier, have much shorter labors, a low incidence of protraction and arrest disorders, and a threefold reduction in the need for operative delivery (both forceps and Caesarean section). As a result, the women who continue exercise have a 30% increase in the rate of spontaneous vaginal delivery with an active phase of labor that is one-third shorter on average.

Postpartum Recovery

While there is no published information on the effect of early postpartum exercise, most women in our study who continue exercise during pregnancy also continue to exercise after childbirth and begin within 2 wk of delivery. At the time of the 6 wk follow-up, they report a more rapid recovery in physical ability, emotional stability, and developing and mastering the new coping skills required (Clapp, 1994). Follow-up for one year indicates that this early resumption of exercise increased $\dot{V}O_2$max and did not contribute to the incidence of poor healing, heavy bleeding, infection, urinary incontinence, sexual malfunction, undue ligamentous laxity, or persistence of diastasis recti. During lactation the rate of loss body weight and fat mass in exercising women is no different from that seen in the matched control populace (Dewey et al., 1994; Little et al., 1994). However, the impact of regular exercise on postpartum weight loss has not been assessed in nonlactating women.

Neurodevelopmental Outcome

In most studies information on neurodevelopmental outcome has been limited to reports of normal Apgar Scores and condition at birth.

However, the issue is extremely important and should be addressed in greater detail in future studies. Recently presented preliminary observations in our exercise populace made at 5 d, 1 y, and 5 y of age have been reassuring (Clapp et al., 1995c), but the populace we have studied is a highly select one.

TRAINING DURING PREGNANCY

Actual and Theoretical Effects

All studies that have examined indices of fitness find that beginning or continuing a regular exercise regimen during pregnancy improves maternal fitness without identifiable risk (Clapp & Capeless, 1991b; Collings & Curet, 1983; Sibley et al., 1981; South-Paul et al., 1988; Wong & McKenzie, 1987). In addition, the physiological effects of exercise on the maternal adaptations to pregnancy suggest that regular physical activity prior to and during pregnancy should be encouraged because it appears to enhance the physiological reserve of a pregnant woman. Theoretically, this should be of benefit to both mother and fetus if complications ensue.

Recommendations for Exercise Prescription during Pregnancy

The data currently available do not support the idea that detailed exercise prescriptions should be viewed as a necessary safety measure for most healthy, physically active, pregnant women. Therefore, this section articulates a common-sense approach to exercise prescription during pregnancy that may be useful in advising otherwise healthy women who have specific questions or wish to begin or maintain a serious, goal-oriented exercise program during pregnancy. Its basic premise is that, save for a few pregnancy-related considerations, the approach should be no different than that used with a nonpregnant individual who desires help developing a goal-oriented exercise plan. A holistic approach is recommended as it is usually most effective; i.e., education, instruction, evaluation, goal setting, monitoring, safety, and interactive components should all be considered.

Education. As knowledge and compliance go hand in hand, exercising women should have a clear understanding of the theoretical concerns and risks that underlie the current sanctioned guidelines as well as the more positive outcome data detailed above. They should also be reasonably versed in the impact that pregnancy has on exercise responses and vice versa, and recognize that pregnancy, like fitness, requires commitment, flexibility, and occasional compromise. Finally, the few common-sense contraindications to exercise during pregnancy should be discussed, and the woman should be given a list of these as a reminder. For an otherwise healthy woman, the minimal list should include: localized pain, hemorrhage, persistent uterine contractions, physician concern that the pregnancy has complications (such as poor fetal growth or twins), and any sudden change in feelings of well-being.

Developing the Training Regimen. The same approach should be used in developing the training regimen for a pregnant woman as would be used if she were not pregnant. The first step is an equally detailed assessment of each woman's fitness level and current training status. Realistic training goals should be developed that will meet her needs within a framework that will avoid boredom, minimize injury risk, and maintain or enhance both fitness and function. The importance of rest-activity cycles, hydration, and nutrition should be stressed, and they should be built into the overall training program. Exercise sessions should be scheduled before or at least three hours after meals and followed with a snack to compensate for the decrease in the counter-regulatory responses to hypoglycemia that occurs in pregnancy. Initially, performance of each activity should be observed to assure that it is being carried out correctly. A log should be kept, and a plan for monitoring the progress of both the training and the pregnancy should also be developed and incorporated into the plan. Finally, consideration should be given to equipment, the training site, and the training environment. Shoes should be replaced frequently, protective gear should be worn, running and walking surfaces should be even, and extremely hot and humid conditions should be avoided.

The initial fitness plan should be assessed periodically to determine if it is achieving its original goals and/or if changes in the type, frequency, and intensity of the exercise are indicated. For example, weight training may become necessary to maintain adequate upper body strength in a gymnast, or water running may be used to replace outdoor running under severe winter conditions.

Modifying the Training Regimen. There are three reasons to modify the training regimen. First, symptoms of under- or overtraining are indications that modification may be necessary. As heart rate is a relatively unreliable parameter during pregnancy, perceived exertion and/or actual oxygen consumption should used to assess intensity. A two-point shift in an individual's level of perceived exertion indicates the need to either increase or decrease the work load (speed, frequency, or range of motion). Additional tests of performance are also useful (strength, speed over distance, etc.). Symptoms of fatigue, localized pain, and poor performance indicate the need for action and suggest worn equipment or overtraining in the pregnant as well as the nonpregnant woman.

Second, if the activity elicits an unusual and/or potentially deleterious physiological response (unusual cardiac activity, pain, hyperthermia, etc.), it should be modified. For example, serious athletes who incorporate extremely intense forms of training such as plyometrics, bounding, and/or vertical climbers in their regimens may overwhelm their abilities to dissipate heat and may raise their rectal temperatures well over 39°C.. A modification of the training program is also in order for women who experience recurrent discomfort associated with a particular activity, or a protracted hypoglycemic response that may be initiated by a prolonged relatively low-intensity workout. Third, if the pregnancy is not entirely normal, modifications may be required. Examples include: multiple pregnancy, uterine malformation, vascular disease, bleeding, anomalous placentation, poor uterine growth, or evidence of early cervical change.

Monitoring. During pregnancy and lactation, maternal well-being, and fetal/infant well-being should be monitored along with the exercise *per se*. In general, the extent of the monitoring should vary directly with the intensity and overall level of the training program. Thus, the monitoring may range from nothing more than routine obstetrical care to periodic evaluation of both maternal and fetal responses in an exercise testing facility. In our experience, the most difficult issues for the mother involve hydration and rest-activity cycles. Simply put, urine in the toilet bowl should have no color, weight loss during a single training session should not exceed 0.8–1 kg, and each hour of exercise should be matched by an hour of daytime rest to avoid signs of dehydration (such as increased uterine contractility) and symptoms of fatigue. In our experience (Clapp, 1994; Clapp & Little, 1995), evidence of progressive fat deposition and weight gain through the seventh month is the best index of adequate energy intake, and weekly self-assessment of discomfort, pain, or undue fatigue should be used to modify the exercise regimen and/or other aspects of an individual's lifestyle.

In terms of the fetus, evidence of normal placental transfer function and growth appear to be the most important variables. When indicated, the former is best monitored by periodically assessing the fetal heart rate response to exercise, a response that should reflect oxygen delivery (Clapp et al., 1993), and the latter by assessing the serial changes in fundal height with or without concomitant ultrasound assessment. Intermittent examination of the cervix is often used as reassurance regarding the possibility of premature labor.

In terms of the exercise, it is important to intermittently assess the thermal, metabolic, and uterine response to a typical exercise session in most competitive athletes adhering to a training regimen, as well as in women who work out at high intensity for more than 30 min per session and in those who engage in over-distance types of workouts that last an hour or more. When indicated, the woman should periodically check her rectal or vaginal temperature immediately before and after exercise and/ or whenever she feels unusually hot, as individual discomfort is usually a good index of a biologically significant increase in core temperature. This is best done using an inexpensive electronic thermometer that can be purchased at most drug stores. Based on current information, a reasonable and practical guideline is that rectal temperature should rise no more than

1.5–1.8°C and not exceed an absolute value of 38.7°C on a regular basis or for a protracted period of time. The latter value is an arbitrary one, picked because it is 0.5°C below the commonly accepted teratogenic level (Clapp, 1989b; Milunsky et al., 1992).

The extent of metabolic monitoring should vary directly with training volume. At the low end, it involves simply an objective rating of perceived exertion, sensations of lightheadedness, or hunger after exercise. At the high end, it should include daily measurement of pulse rate and perceived exertion with periodic measurement of oxygen consumption and substrate levels in a laboratory setting before, during, and after an exercise session at the heart rate and perceived exertion experienced in the field. In these individuals the requisite objective measures of body composition, training session weight loss, fetal heart rate response, etc., can be conveniently obtained at this time.

As premature labor does occur with equal frequency in women who exercise as in those who do not, periodically monitoring subjective uterine activity after a training session may provide a unique opportunity for early risk detection. While symptoms of contractile activity are very common during exercise in middle and late pregnancy, their persistence for 15–30 min after the exercise is completed is distinctly uncommon. Therefore, although currently unproven, it appears prudent to suggest that active women monitor their post-exercise sensations of uterine activity once a week after 20 wk. If contractile activity persists for 30 min, more formal evaluation is indicated.

Limitations and Safety Considerations. Clearly, deficiencies in our knowledge indicate that there is a need to set a few limitations until more information is available in specific areas. For example, although the physiological adaptations to pregnancy may give a woman a competitive edge in early pregnancy (Clapp & Capeless, 1991b; Cohen et al., 1989; Higdon, 1981; Sady & Carpenter, 1989; Villarosa, 1985), it probably is important to avoid serious competition and the all-out, prolonged effort it entails until we learn more about the effect of such exercise on the embryo. Likewise, information from automobile accidents and other sources of trauma clearly demonstrate that there is significant risk associated with both penetrating and blunt abdominal trauma after the 16th week (Sherer & Schenker, 1989). Thus, consideration should be given to modifying or eliminating performance of specific types of recreational exercise that carry similar risk (e.g., horseback riding, gymnastics, water skiing, rock climbing, and hockey). It appears that we do not have the appropriate information to determine if the decompression sequences that are a part of scuba diving are altered by the need for diffusional transfer of gases from the fetus across the placenta to the mother. The same is true for oxygen transfer during sustained exercise at altitudes >3,000 m (U.S.D.H.H.S., 1983). Thus, it seems prudent to avoid high-altitude climbing and skiing as well as scuba diving at or near a depth that requires decompression (or at least extending recommended decompression times by 50% until more is known). Finally, it should be recognized that our collective experience with women who wish to maintain a serious training regimen ($>$400 h/y) is both limited and decentralized. Therefore, if they choose to proceed, such women should be encouraged to have themselves intensively monitored to ensure maximal benefit while minimizing the chance of a poor outcome.

DIRECTIONS FOR FUTURE RESEARCH

The multiple broad areas that warrant further study have been recently reviewed by a task force (Clapp et al., 1992). Three specific areas will be mentioned here. First, the lower and upper levels of rigor (frequency, duration, intensity) for exercise during pregnancy should be determined, and the specific parameters that characterize both threshold and dose-response effects should be identified. In this regard, two important outcome variables that can be precisely and objectively measured are plasma volume and birth weight for gestational age. Another area of interest that has potential therapeutic value would be to assess the physiological effects of introducing training of different types at various time points in the course of pregnancy. For example, it is often stated that swimming may be the ideal training exercise for pregnant women. Is that true? Currently, only limited acute response data comparing swimming to cycle ergometry are available. Finally, the use of exercise training as a therapy for a variety of diseases unique to pregnancy is an exciting and unexplored area. Several potential adverse outcomes of pregnancy that might be positively influenced by the effects of exercise on cardiovascular function and metabolism include gestational diabetes, hypertensive disease, and the history or presence of suboptimal fetal growth. Ironically, the latter two are currently managed by restricting physical activity.

SUMMARY

As a whole, the information currently available does not support a restrictive approach to strenuous recreational physical activity during pregnancy. The data indicate that the discrepancy between the theoretical concern and the observed positive outcome of participation in exercise during pregnancy is probably due to the fact that the physiological adaptations to regular exercise actually enhance adaptations to the pregnancy. In fact, the evidence suggests that regular, sustained physical activity, sufficient to either maintain or improve fitness, has additional physiologic benefits for both the woman and the pregnancy. Therefore, although our knowledge is still incomplete and descriptive, it appears that the inclusion of recreational exercise with specific training objectives as a part of antenatal care for the motivated, healthy woman is reasonable. To be sure that this is the case at a societal as well as an individual level, there is a need for prospective, randomized studies with monitored, quantified, exercise regimens that incorporate objective measures of physiological effects and both short- and long-term outcomes.

ACKNOWLEDGEMENTS

Much of the work discussed in this manuscript was supported by grants # RO1-21268 and # P50-211089 from the National Institutes of Health, several grants from the National Foundation March of Dimes, and the generous support of MetroHealth Medical Center.

In addition, the work would not have been possible without the work of a dedicated staff and the large number of women who gave freely of their time, energy, and sweat, which ultimately made these studies possible.

BIBLIOGRAPHY

Abramson, D., S.M. Robert, and P.D. Wilson (1934). Relaxation of the pelvic joints in pregnancy. *Surg. Gynecol. Obstet.* 58:595–613.

American College of Obstetricians and Gynecologists, (1994). Exercise during pregnancy and the postpartum period. *Technical Bulletin #189* Washington, D.C.: ACOG Press.

Andersen, P., and J. Henriksson (1977). Capillary supply of the quadriceps femoris muscle of man: adaptive response to exercise. *J. Physiol. (London)* 270:677–691.

Artal, R., S. Rutherford, T. Romen, R.K. Kammula, F.J. Dorey, and R.A. Wiswell (1986a). Fetal heart rate responses to maternal exercise. *Am. J. Obstet. Gynecol.* 155:729–733.

Artal, R., R. Wiswell, Y. Romem, and F. Dorey (1986b). Pulmonary responses to exercise in pregnancy. *Am. J. Obstet. Gynecol.* 154:378–383.

Barron, W.M., S.K. Mujais, M. Zinaman, E.L. Bravo, and M.D. Lindheimer (1986). Plasma catacholamine responses to physiological stimuli in normal human pregnancy. *Am. J. Obstet. Gynecol.* 154:80–84.

Barton, D.P.J., M.T. Joy, T.R.J. Lappin, M. Afrasiabi, J.G. Morel, J. O'Riordan, J.F. Murphy, and C. O'Herlihy (1994). Maternal erythropoietin in singleton pregnancies: a randomized trial on the effects of oral hematinic supplementation. *Am. J. Obstet. Gynecol.* 170:896–901.

Beckmann, C.R.B., and C.A. Beckmann (1990). Effect of a structured antepartum exercise program on pregnancy and labor outcome in primiparas. *J. Reprod. Med.* 35:704–709.

Benjamin, F. (1960). Basal body temperature recordings in gynaecology and obstetrics. *J. Obstet. Gynaecol. Brit. Emp.* 67:177–192.

Berg, G., M. Hammer, J. Moller-Neison, U. Linden, and J. Thorblad (1988). Low back pain during pregnancy. *Obstet. Gynecol.* 71:71–74.

Blomqvist, C.G., and B. Saltin (1983). Cardiovascular adaptations to physical training. *Ann. Rev. Physiol.* 45:169–189.

Bonnen, A., P. Campagna, L. Gilchrist, D.C. Young, and P. Beresford (1992). Substrate and endocrine responses during exercise at selected stages of pregnancy. *J. Appl. Physiol.* 73:134–142.

Bullen, B.A., G.S. Skrinar, I.Z. Beitins, G. Von Mering, B.A. Turnbull, and J.W. MacArthur (1985). Induction of menstrual disorders by strenuous exercise in untrained women. *New Eng. J. Med.* 312:1349–1353.

Burt, C. (1949). Periperal skin temperature in normal pregnancy. *Lancet* 2:787–790.

Calganeri, M., H.A. Bird, and V. Wright (1982). Changes in joint laxity occurring during pregnancy. *Ann. Rheum. Dis.* 41:126–128.

Capeless, E.L., and J.F. Clapp (1989). Cardiovascular changes in early phase of pregnancy. *Am. J. Obstet. Gynecol.* 161:1449–1453.

Capeless, E.L., and J.F. Clapp (1991). When do cardiovascular parameters return to their preconception values? *Am. J. Obstet. Gynecol.* 165:883–886.

Carpenter, M.W., S.P. Sady, B. Hoegsberg, M.A. Sady, B. Haydon, E.M. Cullinane, D.R. Coustan, and P.D. Thompson (1988). Fetal heart rate response to maternal exertion. *J.A.M.A.* 259:3000–3009.

Carpenter, M.W., S.P. Sady, M.A. Sady, B. Haydon, D.R. Coustan, and P.D. Thompson (1990). Effect of maternal weight gain during pregnancy on exercise performance. *J. Appl. Physiol.* 68:1173–1176.

Clapp, J.F. (1985). Fetal heart rate response to running in mid and late pregnancy. *Am. J. Obstet. Gynecol.* 153:251–252.

Clapp, J.F. (1989a). Oxygen consumption during treadmill exercise before, during, and after pregnancy. *Am. J. Obstet. Gynecol.* 161:1458–1464.

Clapp, J.F. (1989b). Pregnancy. In: B.A. Franklin, S. Gordon, and G.C. Timmis (eds.) *Exercise in Modern Medicine.* Baltimore: Williams and Wilkins, pp. 268–279.

Clapp, J.F. (1990). The course and outcome of labor following endurance exercise during pregnancy. *Am. J. Obstet. Gynecol.* 163:1799–1805.

Clapp, J.F. (1991a). The changing thermal response to endurance exercise during pregnancy. *Am. J. Obstet. Gynecol.* 165:1684–1689.

Clapp, J.F. (1991b). Exercise and fetal health. *J. Dev. Physiol.* 15:9–14.

Clapp, J.F. (1994). A clinical approach to exercise during pregnancy. *Clin. Sports Med.* 13:443–457.

Clapp, J.F., and E.L. Capeless (1990). Neonatal morphometrics following endurance exercise during pregnancy. *Am. J. Obstet. Gynecol.* 163:1805–1811.

Clapp, J.F., and E.L. Capeless (1991a). The changing glycemic response to exercise during pregnancy. *Am. J. Obstet. Gynecol.* 165:1678–1683.

Clapp, J.F., and E.L. Capeless (1991b). The $\dot{V}O_2$max of recreational athletes before and after pregnancy. *Med. Sci. Sports Exerc.* 23:1128–1133.

Clapp, J.F., and S. Dickstein (1984). Endurance exercise and pregnancy outcome. *Med. Sci. Sports Exerc.* 16:556–562.

Clapp, J.F., and K.D. Little (1995). The effect of endurance exercise on pregnancy weight gain and subcutaneous fat deposition. *Med. Sci. Sports Exerc.* 27:170–177.

Clapp, J.F., E.L. Capeless, K.H. Rizk, and S. Appleby-Wineberg (1995a). The vascular remodelling of pregnancy persists 1 year postpartum. *J. Soc. Gynecol. Invest.* 2:292.

Clapp, J.F., K.D. Little, S.K. Appleby-Wineburg, and J.A. Widness (1995b). The effect of regular maternal exercise on erythropoietin in cord blood and amniotic fluid. *Am. J. Obstet. Gynecol.* 172:1445–1450.

Clapp, J.F., K.D. Little, and E.L. Capeless (1993). Fetal heart rate response to various intensities of recreational exercise during mid and late pregnancy. *Am. J. Obstet. Gynecol.* 168:198–206.

Clapp, J.F., K.D. Little, K.H. Rizk, and S. Appleby-Wineberg (1994). Pregnancy alters the cardiovascular response to mock hemorrhage. *Proc. Soc. Gynecol. Invest.* 41:280.

Clapp, J.F., and K.H. Rizk (1992). Effect of recreational exercise on mid-trimester placental growth. *Am. J. Obstet. Gynecol.* 167:1518–1521.

Clapp, J.F., R. Rokey, J.L. Treadway, M.W. Carpenter, R.M. Artal, and C. Warrnes (1992). Exercise in pregnancy. *Med. Sci. Sports Exerc.* 24:S294–S300.

Clapp, J.F., S.J. Simonian, R.A. Harcar-Sevcik, B. Lopez, and S. Appleby-Wineberg (1995c). Morphometric and neurodevelopmental outcome after exercise during pregnancy. *Med. Sci. Sports Exerc.* 27:S74.

Clapp, J.F., B.L. Seaward, and R.H. Sleamaker (1988). Maternal physiologic adaptations to early human pregnancy. *Am. J. Obstet. Gynecol.* 159:1456–1460.

Clapp, J.F., M. Wesley, and R.H. Sleamaker (1987). Thermoregulatory and metabolic responses to jogging prior to and during pregnancy. *Med. Sci. Sports Exerc.* 19:124–130.

Coggan, A.R., W.M. Kohrt, R.J. Sina, D.M. Bier, and J.O. Holloszy (1990). Endurance training decreases glucose turnover and oxidation during moderate intensity exercise in men. *J. Appl. Physiol.* 68:990–996.

Cohen, G.C., J.C. Prior, Y. Vigna, and S.M. Pride (1989). Intense exercise during the first two trimesters of unapparent pregnancy. *Phys. Sportsmed.* 17:87–94.

Collings, C.A., and L.B. Curet (1985). Fetal heart rate response to maternal exercise. *Am. J. Obstet. Gynecol.* 151:498–501.

Collings, C.A., L.B. Curet, and J.P. Mullen (1983). Maternal and fetal responses to a maternal aerobic exercise program. *Am. J. Obstet. Gynecol.* 146:702–707.

Crandall, M.E., T.M. Keve, and M.K. McLaughlin (1990). Characterization of norepinephrine sensitivity in the maternal splanchnic circulation during pregnancy. *Am. J. Obstet. Gynecol.* 162:1296–1301.

Dale, E., K.M. Mullinax, and D.H. Bryan (1982). Exercise during pregnancy: effects on the fetus. *Can. J. Appl. Sports Sci.* 7:98–102.

Davidge, S.T., and M.K. McLaughlin (1992). Endogenous modulation of the blunted adrenergic response in resistance-sized mesenteric arteries from the pregnant rat. *Am. J. Obstet. Gynecol.* 167:1691–1698.

DeSwiet, M. (1991). The respiratory system. In: F. Hytten and G. Chamberlain (eds.) *Clinical Physiology in Obstetrics.* London: Blackwell Scientific, pp. 83–100.

Dewey, K.G., C.A. Lovelady, L.A. Nommsen-Rivers, M.A. McCrory, and B. Lonnerdal (1994). A randomized study of the effects of aerobic exercise by lactating women on breast-milk volume and composition. *New Eng. J. Med.* 330:449–453.

Dewey, K.G., and M.A. McCrory (1994). Effects of dieting and physical activity on pregnancy and lactation. *Am. J. Clin. Nutr.* 59:446S–453S.

Drinkwater, B.L., and C.H. Chesnut III (1991). Bone density changes during pregnancy and lactation in active women. *Bone Mineral* 14:153–160.

Drinkwater, B.L., K. Milson, C.H. Chestnut, III, W.J. Bremner, S. Shainholtz, and M.B. Southworth (1984). Bone mineral content of amenorrheic and eumenorrheic runners. *N. Engl. J. Med.* 311:277–281.

Durak, E.P., L. Jovanovic-Peterson, and C.M. Peterson (1990). Comparative evaluation of uterine response to exercise on five aerobic machines. *Am. J. Obstet. Gynecol.* 162:754–756.

Duvekot, J.J., E.C. Cheriex, F.A. Pieters, P.P. Menheere, and L.H. Peeters (1993). Early pregnancy changes in hemodynamics and volume homeostasis are consecutive adjustments triggered by a primary fall in vascular tone. *Am. J. Obstet. Gynecol.* 169:1382–1392.

Ellis, M.I., B.B. Seedhom, and V. Wright (1985). Forces in women 36 weeks pregnant and four weeks after delivery. *Engineering Med.* 14:95–99.

Erdelyi, G.J. (1962). Gynecological survey of female athletes. *J. Sports Med. Phys. Fitness* 2:174–179.

Erkkola, R.U., J.P. Pirhonen, and A.K. Kivvijarvi (1992). Flow velocity waveforms in uterine and umbilical arteries during submaximal bicycle exercise in normal pregnancy. *Obstet. Gynecol.* 79:611–615.

Food and Agricultural Organization, WHO, United Nations University (1985). Energy and Protein Requirements. *WHO Tech. Rep. Series* 724:84–85.

Fraser, R.B., F.A. Ford, and G.F. Lawrence (1988). Insulin sensitivity in third trimester pregnancy. A randomized study of dietary effects. *Brit. J. Obstet. Gynaecol.* 95:223–229.

Freinkel, N., B.E. Metzger, M. Nitzan, A. Daniel, B.Z. Surmaczynska, and T. Nagel (1974). Facilitated anabolism in late pregnancy. In: W.J. Malaisse, J. Pirart, and J. Vallance (eds.) *Diabetes Mellitus Proceedings of the Eighth Congress of I.D.F.* Amsterdam: Exerpta Medica, pp. 478–488.

Giraud, G.A., M.J. Morton, L.E. Davis, M.S. Paul, and K.L. Thornburg (1993). Estrogen-induced left ventricular chamber enlargement in ewes. *Am. J. Physiol.* 264:E490–E496.

Goldberg, G.R., A.M. Prentice, W.A. Coward, H.L. Davies, P.R. Murgatroyd, C. Wensing, A.E. Black, M. Harding, and M. Sawyer (1993). Longitudinal assessment of energy expenditure in pregnancy by the doubly labeled water method. *Am. J. Clin. Nutr.* 57:494–505.

Gollnick, P.D. (1985). Metabolism of substrates: energy substrate metabolism during exercise and as modified by training. *Fed. Proc.* 44:353–357.

Gollnick, P.D., B.F. Timson, R.L. Moore, and M. Riedy (1981). Muscular enlargement and number of fibers in skeletal muscles of rat. *J. Appl. Physiol.* 50:936–943.

Hall, D.C., and D.A. Kaufmann (1987). Effects of aerobic strength and conditioning on pregnancy outcomes. *Am. J. Obstet. Gynecol.* 157:1199–1203.

Hart, M.V., J.D. Hosenpud, A.R. Hohimer, and M.J. Morton (1985). Hemodynamics during pregnancy and sex steroid administration in guinea pigs. *Am. J. Physiol.* 249:R179–R185.

Hart, M.V., M.J. Morton, J.D. Hosenpud, and J. Metcalfe (1986). Aortic function during normal human pregnancy. *Am. J. Obstet. Gynecol.* 154:887–891.

Hatch, C.M., X.O. Shu, D.E. McLean, B. Levin, M. Begg, L. Reuss, and M. Susser (1993). Maternal exercise during pregnancy, physical fitness, and fetal growth. *Am. J. Epidemiol.* 137:1105–1114.

Hauth, J.C., L.C. Gilstrap, and K. Widmer (1982). Fetal heart rate reactivity before and after maternal jogging during the third trimester. *Am. J. Obstet. Gynecol.* 142:545–547.

Heaney, R.P., and T.G. Skillman (1971). Calcium metabolism in normal human pregnancy. *J. Clin. Endocr. Metab.* 33:661–676.

Heini, A., Y. Schutz, and E. Jequier (1989). Total daily energy expenditure and heart rate during pregnancy in free-living Gambian women. *Nestle Foundation Annual Report.* Nestle Foundation, Lausanne, Switzerland, pp. 43–54.

Henriksson, J. (1977). Training induced adaptation of skeletal muscle and metabolism during submaximal exercise. *J. Physiol.* 270:661–675.

Higdon, H. (1981). Running through pregnancy. *The Runner* 4(3):46–51.

Hodgen, G.D., and J. Iskovitz (1988). Recognition and maintenance of pregnancy. In: E. Knobil, and J. Neil (eds.) *The Physiology of Reproduction.* New York: Raven Press, pp. 82–108.

Hytten, F.E. (1991). The alimentary system. In: F. Hytten and G. Chamberlain (eds.) *Clinical Physiology in Obstetrics*, 2nd edition, London: Blackwell Scientific, pp. 137–149.

Hytten, F.E., A.M. Thompson, and N. Taggart (1966). Total body water in normal pregnancy. *J. Obstet. Gynaecol. Brit. Comm.* 73:553–561.

Institute of Medicine, Food and Nutrition Board, Committee on Nutritional Status During Pregnancy and Lactation (1990). *Nutrition During Pregnancy*, Parts I and II. Washington: National Academy Press.

Jackson, M.A., P. Gott, S.J. Lye, J.W. Knox Ritchie, and J.F. Clapp (1995). The effect of maternal aerobic exercise on human placental development: placental volumetric composition and surface areas. *Placenta* 16:179–191.

Jones, R.L., J.J. Botti, W.M. Anderson, and N.L. Bennett (1985). Thermoregulation during aerobic exercise in pregnancy. *Obstet. Gynecol.* 65:340–345.

Karasawa, K., J. Suwa, and S. Kimura (1981). Voluntary lactation during pregnancy and lactation and its effects on lactational performance in mice. *J. Nutr. Sci. Vitam.* 27:333–339.

Karzel, R.P., and M.J. Friedman (1991). Orthopedic injuries during pregnancy. In: R.A. Mittlemark, R.A. Wiswell, and B.L. Drinkwater (eds.) *Exercise in Pregnancy*, 2nd edition. Baltimore: Williams and Wilkins, pp. 123–132.

Katz, M., and M.M. Sokal (1980). Skin perfusion in pregnancy. *Am. J. Obstet. Gynecol.* 137:30–33.

Katz, V.L., R. McMurray, M.J. Berry, and R.C. Cefalo (1988). Fetal and uterine responses to immersion and exercise. *Obstet. Gynecol.* 72:225–230.

King, J.C., N.F. Butte, M.N. Bronstein, L.E. Kopp, and S.A. Lindquist (1994). Energy metabolism during pregnancy: influence of maternal energy status. *Am. J. Clin. Nutr.* 59:439S–445S.

Knuttgen, H.G., and K. Emerson (1974). Physiological response to pregnancy at rest and during exercise. *J. Appl. Physiol.* 36:549–553.

Kramer, F.M., A.J. Stunkard, K.A. Marshall, S. McKinney, and J. Liebschutz (1993). Breast-feeding reduces maternal lower body fat. *J. Am. Diet. Assoc.* 93:429–433.

Kulpa, P.J., B.M. White, and R. Visscher (1987). Aerobic exercise in pregnancy. *Am. J. Obstet. Gynecol.* 156:1395–1403.

Lamb, R., M. Anderson, and J. Walters (1979). The effects of forced exercise on two-year old holstein heifers. *J. Dairy Sci.* 62:1791–1797.

Lawrence, M., F. Lawrence, W.A. Coward, T.J. Cole, and R.G. Whitehead (1987). Energy requirements of pregnancy in the gambia. *Lancet* 2:1072–1076.

Lees, M.M., S.H. Taylor, D.B. Scott, and M.G. Kerr (1967). A study of cardiac output at rest throughout pregnancy. *J. Obstet. Gynaecol. Br. Comm.* 74:499–506.

Leibel, R.L., M. Rosenbaum, and J. Hirsch (1995). Changes in energy expenditure resulting from altered body weight. *New Eng. J. Med.* 332:622–628.

Little, K.D., J.F. Clapp, and P.J. Gott (1993). Bone density changes during pregnancy and lactation in exercising women. *Med. Sci. Sports Exerc.* 25:S154.

Little, K.D., J.F. Clapp, and S.E. Ridzon (1994). Effect of exercise on post partum weight loss. *Med. Sci. Sports Exerc.* 26:S15.

Lokey, E.A., Z.V. Tran, C.L. Wells, B.C. Myers, and A.C. Tran (1991). Effect of physical exercise on pregnancy outcomes: a meta-analytic review. *Med. Sci. Sports Exerc.* 23:1234–1239.

Lotgering, F.K., M.B. Van Dorn, P.C. Struijk, J. Pool, and H.C.S. Wallenburg (1991). Maximal aerobic exercise in pregnant women: heart rate, O_2 consumption, CO_2 production and ventilation. *J. Appl. Physiol.* 70:1016–1023.

Loucks, A.B, J.F. Mortola, L. Girton, and S.S.C. Yen (1989). Alterations in the hypothalamic-pituitary-ovarian and the hypothalamic-pituitary-adrenal axes in athletic women. *J. Clin. Endocrin. Metab.* 68:402–411.

Lovelady, C.A., B. Lonnerdal, and K.G. Dewey (1990). Lactation performance of exercising women. *Am. J. Clin. Nutr.* 52:103–109.

Marsal, K., O. Lofgren, and G. Gennser (1979). Fetal breathing movements and maternal exercise. *Acta. Obstet. Gynecol. Scand.* 58:197–201.

McGinnis, J.M. (1992). The public health burden of a sedentary lifestyle. *Med. Sci. Sports Exerc.* 4:S196–S200.

McNitt-Gray, J.L. (1991). Biomechanics related to exercise in pregnancy. In: R.A. Mittlemark, R.A. Wiswell, and B.L. Drinkwater (eds.) *Exercise in Pregnancy*, 2nd edition. Baltimore: Williams and Wilkins, pp. 133–140.

Milunsky, A., M. Ulcickas, K.J. Rothman, W. Willett, S. Jick, and H. Jick (1992) Maternal heat exposure and neural tube defects. *J.A.M.A.* 268:882–885.

Morrow, R.J., J.W.K. Ritchie, and S.B. Bull (1989). Fetal and maternal hemodynamic responses to exercise in pregnancy assessed by doppler. *Am. J. Obstet. Gynecol.* 160:138–140.

Nisell, H., P. Hjemdahl, and B. Linde (1985a). Cardiovascular responses to circulating catacholamines in normal pregnancy and in pregnancy-induced hypertension. *Clin. Physiol.* 5:479–493.

Nisell, H., P. Hjemdahl, B. Linde, and N.-O. Lunell (1985b). Sympatho-adrenal and cardiovascular reactivity in pregnancy induced hypertension. I. Responses to isometric exercise and a cold pressor test. *Brit. J. Obstet. Gynaecol.* 92:722–731.

Palone, A.M., C.H. Wells, and G.T. Kelly (1978). Sexual variations in thermoregulation during heat stress. *Aviat. Space Environ. Med.* 49:715–719.

Pernoll, M.L., J. Metcalfe, P.A. Kovach, R. Watchel, and M.J. Durham (1975a). Ventilation during rest and exercise in pregnancy and postpartum. *Resp. Physiol.* 25:295–310.

Pernoll, M.L., J. Metcalfe, T.L. Schlenker, J.E. Welch, and J.A. Matsumoto (1975b). Oxygen consumption at rest and during exercise in pregnancy. *Resp. Physiol.* 25:285–294.

Pipers, L., J.W. Wladimiroff, and J. McGhie (1984). Effect of short-term maternal exercise on maternal and fetal cardiovascular dynamics. *Brit. J. Obstet. Gynecol.* 91:1081–1086.

Pivarnik, J.M., W. Lee, S.L. Clark, D.B. Cotton, M.T. Spillman, and J.F. Miller (1990). Cardiac output responses of primigravid women during exercise determined by the direct Fick technique. *Obstet. Gynecol.* 75:954–959.

Pivarnik, J.M., W. Lee, T. Spillman, D.B. Cotton, and J.F. Miller (1992). Maternal respiration and blood gases during aerobic exercise performed at moderate altitude. *Med. Sci. Sports Exerc.* 24:868–872.

Pivarnik, J.M., M.B. Mauer, N.A. Ayres, B. Kirshon, G.A. Dildy, and D.B. Cotton (1994). Effect of chronic exercise on blood volume expansion and hematologic indicies during pregnancy. *Obstet. Gynecol.* 83:265–269.

Pomerance, J.J., L. Gluck, and V.A. Lynch (1979). Maternal exercise as a screening test for uteroplacental insufficiency. *Obstet. Gynecol.* 44:383–387.

Prentice, A. (1994). Maternal calcium requirements during pregnancy and lactation. *Am. J. Clin. Nutr.* 59:477S–483S.

Prentice, A.M., G.R. Goldberg, H.L. Davies, P.R. Murgatroyd, and W. Scott (1989). Energy-sparing adaptations in human pregnancy assessed by whole-body calorimetry. *Brit. J. Nutr.* 62:5–22.

Prior, J.C. (1990). Progesterone as a bone trophic hormone. *Endocr. Rev.* 1:386-398.

Roberts, M.F., C.B. Wenger, J.A.J. Stolwijk, and E.R. Nadel (1977). Skin blood flow and sweating changes following exercise training and heat acclimation. *J. Appl. Physiol.* 43:133-137.

Robson, S.C., R. Boys, W. Dunlop, and S. Hunter (1987). Haemodynamic changes during early human pregnancy: an M mode and doppler study. *Br. Heart J.* 57:584-585.

Robson, S.C., S. Hunter, R.J. Boys, and W. Dunlop (1989). Serial study of factors influencing changes in cardiac output during human pregnancy. *Am. J. Physiol.* 256:H1060-H1065.

Rowell, L.B., J.R. Blackmon, R.H. Martin, J.A. Mazzarella, and R.A. Bruce (1965). Hepatic clearances of indocyanine green in man under thermal and exercise stresses. *J. Appl. Physiol.* 20:384-394.

Rozycki, T.J. (1984). Oral and rectal temperature in runners. *Phys. Sportsmed.* 12:105-108.

Rush, D. (1994). Periconceptional folate and neural tube defect. *Am. J. Clin. Nutr.* 59:511S-516S.

Ryan, E.A., M.J. O'Sullivan, and J.S. Skyler (1985). Insulin action during pregnancy. Studies with the euglycemic clamp technique. *Diab.* 34:380-389.

Saar, E., R. Chayoth, and N. Meyerstein (1986). Physical activity and blood presure in normotensive young women. *Eur. J. Appl. Physiol.* 55:64-67.

Sady, S.P., and M.W. Carpenter (1989). Aerobic exercise during pregnancy: special considerations. *Sports Med.* 7:357-375.

Sady, S.P., M.W. Carpenter, P.D. Thompson, M.A. Sady, B. Haydon, and D.R. Coustan (1989). Cardiovascular response to cycle exercise during and after pregnancy. *J. Appl. Physiol.* 66:336-341.

Saltin, B., G. Blomqvist, J.H. Mitchell, R.L. Johnson Jr., K. Wildenthal, and C.B. Chapman (1968). Response to exercise after bed rest and after training: a longitudinal study of adaptive changes in oxygen transport and body composition. *Circulation* 38(suppl 7):VII1-VII78.

Saltin, B., and L. Hermansen (1966). Esophageal, rectal and muscle temperature during exercise. *J. Appl. Physiol.* 21:1757-1762.

Saltin, B. and L.B. Rowell (1980). Functional adaptations to physical activity and inactivity. *Fed. Proc.* 39:1506-1513.

Schultz, L.O., A.I. Harper, J.H. Wilmore, and E. Ravussin (1992). Energy expenditure of elite female runners measured by respiratory chamber and doubly labeled water. *J. Appl. Physiol.* 72:23-28.

Sherer, D.M., and J.G. Schenker (1989). Accidental injury during pregnancy. *Obstet. Gynecol. Survey* 44:-330-338.

Sibley, L., R.O. Ruhling, J. Cameron-Foster, C. Christensen, and T. Bolen (1981). Swimming and physical fitness during pregnancy. *J. Nurse Midwifery* 26:3-12.

Sorensen, K.E., and K.G. Borlum (1986). Fetal heart function in response to short-term maternal exercise. *Brit. J. Obstet Gynaecol.* 93:310-313.

South-Paul, J.E., K.R. Rajagopal, and T.F. Tenholder (1988). The effect of participation in a regular exercise program upon aerobic capacity during pregnancy. *Obstet. Gynecol.* 71:175-178.

Sovia, K., A. Salmi, M. Gronroos, and T. Peltonen (1964). Physical work capacity during pregnancy and effect of physical work tests on foetal heart rate. *Ann. Chir. Gynaecol. Fenniae.* 53:187-196.

Sowers, M., M. Crutchfield, M. Jannausch, S. Updike, and G. Corton (1991). A prospective evaluation of bone mineral change in pregnancy. *Obstet. Gynecol.* 77:841-845.

Steegers, E.A.P., G. Bunnick, R.A. Binkhorst, H.W. Jongsma, P.F.F. Wijn, and P.R. Hein (1988). The influence of maternal exercise on the uteroplacental vascular bed resistance and the fetal heart rate during normal pregnancy. *Eur. J. Obset. Gynecol. Reprod. Biol.* 27:21-27.

Stephanick, M.L. (1993). Exercise and weight control. *Exerc. Sports Sci. Rev.* 21:363-396.

Stephenson, L.A., and M.A. Kolka (1985). Menstrual cycle phase and time of day alter reference signal controlling arm blood flow and sweating. *Am. J. Physiol.* 249:R186-R191.

Tankersley, C.G., W.C. Nicholas, D.R. Deaver, D. Mitka, and W.L. Kenney (1992). Estrogen replacement in middle-aged women: thermoregulatory responses to exercise in the heat. *J. Appl. Physiol.* 73:1238-1245.

Tipton, C.M. (1991). Exercise, training and hypertension: an update. In: J.O. Holloszy (ed.) *Exercise and Sport Sciences Reviews*, Vol. 19. Baltimore, MD.: Williams & Wilkins, pp. 447-505.

Tipton, C.M., A.C. Vailas, and R.D. Matthes (1986). Experimental studies on the influences of physical activity on ligaments, tendons, and joints: a brief review. *Acta. Med. Scand.* Suppl 711:157-168.

Treadway, J.L., and S.A. Lederman (1986). The effects of exercise on milk yield, milk composition, and offspring growth in rats. *Am. J. Clin. Nutr.* 44:481-488.

U.S. Department of Health and Human Services (1983). Adjustment to high altitude. NIH publication # 83-2496, pp. 13-18.

van Doorn, M.B., F.K. Lotgering, P.C. Struijk, J. Pool, and H.C.S. Wallenberg (1992). Maternal and fetal cardiovascular responses to strenuous bicycle exercise. *Am. J. Obstet. Gynecol.* 166:854-859.

van Raaij, J.M.A., C.M. Schonk, S.H. Vermaat-Miedema, M.E.M. Peek, and J.G.A.J. Hautvast (1990). Energy cost of walking at a fixed pace before, during and after pregnancy. *Am. J. Clin. Nutr.* 51:158-161.

Veille, J.C., H.K. Hellerstein, and A.E. Bacevice (1992). Maternal left ventricular performance during bicycle exercise. *Am. J. Cardiol.* 69:1506-1508.

Veille, J.C., H.K. Hellerstein, B. Cherry, and A.E. Bacevice (1994). Effects of advancing pregnancy on left ventricular function during bicycle exercise. *Am. J. Cardiol.* 73:609–610.

Veille, J.C., A.R. Hohimer, K. Burry, and L. Speroff (1985). The effect of exercise on uterine activity in the last 8 weeks of pregnancy. *Am. J. Obstet. Gynecol.* 151:727–730.

Veille, J.C., M.J. Morton, K. Burry, M. Nemeth, and L. Speroff (1986). Estradiol and hemodynamics during ovulation induction. *J. Clin. Endocrin. Metab.* 63:721–724.

Villarosa, L. (1985). Running and pregnancy: having it all. *The Runner* 8(7):25–31.

Wallace, A.M., D.B. Boyer, A. Dan, and K. Holm (1985). Aerobic exercise, maternal self-esteem, and physical discomforts during pregnancy. *J. Nurse Midwifery* 31:255–262.

Wallace, J.P., G. Inbar, and K. Ernsthausen (1992). Infant acceptance of postexercise breast milk. *Pediatrics* 89:1245–1247.

Watson, W.J., V.L. Katz, A.C. Hackney, M.M. Gall, and R.G. McMurray (1991). Fetal responses to maximal swimming and cycling exercise during pregnancy. *Obstet. Gynecol.* 77:382–386.

Wolfe, L.A., and M.F. Mottola (1993). Aerobic exercise in pregnancy: an update. *Can. J. Appl. Physiol.* 18:119–147.

Wolfe, L.A., R.M.C. Walker, A. Bonen, and M.J. McGrath (1994). Respiratory adaptations to acute and chronic exercise in pregnancy. *J. Appl. Physiol.* 76:1928–1936.

Wong, S.C., and D.C. McKenzie (1987). Cardiorespiratory fitness during pregnancy and its effects on outcome. *Int. J. Sports Med.* 8:79–83.

Zaharieva, E. (1972). Olympic participation by women. *J.A.M.A.* 221:92–95.

DISCUSSION

PERRAULT: Is the relative benefit/risk ratio for exercise during pregnancy the same regardless of when in life the pregnancy occurs?

CLAPP: Unfortunately, our data cover a very narrow age range. Recreational exercise requires "free" time, and most women perceive that they don't have such time until the 30s. We have only about 10 subjects under the age of 30. The median age in the study is 32 and we are not allowed to study over the age of 40 because of concerns about risk to the pregnancy.

LOUCKS: One of your recommendations is that we need to establish threshold levels of exercise for the benefits and risks. What is your recommendation for women right now?

CLAPP: It depends on what the woman hopes to achieve. For example, I think if the goal is to grow a big baby, a woman should exercise 3 d/wk for 20 min and then start slowing down at about 30 wk of gestation. Is bigger better? I can't find a pediatrician who will tell me what the best proportions are for a newborn baby. The healthy woman who exercises before pregnancy can exercise during pregnancy to over a 100% of prepregnancy exercise level without apparent harm. To achieve the beneficial goals I've described in the chapter, women who haven't been exercising before they got pregnant need to train for a minimum of 5 d/wk, 60 min/d, at 55% of $\dot{V}O_2$max.

WILMORE: What is known about the effects of training on fertility, especially for the amenorrheic athlete who does a lot of intense training?

CLAPP: There is very little reliable information addressing that topic. It is going to be years before we have the answer to that question.

WISWELL: If a woman is tested for $\dot{V}O_2$max when she is 26 wk of gestational age and retested a week later, reproducibility is poor because of gestational changes that have occurred during that week; thus, any effects of training are confounded by this poor reproducibility. Second, the comparison of fitness data collected during pregnancy with those obtained, e.g., 6 wk after delivery, introduces a lot of confusion to many people who read the literature. Finally, we have little knowledge about first trimester exercise because it is so hard to find subjects. Would you comment on these issues?

CLAPP: Those concerns are exactly why I have chosen to enroll people prior to conception. As an example of the problem, I am completing cardiovascular studies a year after delivery and find that ventricular remodeling and total peripheral resistance are still not back to where they were prior to conception. I'm beginning to think that pregnancy may alter the risk of cardiovascular disease. I'm very suspicious about assuming that postpartum values are the same as pre-pregnancy values. A woman seems to be affected by pregnancy physiologically at least until she stops lactating and perhaps for 3 mo or even longer after she stops lactating; maybe she never returns to her preconception status. Baseline data must be gathered prior to pregnancy. I agree with your concern about reliability of performance tests repeated during pregnancy. Serial tests are critical to resolve this issue, but it is difficult to get human-subject committees to allow such studies because they somehow feel it is not a good thing to exercise pregnant women.

BAR-OR: Is there any information about the rate of children born at very low birth weights in the exercising mother vs. the sedentary mother? We have data showing that kids who are born weighing less than 1,500 g may have cognitive deficiencies, muscular problems, and performance problems.

CLAPP: In the cohorts that we have studied, we haven't seen infants who had extremely low birth weights. As I recall, the lowest birth weight we have seen is 2,200 g, and that baby was premature, not poorly grown. There are many factors that lead to extremely low birth weight that are not present in an exercising populace. I would argue that the introduction of preconceptual exercise and exercise training during pregnancy might well turn out to be a factor that would actually lower risk in an at-risk populace.

KENNEY: You implied that increases in minute ventilation during pregnancy could be a means of thermoregulatory cooling. Even under the most extreme conditions (very cold, very dry environments), those respiratory effects are really negligible with respect to temperature.

CLAPP: I agree.

KENNEY: Is the change in the surface area-to-mass ratio as women get larger during pregnancy quantitatively important? If the ratio of surface area-to-mass decreases through pregnancy, there would be a lower change in body core temperature for a given amount of heat storage.

CLAPP: As far as I know, the answer to the question about the surface area-to-mass ratio for pregnant women is unknown. I think one needs to mummify the pregnant woman briefly to make this measurement.

KNUTTGEN: You have concentrated on aerobic exercise in this chapter. Have you experience with strength-training exercise during pregnancy, with special reference to muscle blood flow retardation, associated blood pressure increases, and intra-abdominal pressure during a Valsalva maneuver?

CLAPP: I have some experience with weight training, specifically in about 10 power lifters who got pregnant. They don't appear to use a Valsalva maneuver as far as I can see. It was an area of great concern to me. These women did not appear to have significant difficulty in maintaining their weight training regimens during pregnancy nor did they seem to have any difficulty with fetal placental growth.

TERJUNG: Is it known what accounts for the insulin resistance that can occur during pregnancy, and can exercise help reverse this insulin resistance?

CLAPP: I think the insulin resistance of pregnancy is partially an artifact of a Western diet, but that is my prejudice. It has always been attributed to the actions of human placental lactogen. However, I have never seen a controlled study that actually documented that fact. In response to ingestion of pure glucose, the area under the blood glucose curve and both the first and second phases of insulin response increase in late pregnancy. Furthermore, if one does hyperinsulinemic glycemic clamps on non-athletic women, there is clear evidence of peripheral insulin resistance, presumably at the level of muscle cell. This appears to be a post-transporter defect in terms of second messenger function. But whether exercise training changes these responses is currently not known.

DAVIS: What underlies the observation that those who exercise during pregnancy produce infants who perform better on standardized tests?

CLAPP: I am having great difficulty getting manuscripts published on neurodevelopment of such children because of a healthy element of skepticism regarding postnatal events and their effect on these children's ability to take tests. We have matched for every variable under the sun, and the reviewers still aren't happy. Thus, we've just completed a subset of 40 matched pairs at one year of age with a Bailey test, and the children of mothers who exercised during pregnancy scored exactly the same on the mental performance part of the test as those whose mothers were inactive, but on the psychomotor part of the test, the children born to exercising women did far better. That still wasn't enough for the reviewers, so we have now completed about 25 babies at 5 d of age using the Brazelton Assessment Scale of Behavioral Development. At 5 d of age, the babies born to the exercising women oriented better and self-quieted better than did the matched controls, presumably as an effect of in-utero stimulation. Thus, infants from exercising mothers don't show any evidence of intellectual impairment. I'm not prepared to say that they are going to have a better general intelligence, but I am prepared to say that they performed better on the standardized testing.

FREEDSON: There may be a slightly lower average birth weight of infants from exercising mothers vs. non-exercising mothers. Does that imply a negative consequence of exercise during pregnancy?

CLAPP: It depends on whom you talk to. There is a whole new area called in-utero imprinting that is arising that says that cardiovascular risk and metabolic risk for the triple x syndrome and diabetes are established in utero. That would suggest that bigger is better. However, this also suggests that leaner may be better, and leaner infants, i.e., 9–10% fat vs. 15–16% fat, are born to exercising mothers. That is the major difference in weight. Unfortunately, it is not known if this difference in fat mass is caused by differences in adipocyte cell number or size, and we can't claim that leaner infants will be leaner adults. In our society, most of the variance in birth weight is caused by variance in fat mass. The variation in lean mass at any gestational age is extremely small, and about 70% of the variance in birth weight for gestational age is related to fat mass. Infants who are too lean can have problems with thermoregulation in the newborn period, and if the mother's breast milk doesn't come in when it is supposed to, the lean infant may receive too little dietary energy. However, we haven't had a single case where either of those things has been a problem.

GREGG: Are race and education potential confounders in interpreting the results of your studies?

CLAPP: I've matched my control and exercising groups for education and family income among other things. The lack of minority participation in similar programs is an extremely difficult one that I've been trying to deal with for the last 4–5 y, and I have only 5 minority women who have completed our program over that period of time after lots of effort at recruitment. Exercise is very low on the totem pole of priorities for most minority women, as perhaps it should be given the other problems that they need to deal with.

SMITH: What recommendations might you have for women on a routine resistance-training program and for those interested in more anaerobically-biased exercise, particularly brief 2–4 min bouts of intense activity?

CLAPP: There is evidence in the literature on small numbers of subjects that circuit-type weight training and machine weight training, not free weight training (there is very little information about free weights), is tolerated well by pregnant women and that they can increase their loads and repetitions and sets in pregnancy without apparent detriment. I can't believe that 2–4 min of anaerobic activity would be detrimental. That is just a little longer than a uterine contraction.

SUTTON: I'd be interested in your general thoughts as to how one can rectify the problem of medical organizations pontificating against exercise during pregnancy when these organizations have no solid data to support their positions? I am particularly concerned about groups such as the American College of Obstetricians and Gynecologists.

CLAPP: I feel very strongly about this issue. When I started this work the clinical research center in which I was working almost didn't get funded because it was judged that I was doing unethical work. All my training studies are limited to training at 55% of measured $\dot{V}O_2$max with, in my view, lots of unnecessary safety precautions that severely limit research output, just because people aren't sure what is safe. I am now conducting a protocol with exercise and diet, and I am being monitored by the FDA as though I were administering medicine. What one must do is ploddingly go ahead one step at a time and satisfy the regulatory agencies before going on to the next step. It is not very efficient.

PERRAULT: Do you feel that we can use data from laboratory animals to extrapolate to the human species on this topic?

CLAPP: Much of the concern about the impact of exercise in human pregnancy comes from animal data that shows striking adverse effects on many variables, including growth and development in the fetus. Unfortunately, these animal studies almost always used forced exercise at very great intensities and or durations in hopes that effects of some kind would be demonstrated. I am not convinced that results from this kind of animal research have any bearing on the types of exercise most women are likely to engage in.

BAR-OR: In your population, would it be ethical to take young women who are pregnant and put them in a climatic chamber under somewhat severe climatic heat stress and test them during exercise? Most of the research so far has been in thermoneutral environments or in water.

CLAPP: I don't think such research would be dangerous because our women can carry electronic thermometers when they train so that they can check their rectal or vaginal temperatures during a protracted exercise bout in early pregnancy. It would be very enlightening to put pregnant women in such an environment and study them, but that has not been possible in this country. However, I think the Scandinavians are probably doing it as we speak.

MURRAY: What evidence is there that lean, hard-working women show an increase in energy efficiency during pregnancy?

CLAPP: There are some very interesting studies with Gambian women who, when engaged in hard work during the wet season deposit virtually no fat when pregnant, but grow 2,500 g babies. The doubly-labeled water studies indicate that they are much more energy efficient under those conditions than they are in the non-pregnant state.

MURRAY: Efficiency as judged by what?

CLAPP: Efficiency was defined as the amount of work done relative to energy intake. An article in the *New England Journal of Medicine* several weeks ago suggested that, although basal metabolic rate doesn't change when losing or gaining body weight, the energy cost of physical activity can increase or decrease by as much as 15–20%. That article would argue that the person who constitutionally is heavy can never stay thin, and the person who is constitutionally thin can never get fat, no matter how much he or she eats.

OLDRIDGE: Women in developing countries spend tremendous amounts of energy throughout pregnancy. Are there epidemiological data suggesting that women in developing countries have increased risks associated with pregnancy?

CLAPP: Absolutely. The data are focused on neonatal and infant mortality, both of which are high and primarily related to infectious disease.

Index

Calcium intake, adulthood, 108–109; BMD, 106–113; during childhood, 106; interpreting studies, 112–113; old age, 112; perimenopausal women, 110–111; postmenopausal women, 111–112; young/premenopausal women, 109–110

Cancer, obesity association, 2

Cardiac rehabilitation, exercise-based, 393–398; exercise-based benefits, 394–395; functional capacity, 394–395; morbidity/mortality effects, 394; nationwide survey, 398; women's participation levels, 395–398

Cardiorespiratory function, 215–248; endurance event female performance, 216–219; maximal aerobic power, 219–224; oxygen transport system, 224–234; physiological factors, 219

Cardiovascular adaptations, exercise, 417–418; pregnancy, 417

Cardiovascular disease (CVD), 366

Cardiovascular health, future research, 398–399

Cardiovascular heat responses, age-related pattern, 271–272; gender-related differences, 270–271

CDC (Centers for Disease Control and Prevention), 3; physical activity definitions, 8; BRFSS (Behavioral Risk Factor Surveillance System), 15–16; YRBS (Youth Risk Behavior Survey), 12

childhood, calcium intake, 106–108

Children, activity level assessments, 10–11; chronic disease associations, 21–28; growth/development documentation, 61; physical activity demographics, 12–14; reproductive system development research, 60

Chronic diseases, physical activity associations, 21–28; sedentary behavior risk factors, 21–22

Circulation, reflex control gender-related differences, 233

Cold, thermoregulation responses, 274–278

Community interventions, future research, 29

Computed tomography (QCT), 77–78, 88–91; bone type, 80–81

Concentric strength, vs eccentric in young adulthood, 312–313; old age, 324–328

Coronary heart disease (CHD), 366; pathobiology, 366–369; preventing, 389–393; risk factors, 369–379; obesity association, 2, 372–374, 386–387

Cortical bone, 74

CT (computed axial tomography), 158–159

CVD (Cardiovascular disease), 366

Demographics, adult physical activity, 14–17; children/adolescents, 12–14; physical activity, 11–17

Determinants, environmental, 20–21; physical activity, 17–21; physiological, 18; psychosocial, 18–20

Diabetes mellitus, CHD risk factor, 372; effect of exercise, 384–386; obesity association, 2

Dimensions, physical activity, 22

Disability, physical activity associations, 21–28

Disordered eating, 178–193; assessment, 178–180; athlete prevalence, 181–186; development of, 186–190; diet adequacy risks,

190–193; DSM-IV (Diagnostic and Statistical Manual), 178; EAT (Eating Aptitude test), 179; EDI (Eating Disorder Inventory), 179; general population prevalence, 180–181; medical/safety concerns, 193–195; MSU Weight Control Survey, 180; predisposing factors, 187

Distance running, physiological factors, 219

DSM-IV (Diagnostic and Statistical Manual), 178

Dual-energy X-ray Absorptiometry, 77–78

Dual-Photon Absorptionometry (DPA), 77–78

Dynamic exercise, cardiac output response, 225–227

EAT (Eating Aptitude test), 179

Eating disorders, 178–180, not otherwise specified, 178

Eccentric strength, vs concentric from young adulthood to old age, 324–328; vs concentric in young adulthood, 312–313

ECW (extracellular water), 152

EDI (Eating Disorder Inventory), 179

Endocrine adaptations, body composition, 422–424; exercise, 422; substrate utilization, 424–425

Endurance events, female performance, 216–219; physiological factors, 219

Energy, feeding frequency/timing of exercise, 432–433; intake during Energy availability, animal experiments, 55–56; as reproductive disorder mechanism, 54

Energy balance, intake/expenditure weight control effects, 163–170

Energy expenditure studies, future research, 28–29

Energy metabolism, adaptations to strength training, 342; pregnancy, 431–432; nutrient content mix during pregnancy, 432

Environmental physical activity determinants, 20–21

Enzyme activities, muscle metabolic capacity, 331–334

Epidemiologic studies, future research, 29

Estrogen, BMD, 103–104; bone mineral mass, 100–103; menstrual irregularities effects, 2

Estrogen replacement therapy, BMD, 105; CHD risk factor, 374–375

EXCALIBUR experiments, menstrual irregularities, 57–59

Exercise, barriers, 5; breast milk composition, 433; cardiovascular adaptations during pregnancy, 417–418; conception/early pregnancy effects, 433; effect on CHD risk factor, 379–389; endocrine adaptations, 422; fetal response, 427–430; health risks effects, 2; infant weight gain, 433; iron deficiency effects on oxygen transport system, 237–238; life span approach, 5; maternal endocrine response, 422–425; maternal metabolic response, 422–425; maternal response during pregnancy, 417–427; menstrual dysfunction, 102–103; menstrual status effects on performance, 343; metabolic adaptations, 171–175; metabolic adaptations, 422; musculoskeletal adaptations, 425; oxygen extraction, 233–234; placental response, 430–431; pregnancy effects, 433–436; pregnancy gestational length effects, 434–435; pregnancy length of labor effects, 435; pregnancy mode of delivery effects, 435; pregnancy neurodevelopmental outcome, 435–436; pregnancy physical/emotional well-being effects, 434; pregnancy postpartum recovery effects, 435; pregnancy prescription recommendations, 436–440; pregnancy respiratory adaptations, 419–420; public knowledge base, 2–4; scientific knowledge base, 4–5; thermoregulatory adaptations during pregnancy, 420

Exercise stress, animal experiments, 55; as reproductive disorder mechanism, 54

Exercise stroke volume, regulation, 227–233

Exogenous hormones, BMD, 104

Fat topography/distribution, gender differences, 158–163

Fetus, body movements during exercise, 429; breathing movements during exercise, 429; cord entanglement, 416; growth rate exercise effects, 429–430; heart rate during exercise, 428–429; hypoxia, 416; maternal exercise response, 427–430; musculoskeletal injury effects, 416; substrate availability, 416; trauma, 416; velocity-flow profiles during exercise, 429

FFM (fat-free mass), 149–155; gender differences, 149–155; mineral content changes, 152; protein/ muscle mass changes, 153; subcomponent changes, 151–155

Fick equation, oxygen transport system, 224

Force-velocity relation, young adulthood, 313–319; to old age, 328

Fractures, adulthood, 119; effects of estrogen replacement therapy, 105–106

Framingham Heart Study, 46

Future research, body composition, 195–197; bone mineralization, 127–129; cardiovascular health, 398–399; oxygen transport system, 239; physical activity, 28–29; pregnancy exercise/training, 440; reproductive system, 60–62; skeletal muscle, 346–348; thermoregulation, 278–279; weight control, 195–197

Gender differences, body fat topography/distribution, 158–163; FFM (fat-free mass), 149–155

Glucose intolerance, CHD risk factor, 372; effect of exercise, 384–386

Glucose metabolism, physical activity risks, 25–26

Glycogen, muscle metabolic capacity, 329–330

HASG (heat-activated sweat glands), 262

Health risks, adiposity, 24; blood pressure, 26; bone growth, 26–27; exercise and nutrition effects, 2; insulin metabolism, 25–26; lipid metabolism, 24–25; menstrual irregularities effects on blood estrogen levels, 2; musculoskeletal function, 27–28; obesity/coronary heart disease association, 2; obesity/diabetes association, 2; overweight, 24

Healthy People 2000 Objectives (U.S. Dept. Health and Human Services), 11

Heat acclimation, age-related pattern, 279; gender-related differences, 272–273

Heat acclimatization, age-related pattern, 273; gender-related differences, 272–273

Heat effectiveness, age-related pattern, 258–259; gender-related differences, 257–258

Heat tolerance, 260–262; age-related pattern, 260–262; gender-related differences, 260

Hemostatic factors, CHD risk factor, 372–373

High impact activity, 116–117

High-velocity concentric strength, childhood to young adulthood, 308–309

Hormone replacement therapy, BMD, 105–106

Hormones, effect on bone mass, 101–103; exogenous, 104

Hperandrogenism, as reproductive disorder mechanism, 53–54

HSL (hormone-sensitive lipase) activity, 172

Human experiments, long-term menstrual irregularities, 56–57; menstrual irregularities, 56–59; short-term menstrual irregularities, 57–59

Hyperprolactinemia, as reproductive disorder mechanism, 53

Hypertension, CHD risk factor, 370–371; effect of exercise, 379–381

Hypoestrogenism, clinical consequence research, 60

Impact loading ; physical activity, 124–125

Insulin metabolism, physical activity risks, 25–26

Iron deficiency, exercise effects, 237–238

Isometric strength, childhood to young adulthood, 306–308; young adulthood to old age, 319–323

LDL-C (low-density lipoprotein cholesterol), 368

Life cycle, body fat gender differences, 155–163; FFM (fat-free mass) gender differences, 149–155; reproductive system changes, 42–44

lifetime losses, BMD, 98–99

Limb studies, preferred, 117

Lipid metabolism, physical activity risks, 24–25

Lipids/lipoproteins, CHD risk factor, 371–372; effect of exercise, 381–383

Longitudinal studies, physical activity, 118–119

Low-density lipoprotein cholesterol (LDL-C), 368

Low-velocity concentric strength, childhood to young adulthood, 306–308; to old age, 319–323

Lumbar spine volumetric bone mineral density, 88–91

Luteal suppression, 44–47; behavioral characterization, 47–48; endocrine characterization, 48–50; mechanism/clinical consequences research, 60–61; prevalence, 47; prevalence, 61

Maximal aerobic power, aging effects, 221–223; body composition influence, 220; growth/maturation effects, 221; oxygen-carrying capacity influence, 220–221; training status effects, 223–224